Pharmacotherapy Principles & Practice Study Guide: A Case-Based Care Plan Approach

Pharmacotherapy Principles & Practice Study Guide: A Case-Based Care Plan Approach

Editors

Michael D. Katz, PharmD
Clinical Associate Professor
Department of Pharmacy Practice and Science
The University of Arizona College of Pharmacy
Tucson, Arizona

Kathryn R. Matthias, PharmD, BCPS
Clinical Assistant Professor
Department of Pharmacy Practice and Science
The University of Arizona College of Pharmacy
Tucson, Arizona

Marie A. Chisholm-Burns, PharmD, MPH, FCCP, FASHP
Professor and Head
Department of Pharmacy Practice and Science
The University of Arizona College of Pharmacy
Professor
Department of Surgery and Division of Health Promotion
    Sciences
The University of Arizona Colleges of Medicine and
    College of Public Health
Tucson, Arizona

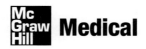

New York   Chicago   San Francisco   Lisbon   London   Madrid   Mexico City   Milan
New Delhi   San Juan   Seoul   Singapore   Sydney   Toronto

Pharmacotherapy Principles & Practice Study Guide: A Case-Based Care Plan Approach

1 2 3 4 5 6 7 8 9 10   QDB/QDB   14 13 12 11

ISBN 978-0-07-170119-8
MHID 0-07-170119-2

This book was set in Minion Pro by Aptara, Inc.
The editors were Michael Weitz and Christie Naglieri.
The production supervisor was Philip Galea.
Project management was provided by Samir Roy, Aptara, Inc.
The designer was Alan Barnett; the cover designer was Pehrsson Design.
Cover image, left to right: 1. Anatomical Travelogue/Photo Researchers, Inc.
2. Image Source. 3. Jim Dowdalls/Photo Researchers, Inc. 4. ER Productions Ltd.
5. John Bavosi/Photo Researchers, Inc.
Quad/Graphics was printer and binder.

This book is printed on acid-free paper.

McGraw-Hill books are available at special quantity discounts to use as premiums and sales promotions, or for use in corporate training programs. To contact a representative please e-mail us at bulksales@mcgraw-hill.com.

CONTENTS

CONTRIBUTORS

Kim Ackerbauer, PharmD
Adjunct Assistant Professor
PGY2 Resident in Cardiology
LAC + USC School of Pharmacy
Los Angeles, California

Sarah Adriance, PharmD
Clinical Pharmacy Specialist, Critical Care
The University of Chicago Medical Center
Chicago, Illinois

Ronda L. Akins, PharmD
Associate Professor, Infectious Diseases
University of Louisiana Monroe
College of Pharmacy
Monroe, Louisiana

Rita Raney Alloway, PharmD, BCPS, FCCP
Research Professor and Director of Transplant
    Clinical Research
University of Cincinnati
Cincinnati, Ohio

David A. Apgar, PharmD
Clinical Assistant Professor
Department of Pharmacy Practice and Science
University of Arizona College of Pharmacy
Tucson, Arizona

Jennifer H. Baggs, PharmD
Clinical Assistant II
University of Arizona College of Pharmacy
Nutrition Specialty Resident
University Medical Center
Tucson, Arizona

Nicole A. Baker, PharmD
Pharmacist, Teton Pharmacy I.V. Home
    Health & Oxygen
Idaho Falls, Idaho

Kim W. Benner, PharmD, BCPS, FASHP
Professor of Pharmacy Practice
Samford University McWhorter School of Pharmacy
Pediatric Clinical Pharmacy Specialist
Children's Hospital
Homewood, Alabama

Kade Birkeland, PharmD
Clinical Pharmacy Specialist in Cardiology
Masters of Pharmaceutical Care Program
Guest Faculty, School of Pharmacy and Biochemistry
San Marcos University
Lima, Peru

**P. Brandon Bookstaver, PharmD, BCPS
(AQ ID), AAHIVE**
Assistant Professor, South Carolina College of Pharmacy
University of South Carolina Campus
Clinical Pharmacy Specialist, Infectious Diseases
Palmetto Health Richland
Columbia, South Carolina

Emily B. Borders, PharmD, BCOP
Clinical Assistant Professor
University of Oklahoma College of Pharmacy
Oklahoma City, Oklahoma

Sheila R. Botts, PharmD, BCPP
Assistant Professor
Department of Pharmacy Practice & Science
College of Pharmacy University of Kentucky
Clinical Pharmacy Specialist, Psychiatry
Lexington Veterans Affairs Medical Center
Lexington, Kentucky

Nicole J. Brandt, PharmD, CGP, BCPP, FASCP
Associate Professor, Geriatric Pharmacotherapy
Department of Pharmacy Practice and Science, UMB School
    of Pharmacy
Director, Clinical and Education Programs of Peter Lamy
    Center Drug Therapy and Aging
Baltimore, Maryland

Gretchen M. Brophy, PharmD, BCPS, FCCP, FCCM
Professor of Pharmacotherapy & Outcomes Science
    and Neurosurgery
Virginia Commonwealth University
Medical College of Virginia Campus
Richmond, Virginia

Susan P. Bruce, PharmD, BCPS
Associate Professor and Chair of Pharmacy Practice
Northeastern Ohio Universities College of Pharmacy
Rootstown, Ohio

Imad Btaiche, BS, PharmD, BCNSP
Clinical Associate Professor of Pharmacy
University of Michigan College of Pharmacy
Clinical Pharmacist, University of Michigan Hospitals and
    Health Centers
Ann Arbor, Michigan

Christopher Jon Campen, PharmD, BCPS
Clinical Oncology Specialist
Arizona Cancer Center at Orange Grove
Tucson, Arizona

Diane M. Cappelletty, PharmD
Associate Professor of Pharmacy Practice
The University of Toledo College of Pharmacy
Toledo, Ohio

Marshall E. Cates, PharmD, BCPP, FASHP
Assistant Dean for Student Affairs & Professor of
    Pharmacy Practice
Samford University McWhorter School of Pharmacy
Birmingham, Alabama

Larisa H. Cavallari, PharmD
Associate Professor
University of Illinois at Chicago
Department of Pharmacy Practice
Chicago, Illinois

Juliana Chan, PharmD
Clinical Assistant Professor
Assistant Director Pharmacy Clinical Services
Department of Pharmacy Practice College of Pharmacy
Department of Medicine, Sections of Digestive Diseases
    and Nutrition and Section of Hepatology
University of Illinois at Chicago
Chicago, Illinois

Jack J. Chen, PharmD, FCCP, BCPS, CGP
Associate Professor (Neurology)
Loma Linda University Schools of Medicine and Pharmacy
Loma Linda, California

Allison Ann Chilipko, PharmD
University of Maryland School of Pharmacy PGY-1
    Pharmacy Practice Resident
Union Memorial Hospital
Baltimore, Maryland

Marie Chisholm-Burns, PharmD, MPH, FCCP, FASHP
Professor & Head, Department of Pharmacy
    Practice & Science
University of Arizona College of Pharmacy
Professor, Department of Surgery and Division of Health
    Promotion Sciences
University of Arizona Colleges of Medicine and
    College of Public Health
Tucson, Arizona

Holly Chiu, PharmD
Pharmacy Practice Resident
Harper University Hospital Detroit Medical Center
Detroit, Michigan

Kevin W. Cleveland, PharmD
Associate Professor of Pharmacy Practice
Idaho State University
Director, Idaho Drug Information Service
Pocatello, Idaho

Amanda H. Corbett, PharmD, BCPS, FCCP
Clinical Assistant Professor
The University of North Carolina
Eshelman School of Pharmacy and The University of
    North Carolina, School of Medicine
Pharmacy Clinical Specialist
Infectious Diseases, Infectious Diseases Clinic
The University of North Carolina Health Systems
Chapel Hill, North Carolina

Susan Cornell, BS, PharmD, CDE, FAPhA, FAADE
Assistant Director of Experiential Education
Assistant Professor of Pharmacy Practice
Midwestern University Chicago College of Pharmacy
Diabetes Pharmacist Educator
DuPage Community Clinic
Downers Grove, Illinois

Brian L. Crabtree, PharmD, BCPP
Associate Professor of Pharmacy Practice
Clinical Associate Professor of Psychiatry
University of Mississippi
Psychopharmacologist, Mississippi State Hospital
Jackson, Mississippi

Jean Ellen Cunningham, PharmD, BSPS
Associate Professor of Pharmacy Practice
University of Findlay College of Pharmacy
Director, Medication Therapy Management Consultation
    Center at the University of Findlay College of Pharmacy
Findlay, Ohio

Clarence E. Curry, Jr., PharmD
Interim Associate Dean
School of Pharmacy CPNAHS, Howard University
Washington, DC

Devra K. Dang, PharmD, BCPS, CDE
Associate Clinical Professor
University of Connecticut School of Pharmacy
Clinical Faculty, Burgdorf Primary Care Clinic
Storrs, Connecticut

Stephanie J. Davis, PharmD
Ambulatory Care Clinical Pharmacy Specialist
Southern Arizona VA Healthcare System
Clinical Assistant Professor
University of Arizona College of Pharmacy
Tucson, Arizona

Kristina De Los Santos, PharmD, BCPS
Assistant Chief, Pharmacy Service Line
Clinical Services and Education
Southern Arizona VA Healthcare System
Clinical Assistant Professor
University of Arizona College of Pharmacy
Tucson, Arizona

Robert J. DiDomenico, PharmD
Clinical Associate Professor
University of Illinois at Chicago College of Pharmacy
Cardiovascular Clinical Pharmacist
University of Illinois Medical Center at Chicago
Chicago, Illinois

Leona Downey, MD
Clinical Assistant Professor of Medicine
University of Arizona
Department of Medicine
Section of Oncology
Tucson, Arizona

Jeremiah J. Duby, PharmD, BCPS
Critical Care Pharmacist
U.C. Davis Medical Center
Assistant Clinical Professor, Touro University
Assistant Clinical Professor, UCSF School of Pharmacy
Sacramento, California

Colleen Dula, PharmD
Clinical Assistant Professor, Pharmacy Practice and
    Administration
The Ohio State University College of Pharmacy
Ambulatory Care Clinical Pharmacist
University Health Connection
The Ohio State University
Columbus, Ohio

Christopher J. Edwards, PharmD, BCPS
Clinical Staff Pharmacist, Emergency Medicine
University Medical Center
Tucson, Arizona

Megan J. Ehret, PharmD, BCPP
Assistant Professor, University of Connecticut
Clinical Pharmacist, Institute of Living
Storrs, Connecticut

Shareen Y. El-Ibiary, PharmD, BCPS
Associate Professor of Pharmacy Practice
Midwestern University College of Pharmacy-Glendale
Glendale, Arizona

John Erramouspe, PharmD, MS
Professor of Pharmacy Practice
Idaho State University
Pocatello, Idaho

Brian L. Erstad, PharmD, BCPS, FASHP
Professor, Department of Pharmacy Practice and Science
University of Arizona College of Pharmacy
Program Director, Critical Care Residency
University Medical Center
Tucson, Arizona

Ema Ferreira, BPharm, MSc, PharmD, FCSHP
Clinical Associate Professor, University of Montreal
Pharmacist, Obstetrics and Gynecology
Centre Hospitalier Sainte-Justine, Montreal
Quebec, Canada

Melanie Foeppel, PharmD
Assistant Professor
Pacific University School of Pharmacy
Hillsboro, Oregon

Patty Ghazvini, PharmD
Associate Professor of Pharmacy Practice
Florida A&M University
Internal Medicine Clinical Preceptor
Tallahassee Memorial Hospital/Family Practice
    Residency Clinic
Tallahassee, Florida

Maqual R. Graham, PharmD
Associate Professor of Pharmacy Practice and
    Administration
University of Missouri-Kansas City
Clinical Pharmacy Specialist, Veterans Affairs
    Medical Center
Kansas City, Missouri

Elaine Marie Greifenstein, MD
Clinical Associate Professor, Internal Medicine
Northeastern Ohio Universities Colleges of
    Medicine & Pharmacy
Rootstown, Ohio

Joshua William Guffey, PharmD
Clinical Assistant Professor
University of Georgia College of Pharmacy
Clinical Pharmacy Specialist
Charlie Norwood VA Medical Center
Athens, Georgia

John G. Gums, PharmD
Professor of Pharmacy and Medicine
Associate Chair, Department of Pharmacotherapy and
    Translational Research
Director of Clinical Research in Family Medicine
University of Florida
Gainesville, Florida

Nancy Heideman, PharmD, BCPS
Clinical Pharmacy Specialist, Pediatrics
University of New Mexico Hospital
Albuquerque, New Mexico

Richard L. Heideman, MD
Professor of Pediatrics
Division of Pediatric Hematology/Oncology
University of New Mexico
Albuquerque, New Mexico

Brett H. Heintz, PharmD, BCPS, (AQ-ID), AAHIVE
Assistant Professor of Clinical Pharmacy
UCSF School of Pharmacy
Pharmacy Specialist, Infectious Diseases
U.C. Davis Medical Center
Sacramento, California

Brian A. Hemstreet, PharmD, BCPS
Associate Professor, Department of Clinical Pharmacy
Director, Pharmaceutical Care Learning Center
University of Colorado School of Pharmacy
Aurora, Colorado

Michelle L. Hilaire, PharmD, CDE, BCPS
Clinical Assistant Professor of Pharmacy Practice
University of Wyoming School of Pharmacy
Faculty Pharmacist, Fort Collins Family Medicine Residency
Fort Collins, Colorado

Marlon Honeywell, PharmD
Associate Dean for Academic Affairs and Professor
Florida A&M University
Ambulatory Care Clinical Preceptor
Bond Community Health Center
Tallahassee, Florida

Alexis Estes Horace, PharmD
Assistant Professor
University of Louisiana at Monroe College of Pharmacy
Baton Rouge, Louisiana

Jaime R. Hornecker, PharmD, BCPS
Clinical Assistant Professor of Pharmacy Practice
University of Wyoming School of Pharmacy
University of Wyoming Family Medicine Residency
    Program/Community Health Center of
    Central Wyoming
Casper, Wyoming

Jamie Hwang, PharmD
Pharmacy Practice Resident
Harper University Hospital Detroit Medical Center
Detroit, Michigan

Cherry W. Jackson, BS, PharmD, BCPP, FASHP
Professor of Pharmacy Practice
Harrison School of Pharmacy, Auburn University
Department of Psychiatry and Neurology
School of Medicine
University of Alabama
Birmingham, Alabama

Jennifer Jordan, PharmD, BCPS
Assistant Professor
Pacific University School of Pharmacy
Hillsboro, Oregon

Michael P. Kane, PharmD, BCPS
Professor, Department of Pharmacy Practice
Albany College of Pharmacy and Health Sciences
Clinical Pharmacy Specialist
The Endocrine Group, LLC
Albany, New York

Michael D. Katz, PharmD
Clinical Associate Professor
Director, International Affairs
Department of Pharmacy Practice and Science
University of Arizona College of Pharmacy
Tucson, Arizona

Deanna L. Kelly, PharmD, BCPP
Director and Chief, Treatment of Research Program
Maryland Psychiatric Research Center
Associate Professor of Psychiatry
University of Maryland Baltimore
Baltimore, Maryland

Jacqueline M. Klootwyk, PharmD, BCPS
Assistant Professor, Thomas Jefferson University
Jefferson School of Pharmacy
Philadelphia, Pennsylvania

Michael D. Kraft, PharmD, BCNSP
Clinical Associate Professor
University of Michigan College of Pharmacy
Clinical Coordinator
University of Michigan Health System
Ann Arbor, Michigan

Thomas E. Lackner, PharmD, CGP, FASCP
Director of Pharmacy Services
Geriatric Care Services
Univita Health
Eden Prairie, Minnesota

Wallace Greg Leader, PharmD (Deceased)
Dean and Professor of Clinical Pharmacy Practice
University of Louisiana at Monroe College of Pharmacy
Monroe, Louisiana

Jeannie Kim Lee, PharmD, BCPS
Clinical Assistant Professor
College of Pharmacy, Department of Pharmacy
    Practice and Science
College of Medicine, Department of Medicine, Section of
    Geriatrics and Gerontology
University of Arizona
Clinical Pharmacy Specialist, Geriatrics
Southern Arizona VA Health Care System
Tucson, Arizona

Mary Lee, PharmD, BCPS, FCCP
Vice President and Chief Academic Officer
Professor of Pharmacy Practice
Midwestern University Chicago College of Pharmacy
Downers Grove, Illinois

Russell E. Lewis, PharmD, FCCP, BCPS
Associate Professor, University of Houston
     College of Pharmacy
Clinical Pharmacy Specialist
Infectious Diseases and Adjunct Associate Professor
The University of Texas M.D. Anderson Cancer Center
Houston, Texas

Raymond A. Lorenz, PharmD, BCPP
Assistant Clinical Professor
Auburn University, Harrison School of Pharmacy
Clinical Pharmacy Specialist
AltaPointe Health Systems
Mobile, Alabama

Amy M. Lugo, PharmD, BCPS, BC-ADM
Clinical Pharmacy Specialist
DoD Pharmacoeconomic Center
Fort Sam Houston, Texas

Leigh V. Maine, PharmD
Ambulatory Care Clinical Pharmacy Specialist
Southern Arizona VA Health Care System
Tucson, Arizona

Mark A. Malesker, PharmD, FCCP, BCPS
Professor of Pharmacy Practice and Medicine
Creighton University
Clinical Pharmacy Specialist
Creighton University Medical Center
Omaha, Nebraska

Michelle T. Martin, PharmD
Clinical Assistant Professor, University of Illinois at
     Chicago College of Pharmacy
Clinical Pharmacist, University of Illinois Medical
     Center at Chicago
Chicago, Illinois

Kathryn R. Matthias, PharmD, BCPS
Clinical Assistant Professor
Department of Pharmacy Practice and Science
University of Arizona College of Pharmacy
Clinical Pharmacist Specialist
Infectious Diseases, University Medical Center
Tucson, Arizona

Lena M. Maynor, PharmD, BCPS
Clinical Assistant Professor
West Virginia University School of Pharmacy
Clinical Specialist, Internal Medicine

West Virginia University Hospitals
Morgantown, West Virginia

Yolanda B. McKoy-Beach, PharmD, R.Ph
Assistant Professor, Howard University College
     of Pharmacy, Nursing and Allied Health
Clinical Pharmacist, La Clinica Del Pueblo
Washington, DC

Patrick J. Medina, PharmD, BCOP
Associate Professor, University of Oklahoma College
     of Pharmacy
Clinical Pharmacist, OU Cancer Institute
Oklahoma City, Oklahoma

April D. Miller, PharmD, BCPS
Assistant Professor, South Carolina College of Pharmacy
University of South Carolina Campus
Clinical Pharmacy Specialist, Critical Care
Palmetto Health Richland
Columbia, South Carolina

Beverly Mims, PharmD
Associate Professor of Pharmacy Practice
Howard University College of Pharmacy,
     Nursing and Allied Health Sciences
Clinical Pharmacist, Howard University Hospital
Washington, DC

Brice Labruzzo Mohondro, PharmD
Assistant Professor of Clinical Pharmacy Practice
University of Louisiana at Monroe College of Pharmacy
Clinical Pharmacist, Baton Rouge General Family Medicine
     Residency Program
Baton Rouge, Louisiana

Caroline Morin, BPharm, MSc
Pharmacist, Obstetrics and Gynecology
CHU Sainte-Justine, Montreal
University of Montreal
Quebec, Canada

Lee E. Morrow, MD, MSc
Associate Professor of Medicine and Associate Professor of
     Pharmacy Practice, Creighton University Medical Center
Pulmonary and Critical Care Fellowship Program Director
     Creighton University Medical Center
Omaha, Nebraska

Keri Naglosky, PharmD, BCPS
Assistant Professor, Pharmacy Practice and Pharmaceutical
     Sciences Department, College of Pharmacy
University of Minnesota, Duluth
Director, Duluth Medication Therapy Management Clinic
Duluth, Minnesota

Rocsanna Namdar, PharmD, BCPS
Assistant Professor, Department of Clinical Pharmacy
University of Colorado School of Pharmacy
Aurora, Colorado

Lynn C. Nelson, PharmD, MBA
Assistant Clinical Professor
UCSD Skaggs School of Pharmacy
San Diego, California

Melinda M. Neuhauser, PharmD, MPH
Clinical Pharmacy Specialist, Infectious Diseases
VA Pharmacy Benefits Management Services
Hines, Illinois

Tien M.H. Ng, PharmD, FCCP, BCPS (AQ-Cardiology)
Associate Professor of Clinical Pharmacy
University of Southern California
Los Angeles, California

Edith A. Nutescu, PharmD, FCCP
Clinical Professor, University of Illinois at Chicago
    College of Pharmacy
Clinical Manager, Antithrombosis Center
University of Illinois Medical Center
Chicago, Illinois

Cara Olsen, PharmD
Instructor of Pharmacy Practice
Creighton University
St. Joseph Hospital Department of Pharmacy
Omaha, Nebraska

David Parra, PharmD, FCCP, BCPS
Clinical Assistant Professor
Department of Experimental and Clinical Pharmacology
University of Minnesota College of Pharmacy
Clinical Pharmacy Specialist in Cardiology
Veterans Affairs Medical Center
West Palm Beach, Florida

Asad Patanwala, PharmD, BCPS
Clinical Assistant Professor
Department of Pharmacy Practice and Science
University of Arizona College of Pharmacy
Clinical Pharmacy Specialist, Emergency Medicine
University Medical Center
Tucson, Arizona

Krina H. Patel, PharmD
Assistant Professor of Pharmacy Practice
Nesbitt College of Pharmacy and Nursing
Wilkes University
Wilkes Barre, Pennsylvania

Susan L. Pendland, PharmD, MS
Adjunct Associate Professor, University of Illinois
    at Chicago

Clinical Staff Pharmacist, St. Joseph Berea Hospital
Berea, Kentucky

Gary Daniel Peksa, PharmD
Pharmacy Practice Resident
Rush University Medical Center
Chicago, Illinois

Hanna Phan, PharmD, BCPS
Clinical Assistant Professor
Department of Pharmacy Practice and Science
    College of Pharmacy
Assistant Professor, Pediatrics, College of Medicine
University of Arizona
Pediatric Pulmonary Medicine
University Medical Center
Tucson, Arizona

Beth Bryles Phillips, PharmD, FCCP, BCPS
Clinical Associate Professor
University of Georgia College of Pharmacy
Clinical Pharmacy Specialist
Charlie Norwood VA Medical Center
Athens, Georgia

Evelyne Rey, MD, MSc
Associate Professor, Department of Medicine and
Adjunct Professor, Department of Obstetrics and
    Gynecology
University of Montreal
Head Obstetric Medicine Division
Department of Obstetrics and Gynecology
CHU Sainte-Justine, Montreal
Quebec, Canada

Leigh Ann Ross, PharmD
Associate Professor and Chair
Department of Pharmacy Practice
Associate Dean for Clinical Affairs
University of Mississippi School of Pharmacy
Jackson, Mississippi

Brendan Sean Ross, MD
Clinical Associate Professor
Department of Pharmacy Practice
University of Mississippi School of Pharmacy
Jackson, Mississippi

Laurajo Ryan, PharmD, MSc, BCPS, CDE
Clinical Assistant Professor, University of Texas
    at Austin College of Pharmacy
Clinical Assistant Professor
University of Texas Health Science
    Center San Antonio
San Antonio, Texas

Lauren S. Schlesselman, PharmD
Assistant Clinical Professor and Director of Assessment
    and Accreditation
University of Connecticut School of Pharmacy
Storrs, Connecticut

Roohollah Sharifi, MD, FACS
Professor of Surgery
University of Illinois at Chicago, College of Medicine
Director, Surgery Clinic
University of Illinois Hospital
Chicago, Illinois

Colin I. Sheffield, PharmD, AAHIVE
Clinical HIV and Infectious Diseases Specialist
Kerr Health Specialty Pharmacy
Raleigh, North Carolina

Angela Singh, PharmD
Associate Professor of Pharmacy Practice
Florida A&M University
Internal Medicine and Oncology Clinical Preceptor
Tallahassee Memorial Hospital
Tallahassee, Florida

Steven M. Smith, PharmD
Postdoctoral Fellow in Family Medicine
University of Florida
Colleges of Pharmacy and Medicine
Gainesville, Florida

Sarah A. Spinler, PharmD, BCPS (AQ Cardiology), FCCP, FAHA, FASHP
Professor of Clinical Pharmacy
Department of Pharmacy Practice and Pharmacy
    Administration
Philadelphia College of Pharmacy
University of the Sciences in Philadelphia
Philadelphia, Pennsylvania

Sara A. Stahle, PharmD, BCPS
Clinical Pharmacist
Oregon Health and Science University
Portland, Oregon

Robert J. Straka, PharmD, FCCP
Professor, Department of Experimental and Clinical
    Pharmacology
University of Minnesota
Minneapolis, Minnesota

Amy L. Stump, PharmD, BCPS
Clinical Assistant Professor of Pharmacy Practice
University of Wyoming School of Pharmacy
Clinical Pharmacist, Family Medicine Residency Training
    Program at Cheyenne
Cheyenne, Wyoming

Janice L. Stumpf, PharmD
Clinical Associate Professor, University of Michigan
    College of Pharmacy
Clinical Pharmacist, Drug Information Service
University of Michigan Health System
Ann Arbor, Michigan

Meghan K. Sullivan, PharmD
Assistant Professor
Deparment of Pharmacy Practice and Science
University of Maryland School of Pharmacy
Rockville, Maryland

Joseph M. Swanson, PharmD, BCPS
Assistant Professor of Clinical Pharmacy
Pharmaceutical Sciences, and Pharmacology
University of Tennessee
Colleges of Pharmacy and Medicine
Memphis, Tennessee

Eljim P. Tesoro, PharmD
Clinical Assistant Professor
University of Illinois at Chicago
Clinical Pharmacist, Neuroscience ICU
University of Illinois Medical Center
Chicago, Illinois

Andrea N. Traina, PharmD
Assistant Professor of Pharmacy Practice
St. John Fisher College
Wegmans School of Pharmacy
Clinical Pharmacy Specialist
Lifetime Health Medical Group
Rochester, New York

Toby C. Trujillo, PharmD, BCPS (AQ-Cardiology)
Associate Professor, University of Colorado Denver
    School of Pharmacy
Clinical Specialist, Anticoagulation/Cardiology
University of Colorado Hospital
Aurora, Colorado

Elena M. Umland, PharmD
Associate Professor of Pharmacy Practice
Associate Dean for Academic Affairs
Jefferson School of Pharmacy
Thomas Jefferson University
Philadelphia, Pennsylvania

Atula Vachhani, PharmD
Primary Care Resident
University of Connecticut School of
    Pharmacy and Burgdorf Primary Care Clinic
Hartford, Connecticut

Heather L. VandenBussche, PharmD
Professor, Department of Pharmacy Practice
Ferris State University College of Pharmacy
Kalamazoo, Michigan

Nicole D. Verkleeren, PharmD, BCPS
Clinical Pharmacist, The Western Pennsylvania
    Hospital—Forbes Regional Campus
Monroeville, Pennsylvania

Geoffrey C. Wall, PharmD, FCCP, BCPS, CGP
Associate Professor of Clinical Sciences
Drake University College of Pharmacy and Health Sciences
Internal Medicine Clinical Pharmacist
Iowa Methodist Medical Center
Des Moines, Iowa

R. Carlin Walsh, PharmD, BCPS
Transplant Pharmacy Fellow
Department of Surgery
Division of Transplantation
University of Cincinnati Medical Center
Cincinnati, Ohio

Heidi Wehring, PharmD, BCPP
Instructor, Maryland Psychiatric Research Center
University of Maryland Baltimore School of Medicine
Baltimore, Maryland

Christy M. Weiland, PharmD, BCPS
Clinical Assistant Professor, University of Wyoming
Family Medicine Faculty
Fort Collins Family Medical Residency/Poudre
    Valley Hospital
Fort Collins, Colorado

Timothy E. Welty, PharmD, FCCP, BCPS
Professor, School of Pharmacy, Adjunct Professor
    Department of Neurology
University of Kansas
Kansas City, Kansas

Teri L. West, PharmD, BCPS
Assistant Professor of Pharmacy Practice
Lake Erie College of Osteopathic Medicine
School of Pharmacy
Bradenton, Florida

Jon P. Wietholter, PharmD, BCPS
Clinical Assistant Professor, West Virginia University
Internal Medicine Clinical Pharmacist
Cabell Huntington Hospital
Huntington, West Virginia

Ann McMahon Wicker, PharmD, BCPS
Assistant Professor, University of Louisiana at
    Monroe College of Pharmacy
Baton Rouge, Louisiana

Sheila M. Wilhelm, PharmD, BCPS
Clinical Assistant Professor
Eugene Applebaum College of Pharmacy and
    Health Sciences
Wayne State University
Clinical Pharmacy Specialist
Harper University Hospital
Detroit, Michigan

Susan R. Winkler, PharmD, BCPS
Professor and Chair, Department of Pharmacy Practice
Midwestern University Chicago College of Pharmacy
Downers Grove, Illinois

**G. Christopher Wood, PharmD, FCCP, BCPS
(AQ-ID)**
Associate Professor of Clinical Pharmacy
University of Tennessee Health Science Center and
    College of Pharmacy
Memphis, Tennessee

PREFACE

Determining and providing organized patient-specific pharmacotherapy recommendations involves a thorough evaluation of the patient's medical problems and medication issues. *Pharmacotherapy Principles and Practice Study Guide: A Case-Based Care Plan Approach* contains 98 patient cases that correspond to chapters published in the second edition of *Pharmacotherapy Principles and Practice*. Our goal for this companion textbook is to be a study guide for today's learners of the clinical application of pharmacotherapy through either self-study or during patient case discussion sessions with other health care professionals. The aim of this study guide is to help students navigate through the process of applying their knowledge of pharmacotherapy to a specific patient case by organizing patient data to logically assess a patient's medication issues and formulate a rational pharmacotherapy care plan.

Using a patient database form as an organized guide, students in the health care profession should learn how to apply their knowledge to evaluate the following key aspects of a patient case:

- *Medical Problem List:* Prioritize and organize each patient's medical problem list and corresponding medications
- *Laboratory Values:* Evaluate provided and missing laboratory values for issues related to each patient's medication and medical problem list
- *Drug Therapy Problem Worksheet:* Assess each patient for drug therapy problems and their causes by specifically focusing on drug dosing, missing medications, medications without an obvious indication, drug interactions, and the social and economical impact of certain pharmacotherapy recommendations
- *Pharmacotherapy Care Plan:* Formulate a comprehensive, rational, and practical patient care plan with pharmacotherapy recommendations that are organized by the prioritized medical problem list
- *Patient Education Summary:* Based on a patient's medical problem list and pharmacotherapy recommendations, summarize brief patient education points that are individualized to the patient case

A guide for reviewing and evaluating patient cases and preparing patient database forms is provided in greater detail in Chapter 1. The cases have been written in a realistic fashion, using terms and abbreviations that would be seen in a real patient's medical record. Definitions of abbreviations can be found in Appendix C. The Online Learning Center at www.PPPstudyguide.com has blank patient database forms that may be downloaded.

We, along with patient case authors, used published literature and our experiences as educators and clinicians to determine the focus of each patient case to be included in this textbook. If upon using this study guide, you feel that anything important has been left out, please let us know your thoughts for future editions.

We acknowledge the commitment of more than 150 patient case authors who dedicated their time and knowledge in the preparation of this first edition study guide. We also thank all of the editors and authors of *Pharmacotherapy Principles and Practice*, 2nd edition, who provided the pharmacotherapy background as reference material for this study guide's patient cases and question hints, and for their thoughts and suggestions as we developed the idea for this book.

We are grateful to everyone at McGraw-Hill who advised us and helped prepare this first edition study guide. We specifically thank Michael Weitz for all of his suggestions and insight in preparing this new textbook. In addition, we thank Christie Naglieri, Samir Roy, and Laura Libretti for guiding us through the publication process and for the hard work related to the copyediting and formatting of each patient case.

At The University of Arizona, we thank Dr. Christina Spivey for her suggestions to provide more consistency between this study guide and the companion *Pharmacotherapy Principles and Practice*, 2nd edition textbook and LeeAnn Landphair for keeping all of the patient case chapter–related materials organized.

Lastly, we sincerely thank Dr. Edward W. Randell for conscientiously checking every laboratory value in each patient case for SI unit conversion.

Michael D. Katz, PharmD
Kathryn R. Matthias, PharmD, BCPS
Marie A. Chisholm-Burns, PharmD, MPH, FCCP, FASHP

1 Applying Pharmacotherapy Principles and Practice: How to Use This Study Guide

Michael D. Katz   Marie A. Chisholm-Burns
Kathryn R. Matthias

As health care becomes more and more complex in the 21st century, the health professional student is increasingly challenged to learn a rapidly expanding amount of information as well as necessary skills to apply that knowledge in a patient care setting. Students of pharmacotherapy quickly learn that the field is rapidly changing as our knowledge of human disease evolves and new drugs are developed to improve patient outcomes. Students also learn that while drug therapy can have tremendous beneficial effects on patient outcomes, such therapy also has the potential to cause harm. The "art" of pharmacotherapy is in applying knowledge and making therapeutic decisions that are most likely to have maximum positive benefit *for a specific patient*. As a companion book to *Pharmacotherapy Principles and Practice*, 2nd ed. (*PPP*), this Study Guide is designed to assist the student in learning to apply didactic knowledge to specific patient situations. Such application requires skills that cannot be learned in lectures or in other passive learning situations, but must be learned by practice and repetition. The more students practice applying their knowledge, using their patient assessment skills, and making therapeutic decisions in their preclinical courses, the more prepared they will be to apply these skills to real patients in their clinical rotations.

This Study Guide is more than a book of patient cases, but it uses patient cases to help students learn to apply pharmacotherapeutic knowledge and skills. Case-based learning is not a new concept in health sciences curricula. As a form of active learning, case-based learning allows the student to practice the skills necessary to provide patient care. The focus of the cases in this Study Guide is, of course, pharmacotherapeutics. A unique feature of this study guide is the expectation that the student will develop a pharmacotherapy care plan as the "output" for each case.

What follows is a general discussion of the patient care process and then specific information regarding the use of the Study Guide and development of the pharmacotherapy care plan.

PHARMACEUTICAL CARE AND THE PATIENT CARE PROCESS

Most pharmacy students are taught about pharmaceutical care early in their pharmacy curriculum. Pharmaceutical care, first described in the late 1980s and early 1990s,[1] can be summarized as "… patient-centered practice in which the practitioner assumes responsibility for a patient's drug-related needs and is held accountable for this commitment."[2] Although the definition of pharmaceutical care does not explicitly state that pharmacists are to perform these tasks, many feel that pharmaceutical care is the central mission of the pharmacy profession.

Although it may seem obvious that health professionals practice in a patient-centered way, all too often, practitioners become distracted by technical or administrative tasks. Pharmacy students, upon graduation, commit to patient-centered practice in the Oath of a Pharmacist:[3]

I promise to devote myself to a lifetime of service to others through the profession of pharmacy. In fulfilling this vow:

- I will consider the welfare of humanity and relief of suffering my primary concerns.
- I will apply my knowledge, experience, and skills to the best of my ability to assure optimal outcomes for my patients.
- I will respect and protect all personal and health information entrusted to me.

- I will accept the lifelong obligation to improve my professional knowledge and competence.
- I will hold myself and my colleagues to the highest principles of our profession's moral, ethical and legal conduct.
- I will embrace and advocate changes that improve patient care.
- I will utilize my knowledge, skills, experiences, and values to prepare the next generation of pharmacists. I take these vows voluntarily with the full realization of the responsibility with which I am entrusted by the public.

A central tenet underlying pharmaceutical care and our desire to improve drug therapy outcomes is the recognition that patients have drug therapy needs. Although sometimes these needs are obvious ("What can I take for my headache?"), in many cases the patient's drug therapy needs are unrecognized. For the practitioner committed to responsibility for a patient's drug-related needs, identifying such needs in an accurate and timely way is paramount. During any pharmaceutical care encounter, the patient must be assessed to determine whether the following drug therapy needs are being met:[2]

1. The medication is appropriate
2. The medication is effective
3. The medication is safe
4. The patient is adherent

The challenge for the beginning pharmacotherapeutic practitioner is in application. How does a student learn to take the scientific and factual information learned in the classroom and in readings and then apply it to patients so that drug therapy outcomes are maximized? The Study Guide is designed for this purpose, to teach the student the patient care process: how to organize patient information, assess patients in a systematic way, and develop a pharmacotherapy care plan.[4]

All clinicians need a structured rational thought process for making clinical decisions. What sets each profession and professional apart is the application of a unique knowledge base and set of clinical skills to identify and solve problems and to prevent problems from occurring. In the context of drug therapy, Cipolle et al. have termed this structured process the "Pharmacotherapy Workup."[2]

There are three steps that comprise the patient care process and constitute the Pharmacotherapy Workup (see Fig. 1-1): patient assessment, development of the pharmacotherapy care plan, and evaluation of the impact or results of the care plan. As Figure 1-1 indicates, each stage of the process is connected to the other stages, and the process is ongoing as the patient's situation changes.

Assessment

The purpose of assessment is to gather patient-specific information and then determine if the patient's drug therapy needs are being met.[5] To develop the best possible pharmacotherapy plan for the patient, the information gathered must be as accurate and complete as possible. Inaccurate or incomplete information may result in bad therapeutic decisions. There are a variety of sources from which such information is gathered. Although the specific sources may differ on the basis of the patient's situation, the clinician must strive to obtain information from all available sources. The patient is a crucial source of information, as are family members, caregivers, and other health professionals. In a health-system setting (hospitals, ambulatory care clinics, etc.), the clinician also will have access to subjective and objective information recorded in the patient's medical record and other institutional databases. For the pharmacotherapy workup, particular attention must be given to obtaining a complete and accurate medication history. Remember that since the patient care process is continuous, the gathering of patient-specific information also must be ongoing. Such information must be documented in an organized and easily

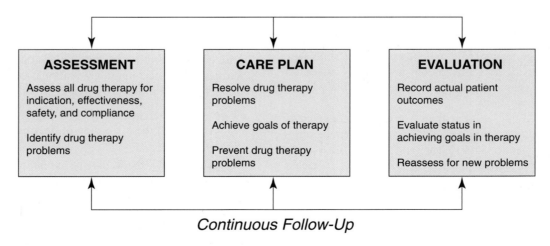

Continuous Follow-Up

FIGURE 1-1. The Patient Care Process. (Reproduced with permission from Cipolle RJ, Strand LM, Morley PC. *Pharmaceutical Care Practice. The Clinician's Guide,* 2nd ed. New York, McGraw-Hill, 2004, p. 246.)

retrievable way that maintains patient confidentiality. Since there may be a large volume of patient-specific information generated, particularly in a hospitalized patient, the use of a standardized patient data form facilitates the organization and retrievability of patient-specific information. Despite the clinician's best effort, in most cases there will be information that is inaccurate and/or incomplete. Never assume that you have all the information you need or that the information you have is correct. The clinician must be mindful of this and seek to "fill in the blanks" by asking appropriate follow-up questions or seeking additional information from other sources.

After all available information is collected, the next step is to develop a problem list.[6] The concept of problem list development is well established in the context of the problem-oriented medical record and the use of the SOAP (Subjective, Objective, Assessment, Plan) method of charting progress notes. The development of an accurate and complete problem list based on the patient's drug therapy needs is crucial in that the development of the pharmacotherapy care plan is derived from the patient's problem list. If a problem is not listed or is not accurate, then the plan will be incomplete or suboptimal. The problem list must be prioritized to ensure that the most important problems are addressed in a timely fashion. For the student learning pharmacotherapy, developing an accurate and complete list of problems is challenging since many pieces of subjective and objective information (findings) have to be interpreted before something can be labeled as a problem. In many cases, problems are medical diagnoses (hypertension, type 2 diabetes, etc.), and in some cases the problem may be a symptom (headache, nausea, pain, etc.). Keep in mind that the definition of a problem may change as more information is gathered. For example, a patient may present with fatigue and, in the absence of other information, that is how the patient's problem is defined at that specific time. However, if the patient is referred to a physician and is found to have hypothyroidism, then the patient's problem list is changed to hypothyroidism, with fatigue as a symptom of the patient's hypothyroidism. A common trap for the beginning student is listing every finding as a problem. With thought and, ultimately, experience, the student will begin to see that the patient's signs and symptoms may be "lumped" into broader problems. If the above-mentioned patient also has cold intolerance, cognitive impairment, weight gain, elevated TSH, and slightly elevated LDL cholesterol, the patient's problem is still hypothyroidism, since each of those findings is a common sign/symptom of hypothyroidism. Although the pharmacotherapy problem list may be very similar to the problem list generated by other clinicians or the problem list present in the patient's medical record, remember that the pharmacist, having a unique body of knowledge, should have a different way of looking at the patient, and the problem list may not be entirely the same. The pharmacotherapy workup must be focused on drug therapy issues, particularly on the presence or risk of drug therapy problems (DTPs). During the entire process, always ask yourself:

- Could the patient's problem(s) be caused by drug therapy?
- Could the patient's problem(s) be managed by a change in drug therapy?

Drug Therapy Problems

The primary focus of the pharmacotherapy workup is the identification and management (treatment and prevention) of DTPs. A DTP is defined as any undesirable event or risk experienced by the patient that involves or is suspected to involve drug therapy and that actually or potentially interferes with a desired patient outcome.[7] Strand et al.'s original list of DTP categories has been expanded to 14 categories:

- Correlation between drug therapy and medical problems
- Need for additional drug therapy
- Unnecessary drug therapy
- Appropriate drug selection
- Wrong drug
- Drug regimen
- Dose too low
- Dose too high
- Therapeutic duplication
- Drug allergy/adverse drug event
- Interactions
- Failure to receive therapy
- Financial impact
- Patient knowledge of drug therapy

Since there are so many categories and specific types of DTPs, and since patients often receive multiple medications, it is important to use an organized, systematic approach to identify actual and potential DTPs. Once a DTP is identified and categorized, it is then necessary to identify the cause of the problem, thereby leading to potential solutions. When multiple DTPs are identified, they need to be prioritized to determine which problems should be addressed first. The patient's concerns must be considered in determining the problems that have the highest priority. Remember that the process of DTP identification is connected to the basic tenets of assessing the patient's drug therapy needs—appropriateness, effectiveness and safety of medications, and the patient's adherence.

Pharmacotherapy Care Plan

The pharmacotherapy care plan[8,9] is the roadmap to achieving improved pharmacotherapy outcomes. It is the action plan developed on the basis of the assessment components described above. Care plans have been an integral component of nursing care, and other professionals or certain health care settings may utilize components of a care plan. However, there is no standard or widely accepted method of care plan development in Pharmacy. Guideline 12.1 of the accreditation standards for pharmacy education in the United States[10] states that "… the college or school must ensure that graduates are competent to provide patient-centered care, through the ability to design, implement, monitor, evaluate and adjust pharmacy care plans that are patient-specific… ."

Ideally, the patient's care plan should be constructed with the patient's involvement and, in a multidisciplinary fashion, developed and altered in a cooperative way by all who are involved with the patient's care. Further, pharmacotherapy care planning should be a component of the patient's overall care plan. Care plans developed in isolation or not shared with the patient or other professionals are less likely to have the desired effect on patient outcomes. A pharmacotherapy care plan must be generated as part of the systematic patient care process and should be a dynamic document that reflects changes in the patient's conditions and drug therapy needs. The care plan is developed in a problem-oriented fashion. Each item in the patient's problem list must be addressed in the care plan, and the care plan should be prioritized in the same way as the problem list.

The pharmacotherapy care plan has several key components for each problem:

- Current drug regimen
- Drug therapy problems
- Therapy goals, desired endpoints
- Therapeutic recommendations
- Rationale
- Therapeutic alternatives
- Monitoring
- Patient education

In patients who have multiple problems, there likely will be some redundancy in the pharmacotherapy care plan in that some problems may be related, and some medications may be used for multiple indications. As the care plan is developed, it is important for the student to see and understand the connections among multiple problems and the pharmacotherapy plan. For example, a patient with hypertension, type 2 diabetes, and chronic kidney disease may be treated with an ACE-I to lower blood pressure, slow progression of renal disease, and reduce risk of cardiovascular events. The student must understand not only that the one drug may be used for several reasons but that the drug could affect the patient's problems in a variety of ways, such as improving blood pressure control while causing an increase in serum potassium or an acute rise in serum creatinine. The risk and significance of these effects must be considered on the basis of the overall clinical picture. In some patients, unintended effects, at least to a defined point, may be acceptable.

Defining therapy goals and endpoints are crucial. You cannot determine whether the patient's desired outcomes are being achieved if you do not know what those desired outcomes are. Think of goals as broad or general outcomes, whereas endpoints are more specific parameters often used as indicators or surrogate markers to indicate that our goals are being achieved. The goals of therapy must be achievable and realistic for the patient. Drug therapy may aim to (1) cure a disease; (2) reduce or eliminate signs and/or symptoms; (3) slow or halt the progression of a disease; (4) prevent a disease; (5) normalize laboratory values; and/or (6) assist in the diagnostic process. Goals and endpoints must be observable, measurable, and describable using specific

parameters. Going back to our diabetic, hypertensive patient mentioned above, the goals of treating those disorders are to prevent cardiovascular disease (stroke, coronary artery disease, peripheral vascular disease), kidney disease, other microvascular complications of diabetes (retinopathy, neuropathy), etc. We also want the patient to feel better and have improved quality of life (QOL). An important goal of any pharmacotherapy care plan is the avoidance of adverse events. We do not want the patient to have side effects or a worsened QOL due to our recommended drug therapy. What would be endpoints for our patient? In our hypertensive diabetic patient, some endpoints would include BP <130/80 mm Hg, glycated hemoglobin <6.5–7% (0.065–0.07), LDL cholesterol <130 mg/dL (<3.36 mmol/L), and weight loss of 10 kg. Goals and endpoints should be associated with a time frame, describing, if possible and realistically, when the goal or endpoint is to be achieved (BP <130/80 mm Hg in 1 month; 22 lb (10 kg) weight loss in 6 months, etc.). The goals and endpoints part of the plan will be directly tied to the monitoring part of the plan, since monitoring is the way we will know if our goals and endpoints have been achieved.

Therapeutic recommendations are the interventions made to meet the patient's drug therapy needs. The recommendations must be specific and individualized to the patient's condition and drug therapy problems. For most problems, there are several ways to intervene to achieve the desired goals and endpoints. The clinician must consider all the possibilities and recommend a therapeutic course that is best for that patient, based on scientific evidence, patient history, cultural and health beliefs, psychosocial issues, health literacy, and cost. Remember that therapeutic recommendations for one problem may have an impact on other problems, so do not lose sight of the big picture.

Although it is important for the clinician to make appropriate therapeutic recommendations, providing a rationale for those recommendations is necessary. The rationale is *why* you are recommending what you are recommending. From an educational standpoint, providing a well-reasoned rationale shows that the student is thinking and understanding, rather than repeating what is in a book, guideline, or said by others. In the clinical practice setting, it is common for pharmacists to be asked to provide their rationale to physicians as part of a discussion about a patient's therapy. Pharmacists need to be adept at providing such a rationale in a succinct way. The rationale should be stated in a way that clearly describes why the recommendation was made for this patient, including why it was chosen over other alternatives, and any evidence available to support the recommendation should be provided.

In determining your therapeutic recommendations, several reasonable alternative regimens typically are available. Even after you have recommended your primary plan, the best alternatives must be kept in mind. The patient or prescriber may not agree with your primary recommendation and request an alternative. Your primary plan may not be effective, or an intolerable adverse event may occur, thereby requiring implementation of an alternative plan. As with your therapeutic recommendations, be specific with your alternative recommendations and base your alternative choices on relative effectiveness and safety based on the best evidence available.

Monitoring and follow-up are important components of the pharmacotherapy care plan and the overall patient care process.[11] Monitoring is how we determine whether our goals and endpoints (achieving positive goals and avoiding negative endpoints) are being reached. An effective monitoring plan must be realistic for the patient setting and include specific monitoring parameters (clinical and laboratory/diagnostic test), frequency of monitoring, and when the patient needs to be seen again for follow-up. Students often struggle with developing a monitoring plan since references often provide only general recommendations for what to monitor and how often. In most patients, the intensity and frequency of monitoring are dynamic. In a critically ill hospitalized patient, some pharmacotherapy monitoring parameters may be assessed multiple times daily. As the patient becomes more stable, leaves the intensive-care unit (ICU), and is, hopefully, discharged home, monitoring becomes less frequent. A patient initiated on warfarin in the hospital may have an INR measured daily. After discharge with a therapeutic INR, monitoring may be done weekly, and as the patient's INR and clinical status remain stable, the frequency is slowly reduced until the INR is measured on a monthly basis. If the INR or the clinical picture changes, the frequency of INR monitoring likely will be increased temporarily. Regardless of the setting, the frequency of monitoring, particularly for those parameters involving blood collection or other invasive tests, must be realistic and based on how often the information truly is needed, what the patient can or is willing to allow, availability of vascular access, and, in the outpatient setting, the ability of the patient to travel to a laboratory or the availability of home care services. In the home setting, some of the monitoring may be done by the patient, such as assessing presence and severity of signs and symptoms, basic physical assessment parameters (e.g., weight, presence of edema), and certain diagnostic or laboratory tests (e.g., blood pressure, blood glucose). The monitoring plan must be specific—what parameters, frequency of monitoring, who will monitor, and when and with whom the patient will follow-up. The results of monitoring naturally will influence the pharmacotherapy care plan, and in many cases, there should be an upfront determination of what action will be taken based on the results of the monitoring plan (e.g., "if the patient's INR is <2, the warfarin dose will be increased from 4 to 5 mg daily").

Patient education is the final piece of the pharmacotherapy care plan. Patient adherence to drug therapy can be improved with effective and ongoing patient education, and ideally, such education should be provided with verbal communication and written materials. Pharmacy students should utilize skills learned in their communications courses and information available in books[12,13] and begin applying those skills in case-based learning, small group discussions, and internship experience in preparation for their pharmacy practice experience rotations and, ultimately, pharmacy practice. The pharmacotherapy care plan must include a summary of what you will tell and provide the patient regarding their drug therapy.

Remember that our model for the patient care process involves continuous follow-up. As the pharmacotherapy care plan is implemented, the patient's response to therapy is monitored, and changes in therapy may be necessary. Changes in previous problems or the development of new signs and symptoms will require the assessment process and changes in the pharmacotherapy care plan. Although the patient care process and the application of your didactic knowledge to the patient care setting may seem daunting, by working through the cases in the Study Guide, your skills can only get better and better. Although this book can be used for self-study, ideally, some of the cases in this Study Guide will be used in a small group discussion setting under the guidance of a group facilitator, so you can see how other students think. Group settings also provide the opportunity to discuss and defend your therapeutic recommendations and practice your verbal communication skills. As you work through the patient cases, you will make mistakes and perhaps choose suboptimal therapy that even could cause harm. Beginners always make mistakes, and you should use the mistakes made by you and your fellow students as powerful learning opportunities. Here are some tips for success in patient care:

- CARE about the patient!
- Know your stuff—be prepared
- Realize that every patient is different
- Review and assess *all* available information
- Be organized and consistent in your approach
- Do not make snap judgments—is your assessment and approach supported by the evidence?
- NEVER make assumptions
- Be skeptical
- Think ahead, and think it through ("… then what?")

HOW THE CASES ARE ORGANIZED

Each patient case in the Study Guide has been prepared in a standard format, similar to how you will see cases presented in a clinical setting. The use of an organized case format will assist you in learning where to find information about the patient and help you get accustomed to the format for when you will be presenting patients yourself in case discussions or rotations. The patient cases in the Study Guide are meant to be realistic. Patients usually will have multiple, sometimes related, problems, though each case will focus on one primary topic or problem. Patients will have DTPs requiring identification and management. The components of each case in the Study Guide will include:

1. *Patient Identification*—name, age, etc.
2. *Chief Complaint*—why the patient is seeking help, in the patient's own words

3. *History of Present Illness* (HPI)—the patient's story about why they are seeking help

4. *Past Medical History* (PMH)—including all significant illnesses, surgical procedures, injuries

5. *Family History*—age and health of immediate family (parents, siblings, children); for deceased relatives, the age and cause of death are included; any hereditary diseases should be noted

6. *Social History*—may include where the patient is from or lives, ethnicity/race, marital status, number of children, educational background, occupation, diet

7. *Tobacco/Alcohol/Substance Use*

8. *Allergy/Intolerances/Adverse Drug Events* (ADEs)—a common area where information from the patient is missing or incomplete

9. *Medication History*—should include current (or medications prior to admission if hospitalized) and previous medications; the list should include what the patient *actually* is taking, not just what is prescribed, and must include OTC drugs and dietary supplements (including herbal and complementary/alternative products).

10. *Review of Systems* (ROS)—systematic, head-to-toe questions asked to elicit symptoms and potential problems not noted by the patient in the HPI. Postitive findings and pertinent negatives (significant absence of a symptom) are included.

11. *Physical Examination* (PE)—nature and completeness of the examination will depend on the patient's history and overall clinical picture. Rarely will a complete PE be done; rather, the examination will be targeted to the situation. Positive and pertinent negative findings will be included in the PE. If you are not familiar with the meaning or significance of some of the examination findings, make sure you look those up. Components of the PE may include:
    - General
    - Vital Signs (include pain as fifth vital sign)
    - Skin
    - HEENT
    - Neck and Lymph Nodes
    - Chest
    - Breasts (in women)
    - Cardiovascular
    - Abdomen
    - Neurology
    - Extremities
    - Genitourinary
    - Rectal

12. *Laboratory and Other Diagnostic Tests*—only data that are common and/or directly relevant to the case will be included. A list of normal laboratory values is included as Appendix B of this Study Guide. All laboratory results will be presented in conventional units typically used in the United States and in Systéme Internationale (SI) units for students using the book in other countries. If you are not familiar with the meaning or significance of some of the laboratory findings, make sure you look those up.

13. *Assessment*—the clinician's impression and/or diagnosis.

14. *Student Workup*—for each case, you will be asked if there is missing information and to evaluate and develop a Patient Database, Drug Therapy Problem Worksheet, and Pharmacotherapy Care Plan. When you are working with actual patients, you will find that the patient's history and information from other sources will be incomplete and/or inaccurate. Patient cases in the Study Guide will have missing information, and it is important that, as you evaluate each case, you recognize what needed information is missing so that you can make an accurate assesment of the patient. One way to remember to assess for missing information is to always create as one of your patient's problems "Inadequate Database," and then list the missing information elements under that problem in your Care Plan. A more detailed description of the Patient Database, Drug Therapy Problem Worksheet, and Pharmacotherapy Care Plan forms will follow.

15. *Targeted Questions*—each case will include a series of questions targeted toward helping you better understand the key elements of the case and the patient's primary problems. A unique feature of this Study Guide is that each question will be followed by a Hint, guiding you to the pages in *Pharmacotherapy Principles and Practice*, 2nd ed. (*PPP*) where you can find the information to answer the question.

16. *Follow-up*—some cases will provide a brief clinical follow-up that may include some outcomes of your initial Care Plan. The Follow-up section may include additional Targeted Questions, with Hints to further assist your studies.

17. *Global Perspective*—another unique feature of this Study Guide is the inclusion of a Global Perspective section that highlights an issue related to the case that is important to countries outside North America or involves different ethnic groups or races. Global Perspectives may highlight differences in disease incidence or manifestations, pharmacokinetics or pharmacodynamics, treatment standards, culturally based beliefs and/or treatments, and drug response.

18. *Case Summary*—a short summary of the key points addressed by the case

19. *References*—will be included in the patient case only if a key reference has been published that is not included in *PPP*. For most cases, the references included in the relevant *PPP* chapters are excellent sources for you to obtain additional information.

STUDENT CASE WORKUP

The desired student workup of each case in this Study Guide is the development of a Pharmacotherapy Care Plan. The principles of the pharmacotherapy workup, patient assessment, and development of a care plan were reviewed earlier in this chapter. Your workup of the Study Guide cases will apply these principles. To facilitate your accomplishing these tasks in a thoughtful, organized and systematic way, you are provided three forms—Patient Database, Drug Therapy Problem Worksheet (DTPW), and Pharmacotherapy Care Plan. The forms used in this Study Guide are adapted with permission from those originally developed by the American Society of Health-System Pharmacists (ASHP) in the early 1990s as part of their Clinical Skills program,[5,6,8,11] and these forms are currently used by particpants in the ASHP Clinical Skills Competition (www.ashp.org/Import/ABOUTUS/Awards/ClinicalSkillsCompetition.aspx).

Different clinicians and institutions use many different types of patient-monitoring forms. Think of the forms used in this Study Guide as a tool to help you learn to provide the best patient care. The forms are designed to help you organize information and to help you organize your thinking. Although you will find the use of such forms helpful, do not obsess about the forms or using them "right." Again, the forms are a tool to help you achieve what you *should* obsess about—making the patient's drug therapy the best it can be.

To help you understand how to best utilize these forms as you workup the Study Guide cases, we have prepared a practice case presented in the same format as other cases in the Study Guide and a completed student workup. Before you embark on your first Study Guide patient case, look over the practice case and the completed forms. We have added some tips in certain places in the practice case forms to help you better understand their application. Learning to effectively assess patients and develop a care plan involves skills that require practice and repetition. As you begin learning pharmacotherapeutics, applying your didactic knowledge to patient situations may seem difficult, and it is likely you will make mistakes. That's OK! The point of this Study Guide is to help you learn and to develop your skills. Through your coursework, reading, and use of this Study Guide, you will see your knowledge and skills increase and you will become a great practitioner who will improve patient drug therapy outcomes.

REFERENCES

1. Hepler CD, Strand LM. Opportunities and responsibilities in pharmaceutical care. Am J Hosp Pharm 1990 47: 533–543.
2. Cipolle RJ, Strand LM, Morley PC. Pharmaceutical Care Practice. The Clinician's Guide, 2nd ed. New York, McGraw-Hill, 2004.
3. American Association of Colleges of Pharmacy. www.aacp. org/resources/academicpolicies/studentaffairspolicies/ Documents/OATHOFAPHARMACIST2008-09.pdf. Accessed June 1, 2010.
4. American Society of Health System Pharmacists. ASHP guidelines on a standardized method for pharmaceutical care. Am J Health-Syst Pharm 1996 53:1713–1716.
5. Mason NA, Shimp LA. Module 2: Building a pharmacist's patient database. In: ASHP Clinical Skills Program—Advancing Pharmaceutical Care. Bethesda, MD, American Society of Health-System Pharmacists, 1993.
6. Shimp LA, Mason NA. Module 3: Constructing a patient's drug therapy problem list. In: ASHP Clinical Skills Program—Advancing Pharmaceutical Care. Bethesda, MD, American Society of Health-System Pharmacists, 1993.
7. Strand LM, Morley PC, Cipolle RJ, et al. Drug-related problems: Their structure and function. DICP 1990 24:1093–1097.
8. Jones W, Campbell S. Module 4: Designing and recommending a pharmacist's care plan. In: ASHP Clinical Skills Program—Advancing Pharmaceutical Care. Bethesda, MD, American Society of Health-System Pharmacists, 1993.
9. Galt K. Developing Clinical Practice Skills for Pharmacists. Bethesda, MD, American Society of Health-System Pharmacists, 2006.
10. American Council for Pharmacy Education. Accreditation Standards and Guidelines for the Professional Program in Pharmacy Leading to the Doctor of Pharmacy Degree, 2006. www.acpe-accredit.org/standards/default.asp. Accessed June 1, 2010.
11. Frye CB. Module 5: Monitoring the pharmacist's care plan. In: ASHP Clinical Skills Program—Advancing Pharmaceutical Care. Bethesda, MD, American Society of Health-System Pharmacists, 1993.
12. Beardsley RS, Kimberlin CL, Tindall WN. Communication Skills in Pharmacy Practice, 5th ed. Philadelphia, PA, Lippincott Williams & Wilkins, 2007.
13. Rantucci ML. Pharmacists Talking with Patients, 2nd ed. Philadelphia, PA, Lippincott Williams & Wilkins, 2007.

PRACTICE CASE

Case Learning Objectives

- Recognize the signs, symptoms, and risk factors for hypovolemia, hypokalemia, and metabolic alkalosis
- Develop an appropriate treatment and monitoring plan for hypovolemia, hypokalemia, and metabolic alkalosis
- Recognize the impact of pregnancy on medication choice and disease management

PATIENT PRESENTATION

Chief Complaint

"I feel so tired and dizzy, and I can't stop throwing up."

History of Present Illness

Susan Jones is a 23-year-old woman brought to the Urgent Care Center c/o severe weakness and dizziness. She states it started 3 days ago when she began to have frequent vomiting. She thinks that "maybe I ate something bad." She also says that her bowel movements have been "a little looser than normal." She states that before she got sick 3 days ago, she felt fine.

Past Medical History

Bulimia with two psychiatric hospitalizations

Depression, s/p suicide attempt × 1 (slashed wrists)

Pelvic inflammatory disease

Family History

Mother died from drug overdose at age 34; she does not know her father.

Social History

Single community college student; no children; works part time in restaurant.

Tobacco/Alcohol/Substance abuse

(+) cigarettes ½ ppd; admits to occasional marijuana use, denies current other illicit or unprescribed drug or alcohol use; used IV heroin until 1 year ago.

Medications

Prozac 20 mg bid PO

Trazodone 50 mg q hs PO

K-DUR 40 mEq q AM PO

Methadone 120 mg q AM PO

Prilosec 20 mg q day PO

Lo-Estrin 1 q AM PO

Review of Systems

(+) Weakness, dizziness, fatigue, nausea, and diarrhea; denies headache, chest pain, or abdominal pain; (+) dysuria; (−) vaginal pain or discharge.

Physical Examination

▶ **General**

Very thin, chronically ill–appearing young woman who fainted when sitting up.

▶ **Vital signs**

BP 105/75 mm Hg lying, 70/0 mm Hg sitting; P 110 lying, 160 sitting; RR 12, T 37.1°C

Weight 47 kg (103.4 lb), height 5′4″ (163 cm)

▶ **Skin**

Dry, poor skin turgor; no rashes or lesions noted

▶ **HEENT**

PERRLA; mouth very dry; poor dentition

▶ **Neck and lymph nodes**

JVD 0 (neck veins flat); thyroid gland normal; no lymphadenopathy

▶ **Chest**

Clear to auscultation and percussion

▶ **Breasts**

Examination deferred

▶ **Cardiovascular**

Tachycardic; normal S_1, S_2; no murmurs, rubs, or gallops

▶ **Abdomen**

No tenderness or organomegaly; bowel sounds slightly hyperactive

▶ **Extremities**

Very thin; trace pedal edema; multiple "tracks" both arms

▶ **Genitourinary**

Normal vaginal discharge; uterus appears to contain approximately 12-week pregnancy

▶ **Rectal**

Mild hemorrhoids; Hemoccult (−)

Laboratory Tests

Fasting, obtained upon admission

	Conventional Units	SI Units
Na	126 mEq/L	126 mmol/L
K	2.1 mEq/L	2.1 mmol/L
Cl	87 mEq/L	87 mmol/L
CO_2	32 mEq/L	32 mmol/L
BUN	8 mg/dL	2.86 mmol/L
SCr	0.5 mg/dL	44.2 µmol/L
Glu	110 mg/dL	6.11 mmol/L
Ca	8.7 mg/dL	2.18 mmol/L
Mg	1.8 mEq/L	0.90 mmol/L
Phosphate	3.6 mg/dL	1.16 mmol/L
WBC	$7.4 \times 10^3/mm^3$	$7.4 \times 10^9/L$
Hgb	11.6 g/dL	116 g/L; 7.2 mmol/L
Hct	34.6%	0.346

Albumin   3.2 g/dL   32 g/L
PT   17 s
INR   1.3

Urine pregnancy test (+)

ABG: pH 7.56, pO_2 98 mm Hg (13.03 kPa), O_2 sat 99%, pCO_2 44 mm Hg (5.85 kPa), HCO_3 31 mEq/L (31 mmol/L)

Urine toxicology screen: (+) cocaine, THC, methamphetamine, nicotine, HCTZ

Electrocardiogram: flat T waves; (+) U wave

Assessment

Twenty-three-year-old pregnant woman with ECF volume depletion, vomiting and ? diarrhea, significant hypokalemia with ECG changes, hyponatremia, and metabolic alkalosis. Urine tox screen indicates active illicit drug use.

Student Workup

Missing Information?

Evaluate: Patient Database
                  Drug Therapy Problems
                  Care Plan (by Problem)

TARGETED QUESTIONS

1. What signs and symptoms of ECF volume depeletion, hypokalemia, and metabolic alkalosis does the patient have?

   Hint: See pp. 255, 480, 487–488, 502–503 in PPP

2. What are the causes of this patient's alkalosis?

   Hint: See pp. 502–503 in PPP

3. What are the risks of administering potassium intravenously?

   Hint: See p. 488 in PPP

4. What are the signs and symptoms of opioid withdrawal, and what drug interactions may occur with methadone?

   Hint: See pp. 615, 620 in PPP

5. What medications have proven teratogenic effects in humans?

   Hint: See p. 824 in PPP

FOLLOW-UP

Three months later, the patient calls you after being discharged from an inpatient substance abuse program. She says she feels great, is staying clean, and her baby is doing well ("Look how fat I am!"). Her obstetrician recently told her that she has low thyroid and wants her to take levothyroxine. She is aftraid that it will hurt her baby and she wants your advice. You look up her laboratory tests in the computer and note that her TSH is 10.1 mU/L (10.1 µU/L). What is your advice to her?

Hint: See p. 772 in PPP

☉ GLOBAL PERSPECTIVE

Depression is a common mental disorder that presents with depressed mood, loss of interest or pleasure, feelings of guilt or low self-worth, disturbed sleep or appetite, low energy, and poor concentration. These problems can become chronic or recurrent and lead to substantial impairments in an individual's ability to take care of his or her everyday responsibilities. At its worst, depression can lead to suicide, with the loss of about 850,000 lives every year.

Depression in the year 2000 was the leading cause of disability worldwide as measured by years lived with disability (YLD) and the fourth-leading contributor to the global burden of disease based on disability-adjusted life-years (DALYs). By the year 2020, depression is projected to reach second place in the ranking of DALYs calculated for all ages, both sexes. Today, depression already is the second cause of DALYs worldwide in the age category 15 to 44 years for both sexes combined. According to the World Health Organization, fewer than 25% of depressed patients have access to care, and in some countries fewer than 10% have access to care. Barriers to effective care include the lack of resources, lack of trained providers, and the social stigma associated with mental disorders, including depression.

REFERENCE

World Health Organization. www.who.int/mental_health/management/depression/definition/en/index1.html. Accessed January 31, 2010.

CASE SUMMARY

- Young pregnant woman with history of depression, eating disorder, and substance abuse who presents with ECF volume depletion, hypokalemia, and metabolic alkalosis due to vomiting and diuretic use. Volume and potassium replacement must be initiated, and the underlying causes addressed to prevent recurrence.

- She is actively abusing drugs, placing her and the fetus at risk for multiple complications. Substance abuse treatment referral is warranted

- The patient needs a referral to an obstetrician for assessment and prenatal care.

For more information on the care plan and facilitator's guide please visit http://www.mhpharmacotherapy.com.

PATIENT DATABASE FORM

Patient Name: Susan Jones	*Real patient names are not used in this Study Guide.*	**Patient ID:**	**Location:** Urgent Care
Physician:		**Pharmacy:**	
Age (or Date of Birth): 23 yo		**Race:** Caucasian	**Sex:** Female
Height: 5'4" (163 cm)		**Weight:** 47 kg (103.4 lb)	
Date of Admission/Initial Visit: 6/1/2010		**Occupation:** Student, restaurant worker	

Allergies/Intolerances/ADRs

❏ No known drug allergies/ADRs

☒ Not known/inadequate information

Drug:	Reaction:

*A common area where information is missing or incomplete. No known drug allergies/ADRs is **NOT** the same as Not known. No known means the patients has been asked and/or chart reviewed, while Not known means there is missing information.*

HPI, PMH, FH, SH, etc...

Weakness, dizziness, vomiting,? diarrhea × 3 days

Hx eating disorder, depression (s/p suicide attempt), PID

Smokes ½ ppd, uses marijuana, Hx IVDU (+) dysuria on ROS

Appears dry—orthostatic, flat neck veins

Evidence of active IVDU

12 wk pregnant

A summary of the key subjective and objective findings from the case.

Prioritized Medical Problem List	Medication Profile	
Hypovolemic hyponatremia, d/t vomiting,? diuretic use		
Hypokalemia with ECG changes	K-Dur 40 mEq q AM PO	*List of medications placed next to problem list to facilitate matching medications with indications. Note that some medications may have multiple indications.*
Metabolic alkalosis due to #1 and #2		
Active substance use with urine (+) cocaine, methamphetamine; no evidence for endocarditis	Methadone 120 mg q day PO	
Tobacco use		
12 wk pregnant by exam, (+) urine HCG	Lo-Estrin PO	
Hx bulimia, appears to be malnourished	Fluoxetine 20 mg bid PO	*Get used to including Inadequate database or Missing Information on your problems list so you will remember to follow-up on all missing information.*
? Diarrhea		
Hx depression, s/p suicide attempt × 1		
Dysuria, R/O UTI		
Inadequate database	? Indications for trazodone, omeprazole	

The form is from *ASHP National Clinical Skills Competition Case Documents*, Copyright 2009, American Society of Health-System Pharmacists, Bethesda, MD (www.ashp.org). Adapted with permission.

Vital Signs, Laboratory Data, and Diagnostic Test Results			
Date	6/1/2010		
Weight (lb/kg)	103.4 (47)		
Temperature (°C)	37.1		
Blood pressure (mm Hg)	105/75 lying, 70/0 sitting		
Pulse	110 lying, 160 sitting		
Respiratory rate	12		
Na 135–145 mEq/L (135–145 mmol/L)	126 (126)		
K 3.3–4.9 mEq/L (3.3–4.9 mmol/L)	2.1 (2.1)		
Cl 97–110 mEq/L (97–110 mmol/L)	87 (87)		
CO_2/HCO_3 22–26 mEq/L (22–26 mmol/L)	32 (32)		
BUN 8–25 mg/dL (2.9–8.9 mmol/L)	8 (2.86)		
Creatinine (adult) Male 0.7–1.3 mg/dL; female 0.6–1.1 mg/dL (male 62–115 µmol/L; female 53–97 µmol/L)	0.5 (44.2)		
Creatinine clearance (adult) 85–135 mL/min (0.82–1.30 mL/s/m^2)	129.9 (1.25)		
Glucose (fasting) 65–109 mg/dL (3.6–6.0 mmol/L)	110 (6.11)		
Total Ca 8.6–10.3 mg/dL (2.15–2.58 mmol/L)	8.7 (2.18)		
Mg 1.3–2.2 mEq/L (0.65–1.10 mmol/L)	1.8 (0.9)		
PO_4 2.5–4.5 mg/dL (0.81–1.45 mmol/L)	3.6 (1.16)		
Hemoglobin Male 13.8–17.2 g/dL; female 12.1–15.1 g/dL (male 138–172 g/L; female 121–151 g/L)	11.6 (116)		
Hematocrit Male 40.7–50.3%; female 36.1–44.3% (male 0.407–0.503; female 0.361–0.443)	34.6 (0.346)		
MCV 80.0–97.6 µm^3 (80.0–97.6 fl)			
WBC 4–10 × 10^3/mm^3 (4–10 × 10^9/L)	7.4 (7.4)		
Differential			
Platelet 140–440 × 10^3/mm^3 (140–440 × 10^9/L)			
Albumin 3.5–5 g/dL (35–50 g/L)	3.2 (32)		
Total bilirubin 0.3–1.1 mg/dL (5.13–18.80 µmol/L)			
Direct bilirubin 0–0.3 mg/dL (0–5.1 µmol/L)			
AST 11–47 IU/L (0.18–0.78 µkat/L)			

Having data in tabular form allows following trends over time (date as column heading).

Vital Signs, Laboratory Data, and Diagnostic Test Results			
ALT 7–53 IU/L (0.12–0.88 μkat/L)			
Alk phos (adult) 38–126 IU/L (0.13–2.10 μkat/L)			
Urine HCG	Positive		
PH 7.35–7.45	7.56		
PO₂ 70–95 mm Hg (9.3–12.6 kPa)	98 (13.03)		
O₂ Saturation (90–110%)	99		
PCO₂ 35–45 mm Hg (4.7–6.0 kPa)	44 (5.85)		

Not every lab test is included on the blank forms, so you will need to add lab tests, normal values and normal values for tests not already on the form. Normal values may be found in Appendix B. Make sure you understand the significance of each lab test.

Notes
Urine tox screen (+) for cocaine, THC, methamphetamine, HCTZ
ECG: NSR, rate 110, flattened T waves, (+) U wave

This is a free text area to add items that do not fit elsewhere or for quick notes to yourself or other clinicians who may be following the patient.

> This Worksheet will help you systematically assess the patient for the presence of and potential for all Drug Therapy Problems. After each problem, is identified, you will then need to assess the significance of each problem, and integrate those problems with your overall Care Plan. Some medications may be associated with multiple problems. Make sure you are as specific as possible in identifying the problem so that appropriate action then can be taken.

DRUG THERAPY PROBLEM WORKSHEET

Type of Problem	Possible Causes		
Correlation between drug therapy and medical problems	Drugs without obvious medical indications	Trazodone, omeprazole	
	Medications unidentified		
	Untreated medical conditions		
Need for additional drug therapy	New medical condition requiring new drug therapy	Pregnancy If dysuria d/t UTI, needs nonteratogenic antimicrobial	Needs prenatal care
	Chronic disorder requiring continued drug therapy		
	Condition best treated with combination drug therapy		
	May develop new medical condition without prophylactic or preventative therapy or premedication		
Unnecessary drug therapy	Medication with no valid indication	Lo-Estrin	Patient is pregnant
	Condition caused by accidental or intentional ingestion of toxic amount of drug or chemical	HCTZ contributed to fluid/electrolyte disorders	
	Medical problem(s) associated with use of or withdrawal from alcohol, drug, or tobacco		
	Condition is better treated with nondrug therapy		
	Taking multiple drugs when single agent as effective		
	Taking drug(s) to treat an avoidable adverse reaction from another medication		
Appropriate drug selection	Current regimen not usually as effective as other choices		
	Current regimen not usually as safe as other choices		
	Therapy not individualized to patient		
Wrong drug	Medical problem for which drug is not effective		
	Patient has risk factors that contraindicate use of drug	Need to assess teratogenic effects of all drugs; hormonal contraceptive in pregnancy	
	Patient has infection with organisms resistant to drug		
	Patient refractory to current drug therapy		
	Taking combination product when single agent appropriate		
	Dosage form inappropriate		
	Medication error		
Drug regimen	PRN use not appropriate for condition		
	Route of administration/dosage form/mode of administration not appropriate for current condition		
	Length or course of therapy not appropriate		
	Drug therapy altered without adequate therapeutic trial		
	Dose or interval flexibility not appropriate		
Dose too low	Dose or frequency too low to produce desired response in this patient		
	Serum drug level below desired therapeutic range		
	Timing of antimicrobial prophylaxis not appropriate		
	Medication not stored properly		
	Medication error		

Identified by comparing problem list and medication list.

Make sure all new problems are addressed (though all may not require drug therapy).

Even if a medication is indicated for the problem, it may not be the BEST therapy for that patient.

DRUG THERAPY PROBLEM WORKSHEET

Type of Problem	Possible Causes	Problem List	Notes
Dose too high	Dose or frequency too high for this patient	Assess methadone dose with substance abuse provider	Make sure all drug doses have been adjusted for the patient's renal and liver function.
	Serum drug level above the desired therapeutic range		
	Dose escalated too quickly		
	Dose or interval flexibility not appropriate for this patient	Need for bid fluoxetine	
	Medication error		
Therapeutic duplication	Receiving multiple agents without added benefit		
Drug allergy/ adverse drug events	History of allergy or ADE to current (or chemically related) agents		
	Allergy or ADE history not in medical records	Need allergy/ADE history	Allergy/ADE information commonly is missing or incomplete.
	Patient not using alert for severe allergy or ADE		
	Symptoms or medical problems that may be drug induced	HCZT and fluid/ electrolyte disorders Fluoxetine and insomnia	
	Drug administered too rapidly		
	Medication error, actual or potential		
Interactions (drug–drug, drug–disease, drug–nutrient, drug–laboratory test)	Effect of drug altered due to enzyme induction/ inhibition from another drug patient is taking	Fluoxetine and methadone	Slight reduction in methadone clearance; watch QTc
	Effect of drug altered due to protein-binding alterations from another drug patient is taking		
	Effect of drug altered due to pharmacodynamic change from another drug patient is taking	Fluoxetine and trazodone	Both serotonin modulators
	Bioavailability of drug altered due to interaction with another drug or food		Assessing for interactions is important, but make sure you assess for the clinical significance of the interaction in the patient.
	Effect of drug altered due to substance in food		
	Patient's laboratory test altered due to interference from a drug the patient is taking		
Failure to receive therapy	Patient did not adhere with the drug regimen	Unknown, but likely is nonadherent; likely not taking methadone since not in urine tox	ALWAYS assess adherence. If adherence problems are identified, find out the reasons for poor adherence and possible solutions.
	Drug not given due to medication error		
	Patient did not take due to high drug cost/lack of insurance	Unknown	
	Patient unable to take oral medication		
	Patient has no IV access for IV medication		Financial or insurance problems are a common reason for poor adherence.
	Drug product not available		
Financial impact	The current regimen is not the most cost-effective		
	Patient unable to purchase medications/no insurance	Unknown	
Patient knowledge of drug therapy	Patient does not understand the purpose, directions, or potential side effects of the drug regimen	Unknown	Patients often have little understanding about their medications. Make sure you develop an educational plan appropriate for the patient.
	Current regimen not consistent with the patient's health beliefs	Unknown	

PHARMACOTHERAPY CARE PLAN

For acute problems, make sure your therapeutic recommendations are carried through to some resolution or stopping point and/or chronic therapy.

Medical Problem List	Current Drug Regimen	Drug Therapy Problems	Therapy Goals, Desired Endpoints	Therapeutic Recommendations	Rationale	Therapeutic Alternatives	Monitoring
Hypovolemic hyponatremia		HCTZ use may be contributing factor	Normal hemodynamics (BP, pulse, JVD), improved symptoms (weakness, dizziness); prevent recurrence by treating underlying cause	Normal saline IV 1 L now over 15 min, then 500 mL/h × 2. Repeat until no longer orthostatic; if able to take PO, add oral rehydration solution (ORS) 250 mL q 30 min; promethazine 25 mg PO/IM/PR q 4 h PRN N/V; pt needs to stop using HCTZ; if pt has diarrhea, order stool culture, R/O laxative abuse; stop using HCTZ	Severe signs and symptoms, presence of vomiting warrant IV fluid; normal saline best for treating ECF depletion, metabolic alkalosis; hyponatremia will correct with volume replacement	If able to take PO or IV access not available, ORS 500–1000 mL/h as tolerated; metoclopramide 10 mg IV q 6 h PRN nausea	VS q 15 min × 2 h, then q 1 h while in urgent care. Recheck basic metabolic panel (BMP) in 4 h; pt to self-monitor symptoms, weight daily after discharge; repeat BMP in 2 d
Hypokalemia	K-Dur 40 mEq q AM PO	HCTZ	Normal serum K; normal ECG; no symptoms; prevent recurrence by treating underlying cause	KCl liquid 40 mEq PO now, repeat in 2 h; if serum K increasing, change to KCl SR 40 mEq bid × 2 d, then reassess; stop using HCTZ	Oral KCl safer than IV if pt able to take; pt has significant K deficit; need K replacement for correction of alkalosis; use liquid KCl for rapid absorption	If unable to take PO, IV KCl 10 mEq/100 mL with 10 mg lidocaine over 1 h × 4 doses	BMP in 2 h (recheck in 6 h if IV KCl given); ECG in 4 h
Metabolic alkalosis, due to decreased ECF, vomiting, ?diuretic use		HCTZ	Normal ABG, electrolytes, ECF volume; prevent recurrence by treating underlying cause	Volume repletion, K replacement, treat vomiting as above; stop using HCTZ; if alkalosis slow to clear or serum Mg drops, provide Mg replacement as MgSO$_4$ 1 g IV in 100 mL NS over 1 h	Alkalosis will resolve with volume and K replacement and with removal of underlying causes; Mg deficiency can prevent resolution of hypokalemia, alkalosis, though serum Mg now normal	Alternatives to volume, K replacement as above; no indication for IV HCl administration; could give Mg replacement even though serum Mg in normal range	BMP, other monitoring as above; recheck serum Mg in 2 h

Annotation notes:

- Drug therapy problems identified on DTPW listed in this column, tied to medical problem.
- Goals and endpoints should be as specific as possible, and should include preventing adverse outcomes as well as seeking positive outcomes.
- Therapeutic recommendations and alternatives must be specific (drug, route, dose, frequency, duration).
- Make sure monitoring plan is specific (parameters, frequency) and realistic for the setting.
- Your rationale should include why you chose your primary therapy (drug, route, etc.) versus the alternative(s); may include why you did not specifically address certain problems.
- Note that some problems are connected to others, and their resolution may be connected to treatment of those related problems.

PHARMACOTHERAPY CARE PLAN

Medical Problem List	Current Drug Regimen	Drug Therapy Problems	Therapy Goals, Desired Endpoints	Therapeutic Recommendations	Rationale	Therapeutic Alternatives	Monitoring
Substance use	Methadone 120 mg q day PO	Urine tox (+) for cocaine, THC, methamphetamine	No use of illicit drugs; avoidance of medical complications of injection use such as skin abscesses endocarditis Not all problems can be addressed or resolved. Some will require referral to other professionals or institutions.	Hold methadone since pt seems not to be taking and no evidence of narcotic withdrawal; if signs of withdrawal develop, begin methadone 20 mg q day inpatient; if methadone used, watch for potential interactions; blood cultures × 3 to R/O endocarditis; refer back to substance abuse provider after discharge; encourage enrollment in smoking cessation program; test for HIV, hepatitis B and C	Since urine tox was not positive for methadone, pt likely not taking; narcotic withdrawal not life-threatening, so best to wait to see if withdrawal signs develop and then treat with low-dose methadone; while no evidence of endocarditis (fever, murmur), best to R/O with blood cultures especially since she is pregnant	Begin methadone 20 mg q day if patient was taking methadone or other opioids chronically	Signs and symptoms of drug withdrawal; temperature q 6 h while in facility, then by pt daily; examine injection sites daily; CBC in 2 d; QTc if on methadone
Pregnancy		Lo-Estrin, drugs of abuse, tobacco	Cessation of behavior that is high risk to the fetus; adequate prenatal care	DC Lo-Estrin; substance abuse program as per substance abuse provider; refer to OB for full assessment, prenatal care; prenatal vitamin 1 q day; nutrition consult; smoking cessation; need to review all current and future drugs for teratogenic effect	Substance abuse and malnutrition will severely compromise development and health of fetus	None	As per substance abuse provider, OB

PHARMACOTHERAPY CARE PLAN

Medical Problem List	Current Drug Regimen	Drug Therapy Problems	Therapy Goals, Desired Endpoints	Therapeutic Recommendations	Rationale	Therapeutic Alternatives	Monitoring
Eating disorder, depression	Fluoxetine 20 mg bid PO	Drugs of abuse; fluoxetine bid ? causing insomnia; HCTZ use, ? laxative use	Normal eating patterns, no use of diuretics or laxatives; normal mood with no s/s depression	If patient has been taking fluoxetine, continue at 20 mg q day; psych consult; if insomnia, withhold hypnotics at this time since may be due to fluoxetine regimen and stimulant use; nutrition consult as above	Avoid SSRI withdrawal syndrome if she has been taking fluoxetine; if insomnia, may resolve with change in fluoxetine regimen, stimulant detox	Change antidepressant to less stimulating agent, i.e., sertraline 50 mg q day	As per psych
Dysuria			No symptoms; cure UTI if present	Urinalysis; if (+) for UTI, send for culture and start cephalexin 250 mg q 8 h × 7 d, start after all three blood cultures drawn	Cephalosporins safe in pregnancy, active against most common organism	Augmentin 500 mg q 8 h × 7 d	UTI s/s daily; repeat UA after antibiotic completed; stool frequency, consistency
Inadequate database				Need allergy/ADE Hx; indications for trazodone, omeprazole; frequency of substance use; adherence with prescribed medications; use of diuretics, laxatives; screen for HIV, viral hepatitis; liver enzymes; previous pregnancies, deliveries			

Therapy may be initiated or altered as missing information is obtained. In such cases make sure that you note that you note that therapy will be started based on obtaining certain information.

For the Study Guide cases, all you can do is list missing information. In a real-life setting, you must try to obtain the missing information from the appropriate sources (patient, family, medical record, other professionals or institutions).

PATIENT EDUCATION SUMMARY

> Summarize your patient education in the type of language you would use with a real patient. Avoid use of medical terms or lingo, and keep in mind the patient's language skills, educational background, and culture.

Notes

- The problems you are having with your fluid and electrolytes are all related and are causing your weakness and dizziness. There are several reasons why these problems developed, including your vomiting and lack of food and fluid intake and your drug abuse. It appears that you are using an unprescribed diuretic, and that is causing or worsening these problems. Although we can easily treat these problems here, it is important that you take steps so that it does not happen again. You can help prevent this in the future by making sure you eat and drink fluids properly, do not use diuretics, and stop abusing drugs. After we give you some IV fluids, we will be giving you some oral fluids, as well as some oral potassium. It is very important that you take these as directed so that we can get your fluid and electrolyte levels back to normal. We have prescribed a medication, promethazine, for nausea and vomiting. Take it only if you need it and are unable to keep down oral fluids. Sometimes this medication can cause you to be a little drowsy or have a dry mouth. Let us know if that happens.

- From your urine screen and looking at your arms we can tell that you are actively abusing drugs. It will be crucial for you and your baby that you stop using immediately. We will refer you back to your substance abuse provider after you are discharged, and we strongly urge that you get involved with a program that will help you stay clean. Since it appears that you have not been using your methadone, we are going to withhold that for the time being. Since injecting drugs can put you (and your baby) at risk for infections like HIV and hepatitis, we are going to test you for those infections. Also, we are going to test you for a bacterial infection of the heart that happens sometimes in people who inject drugs. Smoking tobacco also is very harmful to you and your baby, and we strongly encourage you to stop smoking. Your substance abuse provider can help you with that also.

- We found that you are about 12 wk pregnant. We want to help you have a healthy baby, but the first thing you need to do is stop abusing drugs since they are so harmful to the development of your baby. Also, your nutrition does not appear to be very good, and you need to eat well enough so that your baby can get nutrients. We will refer you to an obstetrician, and we will start you on a prenatal vitamin to be taken every day. Since many medications can harm the baby during pregnancy, make sure all your providers know you are pregnant, and do not take any medication unless you check with your obstetrician or pharmacist. Do not start taking your birth control pills when you get home since you are pregnant.

- You had been prescribed fluoxetine (Prozac) for your depression and bulimia. If you have been taking it on a regular basis, we do not want to stop it suddenly. When you take this medication later in the day, sometimes it can cause problems sleeping, so we will give it to you just in the morning. We are going to have a psychiatrist consult with you so that we can determine the best way to manage these problems, with medications and with counseling.

- We noticed that you are complaining of some pain or burning when you urinate. This may be caused by a urinary tract infection, and we are going to test you for that. If you do have a urine infection, we will give you an antibiotic for that. Make sure you take every dose since a urine infection can harm your baby as well as you. The antibiotic we will give, cephalexin, will not harm your baby. Sometimes it can cause some diarrhea or skin rashes, so if that happens, please let us know.

2 Hypertension: Newly Diagnosed

Keri Naglosky   Kade Birkeland
Robert J. Straka   David Parra

CASE LEARNING OBJECTIVES

- Classify blood pressure levels
- Identify the goals of therapy for HTN
- Select appropriate HTN therapy based on patient's individual characteristics
- Develop an appropriate monitoring and follow-up plan
- Properly educate a patient about antihypertensive treatment

PATIENT PRESENTATION

Chief Complaint

"I need to get my meds renewed."

History of Present Illness

Jose Vasquez is a 57-year-old Mexican American male who lost his job 6 months ago, and had not refilled any of his prescription medications for approximately 5 months because of cost (lost his insurance coverage). He has now started a new job and again has prescription drug coverage. He is concerned because his 52-year-old brother had a heart attack 2 years ago. Jose states his cholesterol was "where it was supposed to be" according to his previous physician while he was on simvastatin 40 mg in the past. Jose also mentions that his blood pressure has been in the 140s/90s at his gym, and he wonders if that is okay. He reports eating a low-fat diet, and exercises (walking, weightlifting) approximately 30 minutes three times/week.

Past Medical History

Dyslipidemia 2003

Gout 2007

Seasonal allergic rhinitis since childhood

Family History

Father died from MVA at the age of 35. Mother's age is 77 with HTN, osteoporosis, and a history of breast cancer. He has a brother (5 years younger) with dyslipidemia, HTN, type 2 DM; MI at age 50. He has two younger sisters, one has HTN, and both have dyslipidemia.

Social History

Born in the United States after his parents emigrated from Mexico. Married and lives with his wife; has three sons aged 35, 32, and 26 (all healthy). Recently started working in a Post Office.

Tobacco/Alcohol/Substance Use

Two to four drinks/week; tobacco use 1 ppd (41 pack-year history), "knows he should quit" but is unwilling to set a quit date given the stress of his new job; (−) illicit drug use.

Allergies/Intolerances/Adverse Drug Events

NKDA

Medications (Current)

Loratadine 10 mg PRN

(Was taking allopurinol 200 mg and simvastatin 40 mg daily prior to losing insurance coverage.)

Review of Systems

Constipation despite fiber-rich diet and at least 64 oz. (1.9 L) water daily. Otherwise unremarkable.

Physical Examination

▶ **General**

Well-appearing, middle-aged, Hispanic male in no acute distress.

▶ **Vital Signs**

BP 146/94 mm Hg, repeat 144/92 mm Hg (right arm, regular cuff), P 56 bpm, RR 12, T 36°C.

Weight 168.4 lb (76.5 kg)

Height 66 in. (168 cm)

Denies pain

▶ **Skin**

Dry

▶ **HEENT**

PERRLA, EOMI intact; TMs appear normal

▶ **Neck and Lymph Nodes**

Thyroid gland smooth; (−) thyroid nodules; (−) lymphadenopathy; (−) carotid bruits

▶ **Chest**

Clear to auscultation

▶ **Cardiovascular**

RRR, normal S_1, S_2; (−) S_3 or S_4

▶ **Abdomen**

Not tender/not distended; (−) organomegaly

▶ **Neurology**

Grossly intact; deep tendon reflexes normal

▶ **Genitourinary**

Examination deferred

▶ **Rectal**

Examination deferred

Laboratory Tests
Fasting from today

	Conventional Units	SI Units
Na	143 mEq/L	143 mmol/L
K	4.2 mEq/L	4.2 mmol/L
Cl	99 mEq/L	99 mmol/L
CO_2	25 mEq/L	25 mEq/L
BUN	13 mg/dL	4.6 mmol/L
SCr	1.2 mg/dL	106 μmol/L
Glu	111 mg/dL	6.2 mmol/L
Total cholesterol	240 mg/dL	6.21 mmol/L
LDL cholesterol	167 mg/dL	4.32 mmol/L
HDL cholesterol	38 mg/dL	0.98 mmol/L
Triglycerides	175 mg/dL	1.98 mmol/L
TSH	2.4 μIU/mL	2.4 mIU/L
Uric acid	9 mg/dL	535 μmol/L

Laboratory Tests from 1 Year Ago
Complete metabolic panel within normal limits

	Conventional Units (mg/dL)	SI Units (mmol/L)
Total cholesterol	170	4.40
LDL cholesterol	99	2.56
HDL cholesterol	42	1.09
Triglycerides	147	1.66

Assessment

Fifty-seven-year-old male with untreated dyslipidemia and gout, impaired fasting glucose, as well as newly diagnosed HTN.

Student Workup

Missing Information?

Evaluate:	Patient Database
	Drug Therapy Problems
	Care Plan (by Problem)

TARGETED QUESTIONS

1. What is the patient's calculated Framingham 10-year coronary heart disease (CHD) risk?

   Hint: See p. 237 in PPP

2. What is the patient's target blood pressure?

   Hint: See p. 52 in PPP

3. Which antihypertensive(s) would you consider initiating based on this patient's specific characteristics? Does he have any compelling indications *for other options*?

   Hint: See pp. 66 and 70 in PPP

4. How would you educate this patient about the medication(s) selected?

   Hint: See Table 5-4 in PPP

5. When and what would you monitor after initiating therapy?

   Hint: See p. 73 in PPP

FOLLOW-UP

The patient returns for follow-up BP check 2 weeks later. BP 132/85 mm Hg, repeat 130/82 mm Hg (right arm, regular cuff). What actions, if any, would you take?

☺ GLOBAL PERSPECTIVE

HTN accounts for significant morbidity and mortality and has a worldwide prevalence estimated to include 1 billion individuals resulting in an estimated 7 million deaths per year. The prevalence of HTN in the United States is among the highest in the world. Efforts to increase awareness, risk factor modification, control, and prevention are essential to reduce the global burden of cardiovascular disease. When designing an effective treatment plan for HTN, individual patient characteristics, comorbidities, the pharmacokinetic and pharmacodynamic properties of antihypertensive agents, and drug costs must be considered.

CASE SUMMARY

- His current clinical picture is consistent with newly diagnosed HTN, and intervention is necessary.
- Lifestyle modification and pharmacotherapy are warranted to achieve target blood pressure and other risk factors for CVD.
- A variety of therapeutic options are available, and the advantages and disadvantages of each should be considered based on the patient's individual characteristics.

For more information on the care plan and facilitator's guide please visit http://www.mhpharmacotherapy.com.

3 Uncontrolled Hypertension

Kade Birkeland   Keri Naglosky

David Parra   Robert J. Straka

CASE LEARNING OBJECTIVES

- Classify blood pressure levels and treatment goals
- Recognize contributing factors in uncontrolled hypertension
- Recommend appropriate lifestyle modifications and pharmacotherapy for patients with uncontrolled hypertension on the basis of individual patient characteristics
- Construct an appropriate monitoring plan to assess hypertension treatment
- Properly educate a patient about antihypertensive treatment

PATIENT PRESENTATION

Chief Complaint

"My blood pressure at home is still high."

History of Present Illness

Gusto Roubaix is a 66-year-old black male who presents with his wife to his health care provider complaining that his home BP readings continue to remain high. He was diagnosed with HTN 10 years ago, and it was well controlled until the past 18 months. He blames this on stress related to a poor real-estate market and a significant [>30 lb (>13.6 kg)] weight gain over the past 5 years (tries to practice portion control but dines out frequently; he does not have salt at the table or cook with salt). He is frustrated as his BP has not improved despite 1 hour of light aerobics (walking and water aerobics) daily over the past 6 months. His home BP log, which he brought with him, reveals resting seated systolic BPs ranging from 130 to 155 mm Hg and diastolic pressures ranging from 70 to 90 mm Hg and a pulse of 50 to 58 bpm in the morning over the past 30 days. In addition, despite restricting his calories, he has not lost any weight. He complains of excessive fatigue, and his wife states she is always tired as well, as his snoring "keeps the whole house up all night long." He denies any dizziness or lightheadedness, edema, chest pain, or shortness of breath.

Past Medical History

HTN (diagnosed 10 years ago)

Impaired fasting glucose

Metabolic syndrome

Dyslipidemia

Osteoarthritis of the knees (unresponsive to high-dose APAP)

History of gout

GERD

Obstructive sleep apnea

BPH

Obesity

"Stress/fatigue"

Family History

Mother deceased, stroke at age 82. Father is alive and well, aged 86. Sister diabetes and CKD, aged 59. Brother alive and well, aged 63.

Social History

Lives in South Florida year round with his wife of 40 years.

Tobacco/Alcohol/Substance Use

Social drinker, one to two glasses of wine nightly, (−) tobacco products, (−) illicit drugs.

Allergies/Intolerances/Adverse Drug Events

Penicillin (angioedema)

Medications (Current)

Aspirin 81 mg PO q AM

Verapamil SA 240 mg PO q 24 h

Metoprolol Succinate SA 200 mg PO q 24 h

Terazosin 5 mg PO q hs

Simvastatin 80 mg PO q hs

Omeprazole 20 mg PO q AM

Ibuprofen 400 mg PO 4 times daily PRN pain

OTC energy supplement PO daily

Review of Systems

Frequent body aches that the patient attributes to exercise and arthritis; wakes up two to three times nightly to urinate with some hesitancy and dribbling; no chest pain at rest or with exercise; no shortness of breath, dizziness, lightheadedness, or edema.

Physical Examination

▶ General

Well-nourished, appears his age, overweight black male in no distress

▶ Vital Signs

BP 152/92 mm Hg, P 56 bpm (left-arm, regular-sized adult cuff), repeat 148/90 mm Hg, P 54 bpm

RR 16, T 37°C

Weight 184 lb (83.6 kg)

Height 68 in. (173 cm)

Currently denies pain

▶ Skin

Dry appearing skin; (−) rashes or lesions

▶ HEENT

PERRLA, EOMI; (−) sinus tenderness; TMs appear normal

▶ Neck and Lymph Nodes

(−) thyroid nodules; (−) lymphadenopathy; (−) carotid bruits

▶ Chest

Clear to auscultation

▶ Cardiovascular

RRR, normal S_1, S_2; (−) S_3 or S_4

▶ Abdomen

Not tender/not distended; (−) organomegaly

▶ Neurology

Grossly intact; deep tendon reflexes normal

▶ Genitourinary

Examination deferred

▶ Rectal

Prostate is enlarged approximately 30 g, no areas of induration or nodularity

Laboratory Tests
(Fasting, obtained 7 days ago)

	Conventional Units	SI Units
Na	142 mEq/L	142 mmol/L
K	4.2 mEq/L	4.2 mmol/L
Cl	98 mEq/L	98 mmol/L
CO_2	24 mEq/L	24 mmol/L
BUN	12 mg/dL	4.3 mmol/L
SCr	1.2 mg/dL	106 μmol/L
Glu	104 mg/dL	5.8 mmol/L
Total cholesterol	146 mg/dL	3.78 mmol/L
LDL cholesterol	79 mg/dL	2.04 mmol/L
HDL cholesterol	36 mg/dL	0.93 mmol/L
Triglycerides	156 mg/dL	1.76 mmol/L

Assessment

Sixty-six-year-old male with uncontrolled hypertension despite three antihypertensive agents.

Student Workup

Missing Information?

Evaluate:	Patient Database
	Drug Therapy Problems
	Care Plan (by Problem)

TARGETED QUESTIONS

1. What stage hypertension does this patient have and what is his target blood pressure?

   Hint: See p. 57 in PPP

2. What are some contributing factors in uncontrolled hypertension?

   Hint: See p. 54 in PPP

3. Based on this patient's individual characteristics, what are the advantages and disadvantages of different therapeutic options?

   Hint: See Table 5-4 in PPP

4. What risks and adverse effects of therapy would you discuss with the patient?

   Hint: See Table 5-4 in PPP

5. What are appropriate follow-up monitoring parameters?

   Hint: See p. 73 in PPP

FOLLOW-UP

Four weeks later, the patient returns for follow-up. He feels much better; his stress has actually improved because he is not nearly as fatigued, "maybe because I don't wake up to go to the bathroom three times per night anymore?" His wife adds, "That CPAP machine works wonders … he quit snoring … I am getting my usual 8 hours of sleep now." His pain is no better or worse on salsalate compared to when he was on ibuprofen; however he is satisfied with the current level of pain relief. He states that his body aches are "the same"; further questioning reveals these are not muscle weakness, cramping, or suggestive of statin myopathy. In addition, total CK was within normal limits. In the office, although improved, his seated blood pressure remains elevated and is consistent with his home blood pressure log (seated systolic blood pressures ranging from 128 to 143 mm Hg and diastolic pressures ranging from 68 to 84 mm Hg and a pulse of 60 to 74 bpm in the morning). The patient's BMP is within normal limits, and he reports no signs or symptoms of intolerance to his new therapeutic regimen. What additional interventions or modifications would you now make to improve the patient's blood pressure control?

○ GLOBAL PERSPECTIVE

Although the global burden of hypertension is growing substantially, it does not affect all groups or populations equally. It is estimated that 1 billion adults (333 million in economically developed and 639 million in economically developing countries) have hypertension, with those who reside in economically developing countries being increasingly affected. Eastern Europe and Latin American/Caribbean regions have the highest prevalence of hypertension, whereas prevalence of age-specific and age-adjusted hypertension continues to increase in China. Efforts to increase awareness, control, and prevention of hypertension are paramount in reducing the global burden of cardiovascular disease. Comprehensive risk-factor modification (tobacco use, cholesterol, obesity, diabetes) are also essential, with special considerations given by region. In addition the pharmacokinetic and pharmacodynamic properties of antihypertensive agents and adverse event profiles may differ among various populations. For example, blacks are more likely to experience angioedema from ACE inhibitors while Chinese are more likely to experience cough. Finally, differences in drug cost, availability, and national resources may influence the approach to treating hypertension.

CASE SUMMARY

- His current clinical picture is consistent with uncontrolled hypertension, and intervention is necessary.

- A thorough investigation of factors contributing to uncontrolled hypertension is warranted in addition to lifestyle and pharmacologic intensification.

- A variety of therapeutic options are available, and the advantages and disadvantages of each should be carefully considered based on the patient's individual characteristics.

For more information on the care plan and facilitator's guide please visit http://www.mhpharmacotherapy.com.

4 Heart Failure

Kimberly A. Ackerbauer
Tien M.H. Ng

CASE LEARNING OBJECTIVES

- Differentiate among the common underlying etiologies of heart failure (HF), including ischemic, nonischemic, and idiopathic causes.
- Identify signs and symptoms of HF and classify a given patient by the New York Heart Association Functional Classification (NYHA FC) and American College of Cardiology/American Heart Association (AHA) HF Staging.
- Develop a specific evidence-based pharmacologic treatment plan for a patient with acute or chronic HF based on disease severity and symptoms.
- Properly educate a patient taking chronic HF medications.

PATIENT PRESENTATION

Chief Complaint

"I was so short of breath this morning I couldn't get out of bed. I have also gained about 15 pounds (~7 kg) over the last few days, but it can't be from food because I haven't been very hungry."

History of Present Illness

DB is a 64-year-old Hispanic male who presents to the emergency department with a 3-day history of shortness of breath, lower extremity swelling, and an 18-lb (8-kg) weight gain. About 4 days ago, he ran out of medications and was unable to make it to the pharmacy to refill his medications. This morning, the shortness of breath persisted at rest to the point he could not get out of bed. This prompted him to come to the hospital. The patient also admits to waking up at night to catch his breath and needing at least three pillows to prop himself up while sleeping because he feels like he is drowning when laying flat. In the emergency room he was placed on oxygen, given his home dose of amlodipine, given intravenous boluses of furosemide without much response, and then started on a fursosemide intravenous infusion at 5 mg/h. After 3 hours, DB had no symptomatic relief and was transferred to the cardiac intensive care unit for further management.

Past Medical History

HTN × 20 years
Bipolar disorder × 6 years

Family History

Father had type 2 diabetes, HTN, and died at age 84 from an unknown cause.
Mother is alive at age 87 with HTN and gout.

Social History

Came to the United States from El Salvador at age 13. Speaks fluent English and Spanish. Divorced and lives alone. He has a son who visits him about once a week for help around the house. Retired, used to work as a travel agent, now mainly sedentary. Eats mainly processed or premade foods.

Tobacco/Alcohol/Substance Use

Denies alcohol use; (−) tobacco or illicit drug use

Allergies/Intolerances/Adverse Drug Events

Benazepril (cough)

Medications (Current)

HCTZ 25 mg PO q AM
Amlodipine 10 mg PO q 24 h
Lithium 300 mg PO q 8 h

Review of Systems

Well-appearing male unable to lie flat in bed. No complaints of pain, headache, fever, or chills. Denies changes in mental status, nausea, or vomiting.

Physical Examination

▶ General

Moderately distressed, obese, middle-aged Hispanic male.

▶ Vital Signs

BP 154/92 mm Hg, P 87, RR 27, T 37.3°C, O_2 saturation 92% (0.92) on 2 L via nasal cannula

Weight 211 lb (96 kg)

Height 68 in. (173 cm)

Denies pain

▶ HEENT

Unremarkable

▶ Neck and Lymph Nodes

Neck supple, (+) JVD

▶ Chest

Crackles bilaterally

▶ Cardiovascular

RRR, normal S_1, S_2, (+) S_3, (+) S_4 heart sounds, no murmurs, PMI displaced laterally

▶ Abdomen

(+) Bowel sounds, hepatomegaly

▶ Neurology

Alert and oriented × 3, no focal deficits

▶ Extremities

Warm, 2+ pulses (pedal/radial), 2+ bilateral lower extremity edema up to knees

▶ Genitourinary

Examination deferred

▶ Rectal

Examination deferred

Laboratory Tests

Fasting, obtained upon admission

	Conventional Units	SI Units
Na	137 mEq/L	137 mmol/L
K	3.6 mEq/L	3.6 mmol/L
Cl	104 mEq/L	104 mmol/L
CO_2	22 mEq/L	22 mmol/L
BUN	28 mg/dL	10 mmol/L
SCr	1.4 mg/dL	124 μmol/L
Glu	189 mg/dL	10.5 mmol/L
Ca	8.7 mg/dL	2.18 mmol/L
Mg	1.8 mEq/L	0.90 mmol/L
Phosphate	3.6 mg/dL	1.16 mmol/L
WBC	$9.4 \times 10^3/mm^3$	$9.4 \times 10^9/L$
Hgb	11.6 g/dL	116 g/L; 7.2 mmol/L
Hct	34.6%	0.346
MCV	88.0 μm³	88.0 fL
Platelet	$213 \times 10^3/mm^3$	$213 \times 10^9/L$
Albumin	3.2 g/dL	32 g/L
Total bilirubin	1.5 mg/dL	25.7 μmol/L
Direct bilirubin	0.8 mg/dL	13.7 μmol/L
AST	89 IU/L	1.48 μkat/L
ALT	96 IU/L	1.60 μkat/L
Alk phos	180 IU/L	3.00 μkat/L
PT	17 s	
INR	1.3	
Total cholesterol	164 mg/dL	4.24 mmol/L
Triglycerides	135 mg/dL	1.53 mmol/L
LDL cholesterol	96 mg/dL	2.48 mmol/L
HDL cholesterol	41 mg/dL	1.06 mmol/L
Lithium	0.8 mEq/L	0.8 mmol/L
B-type natriuretic peptide	9,022 pg/mL	9,022 ng/L

Diagnostic Tests

▶ Electrocardiogram

Left ventricular hypertrophy, no acute ST-segment changes

▶ Chest radiograph

Cardiomegaly, bilateral pleural effusions at the bases, no infiltrates

▶ Echocardiography

Hypertrophied and dilated left ventricle, left ventricular EF 35%

Assessment

Sixty-four-year-old man presenting with new-onset HF.

Student Workup

Missing Information?

Evaluate:	Patient Database
	Drug Therapy Problems
	Care Plan (by Problem)

TARGETED QUESTIONS

1. What signs and symptoms of HF does this patient have?
   Hint: See p. 85 in PPP

2. What NYHA Functional Class is this patient?
   Hint: See pp. 6–5 in PPP

3. How do you determine when the addition of intravenous vasodilatory therapy is desirable in an acute HF patient?
   Hint: See p. 101 in PPP

4. How do ACE-I and β-blockers interfere with the pathophysiology of HF to improve patient survival?
   Hint: See pp. 91–95 in PPP

5. What education would you provide regarding lifestyle changes and self-monitoring for this patient?
   Hint: See p. 105 in PPP

FOLLOW-UP

Six months later, DB returns to the clinic for a routine follow-up and medication refills. He states that he has no major complaints at this time. When prompted, he admits that over the past 3 months his exercise tolerance has decreased. He used to walk about six blocks to the grocery store and is now only able to walk two blocks. He denies any swelling in his legs but still needs three pillows while sleeping at night.

Furosemide 20 mg PO twice daily

Carvedilol 25 mg PO twice daily

Losartan 100 mg PO daily

Amlodipine 10 mg PO daily

Lithium 300 mg PO three times daily

► *Vital Signs*

BP 103/61 mm Hg, P 58, RR 18, T 37.4°C

Weight 204 lb (93 kg)

	Conventional Units	SI Units
Na	136 mEq/L	136 mmol/L
K	3.7 mEq/L	3.7 mmol/L
Cl	109 mEq/L	109 mmol/L
CO_2	21 mEq/L	21 mmol/L
BUN	24 mg/dL	8.6 mmol/L
SCr	1.2 mg/dL	106 μmol/L
Glu	129 mg/dL	7.2 mmol/L

6. Are there any changes that could be made to his outpatient regimen to improve his symptoms?
   Hint: See p. 95 in PPP

⊙ GLOBAL PERSPECTIVE

Although the main etiologies of systolic HF are ischemic heart disease and hypertension in the United States, acquired etiologies can be more prevalent in developing countries. The availability of certain medications also varies from continent to continent. For example, in many countries in Europe and Scandinavia, additional intravenous agents such as levosimendan are available for the treatment of acute HF. Finally, patterns of prescribing may differ among countries. This applies to both acute HF therapies such as inotropes and chronic medications such as β-blockers and ACE-I.

CASE SUMMARY

- His current clinical picture is consistent with being congested, necessitating aggressive diuresis and intravenous vasodilator therapy. It is appropriate to continue the furosemide infusion and start nitroglycerin.

- When clinically stable, this patient should be started on chronic disease-modifying agents that antagonize the renin-angiotensin-aldosterone-system (RAAS) as well as the sympathetic nervous system.

- Prevention of future acute HF exacerbations with the use of diuretics, optimal management of the hypertension, and lifestyle modifications are necessary to improve this patient's long-term prognosis.

For more information on the care plan and facilitator's guide please visit http://www.mhpharmacotherapy.com.

5 Ischemic Heart Disease

Larisa H. Cavallari   Gary Peksa
Robert J. DiDomenico

CASE LEARNING OBJECTIVES

- Recognize the symptoms and diagnostic criteria of ischemic heart disease (IHD)
- Identify risk factors for the development of IHD
- Identify the treatment goals of IHD and appropriate lifestyle modifications and pharmacologic therapy to address each goal
- Design an appropriate therapeutic regimen for the management of IHD based on patient-specific information

PATIENT PRESENTATION

Chief Complaint

"I get pain in my chest and feel dizzy when I exercise. I have to stop exercising and rest for the pain and dizziness to go away."

History of Present Illness

GP is a 58-year-old African American male who presents to his primary care physician complaining of chest pain radiating to his neck and left shoulder, excessive sweating, and dizziness (over the last month) when he attempts to exercise on a treadmill or stair stepper. He describes the pain as "feeling tight" and "pressure-like." The symptoms resolve after resting for a couple of minutes. He denies dyspnea, nausea, or vomiting. He also denies symptoms at rest, with change in body position, or in relation to meals. GP is concerned that he will not be able to exercise, which he is doing to lose weight. He is hoping that he can take something to prevent the chest pain and other symptoms that occur with exercise. He also reports swelling in his ankles that is worse after being on his feet all day and relieved with leg elevation.

Past Medical History

HTN × 10 years

Depression × 6 months

Type 2 DM × 2 years

Bursitis in left hip × 6 months after slipping on the ice

Family History

Mother died at age 47 from MI. Father is alive at age 78 S/P CABG at the age of 50. Daughter, aged 24, alive and well.

Social History

He is a widower as of 6 months ago. GP currently lives at home with his 24-year-old daughter and cat. He is employed as a chemist.

Tobacco/Alcohol/Substance Use

(+) Tobacco; quit smoking 10 years ago, but restarted smoking about ½ ppd 6 months ago when his wife died. Denies illicit drug use; social drinker on the weekends.

Allergies/Intolerances/Adverse Drug Events

Penicillin (develops hives)

Medications (Current)

Fish oil 1,000 mg PO once daily

Sertraline 50 mg PO once daily

Lisinopril 40 mg PO once daily

Chlorthalidone 50 mg PO once daily

Naproxen 500 mg PO twice daily

Glipizide XL 10 mg PO once daily

Review of Systems

Takes naproxen twice daily for bursitis. Denies current dizziness, chest pain, diaphoresis, or dyspnea; (–) history of syncope, loss of consciousness, seizures, or visual changes. Reports that bursitis pain has largely resolved.

Physical Examination

▶ General

Middle-aged, well-developed, African American male in no acute distress; conversant and pleasant

▶ Vital Signs

BP 140/92 mmHg, P 94 bpm, RR 17, T 36.8°C

Weight 185 lb (84.1 kg)

Height 68 in. (173 cm)

(–) Pain

▶ Skin

Warm and dry; (–) pallor, rashes, or lesions

▶ HEENT

PERRLA, EOMI; oral mucosa moist; (–) pharyngeal erythema or exudate

▶ Neck and Lymph Nodes

Supple, no tenderness; (–) carotid bruits; (–) jugular vein distension; normal thyroid

▶ Chest

Clear to auscultation bilaterally

▶ Cardiovascular

RRR; normal S_1, S_2; (–) S_3 or S_4; (–) murmurs, rubs, gallops

▶ Abdomen

Soft, nontender, nondistended; normal bowel sounds

▶ Neurology

Alert and oriented, cranial nerves II–XII intact

▶ Extremities

Bilateral lower extremity edema; warm; normal pulses

▶ Genitourinary

Examination deferred; per patient: (–) dysuria; (–) hematuria; (–) discharge

▶ Rectal

Examination deferred

Laboratory Tests

Fasting, obtained prior to clinic visit

	Conventional Units	SI Units
Na	141 mEq/L	141 mmol/L
K	4.4 mEq/L	4.4 mmol/L
Cl	101 mEq/L	101 mmol/L
CO_2	24 mEq/L	24 mmol/L
BUN	10 mg/dL	3.6 mmol/L
SCr	1.1 mg/dL	97 μmol/L
Glu	130 mg/dL	7.2 mmol/L
Ca	10.0 mg/dL	2.50 mmol/L
Mg	1.7 mEq/L	0.85 mmol/L
Phosphate	4.1 mg/dL	1.32 mmol/L
Hgb	15.1 g/dL	151 g/L; 9.38 mmol/L
Hct	45.3%	0.453
WBC	$8.0 \times 10^3/mm^3$	$8.0 \times 10^9/L$
Platelets	$313 \times 10^3/mm^3$	$313 \times 10^9/L$

Assessment and Plan

Fifty-eight-year-old man with symptoms consistent with chronic stable angina. GP's primary care physician has scheduled a treadmill stress echocardiogram (echo stress test) to evaluate him for IHD and assess his left ventricular systolic function.

Student Workup

Missing Information?

Evaluate:	Patient Database
	Drug Therapy Problems
	Care Plan (by Problem)

TARGETED QUESTIONS

1. What symptoms of chronic stable angina does the patient have?

   Hint: See p. 114 in PPP

2. What are the patient's risk factors for IHD?

   Hint: See p. 111 in PPP

3. What is your assessment of GP's current antihypertensive regimen?

   Hint: See pp. 119–120 in PPP and Hypertension chapter

FOLLOW-UP

One week later, the patient's echo stress test comes back positive for inducible myocardial ischemia (i.e., positive for CAD), and shows normal left ventricular systolic function (i.e., no evidence of left ventricular dysfunction). He is diagnosed with chronic stable angina.

4. A coronary angiogram is recommended, but the patient declines, opting for medical management at this time. What therapy do you recommend to manage the patient's symptoms of angina?

   Hint: See pp. 121–125 in PPP

5. Now that you have addressed the patient's antianginal medications, what additional medications (other than those addressed in question 4) would you consider now that he has been diagnosed with IHD?

   Hint: See pp. 119–120 in PPP

6. What lifestyle modifications are appropriate for this patient?

   Hint: See p. 117 in PPP

GLOBAL PERSPECTIVE

In general, persons of African descent may have lesser antihypertensive response to β-blockers or ACE-I monotherapy than those of other racial groups. However, this is not a reason to avoid these drugs in an African American patient when a compelling indication (e.g., IHD, diabetes) exists for their use. These drugs may still have cardio- and reno-protective effects despite less blood pressure-lowering effect. Concomitant use of these drugs with a thiazide diuretic may significantly enhance blood pressure response.

CASE SUMMARY

- His current clinical picture is consistent with chronic stable angina.
- Therapy to relieve acute symptoms of ischemia and prevent recurrent angina should be initiated.
- Additional drug therapy and lifestyle modifications to address the patient's risk factors for IHD to reduce the risk for an acute coronary syndrome (ACS) is warranted.

For more information on the care plan and facilitator's guide please visit http://www.mhpharmacotherapy.com.

6 Acute Coronary Syndromes

Sarah A. Spinler

CASE LEARNING OBJECTIVES

- List key electrocardiographic and clinical features identifying a patient with non-ST-segment elevation (NSTE) acute coronary syndrome (ACS) who is at high risk of myocardial infarction (MI) or death.
- Devise a pharmacotherapy treatment plan for a patient with ST-segment elevation myocardial infarction (STEMI) given patient-specific data.
- Devise a pharmacotherapy treatment and monitoring plan for a patient with NSTE ACS given patient-specific data.
- Formulate a monitoring plan for a patient with NSTE ACS receiving aspirin, clopidogrel, β-blocker, anticoagulant, and glycoprotein IIb/IIIa receptor inhibitor.
- Devise a pharmacotherapy and risk-factor modification treatment plan for secondary prevention of coronary heart disease (CHD) events in a patient following MI.
- List the quality performance measures of care for MI.

PATIENT PRESENTATION

Chief Complaint

"My chest discomfort is gone now that they put a stent in my coronary artery."

History of Present Illness

JW is a 66-year-old male who presented to the Emergency Department (ED) by ambulance at 14:00 complaining of 4 hours of continuous chest pressure that started while raking leaves. JW developed substernal chest pressure at 10:00 about 30 minutes after starting to rake leaves at his home. He stopped and rested but the chest pressure did not resolve. Local paramedics were summoned, and he was given three 0.4 mg SL NTG tablets by mouth, 325 mg aspirin by mouth, and morphine 2 mg IV push at 13:30 without relief of chest discomfort. He was brought to the ED by ambulance. A 12-lead ECG was performed, and NTG 10 mcg/min IV infusion was initiated at 14:15. The cardiology attending consulted with the interventional cardiologist and the decision was made to bring JW to the cardiac catheterization laboratory for coronary angiography. Bivalirudin was initiated at the time of percutaneous coronary intervention (PCI) and was discontinued in the cardiac catheterization laboratory following successful PCI. The patient is now in the CCU s/p PCI with placement of a bare metal stent in the LAD coronary artery.

Past Medical History

HTN × 5 years

Family History

Father with MI at age 75; Mother and sister alive with type 2 DM

Social History

Retired former newspaper reporter

Tobacco/Alcohol/Substance Use

Nonsmoker. Denies use of alcohol or illicit drugs

Allergies/Intolerances/Adverse Drug Events

None

Medications (Current)

NTG 10 mcg/min IV

Medications Taken Prior to Admission

Amlodipine 10 mg PO once daily

ASA 325 mg PO once daily

Review of Systems

Previous 10/10 chest pressure now 1/10; (−) nausea, abdominal pain, or headache.

Physical Examination

▶ *General*

Elderly male in less distress

▶ *Vital Signs*

BP 140/90 mm Hg, P 88 bpm, RR 17, T 37°C

Weight 198 lb (90 kg)

Height 71 in. (180 cm)

Denies pain, but 1/10 chest pressure

▶ *HEENT*

Normal; (−) AV nicking, (−) papilledema

▶ *Chest*

Clear to A&P, JVD 4 cm, PMI left midclavicular line 4th intercostal space

▶ *Cardiovascular*

RRR, normal S_1, S_2, (−) S_3 or S_4, (−) M/R/G

▶ *Abdomen*

Not tender/not distended, normal bowel sounds

▶ *Neurologic*

A&O × 3, cranial nerves II–XII intact

▶ *Genitourinary*

Deferred

▶ *Rectal*

(−) Occult blood

▶ *Extremities*

No bruits, pulses 2+, (−) edema

Laboratory Tests

Nonfasting, obtained in the ED

	Conventional Units	SI Units
Sodium	140 mEq/L	140 mmol/L
Potassium	4.2 mEq/L	4.2 mmol/L
Chloride	105 mEq/L	105 mmol/L
CO_2	24 mEq/L	24 mmol/L
BUN	16 mg/dL	5.7 mmol/L
	1.0 mg/dL	88 mmol/L
	99 mg/dL	5.5 mmol/L

Hgb	14.7 g/dL	147; 9.12 mmol/L
Hct	44.0%	0.440
Plt	$220 \times 10^3/mm^3$	$220 \times 10^9/L$
WBC	$4.3 \times 10^3/mm^3$	$4.3 \times 10^9/L$
Troponin I	7.5 ng/mL	7.5 mcg/L
LDL cholesterol	110 mg/dL	2.84 mmol/L
Triglycerides	240 mg/dL	2.71 mmol/L
HDL cholesterol	35 mg/dL	0.91 mmol/L
Magnesium	2.0 mEq/L	1.00 mmol/L
AST	30 U/L	0.50 μkat/L
ALT	30 U/L	0.50 μkat/L
aPTT	30 s	
INR	1.0	

O_2 sat = 99% (0.99) on RA

ECG: In ED showed sinus tachycardia with 2 mm ST depression in leads V_2–V_4; normal PR, QRS, and QTc intervals; post-PCI ECG shows NSR with resolution of ST depression, no Q waves.

Assessment

Sixty-six-year-old male with signs, symptoms and laboratory tests consistent with ACS.

Student Workup

Missing Information?

Evaluate: Patient Database

Drug Therapy Problems

Care Plan (by Problem)

TARGETED QUESTIONS

1. What type of ACS is this?

    Hint: See pp. 132–133 in PPP

2. What signs and symptoms of ACS does this patient have?

    Hint: See p. 135 in PPP

3. What are this patient's risk factors for developing CHD?

    Hint: See Table 7-2 in PPP

4. How is the diagnosis of MI made?

    Hint: See pp. 134–135 in PPP

5. What high risk of death or MI characteristics does this patient have?

    Hint: See p. 135 and Table 8-1 in PPP

6. If this patient had chronic kidney disease, how would this influence your choice of anticoagulant and dose?

    Hint: See p. 148 in PPP

7. In which patient subgroups is the benefit of reduction in cardiovascular death, MI, or stroke not greater than the risk of major bleeding in patients treated with prasugrel versus clopidogrel following PCI?

   Hint: See Wiviott SD, Braunwald E, McCabe CH, et al. TRITON-TIMI 38 Investigators. Prasugrel versus clopidogrel in patients with acute coronary syndromes. N Engl J Med 2007 357:2001–2015.

8. What is the minimal duration of time that dual antiplatelet therapy should be continued?

   Hint: See Kushner FG, Hand M, Smith SC Jr, et al. Focused updates: ACC/AHA Guidelines for the Management of Patients with ST-Elevation Myocardial Infarction (updating the 2004 Guideline and 2007 Focused Update) and ACC/AHA/SCAI Guidelines on Percutaneous Coronary Intervention (updating the 2005 Guideline and 2007 Focused Update): A report of the American College of Cardiology Foundation/American Heart Association Task Force on Practice Guidelines. Circulation 2009 20:2271–2306.

9. How is the dose of the β-blocker titrated?

   Hint: See p. 146 and Table 8-2 in PPP

10. How would your selection of pharmacotherapy differ if this patient presented with signs and symptoms of acute heart failure (HF)?

    Hint: See Table 8-2 in PPP

11. What is the single best predictor of mortality in this patient?

    Hint: See p. 139 in PPP

FOLLOW-UP

12. The patient presents to his cardiologist 2 weeks following discharge. His BP is 142/90 mm Hg, pulse 55 bpm, and he is afebrile. His chemistry panel includes potassium of 4.2 mEq/L (4.2 mmol/L) and SCr 1.07 mg/dL (95 μmol/L). What recommendations would you make to the physician regarding his pharmacotherapy regimen?

    Hint: See Table 8-2 in PPP

13. The patient presents to his cardiologist 6 weeks following discharge. The patient's LDL cholesterol is 68 mg/dL (1.76 mmol/L), but his fasting triglycerides are still elevated at 185 mg/dL (2.09 mmol/L) and HDL cholesterol still low at 36 mg/dL (0.93 mmol/L). What recommendations would you make to the physician regarding his pharmacotherapy regimen?

    Hint: See pp. 240–247 in PPP

⊙ GLOBAL PERSPECTIVE

MI is the most common type of CVD. Almost 30% of deaths worldwide are caused by CVD. Almost 80% of CVD deaths occur in low- and middle-income countries. More than 20 million people survive MIs and require secondary preventative care. The World Health Organization estimates that by 2010, CVD will be the leading cause of death in developing countries.

CASE SUMMARY

- His current clinical picture is NSTE ACS, and early PCI restored blood flow through the LAD to myocardium.
- Acute pharmacotherapy should be initiated for management in-hospital.
- Secondary prevention pharmacotherapy should be started prior to hospital discharge.
- Key clinical practice guidelines and performance measures guide pharmacotherapy selection.
- Patients should be monitored for development of MI complications and pharmacotherapy adverse effects.

For more information on the care plan and facilitator's guide please visit http://www.mhpharmacotherapy.com.

7 Atrial Fibrillation

Toby C. Trujillo

CASE LEARNING OBJECTIVES

- Compare and contrast the risk factors for and the features, mechanisms, etiologies, symptoms, and goals of therapy of atrial fibrillation (AF).
- Compare and contrast the mechanisms of action of drugs used for ventricular rate control, conversion to sinus rhythm, and maintenance of sinus rhythm in patients with AF, and explain the importance of anticoagulation for patients with AF.
- Design individualized drug therapy treatment plans for patients with AF.

PATIENT PRESENTATION

Chief Complaint
"I was supposed to come back if I didn't feel right."

History of Present Illness
Linda Leong is a 77-year-old Asian female who approximately 1 month ago presented to the emergency department with complaints of SOB, palpitations, fatigue, lightheadedness, and weakness of unspecified duration. She was found to be in AF with a ventricular rate of 130 bpm. At the time of admission, no atrial thrombus was present via transesophageal echocardiography (TEE). Diltiazem was initiated to control her ventricular rate with good response, and IV heparin for bridging plus long-term warfarin was initiated for stroke prevention. The decision for cardioversion was deferred at that time, and she was discharged on diltiazem, warfarin, and her other chronic medications. During the hospitalization, LL was also noted to have lower extremity edema and an elevated JVD, and she was treated with furosemide. She presents today in the cardiology clinic for follow-up. She states she has been compliant with her medications, still feels tired, and occasionally notices she has a fast heart rate.

Past Medical History
AF

HTN

Heart failure (HF) (EF 50% 1 mo ago)

Glaucoma

Dementia

Heartburn

Family History
Mother had CAD and died of an MI at age 66. Father died of lung cancer at age 81. She has one younger brother and sister who are healthy.

Social History
Married and lives with her husband of 47 years.

Tobacco/Alcohol/Substance Use
Occasional glass of wine with dinner; (−) tobacco or illicit drug use

Allergies/Intolerances/Adverse Drug Events
No known drug allergies

Medications (Current)
Diltiazem XR 240 mg PO once daily

Warfarin 2.5 mg PO once daily

Lisinopril 40 mg PO once daily

Furosemide 20 mg PO once daily

Donepezil 10 mg PO once daily

Ranitidine 150 mg PO once daily

Travoprost Z 0.004% one drop each eye once daily

Centrum Silver vitamin PO once daily

Review of Systems
Still reports fatigue over the last month since discharge from the hospital, difficulty in completing chores in the yard; occasional headaches relieved with nonaspirin pain reliever, (−) changes in vision; occasional palpitations, SOB, and DOE;

(−) heartburn or change in appetite; (−) recent changes in memory or cognition.

Physical Examination

▶ *General*

Well-appearing, elderly Asian woman in no acute distress

▶ *Vital Signs*

BP 135/85 mm Hg, P 90 bpm, RR 14, T 37.1°C

Weight 160.6 lb (73.0 kg)

Height 68 in. (173 cm)

▶ *Skin*

(−) Rashes or lesions

▶ *HEENT*

PERRLA, mucosal membranes dry

▶ *Neck and Lymph Nodes*

(−) JVD; (−) carotid bruits

▶ *Chest*

Clear to auscultation

▶ *Breasts*

Examination deferred

▶ *Cardiovascular*

Irregularly irregular rhythm; slightly tachycardic; no murmurs, rubs, or gallops

▶ *Abdomen*

Not tender, not distended; (−) hepatomegaly

▶ *Neurology*

Alert and oriented × 3

▶ *Genitourinary*

Examination deferred

▶ *Rectal*

Examination deferred

Laboratory Tests

Fasting, drawn today

	Conventional Units	SI Units
Na	140 mEq/L	140 mmol/L
K	4.3 mEq/L	4.3 mmol/L
Cl	104 mEq/L	104 mmol/L
CO$_2$	22 mEq/L	22 mmol/L
BUN	22 mg/dL	7.9 mmol/L
SCr	1.3 mg/dL	115 µmol/L
Glu	84 mg/dL	4.7 mmol/L
Ca	8.9 mg/dL	2.23 mmol/L
Mg	1.8 mEq/L	0.90 mmol/L
Phosphate	3.8 mg/dL	1.23 mmol/L
Triglycerides	175 mg/dL	1.98 mmol/L
Hgb	13.5 g/dL	135 g/L; 8.38 mmol/L
Hct	39.7%	0.397
WBC	7.6 × 10³/mm³	7.6 × 10⁹/L
Albumin	3.8 g/dL	38 g/L
AST	26 U/L	0.43 µkat/L
ALT	24 U/L	0.40 µkat/L
Prothrombin	20 s	
INR	1.5	
Total cholesterol	238 mg/dL	6.15 mmol/L
LDL cholesterol	158 mg/dL	4.09 mmol/L
HDL cholesterol	45 mg/dL	1.16 mmol/L

Assessment

Seventy-seven-year-old Asian female who presents with continuing symptoms of AF, now here for follow-up in the cardiology clinic 1 month after being hospitalized for new-onset AF.

Student Workup

Missing Information?

Evaluate: Patient Database

Drug Therapy Problems

Care Plan (by Problem)

TARGETED QUESTIONS

1. What underlying etiologies are present in this patient for the development of AF?

   Hint: See pp. 165–166 in PPP

2. How should this patient's AF be classified?

   Hint: See p. 167 in PPP

3. Should this patient undergo emergent electrical cardioversion at this time?

   Hint: See pp. 167–168 in PPP

4. Should the patient receive aspirin for the prevention of stroke?

   Hint: See pp. 172–173 in PPP

5. Should the patient receive anti-arrhythmic drug therapy at this time?

   Hint: See pp. 168–172 in PPP

FOLLOW-UP

6. Five weeks later, the patient returns for follow-up. She continues to experience SOB, DOE, and occasional palpitations. Her current vitals reveal a BP of 125/80 mm Hg and a HR of 78 bpm. Today her INR is 2.7 (3 weeks ago, it was 2.2). What anti-arrhythmic agent would be recommended for LL at this time to restore and maintain normal sinus rhythm?

   Hint: See pp. 171–172 in PPP

⊙ GLOBAL PERSPECTIVE

In a majority of patients, therapeutic anticoagulation with warfarin is the preferred treatment strategy to prevent stroke in patients with AF. While warfarin has been used in the United States for many years, it is important to note that different vitamin K antagonists are used in other countries worldwide, including acenocoumarol and phenprocoumon. While the mechanism of action for these agents is similar to that of warfarin, there are major differences in the pharmacokinetics of the compounds, and hence differences in how health care professionals may perform routine dose titration and management of therapy. It is important to clarify which specific coumarin derivative the patient is taking in order to optimally manage their anticoagulation. Also, as of mid-2010, one of the new oral direct thrombin inhibitors, dabigatran[1], is available in several European countries and in Canada. There is some evidence that this agent is at least as safe and effective as warfarin in stroke prevention for patients with AF. As more studies are published and as the true clinical efficacy and safety of this and other new agents is determined, the clinical approach to long-term anticoagulation in AF may change.

REFERENCE

1. Connoly SJ, Ezekowitz MD, Yusuf S, et al. Dabigatran versus warfarin in patients with atrial fibrillation. New Engl J Med 2009 361:1139-1151.

CASE SUMMARY

- LL's current clinical picture is consistent with AF diagnosed 1 month earlier.
- Current rate-control therapy is successful at reducing HR to <100 bpm. However, patient still experiencing symptoms attributable to the disease may need to consider restoration of normal sinus rhythm.
- Patient is currently receiving therapy for stroke prevention, but need to question whether current therapy is appropriate.
- Patient has elevated total and LDL cholesterol and need to assess whether treatment is needed.

For more information on the care plan and facilitator's guide please visit http://www.mhpharmacotherapy.com.

8 Venous Thromboembolism: Deep Vein Thrombosis

Michelle T. Martin   Edith A. Nutescu

CASE LEARNING OBJECTIVES

- Recognize the signs and symptoms of venous thromboembolism (VTE)
- Identify elements needed for a proper diagnosis of deep vein thrombosis (DVT)
- Develop a treatment and monitoring plan for patients with DVT
- Select an appropriate bridging plan to oral anticoagulation
- Educate a patient on anticoagulation therapy

PATIENT PRESENTATION

Chief Complaint

"My left leg hurts so bad I can't handle it anymore."

History of Present Illness

Melinda Smith is a 38-year-old white female who presents to the ED with a 2-day H/O edema, severe pain, and warmth in her LLE. Pt. returned home to Chicago 2 days ago from London, England, where she traveled for a long weekend (a gift from her husband). She reports that these symptoms developed after the flight. She had tried massaging her leg, but it is tender and painful to touch. She tried placing a warm towel on it to alleviate the pain, but she states that her leg has become increasingly warm since the symptoms appeared. She states she hates going to the doctor, so she did not want to have her symptoms evaluated initially 2 days ago.

Past Medical History

Tobacco use × 18 years

Use of contraception × 5 years

Obesity

GERD × 10 years

HTN × 2 years

Occasional aches and pains

Family History

Mother: DVT age 63; per patient, she "took blood thinners"

Sister: varicose veins

Social History

Patient works as a receptionist at a law office.

She is married and lives with her husband of 10 years.

They have two children, aged 8 and 5 years

Tobacco/Alcohol/Substance Use

(+) 1.5 ppd × 18 yr

(+) Social drinker two to three drinks/wk

(−) Denies illicit drug use

Allergies/Intolerances/Adverse Drug Events

Amoxicillin (rash at age 3)

Medications (Current)

HCTZ 25 mg PO daily

Omeprazole 20 mg PO (pt states she takes it PRN)

Ortho-Tri-Cyclen PO daily

Ibuprofen 200 mg PO PRN headache or pain

Multivitamin PO daily

Review of Systems

Occasional headaches and back pain relieved by ibuprofen.

Physical Examination

▶ **General**

Obese, Caucasian woman in pain

▶ **Vital Signs**

BP 162/98 mm Hg, P 68 bpm, RR 16, T 36.4°C

Weight 220 lb (100 kg)

Height 64 in. (163 cm)

Pain 9/10 in LLE

▶ **Skin**

(−) Rashes or lesions; (−) trauma at site of LLE; (+) erythema in LLE

▶ **HEENT**

PERRLA, EOMI

▶ **Neck and Lymph Nodes**

(−) Thyroid nodules; (−) lymphadenopathy; (−) carotid bruits

▶ **Chest**

Clear to auscultation; no wheezes or crackles

▶ **Breasts**

Examination deferred

▶ **Cardiovascular**

RRR, normal S_1, S_2; (−) S_3 or S_4

▶ **Abdomen**

Obese, not tender; not distended; (−) organomegaly; (+) bowel sounds

▶ **Extremities**

1+ pitting edema; tenderness to palpation in LLE; (+) pedal pulses

▶ **Neurology**

Grossly intact; deep tendon reflexes normal

▶ **Genitourinary**

Examination deferred

▶ **Rectal**

Examination deferred

Laboratory Tests/Imaging

	Conventional Units	SI Units
Na	137 mEq/L	137 mmol/L
K	4.4 mEq/L	4.4 mmol/L
Cl	103 mEq/L	103 mmol/L
CO_2	25 mEq/L	25 mmol/L
BUN	13 mg/dL	4.6 mmol/L
SCr	0.7 mg/dL	62 μmol/L
Glu	108 mg/dL	6.0 mmol/L
Ca	10.1 mg/dL	2.53 mmol/L
Mg	2.1 mg/dL	0.86 mmol/L
Phosphate	4.1 mg/dL	1.32 mmol/L
Hgb	12.3 g/dL	123 g/L; 7.63 mmol/L
Hct	37.4%	0.374
WBC	$8.8 \times 10^3/mm^3$	$8.8 \times 10^9/L$
MCV	75 μm³	75 fL
Albumin	3.6 g/dL	36 g/L

Venous Duplex Exam Results:

LLE: Evidence of acute nonoccluding thrombus in the popliteal vein.

RLE: There is no evidence of thrombus.

Assessment

Pt is a 38-year-old obese woman with symptoms and imaging consistent with LLE DVT.

Student Workup

Missing Information?

Evaluate: Patient Database

Drug Therapy Problems

Care Plan (by Problem)

TARGETED QUESTIONS

1. What signs and symptoms of DVT does the patient have?

   HINT: See p. 190 in PPP

2. What are the patient's risk factors for developing a DVT? What are other acquired and inherent risk factors for DVT?

   HINT: See Table 10-1 in PPP

3. What clinical and objective criteria should be used to diagnose this patient's DVT?

   HINT: See pp. 189–190 in PPP

4. What is your plan for managing this patient's recent DVT? What initial treatment should the patient start?

What needs to be monitored? How would you transition this patient to an oral anticoagulant?

> *HINT: See Tables 10-3 and 10-5 in PPP*

5. For how long should this patient be treated with an oral anticoagulant? What laboratory values should be monitored, and what is her goal INR?

> *HINT: See Table 10-11, pp. 210–211 in PPP*

6. What risks and adverse effects of therapy would you discuss with the patient?

> *HINT: See Tables 10-8, 10-9, 10-10 in PPP*

7. What can be done to reduce this patient's risk of recurrent DVT?

> *HINT: See Table 10-1 in PPP*

FOLLOW-UP

8. The patient was hospitalized for three nights. Because of her family history (her mother had a history of DVT), a hypercoagulability panel was ordered, which included laboratory values for factor V Leiden, prothrombin G20210A mutation, proteins C and S activity, anticardiolipin antibodies, antithrombin, and lupus anticoagulant. All results came back negative.

The patient was given warfarin 10 mg nightly for 2 days, then warfarin 5 mg nightly. She was started on enoxaparin 100 mg SC q 12 h upon discharge. Two days after the patient is discharged, she presents to the Antithrombosis Clinic for monitoring of her INR. Her INR is 1.73 (after five doses of warfarin). What changes in her therapy, if any, would you recommend?

> *HINT: See pp. 210–211 in PPP*

⟳ GLOBAL PERSPECTIVE

Hepatic metabolism of warfarin varies greatly among patients, leading to very large interpatient differences in dose requirements. Genetic variations in these isoenzymes, specifically polymorphisms in CYP2C9*2, CYP2C9*3, and VCORC1 genotypes result in a significantly lower warfarin dose requirement to achieve a therapeutic response. Ethnic differences exist in the expression of these phenotypes, but the expression is not adequately uniform to allow consistent dose predictions in various ethnic populations. Genetic polypmorphism can be identified by pharmacogenetic testing; however the utility and cost-effectiveness of such testing is controversial.

CASE SUMMARY

- The patient's clinical picture is consistent with DVT.
- After initial acute therapy with a short-acting parenteral anticoagulant, the patient should be transitioned to and complete a 3-month course of oral anticoagulation therapy.
- Anticoagulation prophylaxis needs to be considered in the future if patient will be exposed to risk of VTE (i.e., surgical procedures, long flights, and pregnancy).
- The patient can make lifestyle adjustments to decrease her risk for future events.

For more information on the care plan and facilitator's guide please visit http://www.mhpharmacotherapy.com.

9 Ischemic Stroke

Susan R. Winkler

CASE LEARNING OBJECTIVES

- Recognize the signs and symptoms of acute ischemic stroke
- Identify risk factors for ischemic stroke in a patient and provide appropriate patient education
- Determine whether thrombolytic therapy is indicated in a patient with acute ischemic stroke
- Develop an appropriate patient-specific therapeutic plan for acute ischemic stroke
- Develop an appropriate therapeutic plan for outpatient management of a patient with ischemic stroke, including an appropriate agent to prevent stroke recurrence

PATIENT PRESENTATION

Chief Complaint

"I just could not get the words out. I tried to speak, but nothing would come out."

History of Present Illness

Catherine Smith is an 81-year-old Caucasian woman who was taken by the paramedics to the local hospital after experiencing weakness in her right hand and difficulty speaking during dinner with her neighbors. Her neighbors noted that she was having difficulty holding her fork and her speech seemed jumbled, so they immediately called the paramedics. She arrived in the emergency department within 60 minutes of the onset of her symptoms. She has been feeling tired and anxious since the death of her husband 4 months ago. Her appetite has been poor and she has lost 11 lb (5 kg) during this time. In the past 2 weeks, she has had several episodes where she experienced tingling in the fingers of her right hand and difficulty speaking; however, these episodes resolved within 15 to 20 minutes. She previously experienced these symptoms in 2004.

Past Medical History

HTN for 18 years
PVD diagnosed in 2003
Anemia diagnosed 6 months ago
Anxiety diagnosed 2 months ago

Family History

Both parents are deceased. She has no siblings. She has two adult sons who are healthy.

Social History

She worked as an administrative assistant, and is retired for 22 years. She has two children aged 51 and 45 years.

Tobacco/Alcohol/Substance Use

Social drinker; (−) tobacco or illicit drug use

Allergies/Intolerances/Adverse Drug Events

NKDA

Medications (Current)

Lisinopril/HCTZ 10/12.5 mg, one tablet PO every morning

Atenolol 25 mg, one tablet PO every evening

Aspirin 325 mg, one tablet PO every morning

Ferrous gluconate 300 mg, one tablet PO every morning with food

Citrucel fiber shake, one shake PO daily

Alprazolam 0.25 mg, one tablet PO three times daily PRN anxiety

Medications (Prior)

Cilostazol 50 mg, one tablet PO twice daily, discontinued due to diarrhea

Review of Systems

Denies headache; (−) blurred vision; (−) dizziness; has had difficulty ambulating in recent months due to generalized weakness; no history of migraine headaches or seizures.

Physical Examination

▶ General

Elderly, Caucasian woman, appearing weak and slightly anxious

▶ Vital Signs

BP 158/94 mm Hg, P 84, RR 14, T 36.9°C

Weight 147.4 lb (67.0 kg)

Height 64 in. (163 cm)

Denies headache or pain

▶ Skin

Warm and dry to touch

▶ HEENT

PERRLA, EOMI; no nystagmus; slight right-sided facial droop

▶ Neck and Lymph Nodes

(+) Carotid bruits on the left side; (−) lymphadenopathy

▶ Chest

Clear to auscultation

▶ Breasts

Examination deferred

▶ Cardiovascular

RRR, normal S_1, S_2; (−) S_3; (+) S_4

▶ Abdomen

Soft, nontender, nondistended; (+) BS; (−) organomegaly

▶ Neurology

A&O × 3; (+) dysarthria; slight right-sided facial droop; strength RUE 2/5; RLE 3/5; LUE 5/5; LLE 4/5 DTRs 2+ throughout; normal Babinski reflex

▶ Extremities

No cyanosis, clubbing, or edema; pulses 1+ bilaterally

▶ Genitourinary

Examination deferred

▶ Rectal

Examination deferred

Laboratory Tests

	Conventional Units	SI Units
Na	145 mEq/L	145 mmol/L
K	4.3 mEq/L	4.3 mmol/L
Cl	100 mEq/L	100 mmol/L
CO_2	28 mEq/L	28 mmol/L
BUN	16 mg/dL	5.7 mmol/L
SCr	1.2 mg/dL	106 μmol/L
Glu	115 mg/dL	6.4 mmol/L
Ca	8.7 mg/dL	2.18 mmol/L
Mg	1.7 mg/dL	0.70 mmol/L
Phosphate	3.2 mg/dL	1.03 mmol/L
Hgb	11.6 g/dL	116 g/L; 7.19 mmol/L
Hct	35.2%	0.352
WBC	$5.6 \times 10^3/mm^3$	$5.6 \times 10^9/L$
Platelets	$264 \times 10^3/mm^3$	$264 \times 10^9/L$
aPTT	24.6 s	
Total cholesterol	223 mg/dL	5.77 mmol/L
LDL cholesterol	121 mg/dL	3.13 mmol/L
HDL cholesterol	46 mg/dL	1.19 mmol/L
Triglycerides	184 mg/dL	2.08 mmol/L

Diagnostic Tests

ECG: NSR

Head CT scan: (−) Hemorrhage; evidence of left-sided infarct (see Figure 9-1)

Carotid Doppler: Decreased flow left carotid; 48% stenosis in left carotid

Assessment

Eighty-one-year-old woman who presents to the emergency department with signs and symptoms consistent with a left-sided ischemic stroke. Diagnostic tests completed in the emergency department confirm the diagnosis of ischemic stroke.

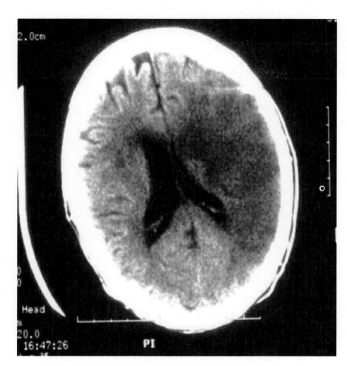

Figure 9-1. CT scan of left-sided stroke. [Reproduced, with permission, from Ropper AH, Samuels MA (eds). Adams and Victor's Principles of Neurology, 9th ed. New York, McGraw-Hill, Inc., 2009.]

Student Workup

Missing Information?

Evaluate: Patient Database

Drug Therapy Problems

Care Plan (by Problem)

TARGETED QUESTIONS

1. What signs, symptoms, and diagnostic tests are consistent with an ischemic stroke in this patient?

    Hint: See p. 218 in PPP

2. What risk factors for ischemic stroke are evident in this patient?

    Hint: See p. 217. Table 11-1 in PPP

3. Would this patient be a candidate for thrombolytic therapy with alteplase or for carotid endarterectomy?

    Hint: See pp. 220–221 in PPP

4. How is alteplase administered and monitored acutely in the clinical setting?

    Hint: See p. 221 and Table 11-5 in PPP

5. What long-term therapy would be appropriate in this patient for secondary stroke prevention, including the management of risk factors?

    Hint: See pp. 223–224 and Table 11-5 in PPP

FOLLOW-UP

6. The patient returns for follow-up 3 weeks after her acute ischemic stroke. Her BP at this visit is 146/84 mm Hg, which is more than the goal of <120/80 mm Hg. How would you manage her BP at this point? Should she continue long-term statin therapy?

    Hint: See p. 224 in PPP

⊙ GLOBAL PERSPECTIVE

Stroke is the third leading cause of death in the United States and a major cause of long-term disability. Strokes occur more commonly in patients 65 years and older, with the stroke risk doubling every decade after age 55 years. Stroke mortality has declined; however, hypertension, atrial fibrillation, and cigarette smoking continue to be important risk factors for stroke. Worldwide, stroke is the second most common cause of death. Approximately 20 million strokes occur globally each year, resulting in 5.7 million deaths annually. In developing countries, stroke mortality has declined due to global efforts to decrease cigarette smoking and manage hypertension. The stroke incidence is expected to increase over the next decade due to the aging of the population.

CASE SUMMARY

- The patient has experienced an acute left-sided ischemic stroke and thrombolytic therapy is indicated in this patient.

- She has risk factors for stroke, including hypertension, hyperlipidemia, previous transient ischemic attacks (TIAs), and PVD that require aggressive management to achieve target endpoints.

For more information on the care plan and facilitator's guide please visit http://www.mhpharmacotherapy.com.

10 Dyslipidemia

Jeannie Kim Lee   Kristina De Los Santos

CASE LEARNING OBJECTIVES

- Determine a patient's coronary heart disease (CHD) risk and corresponding treatment goal according to the National Cholesterol Education Program Adult Treatment Panel (NCEP ATP) III guidelines
- Recommend appropriate therapeutic lifestyle changes and pharmacotherapy interventions for patients with dyslipidemia
- Describe the components of a monitoring plan to assess the effectiveness and adverse effects of pharmacotherapy for patients with dyslipidemia

PATIENT PRESENTATION

Chief Complaint

"My doctor sent me here for you to check my cholesterol."

History of Present Illness

Joe Sanchez is a 68-year-old Hispanic male who is referred to the pharmacy clinic for lipid evaluation and management. He is new to this clinic, having recently been seen by one of the clinic's primary care physicians. He is feeling well with no complaints today. His last medical care was at an emergency department visit 5 years ago, where he was seen for stitches and a Tdap booster. Mr. Sanchez had his baseline laboratory tests drawn 2 weeks ago, as requested by his primary care physician, Dr. Lipidowski, who felt he would benefit from pharmacist evaluation of his cholesterol. Dr. Lipidowski consulted a clinic pharmacist to assess Mr. Sanchez's lipid panel and other pertinent laboratory results, initiate treatment for his lipid management, and follow-up to monitor for the efficacy and safety of the therapy. Mr. Sanchez has recently been diagnosed with HTN and was started on prescription medications, including an aspirin. He questions safety of prescription medications as "they are not natural," and is very resistant to starting any further prescription medications at this time. He drinks four 8 oz (240 mL) glasses of grapefruit juice every day, stating "it keeps me healthy."

Past Medical History

HTN × 1 month
Osteoarthritis
BPH
Obesity

Family History

Father died from complications of CAD at age 52. Mother is alive at 91 with advanced dementia and diabetes.

Social History

Mr. Sanchez is a devout Catholic, who was born in Tucson, Arizona. He speaks Spanish and English. He is married and lives with his wife of 43 years, and they have four children, aged 41, 38, 36, and 35. He is retired from his job at the U.S. Postal Service, and he now works part-time as a handyman.

Tobacco/Alcohol/Substance Use

Current smoker, ½ ppd; drinks six beers each weekend; has never used illicit drugs.

Allergies/Intolerances/Adverse Drug Events

Penicillin (unknown reaction)

Medications (Current)

HCTZ 25 mg daily PO
Doxazosin 4 mg at bedtime PO
Ibuprofen 200 mg PRN PO for knee and low back pain
Aspirin 81 mg daily PO

Review of Systems

(−) Headache, dizziness, light-headedness; (−) chest pain, palpitations; (−) infection; (−) urinary frequency; (+) nocturia one time per night (down from five times since starting doxazosin); (−) constipation, diarrhea, nausea; occasional knee and back pain relieved with ibuprofen.

Physical Examination [from Last Primary Care Provider (PCP) Visit 2 Weeks Ago]

▶ *General*

Well-appearing, elderly, Hispanic male in no acute distress

▶ *Vital Signs*

BP 128/78 mm Hg, P 78, RR 14, T 36.2°C

Weight 245 lb (111 kg)

Height 66 in. (168 cm)

Pain 2/10 today

▶ *Skin*

Dry-appearing skin and scalp; (−) rashes or lesions

▶ *HEENT*

PERRLA, EOMI; trace periorbital edema; (−) sinus tenderness; TMs appear normal

▶ *Neck and Lymph Nodes*

Thyroid gland normal; (−) thyroid nodules; (−) lymphadenopathy; (−) carotid bruits

▶ *Chest*

Clear to auscultation

▶ *Cardiovascular*

RRR, normal S_1, S_2; (−) S_3 or S_4

▶ *Abdomen*

Not tender/not distended; (−) organomegaly

▶ *Neurology*

Grossly intact; deep tendon reflexes normal

▶ *Genitourinary*

Examination deferred

▶ *Rectal*

Examination deferred

Laboratory Tests

Fasting, obtained 2 weeks ago

	Conventional Units	*SI Units*
Na	137 mEq/L	137 mmol/L
K	3.9 mEq/L	3.9 mmol/L
Cl	102 mEq/L	102 mmol/L
CO_2	25 mEq/L	25 mmol/L
BUN	19 mg/dL	6.8 mmol/L
SCr	1.1 mg/dL	97 μmol/L
Total cholesterol	263 mg/dL	6.80 mmol/L
LDL cholesterol	168 mg/dL	4.34 mmol/L
HDL cholesterol	51 mg/dL	1.32 mmol/L
Triglycerides	274 mg/dL	3.10 mmol/L
AST	16 IU/L	0.27 μKat/L
ALT	14 IU/L	0.23 μKat/L

Assessment

Sixty-eight-year-old man with recently diagnosed hypertension, dyslipidemia, and obesity.

Student Workup

Missing Information?

Evaluate: Patient Database

Drug Therapy Problems

Care Plan (by Problem)

TARGETED QUESTIONS

1. What risk factors for CAD does Mr. Sanchez have?

   Hint: See Table 12-4 in PPP

2. What are Mr. Sanchez's 10-year CAD risk, his risk category, and his LDL goal?

   Hint: See Tables 12-5 and 12-6 in PPP

3. Would Mr. Sanchez benefit from any lifestyle modifications? If yes, specify.

   Hint: See Table 12-7 in PPP

4. If pharmacologic treatment is appropriate for Mr. Sanchez, what medication would you choose and how would you plan his monitoring and follow-up?

   Hint: See Tables 12-8 and 12-9 in PPP

5. What education does Mr. Sanchez require to be successful with his treatment plan?

   Hint: See Tables 12-7 and 12-9 and p. 248 in PPP

FOLLOW-UP

6. Five years later, Mr. Sanchez returns for follow-up. He now has diabetes, has suffered a silent MI, and is developing early signs of Alzheimer's disease. He successfully quit smoking 1 year after his silent MI was discovered.

   His fasting laboratory tests include:

   Total cholesterol 270 mg/dL (6.98 mmol/L)

   LDL cholesterol 122 mg/dL (3.15 mmol/L)

   HDL cholesterol 41 mg/dL (1.06 mmol/L)

   Triglycerides 410 mg/dL (4.63 mmol/L)

What is Mr. Sanchez' LDL goal now? How would the treatment plan change? How should the view of Mr. Sanchez' triglycerides be altered given his new diagnoses? How should his cholesterol be managed as his age and Alzheimer's disease progress?

Hint: See Table 12-3 in PPP

⊙ GLOBAL PERSPECTIVE

Dyslipidemia is a global issue. A clinician must be aware that ethnicities may vary in their risk and presentation for CHD. For instance, South Asians, who make up 25% of the global population, have a three- to five-fold increased risk of cardiovascular morbidity and mortality as compared with other ethnic groups. Despite their significantly higher risk of CHD due to a high prevalence of risk factors, they are less likely to receive preventative statin treatment due to their low baseline serum cholesterol levels compared with Caucasian patients. In addition, there is a paucity of data for statin treatment in South Asian patients. The United States (U.S.) Food and Drug Administration (U.S.F.D.A) recommends for South Asians living in the U.S. that the starting dose of rosuvastatin be 5 mg (instead of 10 mg) due to a pharmacokinetic study that showed South Asians had a 1.6- to 2.3-fold increased exposure to rosuvastatin compared with Caucasian patients.

CASE SUMMARY

- Mr. Sanchez's current clinical picture is consistent with newly diagnosed dyslipidemia.
- Initial goals and treatment vary widely on the basis of risk factors. All patients can benefit from lifestyle modifications. Medication therapy is indicated as determined by the NCEP ATP III guidelines.
- Statins are a usual first-line therapy for LDL cholesterol lowering.

For more information on the care plan and facilitator's guide please visit http://www.mhpharmacotherapy.com.

11 Hypovolemic Shock

G. Christopher Wood Joseph M. Swanson

1. Describe the major hemodynamic and metabolic abnormalities that occur in a patient with hypovolemic shock
2. Describe the clinical presentation, including signs, symptoms, and laboratory test measurements, for a typical patient with hypovolemic shock
3. Prepare a treatment plan with clearly defined outcome criteria for a patient with hypovolemic shock, which includes both fluid management and other pharmacologic therapy
4. Compare and contrast the relative advantages and disadvantages of crystalloids, colloids, and blood products in the treatment of hypovolemic shock

PATIENT PRESENTATION

Chief Complaint
"Some guy shot me in the stomach! It hurts really bad!"

History of Present Illness
EM is a 25-year-old male who was at a nightclub and got into an argument with other patrons. During the argument he was shot in the abdomen with a handgun. He was transported to the trauma center by ambulance within approximately 30 minutes of his injury. In the ambulance, he was alert and oriented, and his vital signs were BP 140/95 mm Hg, HR 90, and RR 14. The paramedics reported that the patient had "moderate" blood loss from the bullet entry site. On arrival to the trauma center, he became restless and confused during his interview by the trauma team. His admission BP was 110/70 mm Hg, HR 110, and RR 20. Also at this time, EM was tachypneic and had impaired oxygenation. Subsequently, he was endotracheally intubated and placed on mechanical ventilation. He had two large-bore venous catheters and a urinary catheter placed.

Past Medical History
Noncontributory

Family History
Noncontributory

Social History
Single, employed at a local factory

Tobacco/Alcohol/Substance Use
Social drinker; (−) tobacco; (+) marijuana use

Allergies/Intolerance/Adverse Drug Events
Penicillin (unknown type)

Medications (Current)
None

Review of Systems
Before intubation, the patient complained of generalized weakness. His urine output in the catheter collection system was noted to be very dark yellow.

Physical Examination
▶ *General*

Well-nourished, young, African American male with increasing confusion and restlessness in some distress.

▶ *Vital Signs (10 Minutes After Admission)*

BP 80/45 mm Hg, HR 120, RR 20 (mechanically ventilated), T 36°C

Weight 198 lb (90 kg)

Height 70 in. (178 cm)

▶ *Skin*

Cool

► **HEENT**

PEERLA, EOMI, otherwise normal; oral endotracheal tube in place

► **Neck and Lymph Nodes**

Normal

► **Chest**

(+) Breath sounds and clear to auscultation bilaterally

► **Cardiovascular**

Tachycardic and hypotensive; normal heart sounds

► **Abdomen**

Bullet entry wound (1 cm) in left lower quadrant with active bleeding from the wound; very tender around entry wound.

► **Neurology**

Grossly intact; increasing confusion

► **Genitourinary**

Urinary catheter in place

► **Rectal**

Grossly heme positive

Laboratory Tests (on Admission)

	Conventional Units	SI Units
Na	145 mEq/L	145 mmol/L
K	3.4 mEq/L	3.4 mmol/L
Cl	109 mEq/L	109 mmol/L
CO_2	22 mEq/L	22 mmol/L
BUN	12 mg/dL	4.3 mmol/L
SCr	1.2 mg/dL	106 µmol/L
Glucose	112 mg/dL	6.2 mmol/L
Ca	7.5 mg/dL	1.88 mmol/L
Mg	1.8 mEq/L	0.90 mmol/L
Phosphate	3.2 mg/dL	1.03 mmol/L
Hgb	6.9 g/dL	69 g/L; 4.28 mmol/L
Hct	20.8%	0.208
WBC	$9.5 \times 10^3/mm^3$	$9.5 \times 10^9/L$
Lactate	36 mg/dL	4 mmol/L

Arterial blood gas

pH 7.34

PCO_2 35 mm Hg (4.7 kPa)

PO_2 75 mm Hg (10.0 kPa)

CO_2 22 mEq/L (22 mmol/L)

Base excess −3 mEq/L

Assessment

Twenty-five-year-old male with emerging hemorrhagic hypovolemic shock

Student Workup

Missing Information?

Evaluate: Patient Database

Drug Therapy Problems

Care Plan (by Problem)

TARGETED QUESTIONS

1. What signs and symptoms of hypovolemic shock does the patient have?

   Hint: See Table 13-2 and p. 255 in PPP

2. What alterations of key hemodynamic parameters are occurring in this patient?

   Hint: See Figure 13-1 in PPP

3. What are the immediate treatment goals in the first hour of hypovolemic shock?

   Hint: See Figure 13-4 and pp. 255–257 in PPP

4. What should be administered for initial therapy of hypovolemic shock? Compare the advantages and disadvantages of colloids and crystalloids for fluid resuscitation.

   Hint: See Figure 13-4 and pp. 257–259 in PPP

5. One hour after the initial therapy for hypovolemic shock, what additional therapy is needed?

   Hint: See Figure 13-4 and p. 259 in PPP

FOLLOW-UP

After the initial resuscitation period, an exploratory laparotomy was performed in the operating room. The patient had a penetrating injury to the colon with heavy contamination of colonic contents into the peritoneal space. The sites of acute bleeding were surgically repaired. The following morning, the patient is in the ICU on mechanical ventilation and a pulmonary artery catheter has been placed. The patient's vital signs are BP 85/64 mm Hg, HR 110, pulmonary artery wedge (occlusion) pressure 17 mm Hg, cardiac index 5 L/min/m², and RR 18 (ventilated). Pertinent labs/findings include Hgb 8.4 g/dL (84 g/L; 5.21 mmol/L), lactate 55.9 mg/dL (6.20 mmol/L), and SCr 1.5 mg/dL (133 µmol/L). Within the last hour, the patient's mental status has deteriorated and is now obtunded.

6. What therapy should be administered now for his ongoing shock?

   Hint: See Figure 13-4 and p. 260 in PPP

7. What are the treatment goals for EM's shock within the first 24 hours of onset?

   Hint: See pp. 261–262 in PPP

8. What supportive care pharmacotherapy should be started?

   Hint: See p. 260 in PPP

9. What antimicrobial surgical prophylaxis, if any, should be started?

   Hint: See Table 85-3 in PPP

⊙ GLOBAL PERSPECTIVE

Ideally, management of hypovolemic shock will be similar worldwide. The incidence and causes of hypovolemic shock may vary depending on a number of factors including health care infrastructure (e.g., availability of trauma centers and ability to get the patient transported to a facility within the first "golden" hour) and safety issues (e.g., seat belt use or availability of firearms). A cultural factor in some patients worldwide will be a religious prohibition against receiving blood products (e.g., Jehovah's Witnesses).

CASE SUMMARY

- The clinical picture was consistent with hypovolemic shock and prompt fluid resuscitation was required.
- IV fluids, blood products, and short-term vasopressors were all needed at times in this patient on the basis of his response to therapy. At the end of the case, he was not fully stabilized hemodynamically and would require further therapy.
- Supportive therapies for pain and agitation and prophylactic therapies to prevent DVT, stress ulcers, and intra-abdominal infection are needed in this patient.

For more information on the care plan and facilitator's guide please visit http://www.mhpharmacotherapy.com.

12 Acute Asthma Exacerbation

Ann McMahon Wicker   W. Greg Leader

CASE LEARNING OBJECTIVES

- Classify current asthma severity
- Recognize the clinical signs and symptoms of asthma
- Develop an appropriate treatment and monitoring plan for acute asthma therapy
- List the factors that may affect a patient's adherence to asthma therapy
- Educate a patient who is on asthma medication about the use of inhaled delivery devices, peak flow meters, and asthma education plans

PATIENT PRESENTATION

Chief Complaint

"I am having trouble catching my breath."

History of Present Illness

Jeremy Weber is an 11-year-old African American male who presents to the emergency department complaining of shortness of breath, which has been getting progressively worse over the past 12 hours. His shortness of breath started on the playground at school after a kickball game with his classmates. After the game, in addition to shortness of breath, JW experienced wheezing, coughing, and chest tightness. At this time, he self-treated his breathing difficulty with a Primatene Mist inhaler that he carries in his pocket wherever he goes. Initially, he was having difficulty breathing, but now he is in acute distress. On arrival to the emergency department, his oxygen saturation (SAO_2) was 85% (0.85) and he was able to answer questions only with single words. He was treated with three nebulized albuterol treatments with some relief; repeat SAO_2 was 90% (0.90). JW has had a runny nose and watery eyes for the past 2 weeks, which is not unusual for him.

Past Medical History

Asthma × 8 years with five hospitalizations since diagnosis, but no history of intubation

Perennial allergic rhinitis × 5 years

ADHD × 3 years

Family History

Positive for allergic rhinitis (mother and sister)

Social History/Work History

Currently enrolled in the fifth grade and lives with his mother, father, and sister. There are no animals at home.

Tobacco/Alcohol/Substance Abuse

Denies any tobacco use, but does have exposure to secondhand smoke at home. Also denies any alcohol or drug use.

Allergies/Intolerances/Adverse Drug Events

No known drug allergies

Medications (Prior to Admission)

Primatene Mist inhaler one to two puffs PRN

Albuterol 90 mcg one to two puffs every 4 to 6 hours PRN shortness of breath (has not been filled in over 6 months)

Cetirizine 10 mg PO daily PRN allergies

Methylphenidate 10 mg PO q 9 AM and 3 PM

Review of Systems

Negative, except for above

Physical Examination

▶ General

The patient appears slightly anxious, is in respiratory distress, and looks sick. He is having trouble speaking.

▶ Vital Signs

BP 99/51 mm Hg, P 108, RR 26, T 36.7°C, and O_2 saturation 90% (0.90) on 2L nasal cannula

Weight 78.3 lb (35.6 kg)

Height 58 in. (147 cm)

Denies pain

▶ HEENT

Has boggy, indurated, and edematous nasal mucosa. Red, watery eyes and clear mucoid nasal discharge are noted.

▶ Chest

The patient has significant respiratory distress with marked respiratory effort and use of accessory muscles; diffuse expiratory wheezes bilaterally; no crackles or rhonchi noted.

▶ Cardiovascular

Tachycardic, RRR. No murmurs appreciated

▶ Abdomen

Soft, nontender, and nondistended. Positive bowel sounds

▶ Neurological

Alert and oriented × 3

Laboratory Tests

SAO_2 prenebulizer 85% (0.85)
SAO_2 postnebulizer 90% (0.90)

Diagnostic Studies

CXR shows normal cardiac shadow and clear lung fields.
ECG shows sinus tachycardia.

Assessment

This is an 11-year-old African American male with an acute asthma exacerbation.

Student Workup

Missing Information/Inadequate Data?

Evaluate: Patient Database

Drug Therapy Problems

Care Plan (by Problem)

TARGETED QUESTIONS

1. What is this patient's acute asthma exacerbation severity?
   Hint: See http://www.nhlbi.nih.gov/guidelines/asthma

2. Describe signs and symptoms this patient has that are consistent with an acute asthma exacerbation.
   Hint: See p. 268 in PPP

3. What medications would be most appropriate in an acute asthma exacerbation?
   Hint: See Table 14-4 and Figure 14-4 in PPP

4. When should this patient perform peak flow measurements to determine his personal best?
   Hint: See p. 271 in PPP

5. This patient's mother is concerned about the adverse effects associated with corticosteroid use in children. How would you counsel her regarding her concern?
   Hint: See p. 273 in PPP

FOLLOW-UP

6. JW is admitted to the hospital. On further questioning, he reports awakening about three times per month. He also admits to taking breaks during activity to catch his breath, using his Primatene Mist inhaler about five times per week. What medications should JW be discharged home on? What counseling advice, if any, would you give to him? If he did not respond to the initial therapy, what adjunctive therapies could have been considered?

⟲ GLOBAL PERSPECTIVE

Asthma is a significant public health problem globally, affecting patients in both developed and undeveloped countries. It is estimated that asthma accounts for 1 in 250 deaths worldwide. The majority of asthma deaths worldwide are preventable. Most acute asthma-related deaths are due to the lack of appropriate intensification of therapy because of inappropriate assessment of the severity of the exacerbation causing delays in obtaining medical assistance or lack of access to medical care. Hospitalizations due to asthma are higher and length of asthma-related hospital stays is longer in developing countries than in more affluent countries.

CASE SUMMARY

- His current clinical picture is consistent with a severe acute asthma exacerbation, and medications to manage this exacerbation should be initiated.
- All patients with a diagnosis of asthma, regardless of severity, should have an appropriate rescue inhaler available.

For more information on the care plan and facilitator's guide please visit http://www.mhpharmacotherapy.com.

13 Chronic Asthma

Brice Labruzzo Mohundro   W. Greg Leader

CASE LEARNING OBJECTIVES

- Classify asthma severity
- Assess the existing treatment regimen and proper inhalation technique
- Develop a therapeutic plan (including treatment and monitoring) using patient-specific data that maximize patient response while minimizing adverse drug events and other drug-related problems
- Discuss proper instructions that are to be provided to a patient prescribed asthma medications

PATIENT PRESENTATION

Chief Complaint

DA is a 36-year-old African American female who presents to a family medicine clinic for follow-up after a recent emergency department (ED) visit for an "asthma attack."

History of Present Illness

DA reports having asthma as a child but was told by her mother that she grew out of it. She believes it was around the seventh grade when she stopped using an inhaler. She does not recall the name of the medication she used. On discharge from the ED, the patient was provided with a prescription for prednisone 20 mg daily for 1 week and an albuterol inhaler, but she is not sure if she is using the inhaler correctly. DA reports she finished the 7 days of prednisone a few days ago and is having less difficulty breathing than when she presented to the ED; however, she complains of a cough that she thinks appeared when she began working a second job (about 6 months ago). The patient experiences SOB most days of the week, which is sometimes accompanied by wheezing and a funny feeling in her chest. DA denies any nighttime symptoms. She is concerned because she is not able to run around with her kids when she gets home from work like she used to. She notices on her days off from the drycleaning business, she is usually symptom free unless she is around cats or mowing the yard. In addition to her respiratory complaints, the patient tells you she is experiencing heartburn several times per week, which she has been self-treating with Tums.

Past Medical History

Allergic rhinitis (allergic to cat dander and pollen per intradermal allergy testing) × 20 years

Asthma (diagnosed at age 5 years, no treatment since approximately the age of 12 years)

HTN × 3 years

Family History

Both parents have HTN; father and younger sister have asthma and allergic rhinitis.

Social/Work History

Single mother of three living in a house with no pets. Her primary job is working as a cashier at a grocery store, but she also works a second job at a family-owned drycleaning business.

Tobacco/Alcohol/Substance use

She denies current tobacco and alcohol use.

Allergy/Intolerance/Adverse Event History

Sulfamethoxazole/trimethoprim—rash

Medication History

Albuterol HFA 90 mcg one to two puffs every 4 to 6 hours as needed for shortness of breath

Loratidine 10 mg by mouth daily as needed for allergies

Propranolol extended release 120 mg by mouth daily for hypertension

Ortho Tri-Cyclen-Lo one tablet by mouth daily

Review of Systems

Unremarkable except for what is noted above

Physical Examination

▶ *General*

Well-developed, well-nourished black female in no acute distress

▶ *Vital Signs*

BP 142/90 mm Hg, P 65, RR 20, T 37°C

Weight 180 lb (82 kg)

Higher 65 in. (165 cm)

Denies pain

▶ *Skin*

Red and flaky inside elbows and behind knees

▶ *HEENT*

WNL except for nasal polyps

▶ *Chest*

Clear to auscultation bilaterally

▶ *Cardiovascular*

RRR; S_1 and S_2 normal; no rubs, gallops, or murmurs

Laboratory and Other Diagnostic Tests

Spirometry

	Prealbuterol (% Predicted)	Postalbuterol (% Predicted)
FEV_1	82	96
FVC	98	109
FEV_1/FVC	0.84	0.88

Assessment

Thirty-six-year-old female with signs, symptoms, and diagnostic tests consistent with asthma.

Student Workup

Missing Information/Inadequate Data?

Evaluate: Patient Database
Drug Therapy Problems
Care Plan (by Problem)

TARGETED QUESTIONS

1. How would you classify the patient's asthma severity?
   Hint: See http://www.nhlbi.nih.gov/guidelines/asthma

2. Why are inhaled corticosteroids a preferred therapy for all severities of persistent asthma?
   Hint: See p. 273 in PPP

3. What disease states and medications can potentially worsen asthma?
   Hint: See p. 267 in PPP

4. What adverse effects of inhaled corticosteroids would you discuss with the patient?
   Hint: See p. 273 in PPP

5. Explain the steps involved with proper metered dose inhaler technique.
   Hint: See Figure 14-1 in PPP

FOLLOW-UP

6. Four weeks later, the patient returns for follow-up. The coughing has resolved; however, she is using albuterol three to four times per week for SOB. What level of control is the patient currently experiencing? What changes, if any, would you make to her asthma treatment?
   Hint: See Figure 14-2 in PPP

⊙ GLOBAL PERSPECTIVE

Asthma is a significant public health problem globally, affecting patients in both developed and undeveloped countries. Using conservative criteria, it is estimated that approximately 300 million people worldwide have asthma. International asthma prevalence patterns cannot be explained using current knowledge of asthma pathogenesis; however, asthma prevalence appears to increase in areas that become more urbanized and adopt Western lifestyles. These increases are associated with increases in atopic sensitization and correspond with increases in other atopic disorders, such as allergic rhinitis and eczema. Globally, asthma is responsible for approximately 15 million disability-adjusted life years, a measurement of years of healthy life lost because of the disease, which is similar to that of diabetes mellitus and schizophrenia. Despite the existence of evidence-based guidelines for asthma care, wide variations in the clinical management of asthma exist worldwide.

Major barriers to effective asthma therapy include access to care and cost of therapy. In many areas, patients do not have access to basic asthma medications or medical care, leading to suboptimal long-term therapy and increased risk of death from an acute asthma. One of the primary barriers to appropriate asthma control is the cost of medications, and many patients in countries located in Central America, Africa, South Asia, and the Middle East do not have access to essential asthma medications.

CASE SUMMARY

1. Her presentation is consistent with mild persistent asthma.

2. A daily controller medication should be initiated to improve asthma control.

3. Comorbid conditions that may interfere with asthma control should be managed.

For more information on the care plan and facilitator's guide please visit http://www.mhpharmacotherapy.com.

14 Chronic Obstructive Pulmonary Disease

Nicole D. Verkleeren

CASE LEARNING OBJECTIVES

- Identify the signs and symptoms of a COPD exacerbation
- List the treatment goals for a patient with COPD
- Design an appropriate treatment regimen for a patient with a COPD exacerbation
- Develop a monitoring plan to assess the effectiveness and adverse effects of pharmacotherapy for COPD
- Formulate an appropriate education plan for a patient with COPD

PATIENT PRESENTATION

Chief Complaint

"My breathing just isn't getting better. I'm so tired and out of breath, I couldn't even read a book to my grandson yesterday."

History of Present Illness

Samuel Smarthe is a 67-year-old male who presents to the ED with complaints of increasing SOB over the past 4 to 5 days. He was seen by his primary care physician 3 days ago and was given a prescription for prednisone and told to increase his rescue inhaler use as needed. He comes to the ED this evening because his SOB has continued to worsen and he is increasingly tired and weak. In the last year, he has been hospitalized five times for similar symptoms, most recently 5 weeks ago. He has been using inhalers for his COPD for the past 11 years. About 6 months ago, his ICS dose was increased. He is supposed to use O_2 at home, but he admits to being nonadherent with this.

Past Medical History

COPD diagnosed 12 years ago

HTN diagnosed at age 35

Chronic atrial fibrillation × 5 years

Hyperlipidemia diagnosed at age 45

GERD × 2 years

Osteoarthritis (OA) × 10 years

Family History

Father died at age 70 of lung cancer. Mother died at age 35 in a motor vehicle accident. He has one brother with CAD and an "irregular heartbeat," who is alive.

Social History

The patient is married and lives with his wife of 45 years, his youngest daughter, and his 3-year-old grandson. He has two other children who live out of state. He is a retired steel-mill worker, and he and his wife care for their grandson during the day while his daughter is at work.

Tobacco/Alcohol/Substance Use

Smokes ½ ppd of cigarettes; he cut back about 6 months ago from 1½ ppd for 47 years.

No alcohol or illicit drug use.

Allergies/Intolerances/Adverse Drug Events

None

Medications (Prior to Admission)

Simvastatin 40 mg PO q hs

Atenolol 50 mg PO daily

Warfarin 7.5 mg PO on Mondays and Fridays, 5 mg PO on all other days

Prednisone 30 mg PO daily × 10 days (started 3 days ago)

Fluticasone/salmeterol 500 mcg/50 mcg one inhalation q 12 h

Tiotropium 18 mcg one inhalation q 24 h

Albuterol MDI one to two puffs q 4–6 h PRN SOB (used as often as q 20 min in the hours before presentation)

Famotidine 20 mg PO twice daily

Acetaminophen 500 mg PO q 6 h PRN arthritis pain

Review of Systems

Increasing fatigue over the past week; (−) nasal congestion or drainage; (+) SOB, cough with increased thick, tan, sputum production; (−) fever; (−) chest pain; (−) muscle pain/weakness; (+) moderate arthritis pain in the knees usually relieved by acetaminophen; (−) unusual bleeding/bruising; (−) constipation; (−) sick contacts; (−) recent travel.

Physical Examination

► General

Slightly frail, elderly white man who appears older than his stated age, in moderate respiratory distress since receiving treatment in the ED

► Vital Signs

BP 115/68 mm Hg, P 92, RR 26, T 36.9°C

Weight 134 lb (60.9 kg)

Height 70 in. (178 cm)

2/10 arthritic pain in both knees

► Skin

Warm, dry, and intact

► HEENT

PERRLA, EOMI; TMs appear normal; white patches cover tongue and inside of mouth.

► Neck and Lymph Nodes

(−) Lymphadenopathy; (−) thyromegaly; (−) carotid bruits; (+) mild bilateral JVD ; use of accessory muscles for breathing noted.

► Chest

Barrel-shaped chest; lung sounds distant; (+) rhonchi; (−) rales and crackles; bilateral wheezes on inspiration and expiration.

► Cardiovascular

Irregularly irregular rhythm, normal S_1, S_2; (−) S_3 or S_4; no murmurs, rubs, or gallops

► Abdomen

Nontender, nondistended; (−) organomegaly; paradoxical abdominal motion observed

► Neurology

Alert and oriented × 3; cranial nerves II–XII intact

► Extremities

Cool, slightly cyanotic, no clubbing, 1+ edema of lower extremities; radial and pedal pulses 2+ bilaterally; slightly decreased range of motion in both knees; (−) joint swelling or tenderness.

Laboratory Tests

	Conventional Units	SI Units
Na	139 mEq/L	139 mmol/L
K	3.1 mEq/L	3.1 mmol/L
Cl	107 mEq/L	107 mmol/L
BUN	22 mg/dL	7.9 mmol/L
SCr	1.3 mg/dL	115 μmol/L
Glucose	117 mg/dL	6.5 mmol/L
Hemoglobin	14.1 g/dL	141 g/L; 8.75 mmol/L
Hematocrit	41.1%	0.411
WBC	$9.8 \times 10^3/mm^3$	$9.8 \times 10^9/L$
Platelets	$257 \times 10^3/mm^3$	$257 \times 10^9/L$
PT	28.5 s	
INR	2.6	
ABG		
pH	7.27	
PCO_2	59.1 mm Hg	7.9 kPa
PO_2	58.5 mm Hg	7.8 kPa
HCO_3	28 mEq/L	28 mmol/L
SaO_2	86%	0.86

Diagnostic Tests

CXR shows hyperinflation of the lungs; flattened diaphragm; (−) infiltrates, effusion.

ECG reveals atrial fibrillation with controlled ventricular rate; (−) U-waves, T-waves normal.

Assessment

Sixty-seven-year-old man with signs, symptoms, and laboratory tests consistent with a COPD exacerbation requiring hospitalization and noninvasive mechanical ventilation.

Student Workup

Missing Information?

Evaluate: Patient Database

Drug Therapy Problems

Care Plan (by Problem)

TARGETED QUESTIONS

1. What signs and symptoms of a COPD exacerbation does the patient have?

    Hint: See p. 298 in PPP

2. What are the indications for antibiotic use in the treatment of a COPD exacerbation, and what should be taken into consideration when choosing an antibiotic for this patient?

    Hint: See pp. 298–299 in PPP

3. Why might theophylline be avoided in this patient?

    Hint: What side effect(s) of theophylline might worsen an underlying condition in this patient? See p. 296 in PPP

4. What indications for mechanical ventilation does this patient display?

    Hint: See p. 300 in PPP

FOLLOW-UP

5. Three days later, the patient's blood gases have improved, he remains afebrile, culture results are negative, and he is no longer requiring mechanical ventilation. What changes, if any, would you make to his drug therapy regimen? What considerations regarding his pharmacotherapy regimen should be considered as this patient is being discharged?

    Hint: See p. 299 in PPP for antibiotic duration and the section on immunizations on p. 297 in PPP

☉ GLOBAL PERSPECTIVE

According to US epidemiologic data, Caucasians are more likely than other races and ethnic groups to suffer from COPD; this trend differs from most other lung diseases. Not only are white Americans more prone to COPD, but are also more likely to die from the disease than are African Americans or Hispanics. Although epidemiologic data can be difficult to interpret, particularly when discussing a disease that is underdiagnosed such as COPD, with prevalence rates in whites and African Americans nearly double those seen in Hispanics, a genetic component that is specific to certain ethnicities seems likely. This theory is supported in Asians and Pacific Islanders, in whom some research suggests that they may possess a genetic component that reduces their risk of COPD. In many countries, the prevalence of COPD is increasing, reflecting increased rates of smoking over the past 20 years.

CASE SUMMARY

- His clinical presentation indicates the need for hospitalization, mechanical ventilation, and antibiotics in addition to standard treatment for a COPD exacerbation.

- His underlying medical conditions (atrial fibrillation, for example) and existing medications (warfarin) must be taken into consideration when designing a drug therapy regimen and establishing therapeutic goals and monitoring.

- Unnecessary use of antibiotics should be avoided; therefore, when they are used, they should be discontinued as soon as it is appropriate.

For more information on the care plan and facilitator's guide please visit http://www.mhpharmacotherapy.com.

15 Gastroesophageal Reflux Disease

Jeannie Kim Lee   Stephanie J. Davis

CASE LEARNING OBJECTIVES

- Differentiate between typical, atypical, and complicated symptoms of GERD
- Recommend appropriate lifestyle modifications and pharmacotherapy interventions for patients with GERD
- Formulate a monitoring plan to assess the effectiveness and safety of pharmacotherapy for GERD
- Educate patients on appropriate lifestyle modifications and drug therapy issues, including adherence, adverse effects, and drug interactions

PATIENT PRESENTATION

Chief Complaint

"I have burning in my chest when I am in my recliner after supper watching the evening news."

History of Present Illness

Gertie Burns is a 69-year-old woman who presents to her primary care provider complaining of burning sensation in chest every morning before breakfast and evening after supper. She has also noticed persistent cough and hoarseness develop in the last 2 years. She has had similar symptoms in the distant past but did not pay close attention while busy working multiple shifts as a registered nurse (RN). The burning pain had improved with weight loss, resulting from diet and exercise, when Gertie was in her fifties. After retirement though, she gained her weight back with her new sedentary lifestyle and diet consisting of deep-fried Cajun meals. She has been self-treating her symptoms with Tums and drinking more milk to relieve the burning. The Tums has been working some but not to her satisfaction. She eats dinner around 5:30 PM, so it can be finished by the time the news comes on every evening at 6 PM. She is inquiring if she should purchase Tagamet she saw a commercial on TV about treating stomach acid.

Past Medical History

HTN × 16 years

Osteoarthritis × 9 years

Osteoporosis × 3 months

Onychomycosis of the left big toe × 4 weeks

Impaired renal function

Constipation

Seasonal allergies

Family History

Father had stroke and died at age 74. Mother died of cancer at age 83. Patient has one sister who is 71 and has osteoporosis.

Social History

The patient is an African American woman, originally from Louisiana. She is married and lives with her husband of 47 years, who is a smoker (smoked 1 ppd × 40 years). She and her husband have three daughters, aged 47, 45, and 40. She is a retired RN and works as a volunteer at a local hospital.

Tobacco/Alcohol/Substance Use

Social drinker; (−) tobacco or illicit drug use

Allergies/Intolerances/Adverse Drug Events

NKDA

Medications (Current)

MOM 30 mL PO q 24 h PRN constipation

Alendronate 70 mg PO weekly

Nifedipine XL 30 mg PO q 24 h

Calcium carbonate 1,000 mg PO q 12 h

Terbinafine 250 mg PO q 24 h × 12 weeks

Tums one to two tablets PRN heartburn

Ibuprofen 400 mg PO q 8 h and PRN joint pain and headache

Loratadine 10 mg PO q 24 h PRN allergies

Review of Systems

Occasional sinus headache relieved with ibuprofen and loratadine; (−) tinnitus, vertigo, or infections; occasional cough and hoarseness; burning in the chest nonradiating and no pressure; (−) history cardiac disease; frequent bilateral knee pain; (−) change in urinary frequency; occasional constipation; (−) PUD or IBD; (+) dry skin; (+) toenail fungal infection.

Physical Examination

▶ General

Well-appearing, older and slightly overweight African American woman in no acute distress

▶ Vital Signs

BP 128/76 mm Hg, P 60, RR 14, T 36.2°C

Weight 142.4 lb (64.7 kg); BMI 26.1 kg/m²

Height 62 in. (157 cm)

No pain

▶ Skin

Dry-appearing skin and scalp; (−) rashes or lesions

▶ HEENT

PERRLA, EOMI; trace periorbital edema; (−) sinus tenderness; TMs appear normal

▶ Neck and Lymph Nodes

Thyroid gland normal; (−) thyroid nodules; (−) lymphadenopathy; (−) carotid bruits

▶ Chest

Clear to auscultation

▶ Breasts

Examination deferred

▶ Cardiovascular

RRR, normal S_1, S_2; (−) S_3 or S_4

▶ Abdomen

Not tender/not distended; (−) organomegaly

▶ Neurology

Grossly intact; DTRs normal

▶ Genitourinary

Examination deferred

▶ Rectal

Examination deferred

Laboratory Tests

Fasting, obtained 6 days ago

	Conventional Units	SI Units
Na	140 mEq/L	140 mmol/L
K	4.2 mEq/L	4.2 mmol/L
Cl	101 mEq/L	101 mmol/L
CO_2	22 mEq/L	22 mmol/L
BUN	8.2 mg/dL	2.9 mmol/L
SCr	0.9 mg/dL	80 μmol/L
Glucose	109 mg/dL	6.0 mmol/L
Ca	8.2 mg/dL	2.05 mmol/L
Mg	1.6 mEq/L	0.80 mmol/L
Phosphate	4.0 mg/dL	1.29 mmol/L
Hemoglobin	13.9 g/dL	139 g/L; 8.63 mmol/L
Hematocrit	40.1%	0.401
WBC	7.9 × 103/mm3	7.9 × 109/L
MCV	81 μm³	81 fL
Albumin	4.2 g/dL	42 g/L
AST	18 IU/L	0.30 μkat/L
ALT	18 U/L	0.30 μkat/L

Assessment

Sixty-nine-year-old woman with symptoms consistent with GERD

Student Workup

Missing Information?

Evaluate: Patient Database

Drug Therapy Problems

Care Plan (by Problem)

TARGETED QUESTIONS

1. What typical and atypical symptoms of GERD does the patient have?

   Hint: See p. 318 in PPP

2. Which of the patient's lifestyle and medications may make the GERD symptoms worse?

   Hint: See Table 17-1 in PPP

3. What medications decrease lower esophageal sphincter pressure?

   Hint: See Table 17-1 in PPP

4. How would you answer the patient's question about taking cimetidine for her GERD?

   Hint: Cytochrome p-450 interactions should be explored

5. What would be the drug of choice for the patient's acid suppression therapy, and how long should the patient be treated?

   Hint: See pp. 321–322 and Table 17-2 in PPP

6. What risks and adverse effects of therapy would you discuss with the patient?

   Hint: See pp. 321–322 and Table 17-2 in PPP

FOLLOW-UP

7. Twelve weeks later, Gertie returns for her second follow-up. She has lost 6 lb (2.7 kg) and is adhering to most of the lifestyle modification recommendations provided during the last visit. She is now taking the aldenodrate correctly every Sunday morning. She is no longer having GERD symptoms, except when she goes out to the local BBQ restaurant and eats fried pickles. Would you consider a change in her current acid suppression therapy? If yes, what change would you recommend? What are the potential risks of taking PPIs for long term? What actions, if any, would you take?

   Hint: See pp. 321–322 in PPP

⟳ GLOBAL PERSPECTIVE

Genetic variations among patients may change PPI effectiveness because of an alteration in their ability to metabolize drugs through the cytochrome p-450 (CYP450) enzyme system. It is unclear which patients have a polymorphic gene variation that makes them slow or fast metabolizers. Drug interactions with omeprazole are associated more often with those who are considered "slow metabolizers." Asian populations have a greater number of PPI rapid metabolizers compared to Caucasian populations. Rapid metabolizers may not receive optimal therapeutic effect from PPI therapy. PPIs may differ in the extent of drug–drug interaction related to the CYP450 enzyme system. For example, esomeprazole is metabolized more readily by CYP3A4 enzymes and may be affected less by the patient's genotype. Therefore, patients on PPI therapy should be monitored routinely for drug interactions and associated drug-related problems.

CASE SUMMARY

- Patient's current clinical picture is consistent with GERD, presenting with typical as well as atypical symptoms warranting acid suppression therapy.

- An initial PPI trial (e.g., omeprazole 20 mg daily is reasonable) of 8 weeks, along with lifestyle modification, can determine the diagnosis of GERD.

- Overuse of PPI agents should be avoided, especially in the elderly, with other complications related to prolonged and high-dose PPI use.

For more information on the care plan and facilitator's guide please visit http://www.mhpharmacotherapy.com.

16 Peptic Ulcer Disease

Geoffrey C. Wall

CASE LEARNING OBJECTIVES

- Recognize the signs and symptoms of peptic ulcer disease (PUD)
- Identify the desired therapeutic outcomes for patients with PUD
- Identify factors that guide selection of an appropriate *Helicobacter pylori* eradication regimen
- Formulate a monitoring plan for patients with PUD on follow-up

PATIENT PRESENTATION

Chief Complaint

"I'm been very nauseated lately. My stomach burns after I eat anything."

History of Present Illness

Robert Benton is a 51-year-old man who presents to his local hospital's emergency department complaining of feeling dizzy, with nausea (no vomiting), lethargy, and epigastric pain—described as "burning" off and on during the day, but especially after eating. He has recently moved to this area from another state and has yet to establish a primary care provider. He has never experienced the symptoms described before. He rarely saw his prior primary care physician in the past, although he had visited her for increasing left-knee pain that she ascribed to osteoarthritis. The patient does not like to take "artificial" medications and refused any treatment for his osteoarthritis. He denies any melena, frank blood in stool, throwing up blood, chest pain, or any other symptoms. Because of the nausea he has not eaten or drunk much in the last 3 days.

Past Medical History

Osteoarthritis of left knee.

"High cholesterol" "diagnosed" at a health fair 1 year ago. He had not told his former primary care physician about this.

Family History

His father had a history of HTN and hyperlipidemia, but died of colon cancer at age 72. Mother is alive and well at age 74. He has no siblings.

Social History

The patient is married and lives with his second wife. He has one son from a prior marriage, aged 18. He works as a certified public accountant. He is generally uncomfortable with taking medications, and feels that "natural" medicines are preferable to "artificial pills" (his words).

Tobacco/Alcohol/Substance Use

Social drinker; (–) tobacco or illicit drug use

Allergies/Intolerances/Adverse Drug Events

Penicillin (unknown reaction)

Medications (Current)

A herbal preparation, "some sort of yeast product," for his "high cholesterol"

Review of Systems

Nausea and epigastric pain as listed above; (–) changes in bowel habit or change in color/consistency of stool; dizzy and tired × 2 days, as listed above; anorexia, as listed above; (–) tinnitus, vertigo, or infections; (+) left-knee pain, especially when kneeling or first thing in the morning.

Physical Examination

▶ *General*

Well-appearing white man, with minimal distress

▶ *Vital Signs*

BP 122/79 mm Hg, P 64 (sitting), BP 99/69 mm Hg, P 82 (standing), RR 11, T 37.2°C

Weight 165 lb (75 kg)

Height 70 in. (178 cm)

Pain was 2/10 in knees this morning

Epigastric pain 4/10

▶ **HEENT**

PERRLA, EOMI; (−) sinus tenderness; TMs appear normal

▶ **Skin**

Decreased skin turgor

▶ **Neck and Lymph Nodes**

Thyroid gland smooth; (−) thyroid nodules; (−) lymphadenopathy; (−) carotid bruits; flat neck veins

▶ **Chest**

Clear to auscultation

▶ **Cardiovascular**

RRR, normal S_1, S_2; (−) S_3 or S_4

▶ **Abdomen**

Not tender/not distended; (+) epigastric pain, not worse on palpation

▶ **Neurology**

Grossly intact; DTRs normal

▶ **Genitourinary**

Examination deferred

▶ **Rectal**

Normal rectal tone; smooth prostate with no nodules; minimal stool in rectal vault that is occult blood (−)

Laboratory Tests

Obtained while in ED

	Conventional Units	SI Units
Na	140 mEq/L	140 mmol/L
K	3.9 mEq/L	3.9 mmol/L
Cl	100 mEq/L	100 mmol/L
CO_2	22 mEq/L	22 mmol/L
BUN	40 mg/dL	14.3 mmol/L
SCr	0.7 mg/dL	62 µmol/L
Glucose	89 mg/dL	4.9 mmol/L
Ca	9.4 mg/dL	2.35 mmol/L
Mg	1.8 mEq/L	0.90 mmol/L
Phosphate	3.8 mg/dL	1.23 mmol/L

Hemoglobin	14.1 g/dL	8.75 mmol/L (141 g/L)
Hematocrit	40.1%	0.401
WBC	$8.2 \times 10^3/mm^3$	$8.2 \times 10^9/L$
MCV	88 µm³	88 fL
Platelets	$247 \times 10^3/mm^3$	$247 \times 10^9/L$
H. pylori serology	(+)	
TSH	4.2 µIU/mL	4.2 mIU/L
Stool for occult blood	(−)	
Total cholesterol	220 mg/dL	5.69 mmol/L
LDL cholesterol	122 mg/dL	3.15 mmol/L
HDL cholesterol	46 mg/dL	1.19 mmol/L

Assessment

Fifty-one-year-old man with history, signs, symptoms, and laboratory tests consistent with the following:

1. Probable PUD, without acute GI bleeding
2. Probable *H. pylori* infection
3. Fluid depletion secondary to nausea and decreased intake
4. Osteoarthritis currently untreated
5. Dyslipidemia currently on herbal treatment
6. Health maintenance: colon cancer screening

Student Workup

Missing information?

Evaluate: Patient Database

Drug Therapy Problems

Care Plan (by Problem)

TARGETED QUESTIONS

1. What signs and symptoms of PUD does this patient have?

   Hint: See p. 332 in PPP

2. What treatment regimen for *H. pylori* infection would you select in this patient? What specific parts of the patient database would guide your decision?

   Hint: See pp. 333–335 in PPP

3. What medications should be *avoided* in this patient to treat his osteoarthritis?

   Hint: See p. 329 in PPP

4. What risks and adverse effects of therapy would you discuss with this patient?

   Hint: See pp. 333–335 in PPP

5. How would you initially treat the patient's dehydration?

   Hint: The patient is mildly volume depleted, probably owing to the decreased oral intake he has had over the last several days. He is orthostatic and has a high BUN:creatinine ratio (although a significant GI bleeding can often cause the BUN to rise secondary to partially digested blood). See Chapter 27, Fluids and Electrolytes in PPP for more details on managing fluid status.

FOLLOW-UP

6. The patient is referred to a new primary care physician to establish care and for follow-up. The patient is seen 5 days after completing *H. pylori* eradication therapy. Although he feels somewhat better, he still complains of epigastric pain after meals. However, this pain is diminished and the nausea he felt before has abated. He is eating and drinking normally at this time. The patient is then referred to a gastroenterologist who performs an upper GI endoscopic procedure on him. The endoscopy reveals several shallow duodenal ulcers that are partially healed with no blood or visible blood vessels. Biopsy of one of these ulcers is subjected to a tissue CLO test that reveals *H. pylori* infection. The patient confirms that he was adherent to the original *H. pylori* eradication regimen. What actions, if any, would you take?

   Hint: See p. 335 in PPP

⊙ GLOBAL PERSPECTIVE

H. pylori infection is one of the most common causes of duodenal ulcers worldwide. The organism is a microaerophilic Gram-negative rod that thrives within the low-pH environment of the stomach. Although the host and organism factors that lead to development of peptic ulcers in *H. pylori* infection are becoming better understood, what actually triggers symptomatic disease is still a mystery. Roughly 50% of the world's population is infected with the organism, yet only a small percentage of patients ever develop clinical PUD. Further, *H. pylori* is an inherently resistant organism requiring multiple antimicrobials and antisecretory agents for treatment. Resistance patterns for the organism vary significantly, depending on country with high percentages of metronidazole resistance in Asia and moderate resistance rates to clarithromycin in Europe. As it is not clinically feasible to perform traditional culture and sensitivities on this organism, the results of surveillance programs that outline general resistance patterns by geographic location should be known by the clinicians practicing in that region.

CASE SUMMARY

- This patient has probable *H. pylori* PUD. As he is demonstrating no signs and symptoms of acute GI bleeding, has no alarm symptoms concerning for cancer (i.e., weight loss and night sweats), and is relatively young, he may be treated empirically.

- Normally a standard regimen consisting of amoxicillin, clarithromycin, and a PPI would be initiated. Unfortunately, the patient has a listed allergy to penicillin. Clarification of the reaction would be helpful. In addition, the patient may be taking Chinese red yeast rice for his dyslipidemia. As this compound is essentially a less refined version of HMG CoA reductase inhibitors, the possibility that the clarithromycin may interact with the compound increasing the risk for rhabdomyolysis also exists. Thus, a secondary regimen should be selected.

- The patients' dyslipidemia should be evaluated appropriately by his primary care physician, and if necessary, appropriate nonpharmacologic and/or pharmacologic treatment should be initiated.

- For the patient's osteoarthritis, aspirin or NSAID should be avoided, especially in the immediate post-PUD treatment phase. Scheduled acetaminophen would be a reasonable alternative. If in the future the patient requires chronic use of either aspirin or an NSAID, appropriate gastroprotection could be considered as could a low-potency opioid or a local corticosteroid injection.

- In follow-up it appears that the *H. pylori* infection was not eradicated. Given the patient's allergy and medication history outlined above, the number of salvage regimens that can be used for the patient is limited. A furazolidone, tetracycline, bismuth, and PPI regimen would be one of the few choices left in this situation.

For more information on the care plan and facilitator's guide please visit http://www.mhpharmacotherapy.com.

17 Ulcerative Colitis

Brian A. Hemstreet

CASE LEARNING OBJECTIVES

- Recognize the signs and symptoms of ulcerative colitis (UC)
- Identify the goals of therapy for patients with UC
- Develop an appropriate treatment and monitoring plan for UC
- Select appropriate drug therapy for a patient with active UC
- Properly educate a patient regarding proper use and potential adverse effects associated with drug treatments for UC

PATIENT PRESENTATION

Chief Complaint

"I'm still having abdominal pain and diarrhea when I lower my dose of prednisone."

History of Present Illness

Allison Gentry is a 29-year-old woman who presents to her gastroenterologist complaining of 2 to 4 bloody bowel movements per day, intermittent crampy abdominal pain, low-grade fever, and feeling fatigued. She was initially diagnosed with UC 15 months ago. At that time she was placed on Asacol 4.8 g/d, which initially induced remission of her UC. Five months ago she experienced a flare of her UC, for which she received a course of prednisone 60 mg daily. Since that time she has been unable to taper off the prednisone. Her typical UC symptoms, particularly sharp abdominal pain, bloody diarrhea, and low-grade fever reappear once her daily prednisone dose is lowered below 30 mg daily. She still takes her Asacol and reports adherence to this therapy. Over the last 2 months she has noticed an increase in fatigue as well. She feels like she wants to rest all the time and she is unable to jog as far as she used to when her symptoms were under better control. She has also had a 15 lb (6.8 kg) weight gain over the last 5 months and is experiencing intermittent outbreaks of acne, which she views as very embarrassing. She is frustrated with the fact that her UC was initially under control, but now seems to be less responsive to her Asacol. Since she has recently gotten engaged and is planning her wedding for next year, she would like to be tapered off the prednisone as soon as possible. Likewise, she and her fiancé have also discussed the desire to have children once they are married.

Past Medical History

UC (classified as pancolitis by colonoscopy 15 months ago)
UTI (3 years ago)
GERD

Family History

Father had colon cancer at the age of 54, and is still alive following resection and chemotherapy. Mother is alive at the age of 70 with hypothyroidism. She has two younger sisters, both healthy.

Social History

Engaged and lives with her fiance. No children. Works as a physical therapist at a local hospital. Sexually active.

Tobacco/Alcohol/Substance Use

Occasional alcohol use; (+) tobacco use 1 ppd for 10 years, (−) illicit drug use.

Allergies/Intolerances/Adverse Drug Events

Sulfa (rash after receiving Bactrim DS)

Medications (Current)

Loperamide 2 mg PO as needed for diarrhea

Asacol 400 mg, four tablets PO three times daily

Prednisone 40 mg q day

Prilosec OTC 20 mg PO as needed

Maalox Advanced Maximum Strength liquid one to two teaspoons PO as needed

Ibuprofen 200 mg tablets, three to four tablets PO as needed for pain and headaches

Review of Systems

Occasional H/A and muscle aches relieved with ibuprofen, (+) fatigue, (−) SOB, (+) bloody bowel movements with crampy abdominal pain, (+) acne, (+) weight gain, (−) rash or yellowing of skin, (+) subjective low-grade fever, (+) GERD, partially relieved with Prilosec or antacids.

Physical Examination

▶ General

Well-appearing, young White woman in no acute distress

▶ Vital Signs

BP 130/76 mm Hg, P 85, RR 17, T 37.6°C

Weight 138.6 lb (63.0 kg)

Height 68 in. (173 cm)

Denies pain

▶ Skin

Face appears oily, with acne on upper back and forehead; (+) pallor

▶ HEENT

PERRLA, EOMI; (−) sinus tenderness; TMs appear normal.

▶ Neck and Lymph Nodes

Thyroid gland smooth, no thyromegaly (−) thyroid nodules; (−) lymphadenopathy; (−) carotid bruits.

▶ Chest

Clear to auscultation

▶ Breasts

Examination deferred

▶ Cardiovascular

RRR, normal S_1, S_2; (−) S_3 or S_4

▶ Abdomen

Tender to deep palpation in LLQ/not distended; (−) organomegaly, (−) rebound.

▶ Neurology

Grossly intact; DTRs normal

▶ Genitourinary

Examination deferred

▶ Rectal

(−) Hemorrhoids

Laboratory Tests

Fasting, obtained 2 days ago

	Conventional Units	SI Units
Na	138 mEq/L	138 mmol/L
K	3.1 mEq/L	3.1 mmol/L
Cl	98 mEq/L	98 mmol/L
CO_2	27 mEq/L	27 mmol/L
BUN	15 mg/dL	5.4 mmol/L
SCr	1.0 mg/dL	88 μmol/L
Glu	119 mg/dL	6.6 mmol/L
Ca	9.0 mg/dL	2.25 mmol/L
Mg	1.8 mEq/L	0.90 mmol/L
Phosphate	3.8 mg/dL	1.23 mmol/L
Hgb	10.0 g/dL	100 g/L; 6.21 mmol/L
Hct	30.7%	0.307
WBC	$8.6 \times 10^3/mm^3$	$8.6 \times 10^9/L$
MCV	74 μm³	74 fL
Platelets	$230 \times 10^3/L$	$230 \times 10^9/L$
ALT	25 U/L	0.42 μkat/L
AST	20 U/L	0.33 μkat/L
Bilirubin total	0.9 mg/dL	15.4 μmol/L
TSH	3.8 mIU/L	3.8 μIU/L
Albumin	3.9 g/dL	39 g/L
C-reactive protein (CRP)	5 mg/dL	50 mg/L

Assessment

Twenty-nine-year-old woman with signs, symptoms, and laboratory tests consistent with active UC.

Student Workup

Missing Information?

Evaluate: Patient Database

Drug Therapy Problems

Care Plan (by Problem)

TARGETED QUESTIONS

1. What signs and symptoms of UC does the patient have?

   Hint: See p. 344 in PPP

2. How would you assess the appropriateness of her drug therapy for UC when she was initially diagnosed 15 months ago?

   Hint: See pp. 345–348 in PPP

3. How would you assess and classify this patient's UC at this point in time?

   Hint: See pp. 342–345 in PPP

4. What are potential risks of long-term oral corticosteroid use in this patient?

   Hint: See p. 347 in PPP

5. What are potential pharmacotherapeutic intervention(s) that could be made at this time to manage this patient's UC?

   Hint: See pp. 349–350 in PPP

FOLLOW-UP

6. The patient is seen again in clinic 8 months later. Her symptoms have improved and she has been able to reduce her dose of prednisone to 10 mg daily. She has lost 7 lb (3.2 kg) and her acne is much improved. She inquires about smoking cessation, stating that she wishes to quit in anticipation of beginning to try to conceive within the next year. She knows it is difficult to quit and is willing to try. How will reductions in tobacco use affect her UC? What recommendations would you make regarding smoking cessation therapy for this patient?

⊙ GLOBAL PERSPECTIVE

Treatment of UC may involve many different therapies aimed at suppressing the inflammatory response. Among these therapies are azathioprine and 6-mercaptopurine, which possess potent immunosuppressive properties. Although effective for treatment of UC, thiopurine drugs may be associated with serious toxicities, such as bone marrow suppression and hepatotoxicity. Azathioprine is metabolized to its active form largely by the enzyme thiopurine methyltransferase (TPMT). Genetic polymorphisms in the TPMT enzymes among various ethnic groups may lead to some patients having low enzyme activity. These patients would be at risk for accumulation of azathioprine at standard doses typically used in UC, resulting in severe and prolonged leucopenia and increased risk of hepatotoxicity. TPMT mutations resulting in slower metabolism are more prevalent in Asian and African populations. For this reason the FDA recommends that patients should be tested for TPMT activity prior to initiating therapy to decide if the patient will need dose reductions to prevent toxicity.

CASE SUMMARY

- Her current clinical picture is consistent with UC.
- Initiation of therapy to induce and maintain remission as well as to provide long-term steroid-sparing effects is preferable.
- Appropriate baseline monitoring should be performed prior to initiating therapy with the selected agent(s).

For more information on the care plan and facilitator's guide please visit http://www.mhpharmacotherapy.com.

18 Nausea and Vomiting

Sheila Wilhelm   Jamie Hwang
Holly Chiu

CASE LEARNING OBJECTIVES

- Recognize the causes and risk factors for nausea and vomiting
- Identify the goals of therapy for nausea and vomiting
- Develop and recommend an appropriate treatment for patients with nausea and vomiting associated with cancer chemotherapy and surgery
- Implement a monitoring plan for nausea and vomiting
- Properly educate a patient taking anti-emetics

PATIENT PRESENTATION

Chief Complaint
"I feel nauseated and it feels like I need to vomit."

History of Present Illness
JM is a 45-year-old Caucasian woman with complaints of nausea and vomiting after a laparotomy with total abdominal hysterectomy and bilateral salpingo-oopherectomy for staging and initial treatment of ovarian cancer.

Prior to her procedure, JM had been given dexamethasone 4 mg IV for prophylaxis of nausea and vomiting (N/V) and received the institution's standard anesthesia protocol with thiopental 4.5 mg/kg, atracurium 0.5 mg/kg, and fentanyl 0.05 mg followed by tracheal intubation along with 75% nitrous oxide, 0.5% to 2% isoflurane, and oxygen therapy.

The procedure results indicated stage III ovarian cancer. JM seemed to have tolerated the procedure well except that she felt nauseated and vomited once despite anti-emetic prophylaxis. She has been given hydrocodone/acetaminophen 7.5/750 mg four times a day, which is adequately controlling her pain associated with the procedure. For N/V, she received dexamethasone again postoperatively that failed to control her symptoms. For the new diagnosis of stage III ovarian cancer, she will be started on cisplatin and paclitaxel in the oncology clinic 1 week following surgery.

Past Medical History
HTN × 6 years

DM × 3 years
GERD × 3 years

Family History
Mother died of breast cancer at the age of 65. Father is alive at age 70 with HTN and diabetes. She has one sister who also has diabetes.

Social History
Lives at home with husband and two children. Works as a paralegal.

Tobacco/Alcohol/Substance Use
Drinks one glass of wine every night; (−) tobacco or illicit drug use.

Allergies/Intolerances/Adverse Drug Events
No known drug allergies (NKDA)

Medications Prior to Admission (PTA)
HCTZ 25 mg PO daily

Glyburide 5 mg PO twice daily

Metformin 500 mg PO twice daily

Omeprazole 20 mg PO daily

Acetaminophen 650 mg PO PRN for HA

Medications (Current)

HCTZ 25 mg PO daily

Glyburide 5 mg PO twice daily

Metformin 500 mg PO twice daily

Pantoprazole 40 mg PO daily

Review of Systems

Occasional headaches relieved with non-aspirin pain reliever; (−) tinnitus, vertigo, or infections; frequent body aches that she attributes to lack of exercise; (−) change in urinary frequency, but she has noticed an increase in the number of episodes of constipation in the past year; reports cold extremities; (−) history of seizures, syncope, or loss of consciousness; (+) dry skin.

Physical Examination

▶ General

Well-appearing, middle-aged, Caucasian woman in no acute distress.

▶ Vital Signs

BP 149/85 mm Hg, P 65, RR 19, T 36.1°C

Weight 134 lb (61 kg)

Height 67 in. (170 cm)

Denies pain

▶ Skin

Dry appearing skin and scalp; (−) rashes or lesions

▶ HEENT

PERRLA, EOMI; trace periorbital edema; (−) sinus tenderness; TMs appear normal

▶ Chest

Clear to auscultation

▶ Breasts

Examination deferred

▶ Cardiovascular

RRR, normal S_1, S_2; (−) S_3 or S_4

▶ Abdomen

Not tender/not distended; (−) organomegaly

▶ Neurology

Grossly intact; deep tendon reflexes normal

▶ Genitourinary

Examination deferred

▶ Rectal

Examination deferred

Laboratory Tests

Fasting, obtained 2 days ago

	Conventional Units	SI Units
Na	143 mEq/L	143 mmol/L)
K	4.1 mEq/L	4.1 mmol/L
Cl	100 mEq/L	100 mmol/L
CO_2	24 mEq/L	24 mmol/L
BUN	8 mg/dL	2.9 mmol/L
SCr	0.7 mg/dL	62 μmol/L
Glu	130 mg/dL	7.2 mmol/L
Ca	9.4 mg/dL	2.35 mmol/L
Mg	1.8 mEq/L	0.90 mmol/L
Phosphate	3.8 mg/dL	1.23 mmol/L
Hgb	13 g/dL	130 g/L; 8.07 mmol/L
Hct	40%	0.40
WBC	$6 \times 10^3/mm^3$	$6 \times 10^9/L$
MCV	83 μm³	83 fL
Platelets	$230 \times 10^3/mm^3$	$230 \times 10^9/L$
Albumin	3.8 g/dL	38 g/L
CA-125	90 U/mL	90 kU/L
Total cholesterol	159 mg/dL	4.11 mmol/L
LDL cholesterol	85 mg/dL	2.20 mmol/L
HDL cholesterol	56 mg/dL	1.45 mmol/L
Triglycerides	90 mg/dL	1.02 mmol/L

Assessment

Forty-five-year-old woman with signs, symptoms, and risk factors consistent with postoperative nausea and vomiting (PONV); at risk in future for chemotherapy-induced nausea and vomiting (CINV)

Student Workup

Missing Information?

Evaluate: Patient Database

Drug Therapy Problems

Care Plan (by Problem)

TARGETED QUESTIONS

1. What risk factors does this patient have that contribute to development of PONV?

   Hint: See p. 365 in PPP

2. Why did the patient develop N/V despite the prophylaxis for PONV?

   Hint: See p. 366 in PPP

3. What therapy would be most appropriate to treat the patient's PONV that developed despite prophylaxis?

   Hint: See p. 366 and Table 20-2 in PPP

4. What risks and adverse effects of PONV therapy would you discuss with the patient?

   Hint: See Table 20-2 in PPP

FOLLOW-UP

One week later, patient presents to the oncology clinic. She is to be started on cisplatin and paclitaxel for the management of stage III ovarian cancer.

5. What risk factors does this patient have that contribute to development of CINV?

   Hint: See p. 364–365 in PPP

6. What prevention regimen is recommended for acute CINV?

   Hint: See Table 20-4 in PPP

7. What prevention regimen is recommended for delayed CINV?

   Hint: See Table 20-4 in PPP

8. What breakthrough treatment is recommended for this patient's CINV?

   Hint: See p. 365 in PPP

9. What risks and adverse effects of CINV therapy would you discuss with the patient?

   Hint: See Table 20-2 in PPP

⟳ GLOBAL PERSPECTIVE

Domperidone, which is widely available in many countries (including Mexico) but is not FDA approved in the United States, is pharmacologically similar to metoclopramide but has minimal passage across the blood–brain barrier. It has similar CTZ-mediated anti-emetic efficacy as metoclopramide but is less likely to cause centrally mediated adverse effects (extrapyramidal reactions, tardive dyskinesia, etc.). Patients from other countries or Americans who travel to other countries may be receiving domperidone for N/V, GERD, or gastroparesis. Domperidone can prolong the QT interval and it should not be used in patients who have QT prolongation or are receiving other medications that may cause QT prolongation.

CASE SUMMARY

- Patient has multiple risk factors for N/V and prophylactic therapy for PONV and CINV should be initiated.
- Combinations of anti-emetics are recommended for preventing PONV for high-risk patients.
- Cisplatin is a highly emetogenic chemotherapy. A combination of anti-emetics with different mechanisms of action is recommended for prevention of acute and delayed CINV.

For more information on the care plan and facilitator's guide please visit http://www.mhpharmacotherapy.com.

19 Diarrhea

Yolanda McKoy-Beach   Clarence E. Curry, Jr

CASE LEARNING OBJECTIVES

- Recognize the signs and symptoms of diarrhea
- Distinguish between acute and chronic diarrhea
- Explain how medication use can lead to diarrhea
- Identify the goals of therapy for diarrhea
- Develop an appropriate treatment plan for a patient with diarrhea

PATIENT PRESENTATION

Chief Complaint

"I have diarrhea, I think. I have also been throwing up and I have watery stools at different times."

History of Present Illness

Jose Zapata is a 40-year-old Latino male who is a native of Mexico. The patient complains of symptoms described as abdominal pain, vomiting, and loose watery stools occurring at different times. These symptoms have been occurring for a couple of weeks. He reports that he recently went home to Mexico and "ate a lot of vegetables and fruits" that were grown on his parents' land. He says that he returned to the United States about 2 weeks ago and that he really hasn't noticed a change in the frequency of the bouts of diarrhea.

Jose became a patient at the community clinic approximately 2 months ago. On his initial visit, he described symptoms of polyuria, polydipsia, and weight loss of 10 lb (4.5 kg) over the previous couple of months without trying to lose weight. At that time, a fingerstick was performed in the clinic and the result showed a blood glucose of 190 mg/dL (10.5 mmol/L). He reports that afterward, he came to the clinic on two different occasions to have fingersticks done. The results were 154 mg/dL (9.5 mmol/L) and 172 mg/dL (9.5 mmol/L), respectively. Based on those results, he was started on metformin 500 mg once daily for 7 days, then 500 mg twice daily. He thinks the episodes of diarrhea and vomiting began after the metformin was increased to 1,000 mg twice daily at his last clinic visit. Today he is also feeling "very down" and misses his wife and children.

Past Medical History

Type 2 DM diagnosed 6 weeks ago
HTN diagnosed 1 year ago in Mexico
Dyslipidemia diagnosed at the last clinic visit

Family History

Father (+) Type 2 DM; mother (+) HTN and type 2 DM. His wife and children are all in good health

Social History

Originally a native of Mexico; has been in the United States for 4 years.

The patient has a seventh-grade education; nonsmoker; patient has no health insurance and receives prescription medications through a national chain pharmacy's $4.00 generic drugs.

Tobacco/Alcohol/Substance Use

Denies alcohol use

Medication History (Current)

Metformin 1,000 mg PO twice daily
Lisinopril 10 mg PO daily
Aspirin 81 mg PO daily
Pravastatin 10 mg PO nightly
Preparation-H PRN

Allergies

NKDA

Physical Examination

▶ *General*

Well-nourished male in no acute distress; appears depressed.

▶ *Vital Signs*

BP 146/90 mm Hg, HR 80 bpm, RR 18, T 36.2°C

Weight 220 lb (100 kg)

Height 69 in (179 cm)

BMI 31 kg/m²

Denies pain

▶ *HEENT*

PERRLA, EOMI

▶ *Cardiovascular*

RRR; S_1 and S_2 normal; no S_3 or S_4

▶ *Chest*

Clear to auscultation and percussion

▶ *Abdomen*

No hepatomegaly or splenomegaly; nontender, distended; normoactive bowel sounds

▶ *Genitourinary*

Within normal limits

▶ *Rectal*

No fissures or hemorrhoids; palpable stool; heme (−)

▶ *Neurology*

Alert and oriented × 3; Cranial nerves intact; (−) Babinski

Laboratory and Diagnostic Tests

	Conventional Unit	SI Units
Na	134 mEq/L	134 mmol/L
K	4.1 mEq/L	4.1 mmol/L
Cl	101 mEq/L	101 mmol/L
HCO₃	30.7 mEq/L	30.7 mmol/L
BUN	23 mg/dL	8.2 mmol/L
Scr	0.9 mg/dL	80 µmol/L
Glu	150 mg/dL	8.3 mmol/L
AST	18 IU/L	0.30 µkat/L
ALT	22 IU/L	0.37 µkat/L
Alk phos	80 IU/L	1.33 µkat/L
Ca	9.3 mg/dL	2.33 mmol/L
PO₄	4.6 mg/dL	1.49 mmol/L
Hgb	14.4 g/dL	144 g/L; 8.94 mmol/L
Hct	41%	0.41
WBC	5.98×10^3 mm	5.98×10^9/L
Total cholesterol	213 mg/dL	5.51 mmol/L
HDL cholesterol	39 mg/dL	1.01 mmol/L
LDL cholesterol	124 mg/dL	3.21 mmol/L
Triglyceride	241 mg/dL	2.72 mmol/L
Hemoglobin A_{1C}	8.2%	0.082

Urinalysis

Clear and colorless

Stool

(−) blood; (−) ova and parasites

Stool culture is pending

Assessment

Forty-year-old man with signs and symptoms of diarrhea.

Student Workup

Missing Information/Inadequate Data?

Evaluate: Patient Database
             Drug Therapy Problems
             Care Plan (by Problem)

TARGETED QUESTIONS

1. What signs and symptoms of diarrhea does the patient have?

   Hint: See pp. 377–378 in PPP

2. What medications can cause diarrhea?

   Hint: See Table 21-3 in PPP

3. When should a colonoscopy be performed in a person with chronic diarrhea?

   Hint: See p. 377 in PPP

4. What is/are the primary management for diarrhea?

   Hint: See pp. 378–379 in PPP

5. Should this patient be treated for dehydration? Why or why not?

   Hint: See p. 378 in PPP

FOLLOW-UP

Two weeks later, the patient returns for follow-up. He reports that the diarrhea has resolved. The metformin dose, which was lowered to 500 mg twice daily, will now be gradually increased over the next 4 to 6 weeks to achieve the target dose of 2,000 mg/d.

⊙ GLOBAL PERSPECTIVE

Diarrhea is not a disease, but rather a symptom of another problem. Dehydration is frequently a consequence of diarrhea, and its effect in the very young or the elderly can be significant. Diarrhea is classified as acute or chronic and can be brought on by infectious microorganisms or by noninfectious causes, including medications. In developing countries, diarrhea, often resulting from infectious causes, is a major cause of morbidly and mortality. Lactose intolerance, the result of a deficiency of lactase, is a common cause of diarrhea. It occurs widely throughout the world affecting virtually all racial and ethnic groups, although it is seen less often in northern Europe. Irritable bowel syndrome (IBS) is another condition seen worldwide that is frequently characterized by diarrhea. The availability of clean water is perhaps the single most important way to curb infectious diarrheal illnesses seen in developing countries.

Treatment for diarrhea in the developing world is most often accomplished through the use of oral rehydration therapy. In any part of the world, significantly dehydrated patients and those whose diarrhea is caused by an invasive microorganism, as well as the very young or the elderly and those with co-morbidities, may require more extensive evaluation, treatment, and monitoring.

CASE SUMMARY

- Current clinical picture is consistent with acute or persistent diarrhea that could have been caused by an infectious agent (traveler's diarrhea) or is drug-induced.
- The treatment of suspected traveler's diarrhea is bismuth subsalicylate (Pepto-Bismol), regular strength. The recommended adult dose is 30 ml or 2 tablets, repeated every 30–60 minutes as needed, not to exceed eight doses.
- The treatment of suspected drug-induced diarrhea is to decrease or discontinue the causative agent.

For more information on the care plan and facilitator's guide please visit http://www.mhpharmacotherapy.com.

20 Constipation

Beverly C. Mims   Clarence E. Curry, Jr

CASE LEARNING OBJECTIVES

- Identify the causes of constipation
- Recognize the symptoms of functional constipation
- Identify the goals of therapy for functional constipation
- Recommend lifestyle modifications and therapeutic interventions for the treatment of functional constipation

PATIENT PRESENTATION

Chief Complaint

"I'm constipated. I haven't had a bowel movement in 4 days, and this isn't the first time it has happened."

History of Present Illness

QN is a 48-year-old female who presents to her physician's office complaining of constipation. QN is evaluated every 6 months by her primary-care physician and was last seen 5 months prior to presentation. Upon further questioning by her physician, QN reported that she often has to strain when attempting to have a bowel movement. When she does have a movement, her stools are small, dry, and hard. She had used docusate in the past with some benefit, but recently it seemed to stop working. She has tried psyllium in the past, but she didn't like mixing it with so much water and it made her constipation worse. QN denied abdominal pain. QN has a history of HTN, neuropathic pain, and joint and muscle pain.

Past Medical History

Essential HTN

Neuropathic pain—radiculopathy caused by traumatic injury

Family History

Father is alive at age 72 and has CAD, HTN, osteoarthritis, and type 2 DM. Mother is alive at age 67 with type 2 DM, HTN, osteoarthritis, and hypercholesterolemia. QN has three siblings; all are living. Two siblings are known to have migraine headaches and HTN, and one sibling has type 1 DM.

Social History

QN is a divorced mother of two children aged 19 and 15. She works as a paralegal for the county government.

Tobacco/Alcohol/Substance Use

(−) Alcohol, tobacco, or illicit drug use

Allergies/Intolerances/Adverse Drug Events (ADEs)

Gabapentin (pruritus)

Medications (current)

Lisinopril 40 mg PO q day

HCTZ 25 mg PO q day

Amitriptyline 50 mg PO at bedtime

Multivitamin 1 tablet PO every 24 hours

Ibuprofen 200 mg PO every 8 hours as needed for headaches and joint and muscle pain

Review of Systems

Occasional headaches and joint and muscle aches and pains are relieved with ibuprofen; noticed a change in bowel habits when she started taking amitriptyline for neuropathic pain caused by traumatic injury; feels full

Physical Examination

▶ *General*

Well-developed, well-nourished middle-aged female in no acute distress

▶ *Vital Signs*

BP 120/80 mm Hg, P 70, RR 20, T 37.0°C

Weight 146 lb (66.4 kg)

Height 60 in. (152 cm)

Denies pain

▶ *Skin*

Dry-appearing skin; skin intact; (−) rashes or lesions

▶ *HEENT*

PERRLA, EOMI, (+) sinus tenderness

▶ *Neck and Lymph Nodes*

Supple w/o JVD, bruits, or thyromegaly

▶ *Chest*

Clear to auscultation

▶ *Cardiovascular*

Within normal limits w/o gallop, murmur, rub, click, or irregularity

▶ *Abdomen*

No scars, lesions, or rashes; round, soft, nontender, symmetrical abdomen; hypoactive bowel sounds; no visible pulsations; no bruits; no guarding

▶ *Neurology*

Grossly intact; DTRs normal

▶ *Genitourinary*

Deferred

▶ *Rectal*

Anal sphincter pressure normal; (+) small pieces of hard stool in rectal vault; (−) external hemorrhoids

Laboratory Tests

	Conventional Units	SI Units
Na	139 mEq/L	139 mmol/L
K	4.0 mEq/L	4.0 mmol/L
Cl	100 mEq/L	100 mmol/L
CO_2	24 mEq/L	24 mmol/L
BUN	11 mg/dL	3.9 mmol/L
SCr	0.6 mg/dL	53 μmol/L
Glu	160 mg/dL	8.9 mmol/L
Ca	9.7 mg/dL	2.43 mmol/L
Mg	1.8 mEq/L	0.90 mmol/L
Phosphate	3.2 mg/dL	1.03 mmol/L
Hgb	14.7 g/dL	147 g/L; 9.13 mmol/L
Hct	38.6%	0.386
WBC	$7 \times 10^3/mm^3$	$7 \times 10^9/L$
Albumin	3.9 g/dL	39 g/L
Stool occult blood	(−)	

Assessment

Forty-eight-year-old woman with complaints consistent with constipation.

Student Workup

Missing Information/inadequate data?

Evaluate: Patient Database
Drug Therapy Problems
Care Plan (by Problem)

TARGETED QUESTIONS

1. What symptoms of constipation does the patient have?
   Hint: See pp. 372–373 in PPP

2. What medications and other products can cause or worsen constipation?
   Hint: See Table 21-1 in PPP

3. What risks and/or adverse effects associated with laxative products should be considered as you prepare to recommend a product and discuss its use with the patient?
   Hint: See pp. 372–375 in PPP

FOLLOW-UP

Two weeks later, the patient returns for follow-up. She feels better and reports the absence of small hard stools and the need to strain when defecating. She regularly sets aside time to have a bowel movement and reports a symptom-free experience at least three to four times weekly since being on medication.

4. How long should this patient continue to take medication to sustain a symptom-free bowel movement?

5. Should sugar-containing products be excluded from consideration now or in the future for this patient?

⊙ GLOBAL PERSPECTIVE

Constipation occurs all over the world. Perhaps as much as 12% or more of the world's population suffers from constipation at one time or another. It appears that inhabitants of developed countries have a higher incidence than those living in developing countries, perhaps because the diet in developed countries contains less fiber. Around the world, many people choose to treat constipation without the aid of commercially available laxatives. Some people attempt to self-treat constipation by altering their diet, and herbal remedies are popular in many parts of the world. Among those herbs used are buckthorn, flaxseed, aloe, fenugreek, and beetroot. In many cultures, fruit is favored for constipation relief. These may include pears, mangoes, guava, prunes, and papayas. Some locales favor homeopathic remedies such as bryonia, calcarea carbonica, lycopodium, or nux vomica.

CASE SUMMARY

- Forty-eight-year-old female patient presented to her physician complaining of altered stool form and consistency.

- QN's constipation does not appear to be due to organic causes.

- In the recent past, she used psyllium products and a stool softener to self-treat. However she no longer gets relief from their use.

- QN's presenting medication regimen includes several medications that have been associated with constipation as an adverse effect.

For more information on the care plan and facilitator's guide please visit http://www.mhpharmacotherapy.com.

21 Cirrhosis and Portal Hypertension

Laurajo Ryan

CASE LEARNING OBJECTIVES

- Recognize the signs and symptoms of spontaneous bacterial peritonitis (SBP)
- Identify the criteria for diagnosis of SBP
- Develop a treatment plan for ascites and prophylaxis/treatment of SBP
- List common adverse events caused by SBP and develop/identify an appropriate treatment regimen

PATIENT PRESENTATION

Chief Complaint
"My stomach is killing me—I think I need to be tapped."

History of Present Illness
GE is a 48-year-old white female who presents to the Emergency Department (ED) with complaints of severe abdominal pain and a feeling of fullness. She has a 4-year history of ascites, but is a bit vague about how long her abdomen has been distended; she says that the pain has gotten much worse recently. When questioned more closely about the time frame, she becomes angry and agitated. Although she was diagnosed with alcohol-induced cirrhosis 6 years ago, GE has continued to drink. GE reports subjective fever (she did not take her temperature) this morning and yesterday evening, but says she felt better after she took acetaminophen and ibuprofen. GE says she is mostly compliant with her medications, but has been doubling up on her furosemide for the past few days since she assumed her belly pain was a result of fluid overload.

Past Medical History
Ethanol-induced cirrhosis × 6 years

Esophageal varices 2 years ago, s/p banding

HTN × 13 years

Gravida 2, para 2

OA of hands × 8 years

Family History
Father died at age 54 from alcoholic cirrhosis

Mother alive with CAD

Neither brother nor sister have a history of alcohol abuse; sister has type 2 DM

Son with history of alcohol abuse, daughter healthy

Social History
Lives with husband and adult son

Has worked in her family's restaurant since age 12

Tobacco/Alcohol/Substance Use
No tobacco, no illicit drugs, began drinking alcohol daily at age 13, currently drinks about seven to eight shots of liquor daily, but denies other forms of alcohol

Allergies/Intolerances/Adverse Drug Events (ADEs)
Severe hypotension when given IV morphine

Medications (Current)
Lactulose 15 mL PO twice daily

Propranolol 10 mg PO q 12 h

Furosemide 40 mg PO q AM

Spironolactone 100 mg PO q AM

Acetaminophen 1,000 mg PO PRN

Ibuprofen 600 mg PO PRN

Review of Systems
(–) Nausea, vomiting, constipation

Frequent diarrhea that she attributes to lactulose use

Occasional bright red blood in her stools (BRBPR), unsure about melena

Subjective fever as above, (−) SOB, cough, hemoptysis

Physical Examination

▶ **General**

Ill-looking woman who appears much older than stated age

Rates current pain level at 7 on a scale of 0 to 10

▶ **Vital Signs**

BP 92/54 mmHg, HR 104 bpm, RR 16, T 39.3°C

Weight 142 lb (64.5 kg)

Height 67 in. (170 cm)

▶ **Skin**

Dry and jaundiced, with spider angiomata on the upper trunk

▶ **HEENT**

PERRLA, EOMI, (+) scleral icterus

▶ **Chest**

Clear to auscultation bilaterally; breasts tender

▶ **Cardiovascular**

Regular rhythm, tachycardic; no murmurs, rubs, or gallops

▶ **Abdomen**

Very painful and distended with (+) fluid wave, unable to assess for hepatomegaly/splenomegaly due to pain and guarding with palpation, (+) caput medusae

▶ **Neurology**

Grossly intact, some mild confusion and agitation

▶ **Extremities**

No edema

▶ **Genitourinary**

Examination deferred

▶ **Rectal**

Examination deferred

Laboratory Tests

	Conventional Units	SI Units
Na	125 mEq/L	125 mmol/L
K	4.6 mEq/L	4.6 mmol/L
Cl	106 mEq/L	106 mmol/L
CO$_2$	20 mEq/L	20 mmol/L
BUN	17 mg/dL	6.1 mmol/L
Scr	1.4 mg/dL	124 µmol/L
Glu	96 mg/dL	5.3 mmol/L
Hgb	10.4 g/dL	104 g/L; 6.46 mmol/L
Hct	31%	0.31
MCV	104 µm^3	104 fL
WBC	11.2×10^3/mm^3	11.2×10^9/L
Platelets	102×10^3/mm^3	102×10^9/L
Albumin	2.8 g/dL	28 g/L
Total bilirubin	6.7 mg/dL	114.6 µmol/L
Alk phos	174 IU/L	2.90 µkat/L
AST	317 IU/L	5.28 µkat/L
ALT	142 IU/L	2.37 µkat/L
GGT	167 IU/L	2.78 µkat/L
LDH	206 IU/L	3.47 µkat/L
PT	28 s	
INR	1.9	

(−) urine toxicology screen, (−) blood alcohol

Paracentesis results

PMN count	276 cells/mm^3	276×10^6 cells/L
Gram stain negative		
Albumin	1.3 g/dL	13 g/L

Assessment

Forty-eight-year-old woman with a known history of cirrhosis and ascites presents with a painful abdomen and fever, both suggestive of SBP.

Student Workup

What Information is Missing?

Evaluate: Patient Database

Drug Therapy Problems

Care Plan (by Problem)

TARGETED QUESTIONS

1. What signs and symptoms of SBP does this patient have?

   Hint: See pp. 392–393 in PPP

2. What are the diagnostic criteria for SBP?

   Hint: See Figure 22-5 in PPP

3. In what situations would prophylactic treatment for SBP be appropriate?

   Hint: See p. 397 in PPP

4. What empiric treatment regimen should be initiated for SBP?

   Hint: See p. 397 in PPP

5. What sequelae are associated with SBP? Do any of the patient's laboratory tests indicate that she may be at risk of these complications?

   Hint: See p. 397 in PPP. Also look closely at her drug regimen and recent self-treatment.

FOLLOW-UP

6. GE received empiric antibiotic therapy and her abdominal pain is improving. What treatment would be appropriate if the patient progresses to hepatorenal syndrome?

   Hint: See p. 399 in PPP

7. Is long-term therapy to prevent SBP warranted? If so, what options are available?

   Hint: See p. 399 in PPP

8. What steps can be taken to lower GE's risk of further complications from cirrhosis?

   Hint: See p. 400 in PPP

9. What specific counseling would you provide GE to decrease her risk of complications?

   Hint: See p. 400 in PPP

⟳ GLOBAL PERSPECTIVE

In the United States, the majority of cirrhosis cases are caused by overconsumption of alcohol and/or infection with the hepatitis C virus. Worldwide, the primary cause of cirrhosis is hepatitis B; according to the World Health Organization (WHO), approximately 2 billion people worldwide are infected. Hepatitis B is preventable by vaccination, and in those countries (such as the United States) that have implemented vaccination programs beginning in infancy, rates of hepatitis B have dropped dramatically. Cirrhosis related to alcohol consumption has increased in industrialized countries, and hepatitis C–related cirrhosis is increasing in many countries, since a vaccine is not yet available. In the United States, hepatitis C actually began to decrease in 1992 and has since plateaued despite the lack of a vaccine.

CASE SUMMARY

- Patient presents with presumptive SBP; ascitic fluid PMN count warrants immediate treatment despite negative Gram stain.
- Antibiotic regimen should cover most common bacteria associated with SBP, both Gram negative and Gram positive.
- Albumin administration can decrease the risk of progression to hepatorenal syndrome.
- Long-term antimicrobial prophylaxis is warranted in those with a history of SBP.

For more information on the care plan and facilitator's guide please visit http://www.mhpharmacotherapy.com.

CASE LEARNING OBJECTIVES

- List modes of transmission and risk factors for hepatitis B
- Identify the signs and symptoms of hepatitis B
- Create treatment goals for treatment of hepatitis B
- Develop a nonpharmacological and pharmacological treatment and monitoring plan for hepatitis B

PATIENT PRESENTATION

Chief Complaint

"I have hepatitis B and was told to come and get a second opinion."

History of Present Illness

Mrs. Vivian Lin is a 51-year-old Chinese female referred for further evaluation of her hepatitis B virus (HBV). She is currently being treated for the HBV infection by her primary care physician for the past year. Prior to starting Epivir in March 2006, her HBV DNA quantitative level was 2,422,348 copies/mL and alanine transaminase (ALT) level was 101 IU/L (1.68 μkat/L). She brings her laboratory test results in for review, which indicate a detectable HBV DNA level despite being on Epivir. She was born in Hong Kong and immigrated to the United States at the age of 47. She has no complaints of dark urine, pale stools, or yellow eyes or skin.

Past Medical History

Hepatitis B diagnosed in 2006.

Surgical History

None

Family History

Mother has type 2 diabetes but is alive and well.

Father died of heart disease.

Social History

She is married and has no children. Her husband is on hemodialysis. Her husband has been her only sexual partner in her lifetime. She currently works in data entry.

Tobacco/Alcohol/Substance Use

She does not drink alcohol, smoke tobacco, or use illicit drugs.

Allergies/Intolerances/Adverse Drug Events

She denies any allergies.

Medications (Current)

Multivitamin

Epivir 100 mg daily—started March 2006

Review of Systems

(−) Chest pain, SOB, weight loss, weight gain, dysuria, melena, or hematochezia.

Physical Examination

▶ *General*

The patient is a well-developed, alert and oriented, well-nourished looking woman.

▶ *Vital Signs*

BP 122/80 mm Hg, P 80, RR 20, T 37.1°C

Weight 125 lb (56.8 kg)

Height 69 in. (175 cm)

Pain scale: 0 out of 10

▶ *Skin*

There are no spider angiomata or palmar erythema.

▶ *HEENT*

Eyes anicteric, throat examination normal.

► **Neck and Lymph Nodes**

Thyroid not palpable.

► **Chest**

Clear to auscultation and percussion.

► **Cardiovascular**

RRR, no murmurs or gallops.

► **Abdomen**

(+) Bowel sounds. (−) Ascites. Liver and spleen not palpable.

► **Neurology**

(−) Asterixis

► **Extremities**

(−) Peripheral edema

Laboratory Tests

From 5/11/2008

	Conventional Units	SI Units
Na	139 mEq/L	139 mmol/L
K	4.5 mEq/L	4.5 mmol/L
Cl	103 mEq/L	103 mmol/L
CO_2	24 mEq/L	24 mmol/L
BUN	15 mg/dL	5.4 mmol/L
SCr	0.8 mg/dL	71 μmol/L
Glu	100 mg/dL	5.6 mmol/L
Ca	9.3 mg/dL	2.33 mmol/L
Total protein	8.2 g/dL	82 g/L
Alpha fetoprotein	3 ng/mL	3 μg/L
Total cholesterol	148 mg/dL	3.83 mmol/L
LDL cholesterol	86 mg/dL	2.22 mmol/L
HDL cholesterol	49 mg/dL	1.27 mmol/L
Triglycerides	64 mg/dL	0.72 mmol/L
Hgb	13.4 g/dL	8.34 mmol/L
Hct	39.7%	0.397
WBC	$6.1 \times 10^3/mm^3$	$6.1 \times 10^9/L$
Platelet	$240 \times 10^3/\mu L$	$240 \times 10^9/L$
Albumin	4.4 g/dL	44 g/L
Total bilirubin	1 mg/dL	17.1 μmol/L
AST	22 IU/L	0.37 μkat/L
ALT	19 IU/L	0.32 μkat/L
Alk phos	64 IU/L	1.07 μkat/L

Imaging

Abdominal ultrasound 4/2007:

Liver parenchyma shows unremarkable echogenicity. There is no discrete tumor identified. There is no intra- or extrahepatic ductal dilatation. Small polyp is present in the gallbladder, which is otherwise negative. Images of the pancreatic head demonstrate a rounded hypoechoic focus measuring approximately 1.5 cm, which was not clearly present on the comparison study. The right kidney is not hydronephrotic. No ascites is detected.

Impression:

1. Abnormality within the pancreatic head measuring approximately 1.5 cm and for which contrast-enhanced CT is advised

2. No sonographic abnormality of the liver

3. Small gallbaladder polyp

Assessment

Fifty-one-year-old asymptomatic Chinese woman with normal ALT levels and HBeAg (+) hepatitis B with detectable HBV DNA level suggesting viral resistance.

Student Workup

Missing Information?

Evaluate: Patient Database
              Drug Therapy Problems
              Care Plan (by Problem)

ADDITIONAL PATIENT LABORATORY DATA

	HBV DNA Quant. (Normal Range: <100–5,000,000 copies/mL)	HBsAg	HBcAg	HbeAg	Anti-HBs	Anti-HBe
8/4/2008	2,700	+		+		−
5/11/2008	400	+		+		−
6/21/2007	<100	+	+	+	−	−
1/5/2007	<100	+	+	−	−	+
9/5/2006	<100	+	+	+	−	−
6/7/2006	3,764	+	+	+	−	−
3/5/2006	2,422,348	+	+	+	−	−

TARGETED QUESTIONS

1. What signs and symptoms of hepatitis B does the patient have?

   Hint: See p. 416 in PPP

2. What are the goals of therapy for the treatment of Hepatitis B?

   Hint: See p. 417 in PPP

3. What preventative measure can be taken to prevent the spread of hepatitis B and minimize the progression of the liver disease?

   Hint: See pp. 420–421 in PPP

4. What are the adverse effects of hepatitis B therapy you would need to discuss with the patient prior to starting treatment?

   Hint: See pp. 422–424 in PPP

5. On the basis of these laboratory results, what pharmacological recommendation would you make at this time?

   Hint: See Lok AS, McMahon BJ. Chronic hepatitis B: Update 2009. Hepatology 2009;50:1–36.

FOLLOW-UP

Approximately 1 year later, Mrs. Lin continues to be asymptomatic from her hepatitis B infection. An additional anti-HBV agent, adefovir 10 mg daily was added to the current regimen on 8/5/2008. She had been doing well for the past year and returns for follow-up and results of her laboratory tests.

6. Why is this patient no longer responding to the combination hepatitis B treatment? On the basis of these laboratory results, what pharmacological recommendation would you make at this time?

   Hint: See Lok AS, McMahon BJ. Chronic hepatitis B: Update 2009. Hepatology 2009;50:1–36.

☯ GLOBAL PERSPECTIVE

Despite having an effective vaccine to prevent the spread of hepatitis B infection, this disease continues to affect more than 2 billion people in the world. Each year, approximately 300,000 new hepatitis B cases are diagnosed. Chronic hepatitis B affects close to 400 million people and 500,000 to 700,000 may die due to complications associated with the liver disease. Approximately 75% of chronic HBV cases occur in Asia. The hepatitis B-related mortality rate in Asian immigrants to the United States is seven times greater than individuals who are Caucasian. Although the treatment armamentarium for hepatitis B has grown significantly over the past decade, at present the agents available are only effective in suppressing HBV levels and delaying the progression of liver disease to cirrhosis. These agents may not be readily available to patients in developing countries. Since most of these HBV infections are acquired at birth from mothers infected with HBV, providing the hepatitis B vaccine at birth is the most effective measure to prevent chronic hepatitis B disease.

UPDATED PATIENT LABORATORY DATA

	HBV DNA Quant. (Normal Range: <100–5,000,000 copies/mL)	HBsAg	HBcAg	HBeAg	Anti-HBs	Anti-HBe	Cr mg/dL (µmol/L)	ALT IU/L (µkat/L)
10/5/2009	6316	+		+	−	−	1.4 (124)	50 (0.83)
7/30/2009	500			+			1.3 (115)	39 (0.65)
2/27/2009	< 100	+		+	−	+	1 (88)	17 (0.28)
11/8/2008	< 100	+	+	+	−	−	0.8 (71)	20 (0.33)
8/4/2008	2,700	+		+		−		
5/11/2008	400	+		+		−		19 (0.32)
6/21/2007	< 100	+	+	+	−	−	0.8 (71)	
1/5/2007	< 100	+	+	−	−	+		32 (0.53)
9/5/2006	< 100	+	+	+	−	−		51 (0.85)
6/7/2006	3,764	+	+	+	−	−	0.9 (80)	
3/5/2006	2,422,348	+	+	+	−	−	1 (88)	101 (1.68)

CASE SUMMARY

- The patient developed lamivudine resistance while being treated for HBV. Approximately 70% of the patients treated with lamivudine will develop resistance at 5 years of therapy.

- The treatment for HBV drug resistance may be to add a HBV antiviral agent from another drug class to the existing regimen (i.e., add adefovir to lamivudine) or to discontinue the current regimen and switch to a different class of antiviral agent or switch to a more potent antiviral agent within the same class (i.e., switch lamivudine to high dose entecavir).

- The patient developed adefovir resistance. In addition, the patient's renal function was decreasing. Continued use of adefovir may cause nephrotoxicity.

- Tenofovir has been found to be effective in inhibiting HBV replication in patients who develop lamivudine and adefovir resistance. Therefore, Mrs. Lin's adefovir was discontinued and switched to tenofovir.

For more information on the care plan and facilitator's guide please visit http://www.mhpharmacotherapy.com.

23 Hepatitis C

Juliana Chan

CASE LEARNING OBJECTIVES

- List modes of transmission and risk factors for hepatitis C
- Identify the signs and symptoms of hepatitis C
- Create treatment goals for treatment of hepatitis C
- Develop a nonpharmacological and pharmacological treatment and monitoring plan for hepatitis C

PATIENT PRESENTATION

Chief Complaint

"I had my yearly physical and my physician told me my liver numbers are really high. He sent me to see the liver physician."

History of Present Illness

Ms. Fran Brap is a 56-year-old Caucasian female, with no complaints, whose employer requested that she get a physical for insurance purposes. At that time, her liver enzymes were noted to be elevated and she was referred to see a hepatologist as soon as possible. The earliest appointment to see the hepatologist was in 6 weeks. She states that she feels fine and stress free since returning from her trip from Mexico 3 weeks ago.

Past Medical History

Hypothyroidism 3 years ago

Postmenopause at age 43

Laryngeal cancer—1996

Breast cancer—1996

Depression

Surgical History

Right mastectomy—1996

Laryngectomy requiring a tracheostomy—1997

Cholecystectomy—1973 (blood transfusion was required)

Family History

Mother had HTN and type 2 diabetes, died at age 72.

Father had a 35 pack-year history of smoking and died of lung cancer at the age of 63.

She has one sister and does not know her medical history.

Social History

She was married but now divorced for 12 years. She has two sons who live elsewhere and rarely visit her. She currently works at a grocery store.

Tobacco/Alcohol/Substance Use

She used intravenous drugs including heroin and cocaine starting in her teens and quit in 2001. She was a social drinker and quit in 1993. She smoked tobacco, 1 ppd for 24 years, and quit in 1997 when she was diagnosed with laryngeal cancer.

Allergies/Intolerances/Adverse Drug Events

Ketorolac—seizures

Seasonal allergies to pollen

Medications (Current)

Acetaminophen 500 mg, two tablets three times a day PRN body aches

Levothyroxine 0.137 mg PO daily

Lorazepam 2 mg PO at bedtime

Methadone 75 mg PO daily

Multivitamin one tablet PO daily

Review of Systems

Complains of fatigue frequently with occasional pale color stools.

Physical Examination

▶ *General*

The patient is not in acute distress. She is an obese Caucasian female.

▶ **Vital Signs**

BP 112/77 mm Hg, P 84, RR 20, T 37.1°C

Weight 254 lb (115.5 kg)

Height 69 in. (175 cm)

Pain scale: 2 out of 10

▶ **Skin**

(+) Palmar erythema and some spider angiomas on her anterior chest.

▶ **HEENT**

Normocephalic, atraumatic; sclerae anicteric, no gross lesions.

▶ **Neck and Lymph Nodes**

(+) Tracheostomy; thyroid not enlarged

▶ **Chest**

Clear to auscultation

▶ **Cardiovascular**

RRR, normal S_1, S_2; (−) S_3 or S_4

▶ **Abdomen**

(+) Bowel sounds. She is obese. (+) Scars from her previous cholecystectomy. (−) Hepatomegaly, splenomegaly.

▶ **Neurology**

(−) Asterixis; alert and oriented × 3; DTRs WNL

Extremities: Trace edema bilaterally present.

Laboratory Tests

Fasting, obtained on 4/15/2009

	Conventional Units	SI Units
Na	143 mEq/L	143 mmol/L
K	4.4 mEq/L	4.4 mmol/L
Cl	108 mEq/L	108 mmol/L
CO_2	29 mEq/L	29 mmol/L
BUN	7 mg/dL	2.5 mmol/L
SCr	0.9 mg/dL	80 μmol/L
Glu	86 mg/dL	4.8 mmol/L
Ca	8.6 mg/dL	2.15 mmol/L
TSH	24.59 μIU/mL	24.59 mIU/L
HCV RNA quant.	1,296,980 IU/mL	
Hepatitis C genotype	1a	
Hgb	12.4 g/dL	7.70 mmol/L
Hct	38.5%	0.385
WBC	$2.1 \times 10^3/mm^3$	$2.1 \times 10^9/L$
Platelets	$83 \times 10^3/\mu L$	$83 \times 10^9/L$
Albumin	2.8 g/dL	28 g/L

Total bilirubin	2.2 mg/dL	37.6 μmol/L
AST	90 IU/L	1.50 μkat/L
ALT	105 IU/L	1.75 μkat/L
Total cholesterol	134 mg/dL	3.47 mmol/L
LDL cholesterol	78 mg/dL	2.02 mmol/L
Triglyceride	116 mg/dL	1.31 mmol/L
HDL cholesterol	33 mg/dL	0.85 mmol/L

Imaging and Other Studies

Liver biopsy: 03/2008

Mild chronic hepatitis consistent with HCV infection, grade 2 fibrosis, stage 3 disease.

Histologic activity index:

Portal inflammation: 2, piecemeal necrosis: 2, lobular inflammation: 2, fibrosis: 3.

CT of the abdomen with and without contrast: 10/2008

The liver appears to be heterogeneous. In liver segment 2, there is a hypovascular nonenhancing mass in which hepatocellular carcinoma cannot be excluded, but is unlikely. In segment 5, there is a similar mass that is also hypovascular and nonenhancing. The intrahepatic ducts appear slightly enlarged. The spleen is enlarged with a small cyst present within its parenchyma that is too small to characterize. A duodenal diverticulum is present along with esophageal varices and a hiatal hernia. There is no evidence of ascites. A patent portal vein is present.

Treadmill stress echocardiogram: 4/2009

Global LV function at rest is normal. Rest images could not be reviewed real time. Very limited echo imaging without evidence for significant ischemia.

Assessment

Fifty-six-year-old asymptomatic Caucasian woman with abnormally high ALT levels and confirmed chronic HCV.

Student Workup

Missing Information?

Evaluate:	Patient Database
	Drug Therapy Problems
	Care Plan (by Problem)

TARGETED QUESTIONS

1. What signs and symptoms of HCV does the patient have?

   Hint: See p. 416 in PPP

2. What are the goals of therapy for the treatment of HCV?

   Hint: See p. 417 in PPP

3. What preventative measure can be taken to prevent the spread of HCV and minimize the progression of the liver disease?

   Hint: See pp. 424–425 in PPP

4. What are the adverse effects of HCV therapy you would need to discuss with the patient prior to starting treatment?

   Hint: See pp. 424–425 in PPP

5. Should the patient receive the HCV treatment?

   Hint: This patient has several comorbidities, which include depression, anemia, and hypothyroidism, that must be addressed prior to starting HCV treatment. The HCV medications have many adverse effects that may develop during the course of treatment and could possibly worsen these comorbidities. It would be prudent to treat and stabilize all medical conditions prior to initiating any HCV medications. See p. 424 in PPP.

FOLLOW-UP

The patient's depression is stable and is being followed by a psychiatrist. Her hypothyroidism is stable as well and being followed by an endocrinologist. Her anemia has been ruled out for any oncological causes and she was cleared by an oncologist for initiation of pegylated interferon and ribavirin therapy. She started HCV treatment and returns today for week 12 follow-up. She complains of fatigue and has trouble sleeping at night. She also states that she is more irritable now than prior to starting treatment and wants you to increase her dose of lorazepam.

Laboratory Tests

Fasting, obtained at week 12 of treatment

	Conventional Units	SI Units
Na	141 mEq/L	141 mmol/L
K	4 mEq/L	4 mmol/L
Cl	106 mEq/L	106 mmol/L
CO_2	30 mEq/L	30 mmol/L
BUN	9 mg/dL	3.2 mmol/L
SCr	1 mg/dL	88 µmol/L
Glu	170 mg/dL	9.4 mmol/L
Ca	8.3 mg/dL	2.08 mmol/L
HCV RNA quant.	1,087,341 IU/mL	
Total cholesterol	104 mg/dL	2.69 mmol/L
LDL cholesterol	50 mg/dL	1.29 mmol/L
Hgb	11.4 g/dL	114 g/L; 7.08 mmol/L
Hct	36.7%	0.367
WBC	$3.1 \times 10^3/mm^3$	$3.1 \times 10^9/L$
ANC	$1.2 \times 10^3/mm^3$	$1.2 \times 10^9/L$
Platelets	$61 \times 10^3/\mu L$	$61 \times 10^9/L$
Albumin	2.8 g/dL	28 g/L
Total bilirubin	2.5 mg/dL	42.8 µmol/L
AST	35 IU/L	0.58 µkat/L
ALT	90 IU/L	1.50 µkat/L
Triglyceride	114 mg/dL	1.29 mmol/L
HDL cholesterol	31 mg/dL	0.80 mmol/L

6. Why is the patient complaining of these symptoms? Is the patient responding to the HCV regimen? What action should be taken at this time? What other laboratory test(s) should be obtained at this time?

   Hint: See pp. 424 and 426 in PPP. See also Ref. 1.

⚙ GLOBAL PERSPECTIVE

Hepatitis C may affect anyone in the world. There is a higher prevalence of HCV infections in non-Hispanic blacks vs. non-Hispanic whites. Genotype plays an important role in determining the likelihood of the patient's response to hepatitis C treatment. Approximately 75% of those infected with HCV in the United States have genotype 1, and about 14% and 5% have genotypes 2 and 3, respectively. Genotype 4 is predominately found in the Middle East and genotype 6 in Asia. Research efforts continue to focus on determining reason why non-Hispanic whites are less likely to respond to the hepatitis C treatment when compared with Caucasians, especially if the patient has genotype 1 disease. To improve the patient's rate of sustaining virological response, it is prudent to encourage patients to be compliant with their medication regimens, and not miss any doses or discontinue the therapy without notifying their health care provider.

CASE SUMMARY

- The patient's comorbidities (depression, anemia, hypothyroidism) have been evaluated and cleared by specialists to initiate hepatitis C treatment.
- Treatment would include ribavirin and pegylated interferon. The patient would need to be monitored more frequently for ribavirin-induced hemolytic anemia due to her low baseline hemoglobin levels.
- Treatment response should be re-evaluated at week 4 and week 12 of initiating the hepatitis C medications. If the HCV viral count is positive at week 12, then the treatment should be discontinued, however if the viral count is undetectable, then continue therapy for at least an additional 36 weeks, depending on the week 4 HCV viral level result.

REFERENCE

1. Ghany MG, Strader DB, Thomas DL, Seeff LB; American Association for the Study of Liver Diseases. Diagnosis, management, and treatment of hepatitis C: An update. Hepatology 2009 49(4):1335–1374.

For more information on the care plan and facilitator's guide please visit http://www.mhpharmacotherapy.com.

24 Acute Kidney Injury

Lena M. Maynor

CASE LEARNING OBJECTIVES

- Assess a patient's kidney function based on clinical presentation, laboratory results, and urinary indices
- Identify pharmacotherapeutic outcomes and endpoints of therapy in a patient with acute kidney injury
- Apply knowledge of the pathophysiology of acute kidney injury to the development of a treatment plan
- Select pharmacotherapy to treat complications associated with acute kidney injury (AKI)

PATIENT PRESENTATION

Chief Complaint

"Mom just hasn't been acting like herself for the last few days."

History of Present Illness

Geraldine Lowry is an 84-year-old Caucasian woman with altered mental status who was brought to the emergency department by her daughter. She was discharged from the hospital 1 week ago following treatment for an exacerbation of her chronic heart failure. The patient's history of present illness has been relayed by her daughter, as the patient is unable to provide a history at this time. According to the daughter, GL initially felt less fatigued and short of breath following her hospital discharge, which she attributes to the increased dose of her "water pill" that GL has continued to take since her hospital discharge. Her daughter, who is her primary care giver, has noticed that GL has become progressively more confused and lethargic over the last few days. Today, the patient became very dizzy and lightheaded when trying to stand up, and her daughter decided to bring her to the emergency department.

Past Medical History

Heart failure × 5 years

DM type 2 × 15 years

HTN × 30 years

Osteoarthritis × 35 years

Chronic renal insufficiency × 7 years

Diabetic gastroparesis, diagnosed 6 months ago

Family History

Father died of MI at the age of 67 and mother died of breast cancer at the age of 82. Brother has been diagnosed with CAD and has a history of MI and is alive at age 78.

Social History

Retired, worked as an elementary school teacher for 25 years. Married for 51 years, widowed 7 years ago. Currently lives with daughter.

Tobacco/Alcohol/Substance Use

(−) Alcohol, tobacco, or illicit drug use

Allergies/Intolerances/Adverse Drug Events

Macrolide antibiotics (hives)

Medications (Prior to Admission)

Lisinopril 20 mg PO q 24 h

Metoprolol 50 mg PO q 12 h

Furosemide 40 mg PO twice daily

Metformin 500 mg PO twice daily

Sitagliptin 100 mg PO q 24 h

Ibuprofen 200 mg PO three times daily PRN pain

Multivitamin PO q 24 h

Metoclopramide 10 mg PO with meals and at bedtime

Review of Systems

Patient is currently unable to contribute to review of systems.

Physical Examination

▶ *General*

Elderly female in no apparent distress.

▶ *Vital Signs*

BP 134/82 mm Hg, P 72, RR 16, T 36.6°C

Weight 114.4 lb (52.0 kg)

Height 68 in. (173 cm)

Joint pain 5/10 (knees, according to daughter)

▶ *Skin*

Dry appearing skin; (−) rashes

▶ *HEENT*

Normocephalic, PERRLA

▶ *Chest*

(+) Crackles right lung base

▶ *Cardiovascular*

RRR, (+) S_3

▶ *Abdomen*

(−) Tenderness, distention, organomegaly

▶ *Neurology*

Not fully cooperative with examination

▶ *Genitourinary*

Examination deferred

▶ *Rectal*

Examination deferred

Laboratory Tests

Today

	Conventional Units	SI Units
Na	137 mEq/L	137 mmol/L
K	5.7 mEq/L	5.7 mmol/L
Cl	101 mEq/L	101 mmol/L
CO_2	28 mEq/L	28 mmol/L
BUN	43 mg/dL	15.4 mmol/L
SCr	4.12 mg/dL	364 μmol/L
Glu	119 mg/dL	6.6 mmol/L
Ca	8.6 mg/dL	2.15 mmol/L
Mg	2.1 mEq/L	1.05 mmol/L
Phosphate	4.4 mg/dL	1.42 mmol/L

Hgb	13.9 g/dL	139 g/L; 8.63 mmol/L
Hct	41.3%	0.413
Platelets	$339 \times 10^3/mm^3$	$339 \times 10^9/L$
WBC	$9.2 \times 10^3/mm^3$	$9.2 \times 10^9/L$
Albumin	2.8 g/dL	28 g/L
Urine osmolality	614 mOsm/kg	614 mmol/kg
Urine sodium	15 mEq/L	15 mmol/L
Urine creatinine	113 mg/dL	10.0 mmol/L
Urinalysis		
Character	Cloudy	
Color	Yellow	
Specific gravity	1.011	
Glucose	Negative	
Bilirubin	Negative	
Ketones	10 mg/dL	1.7 mmol/L
Blood	Small	
pH urine	5.5	
Protein	30 mg/dL	300 mg/L
Urobilinogen	Normal	
Nitrite	Negative	
Leukocytes	Negative	
RBC	12/hpf	
WBC	1/hpf	
Bacteria	Occasional	
Squamous epithelial cells	Moderate	

Assessment

Eighty-four-year-old woman with signs, symptoms, and laboratory tests consistent with acute kidney injury

Student Workup

Missing Information?

Evaluate: Patient Database

Drug Therapy Problems

Care Plan (by Problem)

TARGETED QUESTIONS

1. How would this patient's AKI be classified?

   Hint: See pp. 432–433 in PPP

2. Which of the patient's medications could be causing or contributing to the (AKI)?

   Hint: See pp. 440–442 in PPP

3. Which methods of assessing kidney function can be useful in patients with AKI?

   Hint: See pp. 433–434 in PPP

4. What signs and symptoms of AKI does the patient have?

   Hint: See p. 435 in PPP

5. What potential adverse effects could be caused by the patient's current medications, given the patient's AKI?

   Hint: Some medications are eliminated renally, and thus, may accumulate during acute kidney injury. This accumulation may make patients more susceptible to adverse effects from those particular agents. A review of each medication the patient is receiving should be performed to assess the need for dosing adjustment and potential adverse effects that may occur.

FOLLOW-UP

6. One month later, following the resolution of GL's AKI, the patient presents to the emergency department again with complaints of abdominal pain, and her physician orders an abdominal CT scan with IV contrast. What risk factors for contrast-induced nephropathy does this patient have? What measures could be taken to prevent the incidence of contrast-induced nephropathy in this patient?

   Hint: See p. 441 in PPP

☉ GLOBAL PERSPECTIVE

It is estimated that the true incidence of AKI is severely underreported in developing countries, due to lack of data reporting and a lack of a global consensus definition of acute kidney injury. AKI is thought to differ between developed and developing countries in a number of ways. In developed countries or large urban areas, hospital-acquired AKI predominates. Most of these patients are elderly and have multiple comorbidities that contribute to the development of acute kidney injury. Alternatively, patients that acquire AKI in developing areas are generally younger. The AKI in these patients is usually associated with acute, severe volume loss related to a single comorbidity such as gastroenteritis, malaria, leptospirosis, or ingestion of traditional herbal remedies. Reported mortality rates in these patients are generally lower than the reported mortality in developed countries, which is attributed to the younger age and lack of comorbidities in these patients. However, with AKI requiring acute hemodialysis, patients in developing areas are at a definite disadvantage, as access to dialysis is generally limited to only large, urban cities within these countries. In addition, the expense of dialysis generally prohibits the use of dialysis as a treatment option for many patients.

CASE SUMMARY

- Her current clinical picture is consistent with AKI.
- Treatment of AKI is dependent on the etiology of the injury and whether it is prerenal, intrinsic, or postrenal AKI.
- It is important to evaluate current medications to assess for potential causes of AKI and to determine if any medications may be more likely to cause adverse effects due to decreased elimination.

For more information on the care plan and facilitator's guide please visit http://www.mhpharmacotherapy.com.

25 Chronic Kidney Disease

Melanie Foeppel   Jennifer Jordan

LEARNING OBJECTIVES

- List the risk factors for development and progression of chronic kidney disease (CKD)
- Explain the mechanisms associated with progression of CKD
- Outline the desired outcomes for treatment of CKD
- Develop a therapeutic approach to slow the progression of CKD, including lifestyle modifications and pharmacologic therapies
- Recommend an appropriate monitoring plan to assess the effectiveness and safety of pharmacotherapy for slowing the progression of CKD

PATIENT PRESENTATION

Chief Complaint

"I am worried about going fishing with my grandson. I don't feel like eating supper and have just not felt well lately."

History of Present Illness

Alfred Statton is a 70-year-old African-American male who presents with complaints of "not feeling well," loss of appetite, and anxiety about his overall wellness. He has had a lack of energy for the past year, but has attributed it to old age. The patient denies nausea or vomiting, but has noticed over the past 6 months that food "just doesn't taste the same," and he has been eating only two small meals a day. He was last seen by a physician approximately 7 years ago, at which time he was started on HCTZ and amlodipine for HTN. The patient reports that he felt worse on the medications, stopped taking them, and decided never to go back. He is very anxious about taking care of his 5-year-old grandson next Saturday and wants to make sure that he is healthy.

Past Medical History

HTN: diagnosed 20 years ago, untreated

Osteoarthritis: diagnosed 15 years ago

Kidney stones: 1981, 1990, and 1996

Family History

Father: Deceased from MI in his eighties

Mother: Deceased from cervical cancer in her sixties

Social History

The patient is retired but volunteers at the local food bank twice a week as a shelf stocker. Currently, he smokes 1½ ppd of cigarettes and denies alcohol or illicit drug use. His physical activity is limited by osteoarthritis.

Medications

The patient denies taking any prescription, OTC, or herbal medications.

Allergies

No known drug allergies

Physical Examination

▶ *General*

Elderly African-American male in no acute distress

▶ *Vital Signs*

BP 160/98 mm Hg, P 96 bpm, RR 13, T 36.5°C, pain 0

Weight 178 lb (81 kg)

Height 70 in. (178 cm)

► **Skin**

Cool-to-touch, dry-appearing skin and scalp; no rashes/lesions

► **HEENT**

PERRLA; conjunctivae normal; wears bilateral hearing aids

► **Neck and Lymph Nodes**

Thyroid gland smooth, symmetric; (−) thyroid nodules; (−) lymphadenopathy; (−) carotid bruits

► **Chest**

Clear to auscultation

► **Cardiovascular**

RRR, 2/6 systolic murmur heard at apex radiating to axilla

► **Abdomen**

No organomegaly, bruits, or tenderness, (+) bowel sounds

► **Neuro**

Grossly intact; DTRs normal

► **Extremities**

2+ bilateral edema on lower extremities

► **Genitourinary**

Examination deferred

► **Rectal**

(−) Fecal occult blood

Laboratory Tests (Fasting)

	Conventional Units	SI Units
Sodium	135 mEq/L	135 mmol/L
Potassium	4.6 mEq/L	4.6 mmol/L
Chloride	110 mEq/L	110 mmol/L
Bicarbonate	18 mEq/L	18 mmol/L
BUN	45 mg/dL	16.1 mmol/L
Serum creatinine	2.5 mg/dL	221 µmol/L
Estimated GFR	33 mL/min/1.73 m²	0.32 mL/s/m²
Glucose	108 mg/dL	6.0 mmol/L
Total cholesterol	246 mg/dL	6.36 mmol/L
LDL cholesterol	175 mg/dL	4.53 mmol/L
HDL cholesterol	24 mg/dL	0.62 mmol/L
Triglycerides	235 mg/dL	2.66 mmol/L
Urine albumin	435 mg/dL	4.35 g/L

Assessment

Seventy-year-old male with untreated HTN due to poor follow-up and adherence, who is now presenting with signs and symptoms of renal insufficiency

Student Workup

Missing Information?

Evaluate: Patient Database

Drug Therapy Problems

Pharmacotherapy Care Plan (by Problem)

TARGETED QUESTIONS

1. Assuming that the patient's SCr is stable, how would you stage his CKD?

   Hint: See Table 26-1 in PPP. Staging for CKD is based on the MDRD equation, not Cockcroft-Gault

2. What signs and symptoms are consistent with CKD?

   Hint: See p. 449 in PPP

3. Identify the patient's risk factors for developing CKD and explain how his progression factors may contribute to his eventual kidney failure.

   Hint: See Table 26-2 in PPP

4. What nonpharmacologic and pharmacologic treatments are appropriate at this time to slow the patient's progression to ESKD?

   Hint: See pp. 450–452 in PPP

5. What is the goal for each pharmacologic intervention listed above?

   Hint: See pp. 450–452 in PPP

6. The patient is to be started on lisinopril. Describe an appropriate monitoring plan that includes efficacy and medication safety.

   Hint: See p. 452 in PPP

FOLLOW-UP

7. The patient returns to clinic after taking lisinopril for 10 days. His laboratory tests from this morning reveal a serum creatinine of 2.7 mg/dL (239 µmol/L). On the basis of the pharmacologic effects of an ACE-I in CKD, is this an expected result? What symptoms or findings would prompt you to stop his lisinopril immediately?

   Hint: See pp. 442, 452–453 in PPP

⟳ GLOBAL PERSPECTIVE

CKD is increasing in prevalence worldwide. It accounts for a major health care expenditure in the developed world, but accounts for considerable morbidity, mortality, and decreased life expectancy in developing countries. Although hypertension and diabetes are the major causes for CKD worldwide, other causes may be significant based on region. In Southeast Asia, there remains a high prevalence of infection-related glomerulonephritis. HIV-related renal disease plays a major role in South Africa and parts of Sub-Saharan Africa. International movements are under way to identify individuals at risk for CKD and prevent progression; however, there are many obstacles including funding, infrastructure, and access to nephrologists.

CASE SUMMARY

- The patient's presentation and laboratory findings are consistent with CKD.
- Lifestyle and pharmacologic interventions should be initiated to slow the patient's progression to ESKD.
- ACEIs or ARBs are first-line options for decreasing proteinuria. Pharmacists can play a key role in counseling, monitoring, and appropriate titration of these agents.

For more information on the care plan and facilitator's guide please visit http://www.mhpharmacotherapy.com.

26 Euvolemic Hyponatremia

Mark A. Malesker
Lee E. Morrow
Cara M. Olsen

CASE LEARNING OBJECTIVES

- Recognize the signs and symptoms of euvolemic hyponatremia
- List common etiologies of euvolemic hyponatremia
- Identify the goals of therapy for euvolemic hyponatremia
- Develop an appropriate treatment and monitoring plan for euvolemic hyponatremia on the basis of individual patient characteristics

PATIENT PRESENTATION

Chief Complaint
Fall (per family)

History of Present Illness
A–89-year-old Caucasian man fell head-first down five to six concrete steps. His fall was witnessed by his wife and he had no previous history of falls. He initially lost consciousness for about 5 minutes, after which he was confused. He was taken to a local rural hospital where a CT scan demonstrated an intracranial hemorrhage, CXR showed pneumonia, and he became unresponsive. He was then transferred to University Hospital, where his intracranial hemorrhage was managed with IV nicardipine, mechanical ventilation, antibiotics for suspected pneumonia, and hypertonic saline for hyponatremia. On admission, the patient had no evidence of volume depletion or excess on physical examination. The serum sodium on admission was 119 mEq/L (119 mmol/L) and increased to 129 mEq/L (129 mmol/L) within the first 24 hours.

Allergies
Antihistamines: Unspecified
Sulfa: Unspecified
Tramadol: Unspecified
Amitriptyline: Unspecified

Past Medical History
MI, post-percutaneous coronary intervention (PCI)
HTN

Pacemaker for bradycardia
Frequent UTI (enlarged prostate)

Social History
Quit smoking 10 years ago
Denies alcohol and illicit drug use

Medications prior to Admission
HCTZ 50 mg PO daily
Celecoxib 200 mg PO daily
Finasteride 5 mg PO daily
Pantoprazole 40 mg PO daily
Cotrimoxazole PO twice daily
Lorazepam 1 mg PO every 8 hours as needed for anxiety
Latanoprost eyedrops, one drop in both eyes at bedtime

Inpatient Medications
Pantoprazole 40 mg IV daily
Piperacillin/tazobactam 3.375 mg IV every 6 hours
Levofloxacin 500 mg IV q 24 h
Vancomycin 1 g IV q 24 h
3% saline initiated IV at 15 mL/h
Codeine 15 to 30 mg every 8 hours as needed for cough
Metoclopramide 10 mg IV every 6 hours as needed for nausea
Nicardipine IV infusion to keep systolic BP <160 mm Hg
Potassium chloride 40 mEq (40 mmol) IV × 1

Review of Systems

Unattainable as the patient is unresponsive

Physical Examination

▶ General

Frail with some wasting

▶ Vital Signs

BP 148/83 mm Hg, P 120, RR 19, T 99.3°F (37.4°C)

Weight 155.5 lb (70.7 kg)

Height 71 in. (180 cm)

Pain—cannot assess because the patient is unresponsive

▶ HEENT

PERRLA; large bruise on head but no evidence of depressed skull fracture

▶ Neck

Supple; no carotid bruits noted

▶ Cardiac

Tachycardic; RRR, no murmur, rub, or gallop

▶ Respiratory

Clear to auscultation on right side; decreased breath sounds and crackles in the left lower lung fields. Large ecchymosis overlying the left shoulder and upper chest

▶ Abdomen

Soft and nontender; slightly distended; (+) bowel sounds

▶ Extremities

Superficial laceration on the left forearm. Bilateral radial pulses and dorsalis pedis and posterior tibial pulses palpable. Cannot assess ROM due to altered mental state

▶ Neurologic

Unresponsive

Laboratory Tests

	Date		
	6/16 at 0600	6/16 at 2000	6/17 at 0745
Na mEq/L (mmol/L)	119	125	129
K mEq/L (mmol/L)	3.7	3.6	4.1
Cl mEq/L (mmol/L)	84	84	87
CO_2/HCO_3 mEq/L (mmol/L)	27	27	23
BUN mg/dL (mmol/L)	16 (5.7)	26 (9.3)	20 (7.1)
Creatinine mg/dL (μmol/L)	1.0 (88)	1.0 (88)	1.3 (115)

Glucose mg/dL (mmol/L)	186 (10.3)	171(9.5)	160 (8.9)
Total Ca mg/dL (mmol/L)	8.3 (2.08)	8.5 (2.13)	8.6 (2.15)
Hemoglobin g/dL (g/L; mmol/L)	12.9 (129; 8.01)		
Hematocrit %	31.2 (0.312)		
WBC ×10^3/mm³ (×10^9/L)	12.9		
Platelet ×10^3/mm³ (×10^9/L)	182		
Serum osmolality mOsm/kg (mmol/kg)		265	
Urine osmolality mOsm/kg (mmol/kg)	475		
Urine sodium mEq/L (mmol/L)	<20		

Assessment

S/P head trauma, intracranial hemorrhage; significant hyponatremia on admission may have been the cause of fall. The patient appeared to be euvolemic on admission. He will be admitted to the ICU with frequent neuro checks. Hypertonic saline is to be initiated at 15 mL/h and replace potassium.

TARGETED QUESTIONS

1. What are the potential causes of euvolemic hyponatremia in this patient?

    Hint: See p. 485 in PPP

2. What is the sodium deficit in this patient?

    Hint: See p. 486 in PPP

3. Calculate the change in serum sodium following administration of 1 L of 3% NaCl.

    Hint: See p. 486 in PPP

4. What are the safety concerns with sodium replacement?

    Hint: See p. 486 in PPP

5. What other therapeutic options are available to correct the euvolemic hyponatremia in this patient?

    Hint: See p. 486 in PPP

6. After the patient recovers from his acute problems, what therapeutic options exist if he has chronic euvolemic hyponatremia?

    Hint: See p. 486 in PPP

FOLLOW-UP

Despite ICU management, the patient had progressively worsening neurologic function. Following several days of supportive therapy, the family decided to withdraw care.

For more information on the care plan and facilitator's guide please visit http://www.mhpharmacotherapy.com.

27 Hypovolemic Hyponatremia

Mark A. Malesker   Lee E. Morrow
Cara M. Olsen

CASE LEARNING OBJECTIVES

- Recognize the signs and symptoms of hypovolemic hyponatremia
- Identify the goals of therapy for hypovolemic hyponatremia
- Develop an appropriate treatment and monitoring plan for fluid replacement based on individual patient characteristics
- Select an appropriate resuscitation fluid
- Recognize what type of patient may be predisposed to fluid overload

PATIENT PRESENTATION

Chief Complaint
Diarrhea and altered mental status as per neighbor

History of Present Illness
Frank Secretion is a 78-year-old Caucasian man who was found by a neighbor wandering outside his residence with his pants saturated with urine and watery stool. The patient appeared intoxicated but he was oriented to person. He was found to have been falling down repeatedly while walking. The patient lives alone and is a widower. His daughter last spoke to him 4 days ago. The patient was unwillingly taken to University Hospital, where he was seen in the emergency department (ED) and admitted to the intensive care unit for further management. In the ED, the following laboratory results were noted: sodium 121 mEq/L (121 mmol/L), potassium 3.0 mEq/L (3.0 mmol/L), chloride 88 mEq/L (88 mmol/L), BUN 47 mg/dL (16.8 mmol/L), creatinine 2.5 mg/dL (221 μmol/L), ethanol level 150 mg/dL (32.5 mmol/L).

Past Medical History
HTN for 20 years
Alcoholism (18 beers per day)
Leg wound (new)

Family History
Father died of MI in his 50s. Mother died at age 92 from Alzheimer's disease. He has one daughter (46 years), who is healthy.

Social History
Retired carpenter. Completed high school. Married for 50 years. Widower for 1 year. Lives alone.

Tobacco/Alcohol/Substance Use
Long history of alcoholism; (−) tobacco or illicit drug use

Allergies/Intolerances/Adverse Drug Events
No known allergies

Medications (Prior to Admit)
HCTZ 50 mg PO daily
Simvastatin 40 mg PO daily

Medications (ICU list)
Normal saline
IV potassium chloride 40 mEq IV × 1
Piperacillin/tazobactam 2.25 g IV q 6 h

Lorazepam 1 mg IV/PO q 1 h PRN (agitation or tremor) per CIWA alcohol-withdrawal protocol

Folic acid 1 mg PO daily

Thiamine 100 mg PO daily

Multivitamin 1 tablet PO daily

Enoxaparin 40 mg SC q 24 h

Review of Systems

Unobtainable. Patient is extremely drowsy and disoriented.

Physical Examination (in ED)

► General

Unshaven unkempt elderly man with clothing saturated with urine and stool. He is oriented to person only.

► Vital Signs

BP 123/73 mmHg lying; BP 90/74 sitting, P 122 bpm, RR 18, T 36.7°C

Weight 183 lb (83 kg)

Height 72 in. (183 cm)

Denies pain

► Skin

Large open area on left lower extremity, (+) cellulitis

► HEENT

Small pupils, no icterus; mouth appears dry

► Neck and Lymph Nodes

(−) Neck stiffness, lymphadenopathy, thyromegaly; neck veins flat

► Chest

Bibasilar wheezes. Otherwise normal

► Cardiovascular

Tachycardia, nl S_1, S_2; heart sounds distant

► Abdomen

Soft, not distended, (+) bowel sounds, (−) masses, organomegaly

► Neurology

Sedated, disoriented, incoherent speech; DTRs symmetrical, (−) Babinski

► Genitourinary

Examination deferred

► Rectal

Examination deferred

Laboratory Tests

(From ED)

	Conventional Units	SI Units
Na	121 mEq/L	121 mmol/L
K	3.0 mEq/L	3.0 mmol/L
Cl	88 mEq/L	88 mmol/L
CO_2	6 mEq/L	6 mmol/L
BUN	47 mg/dL	16.8 mmol/L
SCr	2.5 mg/dL	221 μmol/L
Glu	128 mg/dL	7.1 mmol/L
Ca	9.4 mg/dL	2.35 mmol/L
Mg	4.5 mEq/L	2.25 mmol/L
Phosphate	9 mg/dL	2.91 mmol/L
Hgb	12.0 g/dL	120 g/L; 7.45 mmol/L
Hct	33.6%	0.336
WBC	$14.4 \times 10^3/mm^3$	$14.4 \times 10^9/L$
Ethanol	150 mg/dL	32.5 mmol/L
Albumin	2.9 g/dL	29 g/L
Total bilirubin	1.0 mg/dL	17.1 μmol/L
AST	13 IU/L	0.22 μkat/L
ALT	10 IU/L	0.17 μkat/L

Assessment

Seventy-eight-year-old man with signs, symptoms, and laboratory tests consistent with hypovolemic hyponatremia

Student Workup

Missing Information?

Evaluate: Patient Database

Drug Therapy Problems

Care Plan (by Problem)

TARGETED QUESTIONS

1. What signs and symptoms of hypovolemic hyponatremia does the patient have?

   Hint: See pp. 485–486 in PPP

2. What are potential causes of hypovolemic hyponatremia in this patient?

   Hint: See p. 486 in PPP

3. How should the hypovolemic hyponatremia be treated?

   Hint: See p. 486 in PPP

4. What type of monitoring should accompany fluid resuscitation?

    Hint: See p. 486 in PPP

5. What type of patient may be predisposed to fluid overload?

    Hint: See p. 486 in PPP

FOLLOW-UP

This 78-year-old male was admitted in a partially responsive state with altered mental status. Initial evaluation revealed hypotonic hyponatremia and left lower leg cellulitis. IV fluid and antibiotics were initiated. Alcohol withdrawal prophylaxis was ordered. His leg cultures were negative. Following fluid resuscitation, the patient's mental status improved. Once the patient was fully alert, he was transferred to the general medical floor and antibiotic treatment was continued. It was later decided to discharge the patient on an alternative regimen for hypertension (lisinopril). The patient was discharged with wound care instructions and plans to live with his daughter. He was instructed to take his medications as prescribed and to refrain from alcohol intake.

CASE SUMMARY

- The patient's clinical picture is consistent with hypovolemic hyponatremia, and replacement fluid should be carefully initiated.
- The use of normal saline as the initial fluid replacement is reasonable, with titration based upon follow-up electrolytes and patient response.
- Overreplacement of IV fluids should be avoided, especially considering the patient's advanced age.

For more information on the care plan and facilitator's guide please visit http://www.mhpharmacotherapy.com.

28 Hyperkalemia

Mark A. Malesker   Lee E. Morrow

Cara M. Olsen

CASE LEARNING OBJECTIVES

- Recognize the signs and symptoms of hyperkalemia
- List the common etiologies of hyperkalemia
- Identify the goals of therapy for hyperkalemia
- Develop an appropriate treatment and monitoring plan for hyperkalemia on the basis of individual patient characteristics

Chief Complaint

N/V, and associated weakness persisting for 4 days

History of Present Illness

Frank N. Stein is a 53-year-old Caucasian male who was brought to the ED via ambulance. The patient was unable to provide an in-depth history, but the patient's family noted that he had been experiencing episodes of N/V/D with associated weakness for approximately 4 days. He began feeling worse yesterday morning and had some increased sleepiness. This morning he was nearly unresponsive, so 911 was called. Upon arrival to the ED, the patient was sleepy but arousable, oriented to person and place, with significant bradycardia and hypotension. An ECG done in the ED showed atrial fibrillation.

Allergies

No known allergies

Past Medical History

Cardiomyopathy

Heart failure

Atrial fibrillation

Chronic renal insufficiency [baseline SCr 1.8 mg/dL (159 μmol/L)]

Social History

Smokes ½ ppd of cigarettes

Occasional alcohol use

Home Medications

Carvedilol 12.5 mg PO daily

Ciclesonide nasal spray (50 mcg/spray) two sprays in each nostril daily

Digoxin 250 mcg PO daily

Enalapril 5 mg PO daily

Potassium chloride 40 mEq PO three times daily

Propoxyphene 100 mg/APAP 650 mg one to two tablets PO every 6 hours as needed

Spironolactone 25 mg PO daily

Torsemide 100 mg PO daily

Warfarin 5 mg PO daily

Salt substitute PRN

Review of Systems

Unattainable due to the patient's decreased mental status

Physical Examination

▶ General

Patient appears to be in moderate distress

▶ Vital Signs

ED arrival: BP 68/36 mm Hg, P 34, RR 16, T 96.1°F (35.6°C)

Weight: 229.9 lb (104.5 kg)

Height: 74 in. (188 cm)

Pain: Unknown because the patient does not respond appropriately to questions

► *HEENT*

PERRLA, NG tube in place

► *Neck*

Supple; (−) carotid bruits noted; (−) JVD

► *Cardiac*

S_1, S_2; pulse irregularly irregular; no murmurs noted

► *Respiratory*

Coarse crackles at both bases; chest expansion equal

► *Abdomen*

Soft and nontender; obese; (+) bowel sounds

► *Extremities*

(−) Clubbing, contusions edema; pulses 2+ in all four extremities

► *Neurologic*

The patient is alert and oriented to person and place; cranial nerves II to XII intact; no focal neurologic findings.

Laboratory Tests

Obtained upon arrival to ED

	Conventional Units	SI Units
Na	135 mEq/L	135 mmol/L
K	9.6 mEq/L	9.6 mmol/L
Cl	112 mEq/L	112 mmol/L
CO_2/HCO_3	6 mEq/L	6 mmol/L
BUN	95 mg/dL	33.9 mmol/L
SCr	4.2 mg/dL	371 µmol/L
Glu	106 mg/dL	5.9 mmol/L
Ca	9.1 mg/dL	2.28 mmol/L
Mg	1.6 mEq/L	0.80 mmol/L
PO_4	7.3 mg/dL	2.36 mmol/L
Hgb	16 g/dL (160 g/L)	9.93 mmol/L
Hct	47%	0.47
WBC	11.2×10^3/mm^3	11.2×10^9/L
INR	7.9	
Digoxin	4.4 ng/mL	5.6 nmol/L
ABG		
pH	7.08	
PO_2	135 mm Hg	18.0 kPa
PCO_2	24.6 mm Hg	3.3 kPa
HCO_3	7 mEq/L	7 mmol/L

ECG

Atrial fibrillation, Ventricular rate 55

Assessment

Fifty-year-old male with s/s, and laboratory values consistent with acidosis, and hyperkalemia

TARGETED QUESTIONS

1. Which s/s of hyperkalemia did this patient present with?

   Hint: See p. 488 in PPP

2. What are the most likely causes of this patient's hyperkalemia?

   Hint: See p. 488 in PPP

3. What medications likely contributed to the development of hyperkalemia in this patient?

   Hint: See p. 488 in PPP

4. What are the treatment options for the management of hyperkalemia?

   Hint: See pp. 488–489 in PPP

5. What is the most likely explanation for this patient's increased serum digoxin level?

   Hint: See p. 429 in PPP

FOLLOW-UP

6. Several days later, the patient is stable and ready to be discharged from the hospital. Important laboratory tests on discharge include INR 2.06, digoxin 0.8 ng/mL (1.0 nmol/L), SCr 1.8 mg/dL (159 µmol/L), and potassium 3.5 mEq/L (3.5 mmol/L). What counseling points should be emphasized on discharge to prevent the patient from presenting in this manner again?

For more information on the care plan and facilitator's guide please visit http://www.mhpharmacotherapy.com.

29 Metabolic Acidosis

Lee E. Morrow   Mark A. Malesker

CASE LEARNING OBJECTIVES

- Systematically interpret laboratory values and correctly identify metabolic acidosis
- Apply routine formulas to clinical data to assess the adequacy of respiratory compensation for metabolic acidosis
- Integrate the concepts of the anion gap and the excess anion gap to better understand a patient's current acid–base status
- Formulate a differential diagnosis for a high-anion-gap metabolic acidosis
- Anticipate the effects of metabolic acidosis on serum electrolyte concentrations
- Incorporate basic concepts of volume resuscitation and appreciate the implications of inadequate volume status in perpetuating an anion gap metabolic acidosis

PATIENT PRESENTATION

Chief Complaint

N/V, HA, and decreased appetite

History of Present Illness

Rachel Willis is a 43-year-old African American female who presented to the ED with the complaints above. On her initial assessment by the ED staff, she was promptly transferred to the ICU for management by the critical care team. The patient reports that she was doing well until 2 days ago, at which time she ran out of her insulin. Since then she has felt dizzy and fatigued. She had two episodes of N/V, and progressive SOB today. The patient is a poor historian who frequently gives conflicting information to different care providers.

Past Medical History

Type 1 DM for 12 years

History of cesarean section

Family History

Father deceased from complications of DM and HTN. Mother is alive but has SLE. Her brother and one of her sisters have "emphysema" and another sister takes medications for HTN. The only other family history she knows is that her grandmother took insulin for diabetes and her grandfather died of metastatic colon cancer.

Social History

She works part time in a local pawn shop and has been intermittently homeless. Because she does not have health care insurance, she does not have a primary care physician and frequently visits the ED for hyperglycemia. The ED records suggest that she does not check her blood sugar at home and that she is not adherent with her insulin therapy.

Tobacco/Alcohol/Substance Use

She has smoked one ppd of cigarettes for 25 years. She drinks alcohol regularly on the weekends (~12 beers a day) and admits to marijuana use when she is "partying hard."

Allergies/Intolerances/Adverse Drug Events

Unknown reaction to codeine

Medications (Outpatient)

Insulin NPH 36 units SC AM and 6 units PM

Insulin regular 15 units SC AM and 6 units PM

Multivitamin PO daily

Loratadine 10 mg PO daily

Omeprazole OTC 10 mg PO as needed

Review of Systems

Decreased appetite for several days and thinks she has lost about 10 lb (4.5 kg); (−) blurring of vision or disturbances in hearing; (−) chest pain or palpitations; (+) shortness of breath; (−) cough, sputum expectoration, or hemoptysis; chronic nausea and bloating after eating; no bowel movement for 2 days; markedly increased urinary frequency for the past week but has had minimal urination in past 24 hours; (−) dysuria, urgency, or incontinence; (+) diffuse weakness and fatigue; (+) numbness and tingling in her feet for several months; (+) diffuse myalgias

Physical Examination

▶ General

African American woman appearing her stated age, uncomfortable appearing, mildly dyspneic, but in no acute respiratory distress

▶ Vital Signs

BP 108/73 mm Hg, P 124, RR 19, T 99.3°F (37.4°C), O_2 sat 99% (0.99) on room air

Weight 115.7 lb (52.6 kg)

Height 66 in. (168 cm)

Headache pain 2/10

▶ Skin

Warm and dry, (−) rash, lesions; (+) decreased turgor with skin tenting, multiple tattoos

▶ HEENT

PERRLA; EOMI; (−) scleral icterus; (−) sinus tenderness; oral mucous membranes dry; TMs normal

▶ Neck and Lymph Nodes

Supple with full ROM; (−) adenopathy, goiter, JVD

▶ Chest

Clear to auscultation bilaterally

▶ Breasts

Examination deferred

▶ Cardiovascular

Tachycardic but regular rhythm; normal S_1, S_2; (−) S_3 or S_4

▶ Abdomen

Soft, mild diffuse tenderness; (−) distention, organomegaly; normally active bowel sounds

▶ Neurology

Awake, alert, and oriented; neurologic examination is grossly intact with normal DTRs.

▶ Genitourinary and Rectal

Examination deferred; however, the nurse notes that the patient has made no urine in the 6 hours she has been in the ED and that catheterization was required to obtain the urine drug screen.

Laboratory Tests

Blood	Day 1—04:35	Day 1—10:20	Day 1—20:00
Na mEq/L (mmol/L)	130	140	139
K mEq/L (mmol/L)	6.0	5.1	3.8
Cl mEq/L (mmol/L)	91	103	117
CO_2 mEq/L (mmol/L)	5	5	16
BUN mg/dL (mmol/L)	19 (6.8)	18 (6.4)	7 (2.5)
SCr mg/dL (μmol/L)	1.7 (150)	1.4 (124)	0.7 (62)
Calcium mg/dL (mmol/L)	9.9 (2.48)	8.0 (2.00)	7.3 (1.83)
Phosphorous mg/dL (mmol/L)			1.5 (0.48)
Glucose mg/dL (mmol/L)	649 (36.0)	352 (19.5)	108 (6.0)
WBC × 10^3/mm³ (×10^9/L)	16.4		7.6
Hemoglobin g/dL (g/L; mmol/L)	14.4 (144; 8.94)		10.7 (107; 6.64)
Hematocrit (%)	43.6 (0.436)		31.0 (0.310)
Platelets × 10^3/mm³ (×10^9/L)	352		221
ABG			
pH	7.05		
PCO_2 mm Hg (kPa)	17 (2.3)		
PO_2 mm Hg (kPa)	157 (20.9)		
HCO_3 mEq/L (mmol/L)	2		
Hgb A_{1C}%	16.6% (0.166)		
INR	1.18		
Alk phos IU/L (μkat/L)	175 (2.92)		
AST IU/L (μkat/L)	16 (0.27)		
ALT IU/L (μkat/L)	16 (0.27)		
Total bilirubin mg/dL (μmol/L)	0.2 (3.4)		
Albumin g/dL (g/L)	4.6 (46)		
Amylase IU/L (μkat/L)			59 (0.98)
Lipase IU/L IU/L (μkat/L)			13 (0.22)
CK IU/L IU/L (μkat/L)	135		91 (1.52)
CK-MB ng/mL (μg/L)	3.3		2.8
Troponin I ng/mL (μg/L)	0.1	0.00	0.00
Urine ketones	Positive (1:16)		
Urine drug screen	(+) cocaine		

Assessment

This 43-year-old woman has DKA, likely caused by noncompliance with her insulin.

Student Workup

Missing Information?

Evaluate: Patient Database

Drug Therapy Problems

Care Plan (by Problem)

TARGETED QUESTIONS

1. What acid–base disturbance does this patient demonstrate on presentation?

   Hint: See pp. 497–498 in PPP

2. Calculate the anion gap in this patient using the initial (04:35) laboratory tests. Is this value abnormal?

   Hint: See p. 499 in PPP

3. What is the likely cause of this patient's acid–base disorder?

   Hint: See p. 501 in PPP

4. What is the best laboratory value to indicate this patient's fluid status? What do you think her fluid status is and why?

   Hint: See p. 480 in PPP

5. Calculate this patient's creatinine clearance (CrCl) at 04:35 and 20:00 using the Cockcroft–Gault equation. Why are the values different? What disorder caused this difference?

   Hint: See p. 484 in PPP

6. Why did the potassium value change in this patient between 04:35 and 20:00? Explain your answer in reference to facts regarding potassium and to total body stores of potassium.

   Hint: See pp. 487–488 in PPP

FOLLOW-UP

7. Upon arrival to the ICU, the patient had a central line placed for fluid resuscitation and hemodynamic monitoring (CVP transduction). She was given 4 L of normal saline as a bolus and is now receiving a continuous infusion at 250 mL/h. She was started on an IV insulin infusion protocol, including hourly glucose measurements, and the infusion rate is being titrated. How quickly should we correct her hyperglycemia? What should be our plan regarding the IV fluids and her electrolytes?

   Hint: See pp. 756–757 in PPP

8. Because she has remained nauseated, metoclopramide 10 mg IV every 6 hours was prescribed. DVT prophylaxis with heparin 5,000 units SC every 8 hours has been initiated. Her home doses of omeprazole and loratadine have been continued. Acetaminophen 325 mg PO every 4 hours as needed was also ordered for her ongoing myalgias and headache. What therapy should be prescribed for her anion gap metabolic acidosis? What additional laboratory tests should be sent? What recommendations can be made regarding her discharge plan?

   Hint: See pp. 501–502 in PPP

CASE SUMMARY

- The patient's clinical presentation and laboratory studies are consistent with DKA, leading to significant volume depletion.

- The presence of severe acidosis affects various electrolytes, particularly potassium, and may have pharmacokinetic and/or pharmacodynamic implications.

- Appropriate treatment of the patient's DKA should resolve her acid–base disorder. Specific therapy for the observed acidosis is typically not required.

For more information on the care plan and facilitator's guide please visit http://www.mhpharmacotherapy.com.

30 Metabolic Alkalosis

Lee E. Morrow   Mark A. Malesker

CASE LEARNING OBJECTIVES

- Correctly interpret ABG values
- Identify risk factors for acid–base and electrolyte disorders
- Develop an appropriate treatment and monitoring plan for a patient with metabolic alkalosis and critical hypokalemia
- Understand the clinical implications of hypophosphatemia
- Integrate magnesium repletion into the care plan of a patient with hypokalemia that is refractory to conventional correction

PATIENT PRESENTATION

Chief Complaint

Altered mental status

History of Present Illness

Helen Baker is a 71-year-old woman transferred from a local nursing home for weakness and confusion. For several days she has had "the flu" according to the nursing home staff. The patient is delirious and unable to provide any history: nursing notes show at least 3 days of N/V/D, and poor oral intake. Several other residents at the nursing home have been ill with similar symptoms. A review of the patient's records shows that she was recently discharged from another hospital after being treated for pneumonia for 7 days. Although she was previously living independently, she had agreed to a temporary stay in the nursing home's acute care area to complete an additional 7 days of intravenous ciprofloxacin and gentamicin for a resistant *Pseudomonas* strain. Her current symptoms began within the first 24 hours of hospital discharge. The hospital discharge note indicates that the only other change to her medications during that hospitalization was the addition of 40 mEq (40 mmol) of oral potassium supplementation taken twice daily for persistent hypokalemia.

Past Medical History

Hyperlipidemia with CAD

MI (1999, 2005); three-vessel CABG (2001)

Angioplasty with stent placement (2009)

Ischemic cardiomyopathy with a left ventricular ejection fraction of 20%

HTN

PVD

CKD: baseline serum creatinine 1.5 mg/dL (133 µmol/L)

GERD

Idiopathic bronchiectasis

Recurrent TIAs

Arthritis

Family History

Unknown, as the patient was adopted

Social History

The patient is a lifelong resident of a rural Iowa farming community. She is a widow and lives with her son. She was employed as a bank teller for 19 years before retiring 5 years ago for health reasons. She has no recent travel history.

Tobacco/Alcohol/Substance Use

The patient is a lifelong nonsmoker. Although she denied alcohol consumption to medical staff during her recent hospitalization and at the time of nursing home admission, her son reports ingestion of a pint of vodka daily for the past 25 years. Her recent hospital records document moderate alcohol withdrawal, requiring short-term benzodiazepine therapy.

Allergies/Intolerances/Adverse Drug Events

NKDA

Medications

Aspirin 81 mg PO daily

Ciprofloxacin 400 mg IV q 8 h

Clopidogrel 75 mg PO daily

Furosemide 40 mg PO bid

Gentamicin 130 mg IV every 24 hours

Isosorbide mononitrate 60 mg PO at bedtime

Nitroglycerin 0.4 mg SL as needed for chest pain

Pantoprazole sodium 40 mg PO bid

KCl 40 mEq PO bid

Prednisone 5 mg PO daily, alternating with 7.5 mg PO daily

Simvastatin 40 mg PO at bedtime

Review of Systems

Unable to obtain a ROS at present given her altered mental status. Although the nursing home staff who accompany her are not particularly familiar with her, they do not remember any symptoms other than those outlined above. Her vaccinations are current.

Physical Examination

▶ General

Elderly Caucasian woman with fluctuating consciousness. She is weak and appears acutely ill.

▶ Vital Signs

BP 103/45 mm Hg; P 121; RR 9; T 97.7°F (36.7°C); SpO$_2$ 100% (0.100) on 2 L via nasal cannulae

Weight 105 lb (47.7 kg)

Height 65 in. (165 cm)

Pain—does not respond to question about her level of pain

▶ Skin

Warm, dry skin without apparent rashes or breakdown; poor turgor with tenting when pinched

▶ HEENT

PERRL; no scleral icterus; TMs appear normal; nares with small amount of old, crusted blood; oropharynx pink and moist without lesions

▶ Neck

Supple with full passive ROM; neck veins flat; no lymphadenopathy or goiter; a soft carotid bruit heard on the right

▶ Chest

Symmetric thoracic movement and resonance to percussion; clear to auscultation throughout

▶ Cardiovascular

Tachycardic with normal S$_1$ and S$_2$; no S$_3$ or S$_4$; PMI not displaced; peripheral pulses diminished

▶ Abdomen

Soft; not tender or distended; no guarding or rebound; no organomegaly; bowel sounds hyperactive

▶ Neurology

Moves all four extremities with intent when stimulated; DTRs normal throughout

▶ Genitourinary

Unremarkable; urinary catheter draining minimal dark-yellow urine

▶ Rectal

No palpable abnormalities; watery stool in rectal vault

Laboratory Tests

	Conventional Unit	SI Units
Na	141 mEq/L	141 mmol/L
K	1.9 mEq/L	1.9 mmol/L
Cl	87 mEq/L	87 mmol/L
CO$_2$	44 mEq/L	44 mmol/L
BUN	55 mg/dL	19.6 mmol/L
SCr	2.1 mg/dL	186 µmol/L
Glu	101 mg/dL	5.6 mmol/L
Ca	8.6 mg/dL	2.15 mmol/L
Mg	1.5 mg/dL	0.75 mmol/L
PO$_4$	1.8 mg/dL	0.58 mmol/L
Troponin I	0.06 ng/mL	0.06 mcg/L
Hgb	15.2 g/dL	152 g/L; 9.43 mmol/L
Hct	46.6%	0.466
WBC	12.7 × 10^3/mm^3	12.7 × 10^9/L
Platelets	519 × 10^3/mm^3	519 × 10^9/L
pH	7.57	
PCO$_2$	50 mm Hg	6.7 kPa
PO$_2$	106 mm Hg	14.1 kPa

Fecal occult blood negative

Stool ova and parasites negative

Clostridium difficile toxin negative

Assessment

Seventy-one-year-old woman receiving antibiotic therapy for pneumonia presents with N/V/D, possibly due to gastroenteritis, antibiotic-associated diarrhea, or *C. difficile*–associated diarrhea. Her poor oral intake coupled with her excessive GI losses and ongoing diuretic therapy has resulted in volume depletion and metabolic alkalosis. She also has critical hypokalemia (despite supplementation) and hypophosphatemia. Given her comorbidities, this combination of metabolic disorders has resulted in delirium.

TARGETED QUESTIONS

1. What medications need to be adjusted on the basis of her calculated creatinine clearance?

    Hint: See p. 434 in PPP and standard drug information reference for renal drug dosing adjustments

2. What acid–base disorder(s) do you recognize?

    Hint: See pp. 497–498 in PPP

3. What electrolyte disorder(s) do you recognize?

    Hint: See Chapter 27 in PPP

4. What factors may have contributed to these disorders?

    Hint: See pp. 502–503 in PPP

5. Why would the admitting team be concerned about the phosphate deficiency?

    Hint: See pp. 490–491 in PPP

6. Describe your treatment plan to correct the patient's electrolyte abnormalities.

    Hint: See Chapter 27 in PPP

7. What medications can contribute to a potential magnesium deficiency?

    Hint: See pp. 502–503 and Chapter 27 in PPP

8. Would you give magnesium to this patient?

    Hint: See pp. 491–492 and 502–503 in PPP

9. What other recommendations do you have to maximize her current medications?

CASE SUMMARY

-   The patient has metabolic alkalosis as a consequence of poor oral intake, excessive GI losses, and inappropriate diuretic therapy.

-   She also has two electrolyte disorders (hypokalemia and hypophosphatemia), which are frequently encountered in this setting. These must be carefully corrected while monitoring serum levels.

-   This patient has risk factors for magnesium deficiency and her suboptimal clinical response to potassium supplementation suggests that magnesium should be given despite the normal serum value.

For more information on the care plan and facilitator's guide please visit http://www.mhpharmacotherapy.com.

31 Epilepsy: Chronic Management

Timothy E. Welty

CASE LEARNING OBJECTIVES

- Differentiate and classify seizure types when provided a description of the clinical presentation of the seizure and EEG
- Identify key therapeutic decision points in the treatment of epilepsy
- Establish therapeutic goals for pharmacotherapy in a patient with epilepsy
- Recommend an appropriate pharmacotherapeutic regimen for the treatment of epilepsy
- Select appropriate monitoring parameters for a pharmacotherapeutic regimen of epilepsy
- Devise a plan for switching a patient from one antiepileptic regimen to a different regimen
- Recognize complications of pharmacotherapy for epilepsy
- Analyze potential drug interactions with antiepileptic drugs
- Determine when and how to discontinue antiepileptic drug (AED) therapy
- Educate a patient or caregiver on epilepsy and pharmacotherapy for this disorder

PATIENT PRESENTATION

Chief Complaint

"I keep having spells where I don't remember things. My friends tell me I act weird at times, but I do not remember this."

History of Present Illness

James Young is a 24-year-old man who presents to his primary care physician complaining of episodes of "lost memory" for the past 3 to 4 months. His last routine visit was 18 months ago, and he had a normal physical examination and laboratory values at that time. He explains that these spells occur randomly and last no longer than a few minutes. From his friends, he has been told that he talks funny, smacks his lips, and his right arm jerks. When asked if he remembers these spells, he insists that he hears people talking but is unable to respond. However, he does not recall anything about what he does during these spells. Immediately after a spell he feels sleepy and somewhat confused. In addition to this description, he volunteers that he awoke a month ago feeling sore and had wet the bed.

Past Medical History

Multiple episodes of otitis media as a child
Fractured arm at age 18

Family History

His father is 58 and has HTN and dyslipidemia. Mother is 54 and has hypothyroidism. He has two siblings in good health.

Social History

He was married a year ago. His wife is 5 months pregnant. He graduated from college and works at a local bank as an assistant branch manager.

Tobacco/Alcohol/Substance Use

Social drinker, but every few months will binge drink on a weekend; (−) tobacco or illicit drug use

Allergies

Sulfa (rash)

Medications (Current)

Multivitamin PO daily

Loratadine 10 mg PO as needed for seasonal allergies

Ibuprofen 200 mg PO PRN headache

Physical Examination

▶ General

WDWN, white male in no acute distress

▶ Vital Signs

BP 118/72 mm Hg, P 70, RR 12, T 37°C

Weight 194 lb (88.2 kg)

Height 73 in. (185 cm)

Denies pain

▶ Skin

Normal color and turgor; (−) rashes or lesions

▶ HEENT

PERRLA, EOMI

▶ Neck and Lymph Nodes

Normal thyroid; (−) lymphadenopathy; (−) carotid bruits

▶ Chest

Clear to auscultation

▶ Cardiovascular

RRR; (−) murmurs or gallops

▶ Abdomen

Not tender or distended; (−) organomegaly

▶ Neurology

Alert and oriented × 3; CN II to XII intact; DTR 3+ and brisk; (−) Romberg; (−) plantar reflex; strength 5/5 in all extremities; normal gait; able to tandem walk; finger to nose intact; normal sensation to touch, pin prick, and vibration.

▶ Genitourinary

Examination deferred

▶ Rectal

Examination deferred

Laboratory Tests

Fasting, obtained the same day

	Conventional Unit	SI Units
Na	140 mEq/L	140 mmol/L
K	4.0 mEq/L	4.0 mmol/L
Cl	105 mEq/L	105 mmol/L
CO_2	24 mEq/L	24 mmol/L
BUN	9 mg/dL	3.2 mmol/L
SCr	0.8 mg/dL	71 μmol/L
Glu	80 mg/dL	4.4 mmol/L
Ca	9.8 mg/dL	2.45 mmol/L
Mg	1.7 mEq/L	0.85 mmol/L
Phos	3.9 mg/dL	1.26 mmol/L
Albumin	4.0 g/dL	40 g/L
AST	35 IU/L	0.58 μkat/L
ALT	32 IU/L	0.53 μkat/L
GGT	25 IU/L	0.42 μkat/L
Hgb	14.2 g/dL	8.81 mmol/L (142 g/L)
Hct	40.2%	0.402
WBC	$6.5 \times 10^3/mm^3$	$6.5 \times 10^9/L$
Platelets	$325 \times 10^3/\mu L$	$325 \times 10^9/L$

Assessment

Twenty-four-year-old man with possible seizures

Student Workup

Missing Information?

Evaluate: Patient Database

Drug Therapy Problems

Care Plan (by Problem)

TARGETED QUESTIONS

1. What s/s of seizures does this patient have?

   Hint: See p. 523 in PPP

2. What information is needed prior to making a decision to starting an AED and selecting the drug to start?

   Hint: See pp. 526–527 in PPP

3. What medications can be used in treating this patient's apparent seizure disorder?

   Hint: See Table 30-2 in PPP

4. For the AEDs most likely to be used in this patient, what are the common starting dose regimens?

   Hint: See Table 30-3 in PPP

5. For the antiepileptic drugs most likely to be used in this patient, what are the most common adverse effects that need to be discussed with the patient?

   Hint: See Table 30-3 and pp. 525–526 in PPP

6. What additional items should be discussed with this patient during this clinic visit?

   Hint: See p. 538 in PPP

FOLLOW-UP

7. Two weeks later, the patient returns to clinic having completed a MRI scan of his head and an EEG. The MRI scan is read as left mesial temporal sclerosis and the EEG is read as left temporal spike waves consistent with a seizure disorder. Should long-term AED therapy be given to this patient? What actions, if any, would you take at this point?

   Hint: See pp. 526–527 in PPP

8. Six years later, the patient returns to clinic for a visit 9 months after a left temporal lobectomy for seizures. He has been seizure free since surgery. Prior to surgery, he continued to have two to three seizures per month despite multiple AEDs and drug combinations. At the time of surgery and currently, he is receiving carbamazepine extended-release capsules 200 mg in the AM and 300 mg in the PM, and levetiracetam 1,000 mg twice daily. Should AEDs be discontinued in this patient? What actions, if any, would you take at this point?

   Hint: See p. 536 in PPP

⟳ GLOBAL PERSPECTIVE

The World Health Organization estimates that there are 40 to 50 million people with epilepsy throughout the world. The annual incidence in third-world nations is twice that of the United States (2/100 compared to 1/100). In many countries the condition remains a stigmatizing condition surrounded with mystical beliefs and social taboos. On a global basis, an astonishing three-fourths of people with epilepsy receive no treatment for their seizures. Such lack of treatment is related to the above-mentioned social stigma as well as lack of access to medical care and medications. Patients may be treated with local traditional remedies in lieu of standard AED therapy. Also, the array of antiepileptic medications available in developing countries is more limited, so patients with seizures who do not respond to older first-line agents may have few options.

CASE SUMMARY

- His clinical presentation, MRI scan, and EEG are consistent with complex partial seizures.
- An AED useful in first-line therapy of partial seizures and with an adverse-effect profile that minimizes the influence of adverse effects on the patient's lifestyle should be selected.
- Ongoing monitoring of efficacy and toxicity is essential to further treatment decisions.

For more information on the care plan and facilitator's guide please visit http://www.mhpharmacotherapy.com.

32 Epilepsy: Status Epilepticus

Eljim P. Tesoro　　　　　　Gretchen M. Brophy

CASE LEARNING OBJECTIVES

- Explain the urgency of diagnosis and treatment of status epilepticus
- Recognize the signs and symptoms of status epilepticus
- Identify the treatment options available for termination of status epilepticus
- Formulate an initial treatment strategy for a patient in generalized convulsive status epilepticus
- Recommend monitoring parameters for a patient in status epilepticus

PATIENT PRESENTATION

History of Present Illness

James Lee is a 48-year-old African American male who was admitted to the hospital 2 days ago for treatment of a subdural hematoma that he incurred after falling down the steps in front of his home and hitting his head. He had surgical evacuation of the hematoma on the day of admission and is recovering in the surgical step-down unit. He had been loaded with phenytoin postoperatively to prevent seizures. The nurse went into his room to take his vital signs and found him unarousable with all his extremities shaking. He was seen talking on the phone 10 minutes before.

Past Medical History

HTN
Type 2 DM
Dyslipidemia
Asthma

Past Surgical History

Cholecystectomy 15 years ago
Appendectomy 21 years ago
Left-knee repair 5 years ago

Family History

HTN in father
DM in mother

Social History

He lives at home with his wife and two children, and works as a city bus driver.

He smokes ½ ppd of cigarettes; he drinks wine socially and denies any illicit drug use.

Allergies/Intolerances

Sulfa (hives)

Current Medications

Lisinopril 20 mg PO daily
Glyburide 5 mg PO daily
HCTZ 25 mg PO daily
Simvastatin 20 mg PO at bedtime
Phenytoin ER 300 mg PO at bedtime
Docusate 100 mg PO twice daily
Acetaminophen 500 mg/hydrocodone 5 mg tablet PO every 4 hours as needed for pain or HA

Review of Systems

Deferred; patient is now unresponsive

Physical Examination

▸ *General*

Slightly overweight, middle-aged male with continuous convulsions of the extremities

► **Vital Signs**

BP 173/98 mm Hg, P 112, RR 20, T 38.0°C

Weight 220 lb (100 kg)

Height 62 in. (157 cm)

Unable to evaluate pain

► **Skin**

Sweaty skin and scalp; (−) rashes or lesions

► **HEENT**

Persistent upward gaze

► **Cardiovascular**

Tachycardic, RRR, normal S_1, S_2; (−) S_3 or S_4

► **Abdomen**

Not tender/not distended; (−) organomegaly

► **Neurology**

Unresponsive; unarousable; actively convulsing

► **Genitourinary**

Incontinent of stool and urine

Laboratory Tests

	Conventional Units	SI Units
Na	142 mEq/L	142 mmol/L
K	4.1 mEq/L	4.1 mmol/L
Cl	100 mEq/L	100 mmol/L
CO_2	24 mEq/L	24 mmol/L
BUN	7 mg/dL	2.5 mmol/L
SCr	0.9 mg/dL	80 μmol/L
Glu	104 mg/dL	5.8 mmol/L
Ca	9.6 mg/dL	2.40 mmol/L
Mg	1.2 mEq/L	0.60 mmol/L
Phosphate	4.1 mg/dL	1.32 mmol/L
Hgb	12.5 g/dL	125 g/L, 7.76 mmol/L
Hct	37.7%	0.377
WBC	$9.6 \times 10^3/mm^3$	$9.6 \times 10^9/L$
MCV	88 μm³	88 fL
Albumin	3.4 g/dL	34 g/L
Phenytoin level	7.8 mcg/mL	31 μmol/L

Assessment

Forty-eight-year-old black male s/p head trauma and evacuation of subdural hematoma with signs of acute status epilepticus

Missing Information?

Evaluate: Patient Database

Drug Therapy Problems

Care Plan (by Problem)

TARGETED QUESTIONS

1. What signs of status epilepticus does this patient have?

   Hint: See p. 543 in PPP

2. What are some possible causes of status epilepticus in this patient?

   Hint: See p. 542 in PPP

3. What medication(s) would you recommend to stop this patient's status epilepticus?

   Hint: See Tables 30-1 and 30-2 in PPP

4. What medication(s) would you recommend for preventing future seizures in this patient?

   Hint: See Table 30-1 in PPP

FOLLOW-UP

Thirty minutes later, the patient continues to have generalized seizures. An endotracheal tube is inserted by Anesthesiology, and the patient is transported to the Neuro-ICU.

5. What therapy for the patient's continued seizures would you recommend now?

6. What if the patient stops convulsing but does not wake up?

7. What if the patient was a 26-year-old female who was 32 weeks pregnant?

   Hint: See p. 550 in PPP (2nd edition)

⟳ GLOBAL PERSPECTIVE

According to the World Health Organization, the incidence of seizures is greater in developing countries compared to the United States, and a large proportion of patients receive no treatment due to social taboos and lack of access to care. Given the higher incidence of seizure disorders and lack of access to therapy in many patients, it is likely that there is a higher incidence of status epilepticus in developing countries. Although the overall therapeutic approach would be the same, patients in developing countries may have poor access to emergency medical care. While first-line medications such as benzodiazepines, phenytoin, and phenobarbital may be available, newer intravenous medications may not be available for refractory status epilepticus.

CASE SUMMARY

- Status epilepticus is a medical emergency and should be assessed and treated immediately.
- Intravenous benzodiazepines (lorazepam or diazepam) are the first drugs of choice to stop seizure activity.
- Anticonvulsants are used after benzodiazepines to prevent future seizures.
- Prolonged status epilepticus can lead to nonconvulsive status epilepticus if not treated.

For more information on the care plan and facilitator's guide please visit http://www.mhpharmacotherapy.com.

33 Parkinson's Disease

Jack J. Chen

CASE LEARNING OBJECTIVES

- Identify motor and nonmotor symptoms of Parkinson's disease (PD) as well as symptoms that indicate disease progression
- Explain the desired therapeutic goals for patients with PD
- Recommend lifestyle modifications and pharmacotherapy interventions for treating motor symptoms of patients with PD
- Recommend drug and nondrug interventions for treating the nonmotor symptoms of patients with PD
- Develop a monitoring plan to assess the effectiveness and adverse effects of nonpharmacologic therapy and pharmacotherapy for PD
- Educate patients about the disease state, appropriate lifestyle modifications, and drug therapy required for effective treatment

PATIENT PRESENTATION

Chief Complaint

"My primary care physician says I might have Parkinson's disease."

History of Present Illness

Oliver Covey is a 62-year-old, right-handed man who is referred to a neurologist by his primary care physician. He was visiting his primary care physician for a routine checkup appointment. At that time, his primary care physician noted that the patient had a mild, right-hand tremor and walked with reduced arm swing. His primary care physician felt that these signs and symptoms were compatible with possible PD and referred him to a neurologist for further assessment. At the neurologist visit, the patient is accompanied by his wife. He states that he is in good spirits. He admits noticing the tremor in his right hand about 1 year ago, but did not think much of it. His wife has also noticed the tremor. The patient states no other problems. However, his wife reports he walks a bit slower and that his "tennis game has gotten worse." She states that he used to be very agile on the tennis court but during the past year, has "slowed considerably and often misses shots." The patient admits this is true. When asked about his employment and work capabilities, he states the movement problems do not interfere. The neurologist asks, "If there is one thing we can make better about your movement, what would it be?" The patient replies, "I want to be able to swing the tennis racket like I used to a year ago." He is willing to start drug therapy to help improve his movement.

Past Medical History

BPH × 1 year

GERD × 1 year

Hyperlipidemia × 5 years

Nephrolithiasis in the past

Tonsillectomy

Family History

He is an only child. His father died of a MI. Mother died of some other type of cardiac problem. No family history of neurologic conditions.

Social History

He was born in Arizona and lives in Los Angeles. He has a college education. He is married and lives with his wife of 32 years, and has two children aged 30 and 25. He works as an agricultural irrigation consultant.

Tobacco/Alcohol/Substance Use

(−) Alcohol, tobacco, or illicit drug use

Allergies/Intolerances/Adverse Drug Events

Sulfonamides (severe rash as a teenager)

Medications (Current)

Omeprazole 20 mg PO q 24 h

Silodosin 8 mg PO q 24 h

Simvastatin 20 mg PO q 24 h

Multivitamin one tablet PO q 24 h

Review of Systems

(−) Cancer, cardiac disease, falls, loss of consciousness, psychiatric conditions, respiratory disease, seizures, stroke, syncope, or vertigo

Physical Examination

▶ **General**

WDWN Caucasian man in no acute distress. Oriented to person, place, and time. Mood and affect appropriate

▶ **Vital Signs**

BP 128/76 mm Hg, P 76, RR 16, T 36.4°C

Weight 180 lb (81.8 kg)

Height 71 in. (180 cm)

Denies pain

▶ **HEENT**

PERRLA, EOMI, (−) nystagmus, (−) gaze palsy, (−) olfactory deficit

▶ **Neck and Lymph Nodes**

Neck supple; (−) adenopathy

▶ **Chest**

Clear to auscultation

▶ **Cardiovascular**

Deferred

▶ **Abdomen**

Deferred

▶ **Extremities**

Pedal pulses are 2+ and equal

▶ **Skin**

Warm and dry; (−) rashes or lesions

▶ **Neurology**

Cranial nerves

II: Normal visual acuity, visual fields, fundi

III, IV, VI: PERRL, EOMI

V: Facial sensation intact

VII: Normal facial asymmetry and strength

VIII: Whisper test normal

IX: Uvula midline with "Ah"

XI: Shoulder shrug strength normal

XII: Tongue midline with protrusion

No masked facies. Mild hypophonia. Slightly stooped posture. DTRs normal. No tremor on finger to nose test

Positive micrographia (Fig. 33-1)

Resting tremor right arm = 2; no tremor in left arm or legs

Rigidity right arm = 2, left arm = 1; no rigidity of lower extremities

Finger taps right = 2, left = 1

Hand movements right = 1, left = 1

Leg agility right = 0, left = 0

Ability to arise from seated position in chair with arms folded across the chest: Normal

Gait normal and steady. Slightly reduced arm swing on right. No postural instability observed upon pull test

▶ **Genitourinary**

Deferred

▶ **Rectal**

Deferred

Laboratory Tests

Fasting, obtained 1 month ago

	Conventional Units	SI Units
Na	140 mEq/L	140 mmol/L
K	4 mEq/L	4 mmol/L
Cl	99 mEq/L	99 mmol/L
CO_2	29 mEq/L	29 mmol/L
BUN	14 mg/dL	5.0 mmol/L
SCr	1 mg/dL	88 μmol/L
Glu	90 mg/dL	5.0 mmol/L
Ca	9.5 mg/dL	2.38 mmol/L
Mg	2.2 mEq/L	1.10 mmol/L
Phosphate	3.5 mg/dL	1.13 mmol/L
Albumin	3.7 g/dL	37 g/L
WBC	$8.5 \times 10^3/mm^3$	$8.5 \times 10^9/L$
RBC	$5.63 \times 10^6/\mu L$	$5.63 \times 10^{12}/L$
Hgb	16.4 g/dL (164 g/L)	10.18 mmol/L
Hct	48.7%	0.487
MCV	$86.4 \ \mu m^3$	86.4 fL
Platelet	$300 \times 10^3/\mu L$	$300 \times 10^9/L$
Total cholesterol	180 mg/dL	4.65 mmol/L
LDL cholesterol	100 mg/dL	2.59 mmol/L
HDL cholesterol	38 mg/dL	0.98 mmol/L

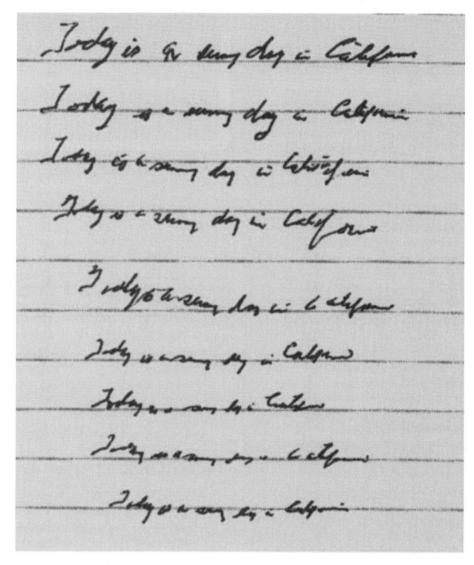

FIGURE 33-1.   Micrographia. (Reprinted with permission from Jack J. Chen, PharmD, Loma Linda University Movement Disorders Center, Loma Linda, CA.)

Assessment

Sixty-two-year-old man with signs and symptoms consistent with idiopathic PD

Student Workup

Missing Information?

Evaluate: Patient Database

Drug Therapy Problems

Care Plan (by Problem)

TARGETED QUESTIONS

1. What motor and nonmotor signs and symptoms of PD does the patient have?

   Hint: See pp. 555–556 in PPP

2. What is the severity of s/s that were rated by the neurologist?

   Hint: See Unified Parkinson's Disease Rating Scale (UPDRS) Section III Motor Examination (see http://www.mdvu.org/ library/ratingscales/pd/updrs.pdf)

3. What are common medications that can cause PD and should be queried during the patient interview?

   Hint: See p. 554 in PPP

4. If pharmacotherapy is desired, what are the classes of medications that can be initiated?

   Hint: See pp. 559–562 in PPP

5. For each class of anti-Parkinson medication, what are the benefits versus risks/adverse effects that you should consider for this specific patient?

   Hint: See pp. 559–562 in PPP

6. Which specific pharmacotherapy regimen would you recommend for this patient and why?

   Hint: See pp. 559–562 in PPP

8. What nonpharmacologic recommendations should this patient receive?

   Hint: See p. 557 in PPP

FOLLOW-UP

9. Eight weeks later, the patient returns for follow-up. He is in good spirits and feels his tremor has improved while on the medication. On examination, his tremor, rigidity, and bradykinesia are still present, but improved. His handwriting is still the same. He also reports that his tennis game seems somewhat improved and is happy about that. He has not experienced any unpleasant side effects. Are any pharmacologic interventions required at this time?

   Hint: See p. 564 in PPP

⊙ GLOBAL PERSPECTIVE

PD affects individuals worldwide. Regional figures showing differences in both incidence and prevalence probably reflect the existence of factors that may be demographic (variations in life expectancy across countries), health care–related (lack of proper and widespread recognition of the disorder, variations in access to health care), genetic, and environmental, together with methodological differences. In addition, early studies had shown variations in prevalence at the international level attributed to ethnic differences across regions. Higher rates were reported for Caucasians in Europe and North America, intermediate rates for Asians in China and Japan, and the lowest rates for blacks in Africa. However, more recent studies from Asia do not show significant differences in prevalence compared with studies in Caucasians (World Health Organization. Neurological Disorders: Public Health Challenges; www. who.int/mental_health/neurology/neurodiso/en/index. html, accessed October 21, 2010).

CASE SUMMARY

- His current clinical picture is consistent with idiopathic PD. The patient desires treatment, so it is justified to initiate pharmacotherapy.

- This patient should be informed that there is no cure of PD and that if left untreated, his movements will likely worsen over time. Several medications are available to make the movements better.

- Several pharmacotherapy options exist for this relatively young patient with early PD, including carbidopa/levodopa, dopamine agonists, and rasagiline. Amantadine and anticholinergics should be avoided due to the patient's history of BPH.

- The advantages, disadvantages, and side effects of amantadine, carbidopa/levodopa, dopamine agonists, and MAO-B inhibitors should be considered when discussing therapeutic options with the patient. An initial trial of rasagiline[1] or a dopamine agonist would be appropriate. However, amantadine and carbidopa/levodopa are also justifiable choices.

- Nonpharmacologic suggestions include encouraging this patient to continue his physical exercise, such as tennis. If the patient and his wife desires, educational material on PD and support groups can be recommended.

- At this stage of his PD, it is unnecessary to provide information about advanced-stage PD or surgical options.

REFERENCE

1. Olanow CW, Rascol O, Hauser R, et al. ADAGIO Study Investigators. A double-blind, delayed-start trial of rasagiline in Parkinson's disease. N Engl J Med 2009 361(13):1268–1278.

For more information on the care plan and facilitator's guide please visit http://www.mhpharmacotherapy.com.

34 Acute Pain Management

Asad E. Patanwala

CASE LEARNING OBJECTIVES

- Recognize components of a comprehensive pain assessment
- Recommend an appropriate choice of analgesic, dose, and monitoring plan for a patient on the basis of type and severity of pain and other patient-specific parameters
- Identify the goals of therapy for the management of acute pain
- Properly educate patients when opioid analgesia is initiated

PATIENT PRESENTATION

Chief Complaint

"This is the worst pain I have ever had. It is like a 10 out of 10."

History of Present Illness

Jose Garcia is a 44-year-old man who is admitted to the hospital after a motorcycle collision. He lost control of his motorcycle and hit a parked vehicle when traveling at approximately 40 mph (64 km/h). He was wearing a helmet at the time of the collision. This occurred at 2 AM today after he left a local bar to go home. According to the paramedics, he did not have any loss of consciousness, was unable to move his right leg, and had a definite odor of alcohol. In the ED, he was given 100 mcg of IV fentanyl for pain and 2 L of IV NS. He was subsequently taken to the OR for an open reduction internal fixation of his right lower extremity fracture. Soon after surgery he was transferred to a general surgical ward for postoperative care.

Past Medical History

PUD × 2 years (had a GI bleed 6 months ago)

Seizure disorder × 10 years

Chronic shoulder pain × 5 years (from previous motorcycle collision)

Family History

His father died at age 60 from alcoholic cirrhosis and mother died at age 50 from a MVA. He has no siblings.

Social History

He is single, has no children, and works at a construction company.

Tobacco/Alcohol/Substance Use

Drinks six beers daily; smokes one ppd; (−) illicit drug use

Allergies/Intolerances/Adverse Drug Events

Morphine (itching); oxycodone (constipation)

Medications (Current)

Famotidine 40 mg PO q hs (home medication)

Promethazine 25 mg IV q 4–6 h PRN

Tramadol 100 mg PO q 4–6 h PRN

Meperidine 50 mg PO q 2–4 h PRN

Phenytoin 100 mg PO q 8 h (home medication)

Ibuprofen 400 mg PO q 6 h PRN (home medication)

Aspirin 325 mg PO q 24 h (home medication)

Docusate 100 mg PO q 12 h

Heparin 5,000 units SC q 24 h

Review of Systems

He has severe leg pain that is not relieved by current therapy; his shoulder is also hurting again from his previous injury; his back is sore from road rash; (+) abdominal distension, constipation, and nausea; vomited twice this morning; feels drowsy.

Physical Examination

▶ **General**

Well-developed, middle-aged, Hispanic male grimacing in pain

▶ **Vital Signs**

BP 160/110 mm Hg, P 102, RR 16, T 37.2°C

Weight 187 lb (85 kg)

Height 70 in. (178 cm)

Pain score 10/10

▶ **Skin**

(+) Road rash on back and right thigh; no penetrating injuries

▶ **HEENT**

PERRLA, EOMI; TMs appear normal, normocephalic, atraumatic

▶ **Neck and Lymph Nodes**

Supple; (−) bruits; (−) thyromegaly; (−) lymphadenopathy; trachea midline

▶ **Chest**

Clear breath sounds bilaterally; (−) crackles

▶ **Cardiovascular**

Tachycardic, RRR, normal S_1, S_2; (−) S_3 or S_4

▶ **Abdomen**

Soft, nontender, distended; (+) bowel sounds; (−) masses; (−) hepatomegaly

▶ **Neurology**

Oriented × 3; neurologic examination grossly intact, DTRs normal

▶ **Extremities**

Right tibia fracture

▶ **Genitourinary**

No abnormalities

▶ **Rectal**

(+) Rectal tone; (−) gross blood

Laboratory Tests

Obtained this morning

	Conventional Units	SI Units
Na	141 mEq/L	141 mmol/L
K	3.9 mEq/L	3.9 mmol/L
Cl	101 mEq/L	101 mmol/L
CO_2	23 mEq/L	23 mmol/L
BUN	11 mg/dL	3.9 mmol/L
SCr	1.1 mg/dL	97 μmol/L
Glu	95 mg/dL	5.3 mmol/L
Ca	8.7 mg/dL	2.18 mmol/L
Mg	0.9 mEq/L	0.45 mmol/L
Phosphate	3.5 mg/dL	1.13 mmol/L
Hgb	14.1 g/dL (141 g/L)	8.75 mmol/L
Hct	42.5%	0.425
WBC	$8.2 \times 10^3/mm^3$	$8.2 \times 10^9/L$
Platelets	$240 \times 10^3/mm^3$	$240 \times 10^9/L$
Albumin	3.7 g/dL	37 g/L
Total bilirubin	1.1 mg/dL	18.8 μmol/L
Direct bilirubin	0.3 mg/dL	5.1 μmol/L
AST	82 IU/L	1.37 μkat/L
ALT	53 IU/L	0.88 μkat/L
Alk phos	96 IU/L	1.60 μkat/L

Assessment

Forty-four-year-old man s/p trauma with right tibia fracture and open reduction/internal fixation, now with s/s of severe acute postoperative pain

Student Workup

Missing Information?

Evaluate: Patient Database

Drug Therapy Problems

Care Plan (by Problem)

TARGETED QUESTIONS

1. What s/s of this patient are consistent with poor pain control?

   Hint: See pp. 569–570 in PPP

2. Why is IV opioid analgesia the treatment of choice for most patients with severe acute pain in the hospital setting?

   Hint: See pp. 575–576 in PPP

3. How does the potency of commonly used opioids differ?

   Hint: See Table 33-2 in PPP

4. What risks and adverse effects of opioid therapy would you discuss with this patient?

   Hint: See p. 577 in PPP

5. Is this patient a candidate for PCA? Explain.

   Hint: See p. 576 in PPP

FOLLOW-UP

6. Three days after surgery the patient is being discharged from the hospital. While in the hospital he was treated only with IV opioids. He now needs to be switched to an oral medication for pain control. What are some of the pertinent pieces of information that you would need to create a regimen that this patient can take at home? What counseling and adjunctive therapy may be required if this patient is sent home with prescriptions for oral opioid analgesia?

   Hint: See pp. 576–577 in PPP

⟳ GLOBAL PERSPECTIVE

Morphine is metabolized in the liver via hepatic conjugation with glucuronic acid. There are significant ethnic differences with regard to morphine metabolism. Morphine clearance is higher in Chinese men compared to Caucasian men. This likely is due to an increase in partial metabolic clearance by glucuronidation in the Chinese population. There is no physiologic or laboratory parameter for accurate pain assessment. Hence, providers must rely on the patient's self-reported pain to make treatment decisions. There are cultural, behavioral, and age-related differences with regard to how patients report their pain. This ranges from expressing their pain in a stoic manner to being very expressive. Also, there is evidence that patients from ethnic minorities or cultures that are different from the health care provider are more likely to receive inadequate analgesia. All of this must be incorporated in the decision-making process with regard to pain assessment and treatment.

CASE SUMMARY

- His clinical picture is consistent with severe acute postoperative pain.
- He is currently on pain medications that are suboptimal and contraindicated due to his seizure disorder and peptic ulcer disease.
- He is experiencing opioid-induced adverse effects, such as sedation, constipation, N/V.

For more information on the care plan and facilitator's guide please visit http://www.mhpharmacotherapy.com.

35 Chronic Pain Management

Michael D. Katz   Jennifer H. Baggs

CASE LEARNING OBJECTIVES

- Recognize the signs and symptoms of various etiologies of pain
- Identify the goals of therapy for chronic pain management
- Identify actual and potential side effects of drugs utilized in pain management
- Develop an appropriate treatment regimen and monitoring plan for chronic pain based on individual patient characteristics
- Select an appropriate drug regimen for chronic pain, including scheduled, as-needed, and adjunctive therapy
- Select appropriate therapy for prevention and treatment of opioid side effects
- Properly educate a patient on pain management therapies

PATIENT PRESENTATION

Chief Complaint
"This back pain is unbearable. What other pain pills are available that won't cause constipation?"

History of Present Illness
Jean Walter is a 58-year-old woman with Stage IV ductal breast carcinoma who presents anxiously to the cancer clinic after having run out of her previous prescription for oxycodone/acetaminophen 1 week prior. Three weeks ago, she was prescribed Oxycontin 10 mg twice daily and Percocet (oxycodone 5 mg/acetaminophen 325 mg) as needed (#120 tablets); however, her insurance did not cover the Oxycontin. After taking all of the Percocet over the course of 2 weeks, she began to supplement her pain regimen with OTC acetaminophen (averaging 12 tablets per day) for her worsening lower back pain. She describes the back pain as throbbing and constant and rates the severity as a 9 on a scale of 1 to 10, but also notes a "pins and needles" sensation that radiates from her lower back down her left leg to her knee and some weakness in her left leg. Ms. Walter was initially diagnosed with breast cancer in 2006 after which she underwent a lumpectomy, radiation therapy, and adjuvant chemotherapy. During the past year, a CT scan showed recurrence of a breast tumor and spinal metastases in the

L4-S2 region, which is consistent with her complaints of increasing back pain and immobility.

Past Medical History
Stage IV ductal breast carcinoma (diagnosed 2006) s/p chemotherapy and radiation

DM type 2 × 12 years

HTN × 17 years

Past Surgical History
Left breast lumpectomy (2006)

Hysterectomy (2000)

Cholecystectomy (1987)

Family History
Father had DM type 2 and CAD and died of a MI at the age of 70. Mother had breast cancer and died at the age of 62 secondary to metastatic disease. She has two brothers who are alive with hypertension and DM type 2.

Social History
Married and lives with her husband of 34 years; has three adult children. She previously worked as a social worker, but had to retire secondary to her disease progression.

Tobacco/Alcohol/Substance Use

(−) Alcohol, tobacco, or illicit drug use

Allergies/Intolerances/Adverse Drug Events

Sulfa (rash), codeine (nausea)

Medications (Current)

Metformin 500 mg PO twice daily

Simvastatin 40 mg PO daily

Lisinopril 20 mg PO daily

Metoprolol 50 mg PO daily

Calcium carbonate/vitamin D 1,000 mg/400 IU PO twice daily

Oxycodone/acetaminophen 5 mg/325 mg, two tablets PO every 4 to 6 hours PRN pain

Acetaminophen 650 mg PO PRN headache

Citalopram 20 mg PO daily

Tamoxifen 20 mg PO daily

Review of Systems

(+) Chronic back pain from metastases, occasionally relieved with Percocet, not relieved with acetaminophen; decreased appetite with some nausea; (+) "pins and needles" sensation in left leg that radiates to the knee; slight weakness upon standing; (+) constipation not relieved with OTC stool softeners.

Physical Examination

► General

WDWN anxious-appearing middle-aged woman in no apparent acute distress

► Vital Signs

BP 132/84 mm Hg, P 82, RR 16, T 37.1°C

Weight 142 lb (64.5 kg)

Height 65 in. (165 cm)

Lower back pain and tingling, which radiates down the back of her left leg to the knee

► Skin

Warm and dry; no evidence of rash

► HEENT

PERRLA, EOMI; TMs clear bilaterally

► Neck and Lymph Nodes

No lymphadenopathy; no tenderness to palpation of the cervical spine

► Chest

Clear to auscultation; no wheezes, crackles, or rhonchi

► Breasts

Well-healed scar on lateral aspect of left breast, and palpable mass on medial side of left breast; no masses or nipple discharge noted on right breast

► Cardiovascular

RRR; no murmurs, rubs, or gallops

► Abdomen

Soft, slight tenderness with mild distension; bowel sounds positive; no organomegaly

► Neurology

Cranial nerves II to XII grossly intact; slight weakness in the left leg upon standing; DTRs are normal; decreased pinprick sensation on posterior aspect of the left thigh

► Genitourinary

Examination deferred

► Rectal

Examination deferred

Laboratory Tests

	Conventional Units	SI Units
Na	139 mEq/L	139 mmol/L
K	3.9 mEq/L	3.9 mmol/L
Cl	104 mEq/L	104 mmol/L
CO_2	23 mEq/L	23 mmol/L
BUN	14 mg/dL	5.0 mmol/L
SCr	1.1 mg/dL	97 μmol/L
Glu	160 mg/dL	8.9 mmol/L
Ca	8.4 mg/dL	2.10 mmol/L
Mg	2.0 mEq/L	1.00 mmol/L
Phosphate	3.6 mg/dL	1.16 mmol/L
Hgb	13.5 g/dL	135 g/L; 8.38 mmol/L
Hct	39.7%	0.397
WBC	6.5×10^3/mm³	6.5×10^9/L
MCV	87 μm³	87 fL
Platelets	178×10^3/mm³	178×10^9/L
Albumin	3.5 g/dL	35 g/L
Alk phos	95 U/L	1.58 μkat/L
AST	37 U/L	0.62 μkat/L
ALT	68 U/L	1.13 μkat/L
Total bilirubin	0.7 mg/dL	12 μmol/L

Assessment

Fifty-eight-year-old woman with ductal breast carcinoma with metastatic lesions on the spine and associated chronic pain and neuropathic pain syndromes

Student Workup

Missing Information?

Evaluate: Patient Database
                  Drug Therapy Problems
                  Care Plan (by Problem)

TARGETED QUESTIONS

1. What other information would be useful in characterizing, assessing, and treating this patient's pain?

   Hint: See pp. 570–572 in PPP

2. What signs and symptoms of neuropathic pain does the patient have, and how does treatment of neuropathic pain differ from other types of chronic pain?

   Hint: See p. 570 in PPP

3. What is the rationale behind the use of both scheduled and PRN medications in chronic pain?

   Hint: See pp. 575–576 in PPP

4. What common adverse effects of opioid medications are dose-dependent, and what are appropriate methods to prevent and treat such adverse effects?

   Hint: See p. 577 in PPP

5. What nonpharmacologic therapies may be useful for this patient?

   Hint: See pp. 573–574 in PPP

FOLLOW-UP

6. Six months later, the patient returns for a follow-up pain visit. She is s/p palliative chemotherapy treatment. Three months ago she developed sepsis from an infected central venous catheter and acute renal failure, and her renal function never fully recovered. Her most recent laboratory work shows a BUN of 41 mg/dL (14.6 mmol/L) and SCr of 2.3 mg/dL (203 μmol/L). At her visit 1 month prior, her pain medication regimen was as follows: MS Contin 100 mg q 8 h, Fentanyl patch 50 mcg/h to be changed every 72 hours, and morphine immediate release (IR) 5 to 10 mg PO every 4 to 6 hours as needed. She presents in a wheelchair with her husband who states that she has been more lethargic, and he is concerned that it may be related to her medications. What changes would you make to her current pain regimen?

   Hint: See p. 577–578 in PPP

⊙ GLOBAL PERSPECTIVE

For over 20 years, the World Health Organization (WHO) has promoted adequate control of cancer-related pain through the application of key therapeutic principles shown to improve pain relief. Opioids are the mainstay of treating moderate to severe pain associated with cancer and other life-threatening conditions associated with chronic pain (e.g., HIV/AIDS). There are a variety of barriers that may interfere with successful pain control in such patients, and one such barrier is availability of and patient access to opioid medications. International research has shown that a country's per capita consumption of opioids is a marker of adequate pain management. There are very large disparities in per capita opioid consumption among regions and individual countries. Some, but not all, of the disparities are related to per capita income. Fifteen percent of the world's population accounts for 87% of the morphine consumption, with the United States, 4.7% of the world's population, accounting for 49% of global morphine consumption (77 mg/capita). Other developed countries consume significantly less morphine: Australia 51 mg/capita, France 37 mg/capita, Germany 22 mg/capita, United Kingdom 21 mg/capita, and Japan 3 mg/capita. Consumption in developing countries is strikingly lower (Brazil 1.7 mg/capita, Thailand 0.8 mg/capita, Kenya 0.6 mg/capita, and Ethiopia 0.0003 mg/capita). There are several reasons for such disparities in opioid consumption beyond simple economics. Because of concerns about opioid addiction and diversion of prescription drugs, many countries have implemented regulations that severely restrict patient access to such drugs. In some countries, potent opioids can be used only in severe cancer-related pain when other agents have failed. Also, there may be cultural or religious differences in how pain and suffering are interpreted and therefore how pain is managed. The WHO and the United Nations are working with countries around the world to develop balanced national policies that deal not only with drug abuse and diversion but also improve the care of patients who are needlessly suffering. However, changes in governmental policies will not by itself improve pain control. Education of health professionals in effective palliative care and changing the attitudes of professionals and patients also will be needed.

REFERENCES

Joranson DE, Ryan KM. Ensuring opioid availability: Methods and resources. J Pain Sympt Manage 2007 33:527–532.

Pain and Policy Studies Group, University of Wisconsin Carbone Cancer Center and WHO. www.painpolicy. wisc.edu/. Accessed March 25, 2010.

CASE SUMMARY

- Her clinical picture is consistent with chronic malignant pain secondary to metastatic disease.

- Her current regimen is not providing adequate pain relief, and she is experiencing adverse effects, including constipation.

- The patient would benefit from an individualized regimen, which includes pharmacologic agents to treat both somatic and neuropathic pain. An appropriate regimen should include scheduled and as-needed medications as part of her opioid pain regimen and bowel regimen to prevent opioid-induced adverse effects.

For more information on the care plan and facilitator's guide please visit http://www.mhpharmacotherapy.com.

36 Headache

Brendan S. Ross   Leigh Ann Ross

CASE LEARNING OBJECTIVES

- Differentiate among types of headaches (HA) based on symptoms and signs
- List underlying causes and precipitating factors of different types of HA disorders
- Recommend appropriate nonpharmacologic measures for HA treatment and prevention
- On the basis of patient-specific data, determine when pharmacologic therapy is indicated for HA
- Propose individualized pharmacologic treatment regimens for the acute and chronic management of HA syndromes
- Construct therapeutic and adverse effect monitoring plans for patients with HA
- Discuss pertinent patient education points for patients with HA disorders

PATIENT PRESENTATION

Chief Complaint

"My headaches just won't go away no matter how many pills I take."

History of Present Illness

A 54-year-old man is evaluated by the outpatient neurology service of an academic medical center because of chronic daily HA that have recently grown more severe. He reports that his HAs are bitemporal and that the pain radiates into his neck and upper back, but that they are not associated with stiffness or weakness: "It feels like a heavy weight on my head and shoulders." The pain is nonpulsating and it grows steadily over hours until it is 8/10 in intensity, and it lasts most of the day, if left untreated. "Almost anything" can bring on a HA, but they are more frequent and more intense when he is under significant "stress." He reports that rumination over recent marital discord makes it difficult for him to fall asleep. Bright lights can make the pain worse, but he has not experienced nausea or any neurologic deficits prior to or during an attack. The pain can make it difficult to concentrate, though he rarely misses business or family obligations. He has experienced HA since his teen years, but they had previously been easy to treat with the use of OTC analgesics. Over the past several years, his HAs have become more difficult to control. His primary care physician (PCP) provided him prescription-strength NSAIDs for PRN use without much relief: "I take them every day; they don't

seem to do much good." His other health issues remain stable, though he is scheduled for a prostate biopsy to further evaluate an elevated screening PSA test.

Past Medical History

Dyslipidemia

Gastritis, status posttreatment for *Helicobacter pylori*

Generalized anxiety disorder, diagnosed at age 44, current medication therapy for 2 years

HTN

Seasonal allergic rhinitis

Family History

Mother aged 79 years is a diabetic who suffers from migraine HA. His father had an open prostatectomy for cancer at age 64 years, and died of a stroke at 84 years. His daughter, age 23 years, is treated for recurrent depression.

Social History

He was divorced from his wife of 25 years, 6 months prior to presentation. He is a retired Naval aviator, currently an attorney. His only child is attending law school. He has few leisure or sports interests, though he used to be an avid golfer.

Tobacco/Alcohol/Substance Use

He smokes half to one ppd of low-tar, filtered cigarettes. He has an occasional beer on weekends. He drinks five to six caffeinated beverages per day. No current or history of illicit drug use.

Medication Allergies

Sulfa (rash)

Medication

Acetaminophen 500 mg 1 to 2 PO PRN headache, to q 6 h ("I pop them around-the-clock.")

Benazepril 10 mg/HCTZ 12.5 mg PO q 24 h

Cetirizine 10 mg PO PRN allergy symptoms q 24 h

Escitalopram 10 mg PO q 24 h

Meloxicam 7.5 mg PO PRN headache to q 12 h ("But 'when needed' means I'm using them everyday.")

Pantoprazole 20 mg PO q 24 h

Simvastatin 40 mg PO q 24 h

Review of Systems

(+) Unintended weight loss of 5 pounds (2.3 kg) over recent months. A recent optometric examination led to an adjustment in his lens prescription, but no evidence of glaucoma was noted. (−) Dizziness or vertigo with HAs reported. (+) Rhinorrhea in spring and autumn. (−) Chest pain or palpitations. (+) Morning "smoker's" cough, but (−) sputum production; (+) dyspnea with strenuous exertion. (−) Reflux complaints on daily antacid medication. (+) Nocturia once each night; (−) hesitancy or dribbling. (+) Left knee arthralgia associated with previous sports injury. (−) Lower extremity edema.

Physical Examination

► General

Well-developed, anxious, middle-aged white male, in no acute distress

► Vital Signs

BP 132/84 mm Hg, HR 78, RR 20, T 37°C

Weight 189 lb (86 kg)

Height 70 in. (178 cm)

Pain 4/10, "mild" neck tenderness

► Skin

No rash or other lesions

► HEENT

PERRLA, EOMI, fundoscopic examination benign, conjunctivae injected, nares with gray, boggy mucosa, (−) mucopurulent nasal discharge, external auditory canals and TMs clear, oropharynx without erythema, (−) temporal artery tenderness, occipital prominences tender bilaterally, without referred pain

► Neck and Lymph Nodes

Tender over trapezius without discrete trigger points, (−) stiffness with passive motion, thyroid without enlargement or nodularity, (−) carotid bruit, (−) JVP elevation, (−) adenopathy

► Chest

Minimal late expiratory wheezes bilaterally, resonant to percussion throughout

► Cardiovascular

RRR, (−) murmur or gallop

► Abdomen

Nontender, (−) organomegaly; normal bowel sounds

► Genitourinary/ Rectal

Examination deferred

► Neurology

Appears nervous, but not agitated. Alert and fully oriented. Cranial nerves intact. Motor and sensory examinations without focality. No cerebellar abnormalities. Speech and thought appropriate to situation.

Laboratory Tests

Nonfasting, obtained at PCP office 2 weeks previously

	Conventional Units	SI Units
Na	139 mEq/L	139 mmol/L
K	4.2 mEq/L	4.2 mmol/L
CL	102 mEq/L	102 mmol/L
CO_2	24 mEq/L	24 mmol/L
BUN	12 mg/dL	4.3 mmol/L
SCr	0.9 mg/dL	80 mmol/L
Glu	96 mg/dL	5.3 mmol/L
Hgb	14.4 g/dL	144 g/L; 8.94 mmol/L
Hct	46.2%	0.462
TSH	2.8 μIU/mL	2.8 mIU/L
Urine toxicology	(+) cotinine	

Assessment

Chronic tension-type headache (TTH) with pericranial muscle tenderness complicated by analgesic medication overuse headache (MOH)

Student Workup

What clinical or diagnostic information is missing?

Evaluate: Patient Database Form

Drug Therapy Problem Worksheet

Pharmacotherapy Care Plan

TARGETED QUESTIONS

1. What signs and symptoms allow the practitioner to differentiate this TTH syndrome from others, such as migraine HA or cluster headache?

   Hint: See pp. 585–587 in PPP

2. What lifestyle issues may be contributing to the development or perpetuation of HA symptoms in this patient, and what nonpharmacologic measures might be recommended to provide pain relief and HA prevention?

   Hint: See pp. 587 and 589 in PPP

3. What medical comorbidities or medication therapies may be contributing to this patient's distress?

   Hint: Uncontrolled HTN and poorly managed emotional distress can precipitate or potentiate HA. Sinusitis and rhinitis can present as HA, so HA sufferers should have such conditions fully addressed. Many drugs list HA as an adverse treatment effect, so any newly added medication therapy should be suspected of contributing to HA pain.

4. Will this patient require prophylactic pharmacologic treatment, as well as acute drug therapy?

   Hint: See pp. 589 and 591 in PPP

5. How will the practitioner assess the outcome of the interventions, assess the need for alterations or additions in the chosen treatment regimen?

   Hint: See p. 592 in PPP

FOLLOW-UP

6. MRI of the patient's brain did not reveal any pathologic lesions, an ESR was within normal limits, and the prostate biopsy only demonstrated benign hyperplasia. Allergy testing revealed reactivity to household dust and anti-allergy treatment was added with good results. Concurrently, the patient was advised to wean caffeine intake and to seek talk therapy for stress reduction. He declined tobacco cessation assistance. A HA diary was completed by the patient, which identified the frequency and severity of his HAs, presumed precipitates and associated symptoms, and his symptomatic response to analgesics. It was believed that acetaminophen and NSAID overuse had "transformed" his episodic TTH into a chronic daily HA syndrome. His use of around-the-clock analgesics was discontinued and, to limit the development of withdrawal HAs, prednisone 50 mg PO per day was added with a rapid taper. He was provided an opiate compound for use, but was instructed that it should be reserved for debilitating pain only. To limit HA recurrence and to improve sleep, amitriptyline 10 mg PO per night was added, with an expected upward dosage titration based on tolerability and treatment benefit. If the patient had been a diabetic, how might this impact the choice of therapies? How can a practitioner tell if an anxiety disorder is adequately treated? What risks are assumed with the concurrent use of a SSRI and a TCA? How would one counsel a patient to monitor and to appropriately react to the development of this potential drug–drug interaction? What is an alternative prevention strategy in a patient who reports headache with muscle pain or stiffness? Are any HTN medications associated with the development or even prevention of headache?

⊙ GLOBAL PERSPECTIVE

Headache is the most common condition seen by neurologists, and TTH is the most prevalent HA syndrome. In a European epidemiologic study, more than 80% of individuals reported having experienced a TTH. The episodic subtype predominates, though most of those affected experience infrequent HAs of mild to moderate intensity; the societal impact of TTH is much less than migraine. Heredity may play an important role in the development of the chronic TTH variant, which places a greater burden on the patient and the health care system. As with migraine, women predominate in chronic TTH cohorts. The peak incidence for TTH is in middle age, with some data suggesting that attacks diminish with age. The distribution of TTH among countries and populations of varying ethnic and socioeconomic groups has not identified clear distinctions, but there is some data to suggest that Caucasians in developed countries and those with advanced educational achievement are more prone to suffer from TTH. Complementary and alternative medicine approaches to HA treatment and prevention are more commonly employed in non-Western societies, with acupuncture demonstrating benefit in limiting headache frequency in clinical trials. Multiple herbal remedies are purported to have analgesic, antispasmodic, and anxiolytic properties that might be beneficial for TTH sufferers: feverfew, valerian, and chamomile are frequently mentioned. Herbal therapies must be used cautiously when prescription drugs are employed, so as to avoid adverse pharmacokinetic or pharmacodynamic interactions, such as the cytochrome (CYP) and serotonin interactions with the concurrent use of St. John's Wort and SSRIs.

CASE SUMMARY

- The clinical presentation is most consistent with TTH, which, due to the frequency of attacks, more than two per week, meets the International Headache Society (IHS) criteria for chronicity; due to the presence of occipital and neck tenderness on manual palpation this pain syndrome can be more fully described as chronic TTH with pericranial tenderness.

- Given the patient's age, family history of prostate cancer and his elevated PSA, increase in pain severity, and analgesic refractoriness, neuroimaging is indicated: a contrasted CT scan or an MRI.

- The daily use of analgesic agents may be complicating definitive diagnostic classification, as unrestrained pain medication use can transform episodic TTH into a chronic daily HA syndrome, the so-called MOH; analgesic withdrawal may be difficult and protracted in either chronic TTH or MOH cases.
- The patient's comorbidities and current medication use may complicate the choice of therapeutic options to limit HA frequency and severity, his HTN and use of an anxiolytic for instance. But they may also serve to direct drug and nonpharmacologic choices, so that the targeted HA therapies chosen benefit the other conditions as well, such as the use of a CCB for his HTN or stress-reducing massage therapy for his GAD.

For more information on the care plan and facilitator's guide please visit http://www.mhpharmacotherapy.com.

37 Alzheimer's Disease

Megan J. Ehret

PATIENT PRESENTATION

Chief Complaint

"I want to die. I hate forgetting all the important things."

History of Present Illness

Barbara O'Neil is a 65-year-old woman who presents with her husband to the primary care clinic. She does not state any other information when asked what has brought her to the clinic for this visit. Her husband describes how over the past several months since their last visit, his wife has had increased memory loss. He notices that she frequently forgets to complete her normal daily activities, such as brushing her teeth, combing her hair, and getting dressed for the day. Several nights ago, he found her wandering down the street looking for their dog that passed away last month. When he tried to bring her home, she became tearful and withdrawn. Additionally, she has always taken her own medications without any help, but the pharmacy has been calling stating that she is late on her refills. He has found multiple bottles of unused medications in their bedroom. Over the past few months, their daughter has also mentioned that her mother appears depressed. She has noticed her decreased appetite, decreased concentration, and a lack of interest in her mother's favorite activities. The husband and daughter are wondering if the patient is suffering from depression.

Past Medical History

Mild cognitive decline diagnosed 6 months ago
HTN
Type 2 DM
Hyperlipidemia

Family History

Mother had dementia and died of pneumonia at age 85. Father died of a MI at age 73. She has one brother, age 62, with HTN and diabetes.

Social History

Married and lives with her husband of 40 years; has one daughter aged 35; retired grade-school teacher

Tobacco/Alcohol/Substance Use

Thirty-three pack-year history; denies alcohol and illicit drug use

Allergies/Intolerance/Adverse Drug Events

Enalapril (cough)

Galantamine (N/V); she self-discontinued the medication at 8 mg twice daily)

Medications (Current)

Amlodipine 10 mg PO daily

Metformin 750 mg PO twice daily

Simvastatin 20 mg PO daily

Multivitamin PO daily

Calcium carbonate 600 mg PO twice daily

Review of Systems

Appears tearful and unable to answer many questions during the mental status examination; (−) history of seizures, head injuries, or loss of consciousness; (+) loss of appetite

Physical Examination

▶ General

Mildly disheveled African American woman who is slightly tearful

▶ Vital Signs

BP 140/90 mm Hg, P 70, RR 14, T 36.4°C

Weight 145 lb (65.9 kg)

Height 68 in. (173 cm)

Denies any physical pain

▶ Skin

Moist skin; (−) rashes or lesions

▶ HEENT

PERRLA, EOMI; (−) sinus tenderness, TMs appear normal

▶ Neck and Lymph Nodes

Normal

▶ Chest

Clear to auscultation

▶ Breasts

Examination deferred

▶ Cardiovascular

RRR, normal S_1, S_2, (−) S_3 or S_4

▶ Abdomen

Not tender/not distended; (−) organomegaly

▶ Neurology

Folstein Mini-Mental Status Examination Score (MMSE) 20/30; unable to count backward from 100 by 7, recalled one out of three items; unable to read paper and follow command; unable to make up a sentence and write it; unable to copy a picture; poor registration with impaired attention and short-term memory

▶ Psychiatry

Tearful expression, mood congruent; (−) auditory and visual hallucinations; (−) delusion; (+) suicidal ideations

▶ Genitourinary

Examination deferred

▶ Rectal

Examination deferred

Laboratory Tests

	Conventional Units	SI Units
Na	140 mEq/L	140 mmol/L
K	4.2 mEq/L	4.2 mmol/L
Cl	100 mEq/L	100 mmol/L
CO_2	24 mEq/L	24 mmol/L
BUN	8 mg/dL	2.9 mmol/L
SCr	0.9 mg/dL	80 μmol/L
Glu	150 mg/dL	8.3 mmol/L
Vitamin B_{12}	600 pg/mL	443 pmol/L
Total cholesterol	240 mg/dL	6.21 mmol/L
LDL cholesterol	200 mg/dL	5.17 mmol/L
HDL cholesterol	30 mg/dL	0.78 mmol/L
Triglycerides	210 mg/dL	2.37 mmol/L
ALT	20 IU/L	0.33 μkat/L
AST	18 IU/L	0.30 μkat/L
TSH	3.1 μIU/mL	3.1 mIU/L
Free T_4	1.1 ng/dL	14.2 pmol/L

CT scan: Mild-to-moderate generalized cerebral atrophy

Assessment

Sixty-five-year-old woman with s/s, and laboratory tests consistent with Alzheimer's disease and depression

---

Student Workup

Missing Information?

Evaluate: Patient Database

Drug Therapy Problems

Care Plan (by Problem)

TARGETED QUESTIONS

1. What signs and symptoms of Alzheimer's disease does the patient have?

   Hint: See pp. 597–598 in PPP

2. What s/s of depression does the patient have?

   Hint: Differentiating between depression and dementia can be difficult, so symptoms of depression should be documented for several months prior to the initiation of therapy for the treatment of depression with Alzheimer's disease. Signs of depression that the patient displays, which make her a candidate for therapy for depression, include suicidal thoughts, anhedonia, withdrawal from activities, and a poor appetite. See pp. 655–656 in PPP

3. Why is a cholinesterase inhibitor in conjunction with nonpharmacologic strategies the treatment of choice for most patients with Alzheimer's disease?

   Hint: See p. 598 in PPP

4. Why are citalopram and sertraline recommended as first-line agents for the treatment of comorbid depression with Alzheimer's disease?

   Hint: See p. 603 in PPP

5. What risks and adverse effects of therapy would you discuss with the patient?

   Hint: See pp. 600–602 in PPP

FOLLOW-UP

6. Four weeks later, the patient returns for a follow-up. She feels somewhat better, with more energy, but still some symptoms of sadness. Her MMSE score is 22/30. Why did her MMSE score not improve more? What actions would you take regarding the residual depressive symptoms and the MMSE score?

   Hint: See p. 600 in PPP

☽ GLOBAL PERSPECTIVE

Overall prevalence rates for dementia have been reported to be substantially higher for African Americans than for Caucasians. Studies have demonstrated prevalence rates from 14% to 500% higher for African Americans than for Caucasians. Preliminary evidence has shown that the relative contributions of several genetic risk factors for the Alzheimer's-type dementia at a molecular level appear to differ between African Americans and Caucasians, particularly with regard to APOE-ε4, which is a potent risk factor in Caucasians, but not in African Americans. However, potential flaws in the research design of the studies may have led to the increased prevalence rates. Cultural factors have led to a relative overreporting of cognitive disability in studies with African Americans, which have utilized self-report or caregiver report of cognitive functioning. Additionally, some investigators have proposed that the lower mean educational level of African American study subjects may account for the difference in cognitive test scores achieved by the older African-American sample versus the Caucasian sample. Research into the actual difference in prevalence rates may affect the clinical practice and future policy planning in the treatment of dementia worldwide.

CASE SUMMARY

- Her current clinical picture is consistent with Stage 4 cognitive decline and mild-to-early stage Alzheimer's disease. Cholinesterase inhibitor therapy should be reinitiated.

- She also has a clinical picture consistent with a major depressive episode, which meets criteria for treatment with an antidepressant.

For more information on the care plan and facilitator's guide please visit http://www.mhpharmacotherapy.com.

38 Alcohol Withdrawal

Krina H. Patel

CASE LEARNING OBJECTIVES

- Identify signs and symptoms associated with alcohol withdrawal
- Recommend appropriate agents for the treatment of alcohol withdrawal on the basis of specific individualized needs
- Design a comprehensive treatment plan and monitoring program to treat alcohol withdrawal, prevent relapse, and maintain abstinence

PATIENT PRESENTATION

Chief Complaint

"My son needs help, he is really sick. He is really shaky and nervous, and he has also been vomiting since last night!"

History of Present Illness

Michael Jones is a 23-year-old male who has a history of alcoholism. His father died 6 months ago and since then he has been drinking on a daily basis. The patient's family states that he is not the same. Recently he has been extremely pessimistic about life, is generally sad, and only gets out of his bed to drink. His mother is getting really frustrated because it has now been 6 months and the patient has still not accepted his father's death and continues to drink. Yesterday afternoon the patient's mother and sister got into an argument with him regarding his drinking. He is tired of all the nagging and wanted to show them that he does not need alcohol and therefore he stopped drinking.

Past Medical History

Perennial allergies × 4 years
Chronic pain × 6 months
Alcohol dependence × 3 years
Bipolar disorder I × 4 years

Family History

Father died at the age of 49 due to a motor vehicle accident. Mother is 51 and has a diagnosis of HTN, generalized anxiety disorder, and migraine. He has an older brother and younger sister; both are healthy.

Social History

The patient has a history of alcohol dependence for 3 years. He had been sober for the past 2 years until recent death of his father. The patient and father were in a motor vehicle accident. The patient survived, but father did not. Currently, he lives with mother and two siblings. He is an elementary school teacher; however, he has not worked since the accident.

Tobacco/Alcohol/Substance Use

Denies tobacco use; drinks one bottle (750 mL) of vodka daily; occasional illicit drug use (marijuana); denies abuse of prescription medications

Allergies/Intolerances/Adverse Drug Events

None

Medications (Prior to Admission)

Cetirizine 10 mg PO daily

Acetaminophen 500 mg PO every 4 to 6 hours PRN pain

Lithium carbonate 300 mg PO in morning and 600 mg at bedtime

Review of Systems

(−) Chest pain, (−) palpitations, (+) nausea since last drink, (+) decreased appetite for past 3 months; (+) Tremors, appeared about 6 hours after last drink, (−) seizures; (+) Anxiety since last drink, (−) hallucinations, (+) headache

Physical Examination

▶ General

Twenty-three-year-old Caucasian male who appears malnourished and thin. Presents with signs of acute distress. The patient is alert and oriented, and is cooperative with clear speech.

▶ Vital Signs

BP 147/98 mm Hg, P 114, RR 20, T 37°C

Weight 120 lb (54.5 kg)

Height 67 in. (170 cm)

Pain level 0/10

▶ Skin

Moist, (−) rash, (−) pruritus

▶ HEENT

PERRLA, EOMI

▶ Neck and Lymph Nodes

(−) Lymphadenopathy

▶ Chest

Lung auscultation clear, (−) crackles, rhonchi, or wheezing

▶ Cardiovascular

Tachycardic, RRR, (−) murmurs

▶ Abdomen

Normal bowel sounds, (+) enlarged liver, (−) abdominal pain

▶ Neurology

Alert and oriented × 3; tremulous; DTRs normal; CN II to XII intact

▶ Extremities

(+) Tremors in fingers and hands

▶ Genitourinary

Examination deferred

▶ Rectal

Examination deferred

Laboratory Tests

	Conventional Units	SI Units
Na	137 mEq/L	137 mmol/L
K	3.5 mEq/L	3.5 mmol/L
Cl	101 mEq/L	101 mmol/L
CO_2	23 mEq/L	23 mmol/L
BUN	9 mg/dL	3.2 mmol/L
SCr	0.8 mg/dL	71 µmol/L
CrCl	110 mL/min	1.84 mL/s
Glu	99 mg/dL	5.5 mmol/L
Ca	9.0 mg/dL	2.25 mmol/L
Mg	1.6 mEq/L	0.80 mmol/L
Phosphate	2.5 mg/dL	0.81 mmol/L
Albumin	3.5 g/dL	35 g/L
PT	12.0 s	
Platelet	$200 \times 10^3/mm^3$	$200 \times 10^9/mm^3$
GGT	122 IU/L	2.03 µkat/L
LDH	200 IU/L	3.33 µkat/L
AST	250 IU/L	4.17 µkat/L
ALT	123 IU/L	2.05 µkat/L
Alk phos	41 IU/L	0.68 µkat/L
Total bilirubin	0.7 mg/dL	12.0 µmol/L
Direct bilirubin	0.2 mg/L	3.4 µmol/L
Ammonia	34.7 mcg/dL	20 µmol/L
Lithium	0.3 mEq/L	0.3 mmol/L

Assessment

Twenty-three-year-old male with history and current signs, symptoms, and laboratory tests consistent with alcohol withdrawal

Student Workup

Missing Information?

Evaluate: Patient Database

Drug Therapy Problems

Care Plan (by Problem)

TARGETED QUESTIONS

1. What signs and symptoms of alcohol withdrawal is this patient presenting with?

   Hint: See Table 36-3 in PPP

2. How should alcohol withdrawal be managed for this patient?

   Hint: See pp. 616–618 in PPP

3. What are some risks of not appropriately managing alcohol withdrawal?

   Hint: See p. 616 in PPP

4. What psychiatric symptoms does this patient present with? How does this psychiatric illness relate to alcohol dependence?

Hint: The patient is presenting with symptoms of depression. The patient appears to have cycled into an acute depressive episode. The prevalence of psychiatric illnesses among the substance-abuse population is quite high. Many patients who have bipolar disorder also have coexisting alcohol dependence. Additionally, alcohol may be a secondary cause for inducing depression. See Bipolar Disorder Chapter 39 in PPP.

FOLLOW-UP

5. A few days later, the patient is doing much better and free of all withdrawal symptoms. However, the patient does mention that he is still experiencing the urge to go out and drink once he is released from the hospital. He states his intention is not to drink; however, he is not sure if can abstain from alcohol. What nonpharmacologic and pharmacologic treatment option would you recommend for this patient?

    HINT: See pp. 623–626 in PPP

⊙ GLOBAL PERSPECTIVE

Substance-related disorders, such as alcohol dependence, are quite prevalent not only in the United States but also in countries around the world. There are some cultures that do tend to have a lower prevalence rate of alcoholism, such as in certain Asian countries. It is believed that genetically determined aldehyde dehydrogenase deficiency may be the reason for the lower prevalence rate among Asian populations. Patients with this type of deficiency may refrain from alcohol intake due to the unwanted effects, such as facial flushing and palpitations, that may occur with alcohol intake. Western countries, in general, tend to have a higher prevalence rate of alcohol dependence. One of the populations in the United States that tends to have a higher prevalence rate of alcohol dependence is the male Latino population. Overall, genetic, environmental, and cultural factors play a significant role in the difference of prevalence rates among different countries and cultures.

CASE SUMMARY

- The patient should be treated for alcohol withdrawal since he is exhibiting signs and symptoms of withdrawal.
- Benzodiazepine treatment should be initiated for alcohol withdrawal. In addition, this patient should also receive thiamine supplementation.

For more information on the care plan and facilitator's guide please visit http://www.mhpharmacotherapy.com.

39 Schizophrenia

Heidi J. Wehring   Deanna L. Kelly

CASE LEARNING OBJECTIVES

- Recognize the signs and symptoms of schizophrenia and be able to distinguish among positive, negative, and cognitive symptoms of the illness
- Identify the treatment goals for a patient with schizophrenia
- Recommend appropriate antipsychotic medications using patient-specific data
- Develop an appropriate treatment and monitoring plan for the treatment of symptoms of schizophrenia
- Educate a patient about antipsychotic medications and the importance of adherence to the treatment

PATIENT PRESENTATION

Chief Complaint

"I'm being poisoned because I'm going to be a TV star."

History of Present Illness

Carla Lee is a 24-year-old woman who presents to the clinic after being brought in by a family member. Her family has noted that she has become more withdrawn within the past 8 months, and she rarely comes out of her room at the family home. Carla has been seen muttering to herself for the past 6 weeks and when questioned, has been telling family members that her "TV agent" has been talking to her all day and all night. By her own report, she is not sleeping as much as usual so that she can get through these important conferences with her agent. Carla's family has become worried since she has been refusing to eat food in the family home. She has been suspicious of all the food that her mother cooks, and complains that her mother and others in the house may be trying to poison her food due to their jealousy over her upcoming celebrity status. She now refuses to eat any food that is not prepackaged or shrink-wrapped, and has started complaining that even that is not a guarantee that her food has not been altered. Carla recently lost her job as a clerk at a convenience store because she missed too many shifts. Other employees saw her as disruptive since she would carry on conversations, apparently with herself, while ringing up customers. Carla stated that she used to like to work at the store, but lately she has noticed people staring at her and talking about her. She attributes this to their jealousy about her role in the TV show "The Carla Show," which is all about her life. Carla presents as unkempt and malodorous, wearing several different layers of clothes and a large hat, which she refuses to take off since it is keeping her fans from recognizing her. She has not showered for several days and has not brought along the correct medical paperwork, although she has brought along her journal, which she uses to track her thoughts for script ideas. Although she complains of being thirsty, she refuses a drink of water as the paper cup may have been tampered with.

Past Medical History

Carla has a history of acne in adolescence, which was treated with oral antibiotics from age 17 to 19. She has been treated for GERD in the past year, first with ranitidine and most currently with esomeprazole, with reportedly good symptom control. She is also prescribed an oral contraceptive, and occasionally, she takes desloratadine 5 mg daily as needed for allergic rhinitis.

Family History

Carla's mother and one of her maternal aunts have type 2 DM, and her paternal grandfather reportedly suffered from an unspecified mental illness.

Social History

Carla is a single, never-married female who lives in her mother's house. She reportedly had some friends and a boyfriend in high school, but over the past several years, she has been seeing fewer people socially, which does not seem to bother her. Carla was a good student in high school and completed several years at a local college before seeming to lose interest in her studies. She left college and worked a series of jobs before the most recent position as a clerk in a convenience store.

Tobacco/Alcohol/Substance Use

Social drinker, generally one to two beers once weekly, although she denies any intake in past month; smokes one ppd of cigarettes since age 16; history of illicit drug use (marijuana)

Allergies/Intolerances/Adverse Drug Events

Intolerance to tetracycline due to GI upset and diarrhea

Medications (Current)

Esomeprazole 20 mg PO daily

Norethindrone and ethinyl estradiol 1 mg/20 mcg PO daily

Desloratadine 5 mg PO daily as needed

Admits to missing doses of her medications "here and there"

Review of Systems

(–) History of head injury or loss of consciousness; (–) tinnitus, vertigo, or infections; (–) history of seizures or syncope

Physical Examination

▶ General

Disheveled and unkempt, young adult woman in no acute distress

▶ Vital Signs

BP 110/84 mm Hg, P 74, RR 14, T 36.8°C

Weight 131 lb (59.5 kg)

Height 64 in. (163 cm)

Denies pain

▶ Skin

Dry-appearing skin and scalp; (–) rashes or lesions

▶ HEENT

PERRLA, EOMI

▶ Neck and Lymph Nodes

(–) Thyroid nodules; (–) lymphadenopathy; (–) carotid bruits

▶ Chest

Clear to auscultation

▶ Breasts

Examination deferred

▶ Cardiovascular

RRR, normal S_1, S_2

▶ Abdomen

Not tender, not distended; (–) organomegaly

▶ Neurology

Grossly intact; DTRs normal

▶ Genitourinary

Examination deferred

▶ Rectal

Examination deferred

Laboratory Tests

Fasting, obtained 2 days ago

	Conventional Units	SI Units
Na	146 mEq/L	146 mmol/L
K	4.8 mEq/L	4.8 mmol/L
Cl	102 mEq/L	102 mmol/L
CO_2	24 mEq/L	24 mmol/L
BUN	9 mg/dL	3.2 mmol/L
SCr	0.9 mg/dL	80 μmol/L
Glu	98 mg/dL	5.4 mmol/L
Ca	9.6 mg/dL	2.40 mmol/L
Mg	1.6 mEq/L	0.66 mmol/L
Phosphate	4.1 mg/dL	1.32 mmol/L
Hgb	12.7 g/dL (127 g/L)	7.88 mmol/L
Hct	40.3%	0.403
WBC	$5.6 \times 10^3/mm^3$	$5.6 \times 10^9/L$
MCV	$80~\mu m^3$	80 fL
Albumin	4.3 g/dL	43 g/L
TSH	2.4 μIU/mL	2.4 mIU/L
Total cholesterol	195 mg/dL	5.04 mmol/L

Mental Status Examination

Carla is a 24-year-old female of average build, appearing stated age, disheveled, unkempt, malodorous, and wearing inappropriately layered clothes. She is somewhat guarded in conversation, but will answer questions when asked. Eye contact is sporadic and she seems to be distracted by and responding to internal stimuli periodically throughout the interview. Carla describes her mood as "just fine." Her range of affect is somewhat blunted, though appropriate. She is alert and oriented to person, place, and time. Intellectual functioning appears average, although, at times, it is difficult to assess due to her tendency to become distracted during the interview. Thought processes are coherent and goal directed; however, her conclusions that people are trying to poison her and her belief in her impending fame are illogical. Prominent delusions are apparent, including her belief that people want to poison her and that she is starring in her own television series. Carla endorses auditory hallucinations of hearing the voice of her "TV agent." She denies suicidal or homicidal ideation. Her insight and judgment are poor.

Assessment

Twenty-four-year-old woman with signs and symptoms consistent with a psychotic disorder such as schizophrenia

---

Student Workup

Missing Information?

Evaluate: Patient Database

                  Drug Therapy Problems

                  Care Plan (by Problem)

TARGETED QUESTIONS

1. What signs and symptoms of schizophrenia does the patient have?

   Hint: See pp. 632–633 in PPP

2. What will be the goals of treatment for Carla?

   Hint: See pp. 634–635 in PPP

3. What types of nonpharmacologic interventions should be implemented in the treatment plan for a person with schizophrenia?

   Hint: See p. 636 in PPP

4. What first-line pharmacologic options are available for the treatment of Carla's symptoms of psychosis?

   Hint: See pp. 636–641 in PPP

5. Which of the options from above would you recommend for Carla, including titration schedule and monitoring plan?

   Hint: See Tables 37-3 and 37-5 in PPP

6. What risks and adverse effects of therapy would you discuss with the patient?

   Hint: See pp. 636–641 and Table 37-4 in PPP

FOLLOW-UP

7. Three months later after Carla's initial visit and her formal diagnosis of schizophrenia, she returns for follow-up. You learn that in the 2 weeks following her initial visit, Carla's symptoms exacerbated to the point that she was hospitalized. During this time, the regimen you selected was discontinued and a regimen of quetiapine

100 mg three times daily was implemented. Carla has now been prescribed this regimen for approximately 2 months. She is complaining that she still hears her agent talking to her and still feels somewhat paranoid about her family. She is upset about the fact that she has gained 12 lb (5.5 kg), and admits to missing several doses of the medication every week because it is hard for her to remember taking the medication several times a day. She states that if she keeps gaining weight, she will stop taking the medication completely. What reason(s) may be contributing to Carla's continuing symptoms? What action would you take?

Hint: See pp. 642–645 in PPP

GLOBAL PERSPECTIVE

Schizophrenia is a disorder that is present worldwide. However, when assessing for the signs and symptoms of schizophrenia (delusions, hallucinations, etc.), it is important to take cultural and religious beliefs into consideration as what is considered within the norm for a certain ethnic group may not be considered within normal limits for another group also. Differences in response to antipsychotic treatment may exist due to differences in genetic makeup of persons with schizophrenia, from both an efficacy and adverse effect standpoint, although information is limited. Antipsychotic medications are the treatment of choice for schizophrenia; however, the particular agents available in various countries may differ. In addition, the treatment algorithms may differ widely depending on the location of treatment.

CASE SUMMARY

- Carla's current clinical picture is consistent with the symptoms of schizophrenia and warrants treatment with antipsychotic medication.

- An initial second-generation antipsychotic such as aripiprazole, risperidone, quetiapine, or ziprasidone at appropriate doses would be appropriate for the treatment of Carla's symptoms.

- Upon her representation to the clinic 3 months later, either an increase in dose of quetiapine (up to 800 mg) or switching to an antipsychotic that may offer once-daily dosing and a lower weight gain burden (such as aripipazole or risperidone) would be appropriate.

For more information on the care plan and facilitator's guide please visit http://www.mhpharmacotherapy.com.

40 Depression

Cherry W. Jackson   Marshall E. Cates
Raymond A. Lorenz

CASE LEARNING OBJECTIVES

- Identify the symptoms and clinical features of major depressive disorder (MDD)
- Outline the goals of therapy for depression
- Develop an appropriate treatment plan for a patient with depression on the basis of individual patient characteristics
- Educate patients and caregivers on the proper use of antidepressants

PATIENT PRESENTATION

Chief Complaint

"I can't keep living like this."

History of Present Illness

Melanie Collie is a 38-year-old female who presents to the primary care clinic for the management of her depression. She was diagnosed with MDD by her primary care physician and is presenting for initiation of medication treatment. During the past month, she experienced a depressed mood, anhedonia, poor sleep and appetite, isolative behavior, and crying spells. In addition, she reports having a passive death wish. There have been no precipitating events and she states "I felt like this two years ago." She states that she initially took an over-the-counter medication for depression, but it did not work. She states that at that point she went to see her physician; he diagnosed her with depression and she has been taking sertraline 50 mg faithfully since then. She states that initially she felt better, but then the medication seemed to stop working and her original symptoms returned. She also states that her friend said that she gained weight on her antidepressant and that she does not want to take any medications that will make her gain weight.

Past Medical History

Depression diagnosed 2 years ago

Chronic migraine headaches since age 18 years

Tonsillectomy age 14 years

Right-knee arthroscopy in 2002

C-section in 1992

Family History

Mother suffers from depression, and alcohol and cocaine dependence. Father died from suicide at age 57 years.

Social History

Thirty-eight-year-old female who is divorced. Has one son in high school. Works in customer service at a local business.

Tobacco/Alcohol/Substance Abuse

Smokes 1½ packs of cigarettes per week; Recently increased alcohol intake (6–8 beers daily); no current illicit drug use, smoked marijuana in high school

Allergies/Intolerances/Adverse Drug Events

Penicillin (pruritus, last exposure at age 4)

Medications (Current)

Ortho Tri-Cyclen Lo one tablet PO daily

Centrum multivitamin one tablet PO daily

Sertraline 50 mg PO daily

Ibuprofen 200 mg two tablets PO as needed for migraine headaches

Sumatriptan 100 mg PO PRN severe migraine headaches; may repeat once after 2 hours, if needed. Do not take more than two tablets in a 24-hour period

Prior Medication Use

St. John's wort 300 mg PO tid for 3 months, with no effect

Review of Systems

Chronic migraine headaches, currently using ibuprofen 200 mg two tablets as needed, but the patient complains that this frequently does not help with her headache pain and she needs to take the sumatriptan to relieve the headache. She also reports an increased frequency of migraine headache from once per month to once every week. (+) Depressed mood, anhedonia, poor sleep and appetite, isolative behavior, crying spells, and suicidal ideation.

Physical Examination

▶ *Vital Signs*

BP 130/87 mm Hg, P 70, RR 12, T 36.0°C

Weight 217 lb (98.6 kg)

Height 68 in. (173 cm)

Denies physical pain

   Physical examination 2 days ago by primary care physician was entirely normal (pelvic examination was deferred) and is not repeated today.

Mental Status Examination

Appearance: The patient is a 38-year-old white female, who appears older than stated age; clothing is wrinkled. No makeup; hair appears disheveled.

Movement/behavior: The patient has poor eye contact and is intermittently tearful. (+) Psychomotor retardation.

Speech: The patient has slow rate and prosody, and she speaks very softly. She was asked to repeat answers several times because of the volume. She clearly understands the questions, and her answers are appropriate.

Affect: Restricted, tearful.

Mood: "Sad." The patient appears withdrawn and isolative. She reports poor sleep and appetite as well as anhedonia.

Thought content: The patient denies paranoia, delusions, hallucinations, obsessions, compulsions, or strange impulses. She reports thinking about her father's suicide. She states that it used to make her angry, but now she understands why he did it. She reports having a passive death wish. She does not have a plan to commit suicide at this time.

Thought process: The patient is logical and coherent, but has some thought blocking.

Cognition: A+O × 3. The patient has poor concentration, and is tearful and distracted throughout the interview, but she could perform serial 7s. Her memory is intact. She has average intellect, evidenced by her response to the interviewer, but not thoroughly assessed. Abstract reasoning is intact, evidenced by, How are an apple and orange similar? "Both are fruit." Different? "One is red and one is orange, they taste different, and they grow in different parts of the country."

Judgment/insight: The patient has some understanding of her illness. She has poor insight and judgment, feeling that "suicide may be the only way out."

Laboratory Tests

	Conventional Units	SI Units
Na	140 mEq/L	140 mmol/L
K	3.9 mEq/L	3.9 mmol/L
Cl	103 mEq/L	103 mmol/L
CO_2	24 mEq/L	24 mmol/L
BUN	11 mg/dL	3.9 mmol/L
SCr	0.93 mg/dL	82 μmol/L
Glu	72 mg/dL	4.0 mmol/L
Ca	9.7 mg/dL	2.43 mmol/L
Mg	2.4 mEq/L	1.20 mmol/L
Phosphate	4.3 mg/dL	1.39 mmol/L
Hgb	14.3 g/dL (143 g/L)	8.88 mmol/L
Hct	42.6%	0.426
WBC	$4.0 \times 10^3/mm^3$	$4.0 \times 10^9/L$
MCV	90.6 μm³	90.6 fL
Albumin	4.6 g/dL	46 g/L
Total cholesterol	191 mg/dL	4.94 mmol/L
LDL cholesterol	83 mg/dL	2.15 mmol/L
HDL cholesterol	97 mg/dL	2.51 mmol/L

Assessment

A 38-year-old woman with symptoms indicative of MDD.

Student Workup

Missing Information?

Evaluate: Patient Database

                   Drug Therapy Problems

                   Care Plan (by Problem)

TARGETED QUESTIONS

1. What symptoms and clinical features of MDD does the patient have?

    Hint: See p. 655 in PPP

2. What is the time course of response for antidepressant therapy and what is the response rate with antidepressants?

    Hint: See p. 662 in PPP

3. What medication therapy might the patient use to treat chronic migraines and depression?

    Hint: See Table 38-6 in PPP

4. How do you treat partial response to an antidepressant?

    Hint: See pp. 662–664 in PPP

5. What risks and adverse effects of antidepressants would you discuss with the patient?

   Hint: See pp. 668–670 in PPP

What If's?

6. What if the patient complained of sexual dysfunction with her antidepressant?

   Hint: See Table 38-4 in PPP

7. What if the patient was receiving her Ortho Tri-Cyclen Lo in addition to St. John's wort?

   Hint: See Table 38-6 in PPP

8. What if the patient was taking an SSRI and needed to be transitioned to an MAOI?

   Hint: See pp. 662–663 in PPP

9. What if the patient was initiated on propranolol for migraine headaches?

   Hint: See Table 38-6 in PPP

10. What if the patient was concerned about all of the media attention about antidepressants making you "want to kill yourself"?

    Hint: See p. 666 in PPP

⟳ GLOBAL PERSPECTIVE

Depression is a common mental disorder that presents with depressed mood, loss of interest or pleasure, feelings of guilt or low self-worth, disturbed sleep or appetite, low energy, and poor concentration. These problems can become chronic or recurrent, and may lead to substantial impairment in an individual's ability to take care of his or her everyday responsibilities. At its worst, depression can lead to suicide, with the loss of about 850,000 lives every year.

Depression in the year 2000 was the leading cause of disability worldwide as measured by years lived with disability (YLD) and the fourth leading contributor to the global burden of disease on the basis of disability-adjusted life-years (DALYs).[1] By the year 2020, depression is projected to reach second place of the ranking of DALYs calculated for all ages, both sexes. Today, depression is already the second cause of DALYs worldwide in the age category 15 to 44 years for both sexes combined. According to the World Health Organization, fewer than 25% of depressed patients have access to care and in some countries, fewer than 10%. Barriers to effective care include the lack of resources, lack of trained providers, and the social stigma associated with mental disorders, including depression.

REFERENCE

1. World Health Organization. www.who.int/mental_health/management/depression/definition/en/index1.html. Accessed January 31, 2010.

CASE SUMMARY

- The patient's clinical picture is consistent with MDD, and an antidepressant medication should be used.

- Sertraline 50 mg is a reasonable initial dose, but the dose needed is to be maximized to a therapeutic dose, especially in the case of partial response.

- Tricyclic antidepressants are one of the treatments of choice for chronic migraine and should be considered in patients who need treatment for both chronic migraine and depression.

For more information on the care plan and facilitator's guide please visit http://www.mhpharmacotherapy.com.

41 Bipolar Disorder

Brian L. Crabtree

CASE LEARNING OBJECTIVES

- Recognize the signs and symptoms of an acute manic episode and bipolar disorder
- Identify the goals of therapy for an acute manic episode and bipolar disorder
- Develop an appropriate treatment and monitoring plan for the pharmacotherapy of bipolar disorder using a specific patient presentation
- Educate a patient on taking medications for bipolar disorder

PATIENT PRESENTATION

Chief Complaint

"My mind's going too fast."

History of Present Illness

Lisa W. is a 34-year-old woman who has been admitted to a public psychiatric hospital. She was brought to the hospital by her husband after she stopped sleeping, would stay up all night praying, could not be redirected, and would say simply, "I am communicating with God." The husband reports Lisa had become more agitated during the past week with rapid speech, irritability, and now bizarre ideas about special powers and abilities. He indicates that "she explodes, anything sets her off, she was talking to people who are not there." She has poor insight into why she was brought to the hospital, but states, "I have problems with nerves and I don't sleep." She is seen on team rounds by a psychiatrist, nurse, pharmacist, psychologist, and social worker.

Past Medical History

Lisa had all of the usual childhood illnesses.

She has a history of psychiatric illness with four hospitalizations dating to 1990, but this is the first admission to this hospital and none of the previous records are immediately available. She is followed on an outpatient basis at a community mental health center.

She has a history of HTN. The husband reports that the patient had "low blood" on her previous medication and this was one reason she stopped taking it.

Family History

Father healthy, except HTN, well controlled on medication. Mother has depression, takes paroxetine. She has three siblings, two brothers and one sister. One brother is alcoholic. She has no children.

Social History

Married, lives with husband. Unemployed; worked previously as a checkout clerk at a supermarket, but has not worked in over a year. High school graduate, but has difficulty with reading and writing. Receives supplemental security income payments and supported by husband. Receives Medicaid coverage. No pending legal problems. No special diet. No regular exercise program.

Tobacco/Alcohol/Substance Use

Occasional binge-drinking episodes. Smokes 1 ppd with approximately 20 pack-year history. Denies illicit substances. Drinks several cups of caffeinated coffee daily.

Allergies/Intolerances/Adverse Drug Events

Diazepam (nausea and vomiting after injection) during a previous hospitalization.

Medications

Paroxetine 20 mg PO daily × 3 months, started during previous hospitalization

Clonazepam 0.5 mg PO three times daily × 3 months, started during previous hospitalization

HCTZ 25 mg PO daily × 4 years

Acetaminophen 500 mg PO as needed, about twice weekly

Previously treated with olanzapine 20 mg PO at bedtime, divalproex 750 mg PO twice daily, stopped approximately 3 months prior to current admission. Denies other prescription and nonprescription medication

Denies herbal or other complementary and alternative therapies

Review of Systems

The patient states she feels "energized" and is impatient with people who do not listen to her ideas. (−) Headaches or dizziness, but states dizziness was a problem when she was taking divalproex. No history of asthma or other lung disease. Says she had a TB skin test recently, but does not know results. (−) Chest pain, palpitations, or heart disease other than HTN. Appetite has been less lately. "I don't need to eat. God will provide." Denies weight loss. (−) Genitourinary complaints. Says some of the medications interfere with her sex drive. Has regular menses. (−) History of sexually transmitted diseases. (−) Neuromuscular complaints. Says "strength is getting better every day."

Physical Examination

▶ General

Well-developed, well-nourished Caucasian female in no acute distress; appears stated age, disheveled, and mildly obese

▶ Vital Signs

BP 154/105 mm Hg sitting, P 102, RR 22, T 97.9°F (36.6°C)

Weight 197 lb (89.5 kg)

Height 66 in. (168 cm)

Denies pain

▶ Skin

Unremarkable

▶ HEENT

PERRLA, EOMI, periorbital bruising apparent, husband says she struck herself; discs sharp, AV nicking noted; TMs normal, normal hearing to conversational volume; several missing teeth, poor oral hygiene

▶ Neck and Lymph Nodes

Supple; (−) thyromegaly, JVD, or lymphadenopathy

▶ Chest

Clear to auscultation

▶ Breasts

No tenderness, no lumps or masses, no discharge

▶ Cardiovascular

Tachycardia, RRR, no murmurs, rubs, or gallops

▶ Abdomen

Nontender, nondistended, (+) bowel sounds, (−) hepatosplenomegaly

▶ Neurology

Mental status—behavior is childlike, mood is elevated and irritable, affect is animated; speech is loud and pressured; thoughts indicate flight of ideas, looseness of associations, ideas of reference, delusions; reports she feels others plot against her because of jealousy over her superior intellectual and physical powers and her ability to receive special messages from God; denies auditory and visual hallucinations; denies suicidal and homicidal ideas; alert and oriented to person, year, not place; shows deficits in long- and short-term memory; concentration poor; judgment poor; insight poor.

Cranial nerves II to XII grossly intact; normal gait; (−) nystagmus, facial weakness, tremor; DTRs normal.

▶ Genitourinary

Deferred

▶ Rectal

Deferred

Laboratory Tests

Urine for toxicology collected the day of hospital admission; ECG and blood obtained fasting at 6:30 AM day after admission.

	Conventional Units	SI Units
Na	137 mEq/L	137 mmol/L
K	3.5 mEq/L	3.5 mmol/L
Cl	100 mEq/L	100 mmol/L
CO_2	24 mEq/L	24 mmol/L
BUN	12 mg/dL	4.3 mmol/L
SCr	0.9 mg/dL	80 μmol/L
Glu	108 mg/dL	6.0 mmol/L
Mg	1.6 mEq/L	0.80 mmol/L
Ca	10.2 mg/dL	2.55 mmol/L
Phos	3.8 mg/dL	1.23 mmol/L
Total protein	7.7 g/dL	77 g/L
Albumin	4.2 g/dL	42 g/L
ALT	54 IU/L	0.90 μkat/L
AST	48 IU/L	0.80 μkat/L
TSH	0.97 μIU/mL	0.97 mIU/L
Total cholesterol	168 mg/dL	4.34 mmol/L
Triglycerides	72 mg/dL	0.81 mmol/L
HDL cholesterol	35 mg/dL	0.91 mmol/L
LDL cholesterol	119 mg/dL	3.08 mmol/L
Serum pregnancy test	(−)	
RBC	$5.3 \times 10^6/mm^3$	$5.3 \times 10^{12}/L$
WBC	$9.7 \times 10^3/mm^3$	$9.7 \times 10^9/L$

Hgb	15.9 g/dL	9.87 mmol/L (159 g/L)
Hct	46.7%	0.467
MCV	88 μm³	88 fL
MCH	29 pg	
Platelets	283 × 10³/mm³	283 × 10⁹/L

Urinalysis

Glucose	(–)
Ketone	Trace +
pH	5.5
Specific gravity	1.013
Protein	1+
Blood	(–)

Toxicology screen

Cannabinoids	(–)
Opiates	(–)
Phencyclidine	(–)
Amphetamines	(–)
Cocaine	(–)
Benzodiazepines	(+)
Other substances	(+) cotinine

ECG

Sinus tachycardia, otherwise normal

Assessment

Bipolar I disorder, most recent episode was manic, with psychotic features; hx of HTN

Student Workup

Missing Information?

Evaluate: Patient Database
Drug Therapy Problems
Care Plan (by Problem)

TARGETED QUESTIONS

1. What signs and symptoms of bipolar disorder does this patient have?
   Hint: See pp. 670–672 in PPP

2. What prescribed or nonprescribed drugs could be exacerbating this patient's illness?
   Hint: See Table 39-3 in PPP

3. What is the purpose of the laboratory examination?
   Hint: See Table 39-1 in PPP

4. Should drug therapy be initiated with mood-stabilizing monotherapy, antipsychotic drug monotherapy, or mood-stabilizing and antipsychotic drug combination therapy?
   Hint: See Table 39-2 in PPP

5. What risks of drug therapy would you discuss with this patient when she is appropriate for patient education?
   Hint: See Table 39-4 in PPP

FOLLOW-UP

6. Drug therapy is initiated with the combination of lithium, titrated to a dosage of 900 mg PO at bedtime and a serum concentration of 1.02 mEq/L (1.02 mmol/L), aripiprazole 20 mg PO at bedtime, and clonazepam 2 mg PO twice daily. The clonazepam is tapered and discontinued prior to hospital discharge. She is continued on HCTZ 25 mg PO daily, and amlodipine 5 mg PO daily is added. She responded well to this regimen, but experienced polyuria, including bothersome nocturia, and a mild tremor. The polyuria improved with consolidating lithium to single-daily dosing instead of divided dosing. The tremor was treated with the addition of propranolol 10 mg PO twice daily. Her hospital discharge drug therapy regimen was lithium 900 mg PO at bedtime, aripiprazole 20 mg PO at bedtime, HCTZ 25 mg PO in the morning, and amlodipine 5 mg PO in the morning. She was counseled to moderate her caffeine intake. Her length of stay in the hospital was 17 days. After 6 months, still feeling well with a generally euthymic mood state, she and her husband are interested in starting a family. During a routine outpatient follow-up visit, she asks about the risks of medications for bipolar disorder and pregnancy. How should she be advised about this issue?
   Hint: See p. 686 in PPP

☉ GLOBAL PERSPECTIVE

The assessment and treatment of bipolar disorder has been largely standardized through the use of common diagnostic criteria and widely available mood-stabilizing and antipsychotic medication. In all countries, financial considerations influence the choice of treatment. Hospital care may not be readily available and length of stay restricted. In rural or poorly developed regions where access to frequent outpatient follow-up may be limited, use of medications with a narrow therapeutic index, such as lithium or drugs that require regular laboratory monitoring, may be less practical. Additionally, although this case presents as a patient experiencing a manic episode, her history indicates a likely prior history of depressive episodes. Epidemiologic data indicate that depressive episodes are more common than manic episodes, in both bipolar disorders I and II. Although research data sometimes conflict, activation of manic episodes by antidepressant drugs may be a risk, as may have happened in this patient's case, and appears as a risk in prescribing information for antidepressant drugs. Teratogenic risks of drug therapy during pregnancy are significant, especially with antiepileptic mood-stabilizing drugs and, to a lesser extent, with lithium. Careful education of the patient about risks and benefits and whether pregnancy is planned or unplanned is an important consideration. The judgment about continuing or stopping drug therapy will be influenced by these factors, the history of the individual patient, and the risk to the fetus in the medicated versus unmedicated condition.

CASE SUMMARY

- This patient's clinical presentation and history are consistent with bipolar disorder I in a manic episode.
- Treatment with mood-stabilizing and antipsychotic medication is appropriate for the acute manic episode. Maintenance therapy may attempt consolidating to mood-stabilizing monotherapy, but research supports reduced relapse with continued combination therapy.
- Antidepressant therapy should be avoided if possible in this patient as she appears to have a history of a pharmacologically induced mood switch.
- Treatment of bipolar disorder during pregnancy must balance the risks of exposure of prescribed drugs to the developing fetus with the risks of relapse of bipolar disorder if not adequately treated. Antiepileptic mood-stabilizing drugs such as divalproex and carbamazepine carry the greatest teratogenic risks.

For more information on the care plan and facilitator's guide please visit http://www.mhpharmacotherapy.com.

42 Anxiety

Sheila R. Botts

CASE LEARNING OBJECTIVES

- List common presenting symptoms of panic disorder (PD)
- Identify the desired therapeutic outcomes for patients with PD
- Discuss appropriate lifestyle modifications and over-the-counter medication use
- Recommend psychotherapy and pharmacotherapy interventions for patients with PD
- Develop a monitoring plan for anxiety patients placed on specific medications
- Educate patients about their disease state and appropriate lifestyle modifications, psychotherapy, and pharmacotherapy for effective treatment

PATIENT PRESENTATION

Chief Complaint

"I think I'm going crazy. I get this tightness in my chest, my heart races and I feel like I am going to die."

History of Present Illness

Angela Brown is a 32-year-old woman who presents to her primary care physician complaining of sudden episodes of fearfulness accompanied by a tightening in her chest and intense anxiety. During these episodes, she has heart palpitations, nausea, sweating, and a fear "that I'm going to die." They "just come out of nowhere" and last 10 to 15 minutes. She reports experiencing two to three episodes a week for the past few months. She recalls having her first episode like this approximately 3 years ago after the death of her father. Over the past 6 to 8 months they have increased in frequency and intensity. She has gone to the emergency department twice in the past 6 months as she felt something was wrong with her heart, but was told her heart was fine and it was probably stress. Her "ECG and blood tests" were normal. She was given a prescription for diazepam 5 mg PO as needed and told that she should schedule an appointment with her regular physician.

She reports worrying a lot about her job, finances, children, and health. She reports feeling sad, irritable, and tense, and has difficulty sleeping. She is very fearful of having another episode and has started to avoid places like Walmart and the mall, where these have occurred. She has difficulty attending after-school events where "everyone is in the gymnasium and I'm afraid I can't get out." She called in sick the day of the holiday performance but fears she will be in trouble at work if this continues.

Past Medical History

Migraine headaches diagnosed 5 years ago

Depression 3 years ago following father's death; resolved with psychotherapy

Family History

Father died at age 54 in a MVA. Mother diagnosed stage 1 breast cancer 14 months ago, s/p lumpectomy with good prognosis. She has one sister who has "anxiety" and is on citalopram.

Social/Work History

Grew up in northern Kentucky with both parents and one younger sibling. College graduate with a degree in secondary education. Currently, employed as an art teacher at the local high school. Happily married with a 2-year-old daughter. Few social activities outside of work.

Tobacco/Alcohol/Substance use

Drinks two to three glasses of wine each evening to relax and help with sleep. Denies tobacco or illicit substance use. Avoids caffeine.

Allergy/Intolerance/Adverse Event History

Fluoxetine (was started on 20 mg daily for depressive episode 3 years ago; stopped after three doses due to extreme agitation and anxiety)

Medications (Current)

Zolmitriptan 2.5 mg PO PRN for migraine headaches

Diazepam 5 mg PO PRN anxiety

Ibuprofen 400 mg PO PRN headache, menstrual pain

Multivitamin with iron PO daily

Review of Systems

Frequent nonmigraine-type headaches relieved by ibuprofen; migraine headaches two to three per month; soreness in the jaw, which she attributes to grinding her teeth; muscle ache in shoulders

Physical Examination

▶ **General**

Mildly anxious 32-year-old woman in no acute distress

▶ **Vital Signs**

BP 118/76 mm Hg, P 88, RR 18, T 37.1°C

Weight 145 lb (65.9 kg)

Height 65 in. (165 cm)

Denies pain

▶ **Skin**

(−) Rashes or lesions

▶ **HEENT**

PERRLA, EOMI; normal fundi; TMs appear normal

▶ **Neck and Lymph Nodes**

Supple, thyroid normal size without nodules; (−) adenopathy

▶ **Chest**

Clear to auscultation

▶ **Breasts**

Examination deferred

▶ **Cardiovascular**

Tachycardia, normal S_1, S_2

▶ **Abdomen**

Not tender/not distended; (−) organomegaly

▶ **Neurology**

Grossly intact; mild tremor in hands; DTRs normal

Mental Status Examination

A 32-year-old cooperative, casually dressed, well-groomed female. Appears anxious and has moderate psychomotor agitation. Speech normal in rate and volume. Mood "worried" and "sometimes sad," affect congruent to mood. No apparent delusions or hallucinations. Denies suicidal or homicidal ideation. Appears to have good attention and concentration.

▶ **Genitourinary**

Examination deferred

▶ **Rectal**

Examination deferred

Laboratory Tests

	Conventional Units	SI Units
Na	142 mEq/L	142 mmol/L
K	4.1 mEq/L	4.1 mmol/L
Cl	100 mEq/L	100 mmol/L
CO_2	24 mEq/L	24 mmol/L
BUN	10 mg/dL	3.6 mmol/L
SCr	0.7 mg/dL	62 μmol/L
Glu	98 mg/dL	5.4 mmol/L
AST	22 IU/L	0.37 μkat/L
ALT	28 IU/L	0.47 μkat/L
Alk phos	40 IU/L	0.67 μkat/L
Hgb	14.5 g/dL	9.00 mmol/L (145 g/L)
Hct	42%	0.42
WBC	$6.8 \times 10^3/mm^3$	$6.8 \times 10^9/L$
Albumin	3.8 g/dL	38 g/L
TSH	1.2 μIU/mL	1.2 mIU/L
Total cholesterol	178 mg/dL	4.60 mmol/L
LDL cholesterol	89 mg/dL	2.30 mmol/L
HDL cholesterol	36 mg/dL	0.93 mmol/L
Urine pregnancy test	(−)	
Urine drug screen	(+) benzodiazepine	
ECG	Sinus tachycardia	

Assessment

PD with agoraphobia

Student Workup

Missing Information?

Evaluate: Patient Database

Drug Therapy Problems

Care Plan (by Problem)

TARGETED QUESTIONS

1. What signs and symptoms of PD does this patient have?

   Hint: See p. 700 in PPP

2. What nonpharmacologic interventions might be useful for this patient?

   Hint: See p. 700 in PPP

3. Why is an antidepressant the drug therapy of choice in PD?

   Hint: See pp. 700–701 in PPP

4. What adverse effects of therapy would you discuss with this patient?

   Hint: See pp. 700–701 in PPP

5. What if this patient fails the first choice of antidepressant treatment?

   Hint: When initial SSRI therapy fails, it is reasonable to try another SSRI or SNRI antidepressant (e.g., venlafaxine XR). Cognitive behavioral therapy (CBT) may also be considered and is expected to result in similar outcomes as medication treatment during acute treatment. CBT combined with antidepressant therapy is associated with the greatest improvement during continuation treatment (e.g., beyond 6 mo). See p. 702 in PPP

FOLLOW-UP

6. The patient returns 8 weeks later and reports a significant reduction in panic attacks, but she still worries she will have another one. She continues to avoid shopping malls and Walmart. What is the expected time frame for improvement in anticipatory anxiety and phobic avoidance? How long should the patient be maintained on drug therapy for her PD?

   Hint: See p. 702 in PPP

○ GLOBAL PERSPECTIVE

Treatment guidelines for PD are similar worldwide to that used in the United States. Culture is expected to play a role in clinical presentation of panic symptoms and should be considered when individualizing CBT. Panic symptoms are reported in other cultures but not always referred to as "panic." For example, Cambodian and Vietnamese cultures often refer to panic as "sore neck" and "wind overload" respectively. In the United States, African Americans seem to have a higher prevalence of agoraphobia and are more likely to seek treatment in primary care settings.

CASE SUMMARY

- The patient's clinical presentation includes panic attacks, anticipatory anxiety, and agoraphobic avoidance resulting in functional impairment, and treatment should be initiated.

- SSRI antidepressants reduce panic attack frequency and severity, anticipatory anxiety, and agoraphobia. Initial doses should be much lower than that used in depression but titrated to a similar target daily dose.

- Antidepressant therapy should be continued for at least 1 year after achieving response to minimize the risk of relapse.

For more information on the care plan and facilitator's guide please visit http://www.mhpharmacotherapy.com.

43 Sleep Disorders

Amy M. Lugo   Amy L. Stump

CASE LEARNING OBJECTIVES

- Recommend and optimize appropriate sleep hygiene and nonpharmacologic therapies for the management and prevention of sleep disorders
- Recommend and optimize appropriate pharmacotherapy for sleep disorders
- Describe the components of a monitoring plan to assess safety and efficacy of pharmacotherapy for common sleep disorders
- Educate patients about preventive behavior, appropriate lifestyle modifications, and drug therapy required for effective treatment and control of sleep disorders

PATIENT PRESENTATION

Chief Complaint

"I'm so tired, can't talk right, feel shaky and my arms and legs don't want to work."

History of Present Illness

Miriam Weber is a 61-year-old woman who presents to the pharmacotherapy clinic complaining of feeling tired, uncoordinated, shaky, anxious, and mentally "foggy" for the past 4 days. In addition, she states that her speech has become slurred, which prompted her to go to the ED earlier today. At the ED, she was told to make an appointment with her regular physician as there were no urgent problems identified, but she has no medical insurance and typically receives all of her care and medications from the local free clinic, which is not open until tomorrow. On hearing of the situation, the physician in charge of the free clinic directed her to you for a medication evaluation. She presents with her husband and a basket full of medications. She asks you if you can recommend something for her to take for sleep. She has been taking a new medication, amitriptyline, for the past week and it does not seem to be working as she still cannot fall asleep at night.

Past Medical History

Hypothyroidism

GERD

Depression

HTN

Gastritis/duodenitis

Migraine headache

Insomnia

Past Surgical History

Total hysterectomy 20 years ago

Family History

Father had a history of DM and stroke. Mother has unknown cancer. Brother has "kidney problems" and alcoholism.

Social History

The patient is married and lives with and cares for her disabled husband and son as well as her elderly mother. She is currently unemployed. Family income consists of social security benefits from husband, son, and mother. She has no medical or prescription drug insurance.

Tobacco/Alcohol/Substance Use

(−) Tobacco and alcohol; (+) methamphetamine, patient has not used in 10 years after going through rehabilitation program.

Allergies/Intolerances/Adverse Drug Events

Cephalexin—hives; Latex—rash

Medications (Current)

Citalopram 20 mg PO daily

Amitriptyline 25 mg PO q hs

Estradiol 1 mg PO daily

Quinapril 20 mg PO daily

HCTZ 25 mg PO daily

Levothyroxine 100 mcg PO daily

Rizatriptan 10 mg PO PRN headache

Dicyclomine 20 mg PO daily

Review of Systems

Complains of fatigue and sleep disorder; (−) fever and sweats; (−) chest pain, racing heart, or light-headedness; (−) cough and SOB; (+) falling down, poor balance, disturbances in coordination, tremors, and slurred speech; (−) fainting, seizures, and numbness; (+) anxiety; (−) depressed mood; (−) nocturia, urinary urgency, and urinary frequency.

Physical Examination

▶ General

Well-developed patient in mild distress, unkempt, noticeable slurred speech, looks older than stated age

▶ Vital Signs

BP 117/73 mm Hg, P 86, RR 20, T 36.9°C

Weight 185 lb (84 kg)

Height 62 in. (157 cm)

Denies pain

▶ Skin

No clubbing, cyanosis, edema, or lesions noted

▶ HEENT

PERRLA, pupils slightly enlarged; EOMI; dry oral mucosa

▶ Neck and Lymph Nodes

No thyromegaly

▶ Chest

Lungs clear to auscultation bilaterally

▶ Breasts

Examination deferred

▶ Cardiovascular

RRR, no murmurs, rubs, or gallops

▶ Abdomen

Examination deferred

▶ Neurology

(+) Ataxia; no hyperreflexia noted

▶ Genitourinary

Examination deferred

▶ Rectal

Examination deferred

Laboratory Tests

From her ED visit this morning

	Conventional Units	SI Units
Na	137 mEq/L	137 mmol/L
K	4.2 mEq/L	4.2 mmol/L
Cl	105 mEq/L	105 mmol/L
CO_2	22 mEq/L	22 mmol/L
BUN	18 mg/dL	6.4 mmol/L
SCr	0.82 mg/dL	72 mmol/L
Glu	104 mg/dL	5.8 mmol/L
WBC	$6.6 \times 10^3/mm^3$	$6.6 \times 10^9/L$
Hgb	14.2 g/dL	8.81 mmol/L (142 g/L)
Hct	42.6%	0.426
Plt	$428 \times 10^3/mm^3$	$428 \times 10^9/L$
MCV	$84 \mu m^3$	84 fL
TSH	0.05 μIU/mL	0.05 mIU/L
Acetaminophen	<1 mcg/mL	<7 μmol/L
Salicylate	<4 mcg/mL	<0.03 mmol/L
Ethanol	<10 mg/dL	<2.2 mmol/L
Urine drug screen	(−)	

Assessment

Sixty-one-year-old female with signs, symptoms, and laboratory tests consistent with possible anticholinergic delirium due to initiation of amitriptyline for insomnia

Student Workup

Missing Information?

Evaluate: Patient Database

Drug Therapy Problems

Care Plan (by Problem)

TARGETED QUESTIONS: COMORBID INSOMNIA

1. What signs and symptoms of anticholinergic delirium does this patient have?

   Hint: Older patients are much more susceptible to the anticholinergic effects of medications.[1] Pharmacists can play a key role in recognizing these drug-induced problems and preventing the addition of a new drug to the patient's regimen to treat the adverse effect. See p. 480 in PPP

2. Why is amitriptyline the most likely cause of anticholinergic delirium in this patient?

   Hint: See pp. 714–715 in PPP

3. What medication would be the best choice to recommend for this patient to treat her insomnia?

   Hint: See Table 41-2 in PPP

4. How might you counsel this patient on nonpharmacologic management of her insomnia?

   Hint: See Table 41-1 in PPP

FOLLOW-UP

5. Two weeks later, the patient returns for follow-up. She feels "back to normal," with no tremor, slurred speech, or coordination problems. However, she is still having trouble falling asleep. She has not taken anything for sleep since her last physician visit because she is scared that she will have another adverse effect to the medication. The patient wishes to use an OTC or herbal product to help her sleep, stating that she feels they are safer because they are not as strong as prescription medications. How will you respond to the patient? What OTC or herbal product(s), if any, would you tell her not to use? What product(s), if any, would you recommend?

   Hint: See p. 715 in PPP

⟳ GLOBAL PERSPECTIVE

Melatonin is a naturally occurring endogenous hormone produced by the pineal gland. Exogenous melatonin has been shown to help regulate circadian rhythm sleep disorders. Many travelers experience a circadian rhythm disorder, commonly known as jet lag. When traveling across time zones, the traveler's sleep–wake cycle becomes out of sync with the time of day. Jet lag severity is determined by direction of travel (traveling east is often worse than traveling west), age of the traveler, and number of time zones crossed. Manipulating factors such as exposure to bright light, social contact, and activity are nonpharmacologic options to improve jet lag. Supplementing with 3 to 5 mg of exogenous melatonin hormone 30 minutes prior to the local bedtime can expedite sleep–cycle normalization.

CASE SUMMARY

- The patient is experiencing anticholinergic adverse effects likely due to the addition of amitriptyline to her medication regimen for the treatment of insomnia. All anticholinergic medications should be discontinued (amitriptyline and dicyclomine).

- A thorough sleep history should be taken from the patient and she should be counseled about nonpharmacologic treatments for insomnia.

- Product selection for sleep aids, both prescription and OTC, should be made with care. Patient-specific factors such as age, comorbid conditions, concomitant medications, and pharmacoeconomic issues should be considered.[1]

REFERENCE

1. Fick DM, Cooper JW, Wade WE, Waller JL, Maclean RJ, Beers MH. Updating the Beers criteria for potentially inappropriate medication use in older adults. Arch Intern Med 2003 163:2716–2724.

For more information on the care plan and facilitator's guide please visit http://www.mhpharmacotherapy.com.

44 Attention Deficit/ Hyperactivity Disorder

John Erramouspe   Nicole A. Baker
Kevin W. Cleveland

CASE LEARNING OBJECTIVES

- Recognize the signs and symptoms of attention deficit/hyperactivity disorder (ADHD) that respond to therapy
- Select appropriate stimulant preparations for a patient with ADHD displaying an adverse effect to another stimulant preparation
- Propose ways of improving the effectiveness and/or minimizing the cost of medications used for ADHD and other common comorbid childhood problems (i.e., encopresis/constipation, sleep latency problems, allergic rhinitis, and asthma)
- Recommend an appropriate monitoring plan for stimulant therapy on the basis of individual patient characteristics and past adverse side-effect profile
- Properly educate a patient taking stimulants for ADHD therapy

PATIENT PRESENTATION

Chief Complaint

"I still have this rash where I stick my Daytrana patch. Using my hay fever spray before I stick on the patch helps a lot but my mom says it is getting kind of expensive."

History of Present Illness

Rev Williams is a 12½-year-old male who presents with his mother to the pediatrician's clinic office for a refill request of Nasonex. His mother works as a receptionist at an adult medicine clinic in a neighboring town. One month ago, after reading a magazine advertisement for Daytrana and talking with various medical staff at her clinic, she requested that her pediatrician switch RW from Vyvanse to the patch. Her reasons for switching were that RW was a little more fidgety on Vyvanse (although this was tolerable), to take advantage of the flexibility in dosing of Daytrana according to her son's schedule, and that Daytrana costs about the same as Vyvanse. She incurs the same monthly $50 co-pay for both ADHD medications since they both are available only as brand-name and nonpreferred tier 3 agents on her current prescription insurance plan. RW was switched to Daytrana and soon afterward began manifesting a bumpy red rash with slight swelling at the application site. RW's mother began applying Nasonex (also nonpreferred tier 3 agent on RW's prescription plan with a $50 co-pay) to her son's application site for the patch as a temporary measure until she could talk to her pediatrician. RW just finished the sixth grade and did very well in his charter school. His teacher says he has a high IQ, is on task, finishes his work quickly, and might benefit from the gifted program. Since beginning stimulant therapy over the last 4½ years (Ritalin LA → Concerta → Vyvanse → Daytrana + methylphenidate PRN), there has been a marked decrease in his level of forgetfulness (e.g., homework and lunchbox), aggressiveness, temper tantrums, anger, frustration, and in hitting and kicking fellow classmates. Prior to stimulant therapy, RW hated to read but now has acquired a desire to read after years of treatment for ADHD and continues to read avidly at almost a ninth-grade level. His favorite class is physical education, especially when they play soccer. This occurs the first hour of the day, immediately after arriving at school. He will be changing to a public junior high school next year due to his parents' desire to increase his range of friends. RW feels like he presently has a sufficient number of friends but seems okay with this change. Some teachers have noted a slight oddity to his behavior and social interactions. He feels like his mood is fine and things are going well within his family. RW states that Daytrana helps him focus and remember better and that the only side effect he has is the bumpy red rash with slight swelling, but that Nasonex has helped lessen this problem. He states that he takes an ADHD pill every weekday at about 5 PM, so he can complete his homework after dinner. RW's pediatrician contacts you, the pharmacist, and asks you if it is okay to continue both the Nasonex and the Daytrana as they are presently being used.

Past Medical History

ADHD for 4½ years

Encopresis/constipation for 8 years

Sleep problems (difficulty falling asleep)

Allergic rhinitis and mild asthma for 7 years

Migraine headache with aura in last month

Chest pain occurred at 9 years (likely musculoskeletal in origin and not cardiac per pediatric cardiologist)—resolved

Sporadic high blood pressure on three occasions at 6 to 8 years—resolved

Nummular eczema on shoulder at 4 years—resolved following use of Eucerin and triamcinolone 0.025% cream for 1 month

Secondarily infected molluscum contagiosum at 4 years—resolved

Meatal stenosis at 4 years—surgically resolved with meatotomy and cystoscopy

Family History

Biological parents are alive and healthy. Mother has migraines and father displays inattentiveness concurrent with ADHD but has never been medically evaluated for ADHD. RW has a biological 8-year-old sister who is comanaged by RW's pediatrician and a pediatric psychologist for ADHD (on Concerta).

Social History

Lives with biological parents (married) and younger sister. Presently attends a charter school, but will be changing to a public junior high school next year in an effort to increase his range of friends.

Tobacco/Alcohol/Substance Use

None

Allergies/Intolerances/Adverse Drug Events

Daytrana—rash (local contact rash vs. sensitivity?)

Medications (Current)

Daytrana 30 mg patch applied daily in the morning with breakfast at 7 AM (remove by 4 PM)

Methylphenidate 5 mg tablet PO in the late afternoon PRN

Lactulose 30 mL PO twice daily (RW does not like the sweet/syrupy taste and admits to frequently taking the product on a PRN basis due to taste and forgetfulness.)

Melatonex 3 mg tablet PO in the evening PRN

Zyrtec 5 mg tablet PO daily

Nasonex two sprays in each nostril once daily

Naproxen sodium 220 mg tablets, one to two tablet(s) PO initially and then one tablet q 8 h until migraine resolves (do not exceed three tablets per day)

Review of Systems

(−) Migraine or other headache symptoms since 1 month ago; (−) vision changes; (−) appetite problems, normal at breakfast, lunch, and dinner (feels hungrier around bedtime), weight is stable; (+) chronic constipation symptoms with infrequent, slightly hard, mildly painful bowel movements every other day; minimal to no complaints of pruritus with rash; (+) difficulty falling asleep often until midnight (plays Pokémon and watches television in his bedroom following completion of homework until he feels sleepy enough to fall asleep); denies any inability to concentrate on school assignment while at school.

Physical Examination

▶ *General*

Well-appearing 12½-year-old male who is not very interested in talking with the pediatrician today

▶ *Vital Signs*

BP 110/70 mm Hg, P 85, RR 16, T 37°C

Weight 94 lb (42.7 kg)

Height 61.4 in. (156 cm)

▶ *Skin*

Faint circumferential erythematous raised rash on left hip where Daytrana patch was located from yesterday; same rash with slight swelling evident beneath patch located on right hip today

▶ *HEENT*

Normocephalic, atraumatic, tympanic membranes and oropharynx WNL, conjunctivae clear

▶ *Neck and Lymph Nodes*

Supple without lymphadenopathy

▶ *Chest*

Clear to auscultation bilaterally

▶ *Cardiovascular*

Heart: RRR without murmurs

Extremities: Normal pulses

▶ **Abdomen**

Soft, nontender without hepatosplenomegaly

▶ **Neurology**

WNL

▶ **Genitourinary**

Normal Tanner stage III male, both testes descended

▶ **Rectal**

Examination deferred

Laboratory Tests

Last assessed at 9 years of age when evaluated by pediatric cardiologist

	Conventional Units	SI Units
Na	140 mEq/L	140 mmol/L
K	4.2 mEq/L	4.2 mmol/L
Cl	100 mEq/L	100 mmol/L
Total CO$_2$	28 mEq/L	28 mmol/L
BUN	14 mg/dL	5.0 mmol/L
SCr	0.7 mg/dL	62 μmol/L
Glu	101 mg/dL	5.6 mmol/L
Ca	9.6 mg/dL	2.40 mmol/L
Mg	1.9 mEq/L	0.95 mmol/L
Phosphate	4.1 mg/dL	1.32 mmol/L
Hgb	13.1 g/dL	8.13 mmol/L (131 g/L)
Hct	39.0%	0.390
WBC	9.1 × 10^3/mm^3	9.1 × 10^9/L
MCV	83 μm^3	83 fL
Albumin	4.5 g/dL	45 g/L
TSH	1.9 μIU/mL	1.9 mIU/L
Free T$_4$	1.07 ng/dL	13.8 pmol/L
Total cholesterol	161 mg/dL	4.16 mmol/L
LDL cholesterol	94 mg/dL	2.43 mmol/L
HDL cholesterol	55 mg/dL	1.42 mmol/L

Assessment

A 12½-year-old preadolescent male with probable local Daytrana-induced contact dermatitis

Student Workup

Missing Information?

Evaluate: Patient Database

Drug Therapy Problems

Care Plan (by Problem)

TARGETED QUESTIONS

1. What signs and symptoms of ADHD has this patient manifested in the past and which ones does he presently display that may respond to stimulant therapy?

   Hint: See pp. 724–725 in PPP

2. Why are stimulants the treatment of choice for most patients with ADHD?

   Hint: See p. 725 in PPP

3. What adverse effects of stimulant therapy would you discuss with this patient and his parent(s) and what remedies would you offer to decrease them?

   Hint: See Table 42-3 in PPP

4. If this patient was to be switched from Daytrana to a different stimulant formulation, what should it be?

   Hint: The patient probably does not require a stimulant preparation with both a rapid onset and an extended duration because his ADHD symptoms have been responding well to Daytrana (an extended-acting stimulant with slow onset) and his first class of the school day, physical education, may not require as much attentiveness as classes later in the school day. Therefore, a less expensive intermediate-acting stimlant might be the best replacement for Daytrana (see Table 42-4 in PPP). In the future, the patient's schedule could change so that more attention would be required earlier in the school day. A stimulant formulation with both rapid- and extended action might be necessary at this point.

5. Are any laxatives that are used chronically for children with encopresis more palatable and less frequently administered than lactulose?

   Hint: Many laxatives are considered to have an unpleasant taste by children and/or require dosing multiple times per day (e.g., lactulose, mineral oil, magnesium hydroxide, sorbitol 70%). Polyethylene glycol (PEG) 3350 (MiraLax) was approved as a prescription laxative in the United States in 1999 and subsequently changed to OTC in 2006. PEG 3350 is currently available both OTC and by prescription. Over the last decade it has been investigated in a variety of childhood constipation disorders and found to consistently have good outcomes. In some childhood studies, it has demonstrated greater efficacy than lactulose or improved tolerability compared to magnesium hydroxide.[1] Many providers consider PEG 3350 a preferred laxative for chronic use in children owing to the fact that it has no taste, can be mixed with a child's preferred beverage, and typically requires dosing only once daily.

6. Is there a preferred medication for treating ADHD children who have difficulty falling asleep despite proper adjustment of their stimulant therapy and an adequate trial of behavioral therapy?

   Hint: Benzodiazepines are frequently avoided in children with chronic sleep disorders due to concerns of excessive sedation and addiction. In randomized controlled trials of children with various sleep disorders, diphenhydramine and zolpidem were shown to have no difference from placebo.[2] Other newer nonbenzodiazepine hypnotics (i.e., zaleplon, eszopiclone, and ramelteon) have not been rigorously investigated in children.[2] Clonidine or guanfacine are sometimes added to existing stimulant therapy in an effort to facilitate proper nightime sleep and improve control of ADHD symptoms (see Table 42-3 in PPP). Melatonin has been shown to be effective in children with sleep problems and various comorbid problems including ADHD (e.g., learning difficulties, visual impairment, and neurodevelopmental disabilities).[2,3]

FOLLOW-UP

7. RW was switched to methylphenidate ER in the morning plus methylphenidate RR in the afternoon prior to 3 PM as needed for his ADHD. At 1-month follow-up, the local reaction he experienced with Daytrana has resolved and he continues to do well in school and in completing his homework. His transition to public school initially was somewhat traumatic due to some bullying behavior he encountered from one classmate. However, now he has established a group of three good friends who play soccer together and the bullying no longer occurs. His bowel function is much improved, and he has been faithfully adhering to laxative therapy on a daily basis and his stool pattern has become more normal with a daily soft bowel movement every morning just following breakfast. He does not like the new nasal spray quite as well as the Nasonex (says it causes his nose to bleed approximately once every couple of months). However, his hay fever symptoms remain adequately controlled. RW's mother is ecstatic about the savings in medications since she now incurs only a $5 co-pay for each methylphenidate prescription. What action, if any, would you take?

☯ GLOBAL PERSPECTIVE

ADHD is a behavioral disorder that affects up to 1 in 20 children in the United States. The predominance of American research into this disorder over the past 40 years has led to the impression that ADHD is largely an American disorder and much less prevalent elsewhere. This impression was reinforced by the perception that ADHD may stem from social and cultural factors that are most common in American society. However, another school of thought suggested that ADHD is a behavioral disorder common to children of many different races and societies worldwide, but that is not recognized by the medical community, perhaps due to confusion regarding its diagnosis and/or misconceptions regarding its adverse impact on children, their families, and society as a whole.

Studies performed in United States and non-United States populations suggest that the prevalence of ADHD is at least as high in many non-United States children as in United States children, with the highest prevalence rates being seen when using DSM-IV diagnostic criteria. Recognition that ADHD is not purely an American disorder and that the prevalence of this behavioral disorder in many countries is in the same range as that in the United States will have important implications for the psychiatric care of children. Although the treatment strategies and medication availability may differ among countries, most published ADHD treatment guidelines from Europe and other parts of the world show similar approaches to managing this disorder.[4]

CASE SUMMARY

- RW's current clinical picture is consistent with a probable local drug–induced contact dermatitis to Daytrana that is being mismanaged by continuance of the patch and misuse of the Nasonex.

- It is reasonable to replace Daytrana with a single 7 AM dose of generic methylphenidate extended release.

- The as-needed afternoon dose of methylphenidate regular-release 5 mg tablet should be continued but given no later than 3 PM in an effort to avoid possible drug-induced difficulties in falling asleep from the afternoon stimulant dose.

- RW's chronic laxative needs to be changed to a more palatable, less frequently administered preparation.

- RW's treatment of migraine with naproxen sodium is appropriate and should be continued. He does not yet require a maintenance medication.

REFERENCES

1. Candy D, Belsey J. Macrogol (polyethylene glycol) laxatives in children with functional constipation and faecal impaction: A systematic review. Arch Dis Child 2009 Feb 94(2):156–160.
2. Gringras P. When to use drugs to help sleep. Arch Dis Child 2008 Nov 93(11):976–981.
3. Sweis D. The uses of melatonin. Arch Dis Child Educ Pract Ed 2005 90:ep74–ep77.
4. Faraone SV, Sergeant J, Gillberg C, Biederman J. The worldwide prevalence of ADHD: Is it an American condition? World Psychiatr 2003 2(2):104–113.

For more information on the care plan and facilitator's guide please visit http://www.mhpharmacotherapy.com.

45 Type 1 Diabetes/ Diabetic Ketoacidosis

Hanna Phan   Christopher J. Edwards

- Recognize the signs and symptoms of diabetic ketoacidosis (DKA)
- Identify the goals of therapy for the treatment of DKA and type 1 diabetes mellitus (T1DM)
- Develop an appropriate treatment and monitoring plan for DKA using individual patient characteristics
- Properly educate a patient newly diagnosed with T1DM to prevent possible future incidents of DKA

PATIENT PRESENTATION

Chief Complaint

"I've been vomiting for two days."

History of Present Illness

Jimmy D. Wilkinson is a 20-year-old Caucasian male university student with known T1DM who comes into the emergency department with a 2-day history of N/V. Two weeks ago, he noticed that he was drinking water and urinating more frequently than usual. He also mentions that recently he has been having some difficulty waking up in the morning and staying awake and alert throughout the day. These symptoms also began about 2 weeks ago and have gotten progressively worse. He mentions that he has been feeling "a bit down" since his last round of final examinations approximately 3 weeks ago. When asked about his insulin therapy, he states that he "has not felt like using it for a while." His came to the emergency department after he missed 2 days of school and work due to N/V. He states that he has not been able to eat or drink without vomiting for about 36 hours. He reports that he has not seen his home physician in 8 months, and he does not currently have a primary care provider on campus. He is currently insured through the university's campus insurance plan. He denies any recent history of weight loss, diarrhea, changes in vision, or dysuria.

Past Medical History

T1DM

Major depressive disorder

Seasonal allergic rhinitis

Tonsillectomy at age 4 years

Family History

Father is alive at age 43 and has a history of T1DM, hypertension, and hyperlipidemia. Uncle on father's side is alive at age 50 and has a history of T1DM and stroke. Grandfather on father's side died at age 63 of a myocardial infarction. He had a history of T1DM. Mother is alive at age 38 with a major depressive disorder and systemic lupus erythematous.

Social History

Currently a junior in college and has a part-time job at a book store.

Tobacco/Alcohol/Substance Use

Admits to occasional alcohol and marijuana use at social gatherings; denies use of tobacco and other illicit drugs.

Allergies/Intolerances/Adverse Drug Events

NKDA

Medications Prior to Admission

Loratadine 10 mg PO daily

Diphenhydramine 50 mg PO every 6 to 8 hours PRN allergies

Fluticasone one spray each nostril daily

Escitalopram 10 mg PO daily

Insulin glargine 20 units SC at bedtime

Insulin lispro 5 units SC with meals (e.g., three times a day)

Review of Systems

General: (−) fevers, chills, rigors, or weight loss

HEENT: (−) visual changes, diplopia, tinnitus, vertigo

Respiratory: (+) tachypnea; (−) SOB and cough

Cardiovascular: (−) rapid heartbeat or palpitations, chest pain

Gastrointestinal: (+) polydipsia, nausea, and vomiting; (−) abdominal pain

Genitourinary: (+) urinary frequency, urgency, polyuria; (−) dysuria

Musculoskeletal: (−) joint or muscle pain

Neurological: (+) fatigue; (−) HA, numbness, weakness, or tingling

Physical Examination

▶ General

Thin, healthy looking young male in no acute distress. Acetone breath noted during examination

▶ Vital Signs

BP 87/62, P 124, RR 27, T 37.2°C

Weight 139 lb (63.2 kg)

Height 68 in. (173 cm)

Denies pain

▶ Skin

Warm and dry, mild acne on face and back. No rashes, petechiae, ecchymosis, or jaundice

▶ HEENT

Normocephalic; PERRLA, EOMI intact; TMs benign bilaterally; oropharynx benign; mucous membranes dry

▶ Neck and Lymph Nodes

Supple; no thyroid nodules, lymphadenopathy, or carotid bruits; neck veins flat

▶ Chest

Breathing unlabored; mild tachypnea; breath sounds equal bilaterally; no wheezes, crackles, or rhonchi

▶ Cardiovascular

RRR, normal S_1, S_2; no S_3 or S_4 detected

▶ Abdomen

Nontender, nondistended; no organomegaly; bowel sounds present

▶ Neurology

No deficits appreciated

▶ Genitourinary

Examination deferred

▶ Rectal

Examination deferred

Laboratory Tests

Fasting, obtained on admission

	Conventional Units	SI Units
Na	130 mEq/L	130 mmol/L
K	3.0 mEq/L	3.0 mmol/L
Cl	104 mEq/L	104 mmol/L
HCO_3	11 mEq/L	11 mmol/L
BUN	40 mg/dL	14.3 mmol/L
SCr	1.5 mg/dL	133 μmol/L
Glu	550 mg/dL	30.5 mmol/L
Ca	9.3 mg/dL	2.33 mmol/L
Mg	2.1 mEq/L	1.05 mmol/L
Phosphate	2.0 mg/dL	0.65 mmol/L
Hgb	15.5 g/dL	9.62 mmol/L (155 g/L)
Hct	44.7%	0.447
WBC	$8.2 \times 10^3/mm^3$	$8.2 \times 10^9/L$
AST	29 IU/L	0.48 μkat/L
ALT	20 IU/L	0.33 μkat/L
Alk phos	516 IU/L	8.60 μkat/L
T bili	2 mg/dL	34.2 mmol/L
D bili	0.2 mg/dL	3.4 mmol/L
HbA_{1c}	10.3%	0.103

Venous blood gas

pH	7.17	
pCO_2	25 mm Hg	3.3 kPa
pO_2	58 mm Hg	7.7 kPa
Calculated HCO_3	9.1 mEq/L	9.1 mmol/L

Urinalysis	urine dark yellow	
pH	5	
Specific gravity	1.017	
White blood cells	(−)	
Nitrite	(−)	
Glucose	890 mg/dL	49.4 mmol/L
Ketone	150 mg/dL	14.7 mmol/L
Red blood cells	(−)	
Protein	(−)	

Assessment

The patient is a 20-year-old male with signs, symptoms, and laboratory tests consistent with DKA secondary to T1DM. He is currently awaiting treatment in a room in the emergency department. The nurse is currently placing a peripheral IV line.

Student Workup

Missing Information?

Evaluate:	Patient Database
	Drug Therapy Problems
	Care Plan (by Problem)

TARGETED QUESTIONS

1. What signs and symptoms of DKA does the patient have?

   Hint: See p. 756 in PPP

2. What happens at the cellular level when insulin is given to a patient with DKA?

   Hint: Consider how insulin treats hyperglycemia and how this may effect ketone production. See p. 756 in PPP

3. What electrolyte changes are likely to occur as the patient's blood glucose levels normalize following insulin therapy?

   Hint: Consider side effects of insulin and glucose metabolism end product. Also see pp. 756–757 and Table 43-11 in PPP

4. What potential adverse effects of insulin therapy during treatment of DKA and as part of T1DM maintenance therapy would you discuss with the patient?

   Hint: See pp. 756–757 in PPP

5. What long-term complications will be avoided with better glycemic control?

   Hint: See pp. 741–743 in PPP

FOLLOW-UP

6. Three months after the patient is discharged from the hospital, he returns to the emergency department. He states that has been feeling much better lately, until he became light-headed, tachycardic, and began to sweat profusely while working out in the gym earlier that day. He was found to have a blood glucose level of 54 mg/dL (3.0 mmol/L) on admission to the emergency department. What should be discussed with the patient to help him recognize, prevent, and treat hypoglycemia?

   Hint: See p. 756 in PPP

GLOBAL PERSPECTIVE

According to global statistics released in the 2007 edition of the International Diabetes Federation's *Diabetes Atlas*, there are 440,000 people younger than 14 years of age worldwide who have been diagnosed with T1DM.[1] This statistic is a fairly conservative estimate as data were not available from several countries. This study reports some interesting information regarding the global incidence of T1DM. The incidence rate seems to vary greatly among different populations. In parts of Asia, Central America, and South America, the incidence is as low as 4 cases per 100,000 in people younger than 14 years. In Scandinavia and some parts of Europe, the incidence is closer to 20 cases per 100,000 in people younger than 14 years. About 0.2% of people younger than 20 years in the United States of America have been diagnosed with T1DM.[2] The exact cause of T1DM is not fully understood. Current theories involve genetic predisposition for the disease coupled with viral-induced autoimmune response to insulin-producing β-cells.[3] These genetic and environmental factors may help to explain variations in the global incidence and prevalence of this disease.

REFERENCES

1. Daneman D. State of the world's children with diabetes. Pediatr Diabetes. 2009 10(2):120–126.
2. US Department of Health and Human Services. National Diabetes Statistics, 2007. National Diabetes Information Clearinghouse Web site. http://diabetes.niddk.nih.gov/DM/PUBS/statistics/. Accessed October 6, 2009.
3. Achenbach P, Bonifacio E, Koczwara K, Ziegler AG. Natural history of type 1 diabetes. Diabetes 2005 54: S25–S31.

CASE SUMMARY

- The patient's current clinical picture is consistent with DKA and he should be started on an insulin drip, with dextrose, fluid, and electrolyte replacement as needed.

- Care should be taken to avoid rapid fluctuations in serum electrolyte levels when correcting the patient's serum glucose level.

- The patient will require extensive education on diabetes, the proper use of insulin, and the importance of adherence with insulin therapy.

For more information on the care plan and facilitator's guide please visit http://www.mhpharmacotherapy.com.

46 Type 2 Diabetes Mellitus

Susan Cornell

CASE LEARNING OBJECTIVES

- Assess the signs and symptoms of hyperglycemia
- Differentiate diabetes-related complications
- Evaluate the goals of therapy for type 2 diabetes (T2DM) mellitus
- Develop an appropriate diabetes self-management education, treatment, and monitoring plan for a patient with T2DM and its related conditions

PATIENT PRESENTATION

Chief Complaint

"My physician told me I need to control my sugar better. I'm feeling okay, but I think I have another urinary infection. I am going to the bathroom more frequently and sometimes it burns. Will cranberry juice help?"

History of Present Illness

AL is a 36-year-old woman who presents to the community pharmacy/clinic complaining of frequent and burning urination. She reports having recurrent UTIs and vaginal yeast infections for the past 8 years, ever since the birth of her second child. She is adherent to her physician appointments every 3 months since she was diagnosed with T2DM 3 years ago. She is aware that her glucose and A_{1c} are not at goal and she needs to control her diabetes. She states that she takes her medications daily as prescribed and only misses an occasional dose. She checks her fasting blood glucose almost every day. She tries to monitor the amount and type of food she eats; but often "cheats," especially during tax season when she and her husband are very busy with their business. She walks 3 to 4 days per week for 20 to 30 minutes, depending on the weather. She denies any feelings of dizziness, lightheadedness, or fatigue.

Past Medical History

Dyslipidemia × 5 years

T2DM × 3 years

Obesity × 20 years

Recurrent UTI and yeast infections × 8 years

Gestational DM in two pregnancies (10 and 8 years ago)

Family History

Father had T2DM, dyslipidemia, and hypertension, and died from a myocardial infarction at the age of 56. Mother is alive at age 60 and has T2DM, dyslipidemia, sleep apnea, and GERD. Brother is alive at age 40 and has T2DM and HTN. Sister is alive at age 33 and is healthy.

Social History

She came to the United States from Puerto Rico at the age of 6, speaks Spanish and English. She is married for 13 years and lives with husband and two children aged 9 and 7. Works as an administrative assistant for her husband's accounting business. He is self-employed.

Tobacco/Alcohol/Substance Use

Social drinker (one to two glasses of wine two to three times per week); (−) tobacco or illicit drug use.

Allergies/Intolerances/Adverse Drug Events

No known drug or food allergies

Medications (Current)

Metformin 1,000 mg PO q 24 h (with dinner)

Atorvastatin 20 mg PO q 24 h (at bedtime)

ASA 81 mg PO q 24 h (with dinner)

Ortho Tri-Cyclen-28 PO q day (at bedtime)

Tylenol 500 mg PRN

Review of Systems

Occasional body aches relieved with acetaminophen. (+) Increased frequency and burning upon urination. (−) Vaginal discharge or dyspareunia; (−) tinnitus, vertigo, dizziness, lightheadedness, or fatigue. (+) Dry skin, minor bruises on (r) upper arm.

Physical Examination

▶ *General*

Well-appearing, young Hispanic woman in no acute distress

▶ *Vital Signs*

BP 136/78 mm Hg, P 68, RR 14, T 36.8°C

Weight 225.5 lb (102.5 kg)

Height 63 in. (160 cm)

BMI 5 kg/m²

Waist circumference 37 inch (94 cm)

Denies pain other than burning on urination

▶ *Skin*

Dry appearing skin, two visible bruises on right upper arm which patient states have been there for several weeks after "bumping into a door"

▶ *HEENT*

PERRLA, (−) sinus tenderness, TMs normal

▶ *Chest*

Clear to auscultation

▶ *Breast*

Examination deferred

▶ *Cardiovascular*

RRR, normal S_1, S_2, (−) S_3 or S_4

▶ *Abdomen*

Not tender/not distended; (−) organomegaly

▶ *Extremities*

No edema, (+) pedal pulses, (−) lesions or callus, (+) hair on first toe at the interphalangeal joint on both feet; normal monofilament examination bilaterally

▶ *Genitourinary*

Examination deferred

▶ *Rectal*

Examination deferred

Laboratory Tests

Fasting

	Conventional Units	SI Units
Na	137 mEq/L	137 mmol/L
K	4.7 mEq/L	4.7 mmol/L
Cl	101 mEq/L	101 mmol/L
CO_2	22 mEq/L	22 mmol/L
BUN	9 mg/dL	3.2 mmol/L
SCr	0.8 mg/dL	71 mmol/L
Glu	168 mg/dL	9.3 mmol/l
HbA_{1c}	8.2%	0.082
AST	22 U/L	0.37 μkat/L
ALT	44 U/L	0.73 μkat/L
Total cholesterol	184 mg/dL	4.76 mmol/L
LDL cholesterol	112 mg/dL	2.90 mmol/L
HDL cholesterol	29 mg/dL	0.75 mmol/L
Triglycerides	217 mg/dL	2.45 mmol/l
Hgb	13.5 g/dL	135 g/L; 8.38 mmol/L
Hct	37.7%	0.377
RBC	$4.47 \times 10^6/mm^3$	$4.47 \times 10^{12}/L$
WBC	$11.2 \times 10^3/mm^3$	$4.47 \times 10^9/L$
Platelets	$172 \times 10^3/mm^3$	$172 \times 10^9/L$

Urinalysis: Trace (+) protein, (−) heme, (+) nitrite, WBC 10–20/HPF

Assessment

Thirty-six-year old woman with obesity, T2DM and inadequate glycemic control, dyslipidemia, and dietary nonadherence. She has signs and symptoms suggestive of UTI, and she has a history of recurrent UTIs and vaginal infections.

Student Workup

Missing Information?

Evaluate: Patient Database

  Drug Therapy Problems

  Care Plan (by Problem)

TARGETED QUESTIONS

1. What signs and symptoms is the patient experiencing that indicate her diabetes in not controlled?

   HINT: See pp. 739–740 and Table 43-7 in PPP

2. What diabetes-related complications does the patient have?

   HINT: See pp. 743 in PPP

3. What are the therapeutic goals for this patient?

    HINT: *See Table 43-7 in PPP*

4. What modifications should be made to her drug therapy and diabetes self-management plans?

    HINT: *See Tables 43-8, 9, 10 in PPP*

5. How should the patient's therapeutic plan be monitored?

    HINT: *See Figure 43-2 and Tables 43-7, 43-8, 10 in PPP*

🌐 GLOBAL PERSPECTIVE

T2DM is growing at an epidemic rate. Worldwide more than 240 million people have diabetes, and more than 3.2 million people die each year from diabetes-related problems. Almost 80% of deaths due to diabetes occur in low- to middle-income countries. Almost half of the deaths (mostly from heart disease and stroke) occur in people younger than 70 years, and it is projected that diabetes deaths will double between 2005 and 2030. As many developing countries adopt a Western diet and lifestyle, increased rates of obesity are associated with increased diabetes morbidity and mortality. The approach to T2DM is similar in all countries, including eating a healthy diet and exercise. However, low-income patients may have poor access to health care and may not be able to afford or have access to healthier foods and medications.[1]

REFERENCE

1. World Health Organization. www.who.int/diabetes/facts/en/index.html. Accessed February 6, 2010.

CASE SUMMARY

- The patient needs diabetes self-management education. She is unaware of the relationship between her recurrent UTIs, delayed wound healing, and cardiovascular complications and her type 2 diabetes.

- If the patient's BP stays above the desired target, starting the patient on hypertension pharmacotherapy is warranted. Adding a second blood glucose-lowering agent may be warranted. Considerations regarding adverse effects and drug/disease interactions must be addressed.

- Lifestyle modifications must be aggressively addressed to achieve improved control of diabetes, hypertension, cholesterol, and weight.

For more information on the care plan and facilitator's guide please visit http://www.mhpharmacotherapy.com.

47 Hyperthyroidism— Graves' Disease Case

Andrea N. Traina   Michael P. Kane

CASE LEARNING OBJECTIVES

- Recognize the signs and symptoms of subclinical and overt hyperthyroidism
- Identify the goals of treatment for hyperthyroidism
- Develop an appropriate pharmacotherapy care plan for the management of hyperthyroidism based on individual patient characteristics and appropriate clinical judgment
- Properly educate a patient being treated for hyperthyroidism

PATIENT PRESENTATION

Chief Complaint

"My neck is swollen and I am having a hard time swallowing!"

History of Present Illness

MV is a 60-year-old female who presents to the clinic complaining of swelling and tenderness in her neck with difficulties swallowing solids and liquids, as well as 5 days of watery diarrhea. She appears anxious and is having a hard time sitting still during the interview. She explains that she has not felt like herself in well over a year, but things have gotten significantly worse over the last 4 months. She has had an unintentional weight loss of approximately 70 lb (32 kg) over the past year despite an increase in appetite. She attributes this weight loss to be the reason she is so exhausted and why her muscles have felt so weak of late. She also complains that she is heat intolerant and perspires with very little activity. Finally, she inquires about allergy eye drops as her eyes have been bothering her for the last several months and are so itchy and watery lately, "feeling as if they are ready to pop out of my head."

Past Medical History

Seasonal allergies

Systolic hypertension × 1 year

Atrial fibrillation × 6 months

s/p total abdominal hysterectomy/bilateral salpingo-oophorectomy (TAH/BSO) at age 45

Family History

Maternal grandmother with goiter and subsequent thyroidectomy. Mother with hyperthyroidism (treated with medication) and osteoporosis. Father with coronary artery disease and type 2 diabetes mellitus.

Social History

Married and lives with her husband of 37 years; has two dogs, and no children. She works as a kindergarten teacher at the local elementary school.

Tobacco/Alcohol/Substance Use

(+) Tobacco 45-pack year history (currently 1.5 ppd); (−) alcohol or illicit drug use.

Allergies/Intolerances/Adverse Drug Events

NKDA

Medications (Current)

Loratadine 10 mg PO daily PRN

Verapamil 240 mg PO daily

Digoxin 0.125 mg PO daily

Warfarin 2.5 mg PO daily

Calcium citrate with D (315 mg calcium with 200 IU Vitamin D_3) two tablets PO three times daily

Review of Systems

Denies chest pain, shortness or breath, abdominal pain, hematochezia, dysuria, hematuria, changes in urinary frequency or urgency.

Physical Examination

▶ General

Pleasant, middle-aged, Caucasian woman in no acute distress

▶ Vital Signs

BP 140/80 mm Hg, P 110, RR 18

Weight 118 lb (53.6 kg)

Height 63 in. (160 cm)

Denies pain

▶ Skin

Warm, moist to touch; (−) rashes or lesions

▶ HEENT

PERRLA, EOMI; (+) lid lag; mild proptosis without diplopia on upper outward gaze

▶ Neck and Lymph Nodes

Thyroid gland approximately 3 × normal size; minimally tender; (+) bruit versus radiated murmur over thyroid; symmetric and non-nodular

▶ Chest

Clear

▶ Cardiovascular

Tachycardia, irregular rate regular rhythm, 1/6 systolic murmur, (−) gallop or rub

▶ Abdomen

Soft, nontender; (−) organomegaly

▶ Neurology

Nonfocal; (+) bilateral resting tremor; increased DTRs

▶ Extremities

(−) Cyanosis, clubbing or edema

Laboratory Tests

Fasting, obtained yesterday

	Conventional Units	SI Units
Na	138 mEq/L	138 mmol/L
K	4.3 mEq/L	4.3 mmol/L
Cl	98 mEq/L	98 mmol/L
CO_2	25 mEq/L	25 mmol/L
BUN	9 mg/dL	3.2 mmol/L
SCr	0.9 mg/dL	80 μmol/L
Glu	84 mg/dL	4.7 mmol/L
Ca	9.2 mg/dL	2.30 mmol/L
Mg	2.0 mEq/L	1.00 mmol/L
Phosphate	3.0 mg/dL	0.97 mmol/L
ALP	123 IU/L	2.05 μkat/L
AST	24 IU/L	0.40 μkat/L
ALT	64 IU/L	1.07 μkat/L
25-OH vitamin D	4.8 ng/mL	12 nmol/L
INR	2.7	
Hgb	12.2 g/dL	122 g/L; 7.57 mmol/L
Hct	39.4%	0.394
WBC	$10.4 \times 10^3/mm^3$	$10.4 \times 10^9/L$
Neutrophils	57%	0.57
MCV	83 μm³	83 fL
PLT	$305 \times 10^3/mm^3$	$305 \times 10^9/L$
Albumin	3.6 g/dL	36 g/L
Anti-thyroid peroxidase (TPO) antibody	(+)	
Thyrotropin receptor (TSHR)-S antibody	(+)	
TSH	<0.01 μU/mL	<0.01 mU/L
T_3	876 ng/dL	13.5 nmol/L
Free T_4	6.71 ng/dL	86.4 pmol/L
Total cholesterol	110 mg/dL	2.84 mmol/L
LDL cholesterol	42 mg/dL	1.09 mmol/L
HDL cholesterol	38 mg/dL	0.98 mmol/L

Assessment

Sixty-year-old woman with signs, symptoms, and laboratory tests consistent with severe Graves' disease

Student Workup

Missing Information?

Evaluate:	Patient Database
	Drug Therapy Problems
	Care Plan (by Problem)

TARGETED QUESTIONS

1. What signs and symptoms of hyperthyroidism does the patient have?

   Hint: See p. 773 in PPP

2. What are the advantages versus disadvantages of thioamide, radioactive iodine (RAI), or surgery for Graves' disease treatment?

   Hint: See pp. 775–777 in PPP

3. What medications can cause hyperthyroidism?

   Hint: See Table 44-6 and p. 777 in PPP

4. What risks and adverse effects of thioamide therapy would you discuss with the patient?

   Hint: See pp. 776 and 777 in PPP

5. What complications of hyperthyroidism is this patient experiencing or at risk for?

   Hint: See p. 774 in PPP

FOLLOW-UP

6. Three weeks later, the patient returns for follow-up. She feels much better, she has regained a bit of weight [4 lb (1.8 kg)], notes improved energy, less weakness, and tremulousness, and denies palpitations. She is no longer having difficulty swallowing and denies neck pain. Her TSH, drawn today, is still undetectable at <0.01 µU/mL (<0.01 mU/L); however, her T_3 and free T_4 have markedly improved at 213 ng/dL (3.3 nmol/L) and 1.48 ng/dL (19.0 pmol/L), respectively. At what point would you recheck thyroid function tests? When would you expect her to reach a euthyroid state? Once a euthyroid state is achieved what, if any, dosage changes would you recommend in her thioamide therapy? At what point would you consider RAI? What medication changes need to be considered prior to RAI therapy?

   Hint: See p. 776 in PPP

⚙ GLOBAL PERSPECTIVE

Iodine deficiency is a common cause of thyroid disease in developing countries. Percentages of hyperthyroid patients treated with RAI, surgery, or drug therapy vary among countries. Several drugs are associated with thyroid disease.

CASE SUMMARY

- Patient's current clinical picture is consistent with severe Graves' disease and treatment needs to be initiated.

- Given the severity of disease methimazole 20 mg PO every 8 hours should be initiated. The patient should return in 1 to 2 weeks and thyroid function tests should be drawn with the methimazole dose titrated accordingly. Once euthyroid state has been reached (approximately 6–8 weeks) a maintenance dose of 5 to 15 mg/d should be given to avoid hypothyroidism.

- Symptomatic relief should also be provided by initiating propranolol 20 mg PO four times daily. Discontinuation of verapamil and digoxin can be considered (with monitoring) after adequate treatment of her hyperthyroidism (the systolic hypertension and atrial fibrillation will likely resolve). In anticipation of reaching a euthyroid state, a discussion of the pros and cons of definitive treatment should take place.

- Patient needs to follow-up with ophthalmology for evaluation, and urged to quit smoking prior to considering RAI therapy as to avoid or minimize the risk of exacerbating Graves' eye disease.

For more information on the care plan and facilitator's guide please visit http://www.mhpharmacotherapy.com.

48 Hypothyroidism

Michael D. Katz

CASE LEARNING OBJECTIVES

- Recognize the signs and symptoms of mild and overt hypothyroidism
- Identify the goals of therapy for hypothyroidism
- Develop an appropriate treatment and monitoring plan for thyroid replacement using individual patient characteristics
- Select an appropriate product for thyroid replacement therapy
- Properly educate a patient taking thyroid replacement therapy

PATIENT PRESENTATION

Chief Complaint

"I'm so tired lately. I have no energy. Maybe I need some vitamins or something."

History of Present Illness

Yi-Ling Wang is a 49-year-old woman who presents to her new physician complaining of feeling tired, lethargic, and "not thinking straight" for the last 6 months. She has seen her previous primary care physician several times and has been told that her symptoms are probably due to anemia from menorrhagia, stress, depression, and/or impending menopause. Despite treatment with iron (and resultant improvement of her anemia), a hormonal contraceptive to help regulate her menstrual cycle, and an antidepressant, her symptoms have slowly worsened. Two years ago at a health fair, she was told her TSH was 6.2 µU/mL (6.2 mU/L) and total cholesterol was 246 mg/dL (6.36 mmol/L). Her primary care physician felt the TSH value was compatible with subclinical hypothyroidism and therefore could not explain her symptoms at that time. She has been wondering if she really is depressed and why the depression medication is not helping. Over the past few months, she has also noticed that her skin seems a little more dry and itchy and that she has difficulty keeping warm even in warm weather. Finally, she asks you what is good for constipation since the Chinese herbs her mother gave her are not helping.

Past Medical History

Iron-deficiency anemia diagnosed 6 months ago

Depression × 6 months

Menorrhagia diagnosed 6 months ago

Osteopenia × 1 year

Family History

Father had CAD and died of gastric cancer at age 74. Mother is alive at age 70 with osteoporosis and hypothyroidism. She has one brother who is healthy.

Social History

Came to the United States from China at age 15. Speaks Mandarin and English. Married and lives with her husband of 24 years; has two children, aged 22 and 19. Works as a language instructor at a local college.

Tobacco/Alcohol/Substance Use

Social drinker; (−) tobacco or illicit drug use

Allergies/Intolerances/Adverse Drug Events

Penicillin (rash as child)

Medications (Current)

MOM 30 mL PO q 24 h PRN constipation

Chinese herb PO PRN constipation

Sertraline 50 mg PO q 24 h

Ortho Tri-Cyclen 28 PO q day

FeSO$_4$ 300 mg PO q 24 h

Calcium carbonate 1,000 mg PO q 12 h

Alendronate 35 mg PO weekly

Acetaminophen 650 mg PO PRN headache, body aches

Review of Systems

Occasional HA relieved with nonaspirin pain reliever; (−) tinnitus, vertigo, or infections; frequent body aches, which she attributes to lack of exercise; (−) change in urinary frequency, but she has noticed an increase in the number of episodes of constipation in the past year; reports cold extremities; (−) history of seizures, syncope, or loss of consciousness; (+) dry skin.

Physical Examination

▶ General

Well-appearing, middle-aged Asian woman in no acute distress

▶ Vital Signs

BP 112/76 mm Hg, P 64, RR 12, T 36.2°C

Weight 127.6 lb (58 kg)

Height 62 in. (157.5 cm)

Denies pain

▶ Skin

Dry-appearing skin and scalp; (−) rashes or lesions

▶ HEENT

PERRLA, EOMI; trace periorbital edema; (−) sinus tenderness; TMs appear normal

▶ Neck and Lymph Nodes

Thyroid gland smooth, slightly enlarged symmetrically; (−) thyroid nodules; (−) lymphadenopathy; (−) carotid bruits

▶ Chest

Clear to auscultation

▶ Breasts

Examination deferred

▶ Cardiovascular

RRR, normal S_1, S_2; (−) S_3 or S_4

▶ Abdomen

Not tender/not distended; (−) organomegaly

▶ Neurology

Grossly intact; DTRs normal

▶ Genitourinary

Examination deferred

▶ Rectal

Examination deferred

Laboratory Tests

Fasting, obtained 2 days ago

	Conventional Units	SI Units
Na	142 mEq/L	142 mmol/L
K	4.1 mEq/L	4.1 mmol/L
Cl	100 mEq/L	100 mmol/L
CO_2	24 mEq/L	24 mmol/L
BUN	7 mg/dL	2.5 mmol/L
SCr	0.7 mg/dL	62 μmol/L
Glu	104 mg/dL	5.8 mmol/L
Ca	9.4 mg/dL	2.35 mmol/L
Mg	1.8 mg/dL	0.90 mmol/L
Phosphate	3.8 mg/dL	1.23 mmol/L
Hgb	13.5 g/dL	135 g/L; 8.38 mmol/L
Hct	39.7%	0.397
WBC	$7.6 \times 10^3/mm^3$	$7.6 \times 10^9/L$
MCV	83 μm³	83 fL
Albumin	3.8 g/dL	38 g/L
Anti-TPO antibody	(+)	
TSH	12.8 μU/mL	12.8 mU/L
Free T_4	0.71 ng/dL	9.1 pmol/L
Total cholesterol	268 mg/dL	6.93 mmol/L
LDL cholesterol	142 mg/dL	3.67 mmol/L
HDL cholesterol	36 mg/dL	0.93 mmol/L

Assessment

Forty-nine-year-old woman with signs, symptoms, and laboratory tests consistent with hypothyroidism

Student Workup

Missing Information?

Evaluate: Patient Database

Drug Therapy Problems

Care Plan (by Problem)

TARGETED QUESTIONS

1. What s/s of hypothyroidism does the patient have?

   Hint: See p. 768 in PPP

2. Why is levothyroxine (LT_4) the treatment of choice for most patients with hypothyroidism?

   Hint: See p. 769 in PPP

3. What medications can cause hypothyroidism?

   Hint: See Table 44-6 in PPP

4. What risks and adverse effects of therapy would you discuss with the patient?

   Hint: See p. 771 in PPP

5. Should the patient receive specific lipid-lowering pharmacotherapy?

   Hint: Hypothyroidism is commonly associated with elevated LDL cholesterol, and adequate LT₄ replacement may significantly lower LDL. Since the patient has no other cardiovascular risk factors, it would be reasonable to withhold specific lipid-lowering pharmacotherapy until she has been euthyroid for several months. See p. 771 in PPP

FOLLOW-UP

6. Eight weeks later, the patient returns for follow-up. She feels much better, with more energy and less depressed feelings. Her TSH, drawn yesterday, is 0.2 μU/mL (0.2 mU/L). What are some reasons why her TSH might now be low, and what are the risks associated with a suppressed TSH? What actions, if any, would you take?

   Hint: See pp. 770–771 in PPP

⊙ GLOBAL PERSPECTIVE

Goiter, an enlargement of the thyroid gland, is caused by a variety of conditions, and can be associated with normal, excessive, or deficient thyroid function (Fig. 48-1). In developed countries, enlargement of the thyroid gland is most often associated with nodular goiter, autoimmune thyroiditis, and Grave's disease. However, in developing countries, iodine-deficient diet is commonly associated with goiter. Iodine deficiency and endemic goiter are especially common in women of childbearing age since pregnancy increases iodine requirements. Substances in the diet can also serve as goitrogens. Diets high in foods containing cyanoglucosides (cassava, lima beans, maize, bamboo shoots, and sweet potatoes) release cyanide, which is then metabolized to thiocyanate, an agent that

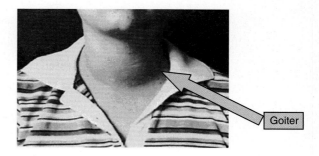

FIGURE 48-1. Goiter. (Adapted, with permission, from Gardner DG, Shoback D. Greenspan's Clinical & Basic Endocrinology, 8th ed. New York, McGraw-Hill, 2007, Fig. 8-27A.)

inhibits iodine transport. Foods high in thioglucosides (cruciferous vegetables) can have a thionamide-like effect on the thyroid gland. Endemic goiter is easily treated with iodine supplementation (often in the form of iodized salt) and avoidance of dietary goitrogens.

CASE SUMMARY

- The patient's current clinical picture is consistent with overt hypothyroidism, and thyroid replacement therapy should be initiated.

- An initial levothyroxine dose of 50 mcg daily is reasonable, with dose titration to target TSH [0.5–2.5 μU/mL (0.5–2.5 mU/L)] using TSH values obtained at least 6 weeks after any change in the dose.

- Overreplacement of thyroid hormone should be avoided, especially with her history of osteopenia.

For more information on the care plan and facilitator's guide please visit http://www.mhpharmacotherapy.com.

49 Cushing Syndrome

Atula Vachhani   Devra Dang

CASE LEARNING OBJECTIVES

- Recognize the clinical presentation of Cushing syndrome and the physiologic consequences of cortisol excess
- Describe the pharmacologic and nonpharmacologic management of patients with Cushing syndrome
- Recommend strategies to prevent the development of Cushing syndrome associated with exogenous glucocorticoid administration
- Recommend therapy-monitoring parameters for patients with Cushing syndrome

PATIENT PRESENTATION

Chief Complaint

"Doctor, something is wrong with me. I'm gaining so much weight and I'm always so tired and weak."

History of Present Illness

JT is a 45-year-old female who presents to her primary care physician's (PCP) office with complaints of increasing fatigue and muscle weakness over the last 3 months. She states that she feels so tired and weak some mornings that she is not able to get herself out of bed. She also reports having gained about 10 lb (~4.5 kg) over the last 3 months and has been experiencing menstrual irregularity since then. She is not pregnant and not currently attempting to become pregnant. JT was diagnosed with RA 2 years ago, at which point she was placed on hydroxychloroquine 400 mg daily and celecoxib 200 mg daily to relieve joint pain and stiffness. Within the last year, she had been experiencing more flare-ups of her RA. Hydroxychloroquine and celecoxib were discontinued and she was placed on prednisone approximately 4 months ago. Since being diagnosed with RA, the patient also reports having episodes of depressed mood. Her depression had been well controlled on sertraline 50 mg PO daily, but she reports increasing number of depressive episodes recently.

Past Medical History

RA × 2 years

Depression × 1½ years

HTN × 1 year

Dyslipidemia × 1 year

Family History

Mother is alive at age 66 with type 2 DM; father is alive at age 69 with type 2 DM and HTN. She has one sister, who is healthy.

Social History

Married and lives with husband. Has a healthy 19-year-old son in college. Works as an assistant manager at a local grocery store

Tobacco/Alcohol/Substance Use

(−) Alcohol, tobacco, or illicit drug use

Allergies/Intolerances/Adverse Drug Events

No known drug/food allergies/intolerances/ADEs

Medications (Current)

Prednisone 10 mg PO q AM

Sertraline 50 mg PO q AM

Lisinopril/HCTZ 20 mg/12.5 mg PO q AM

Atorvastatin 20 mg PO q AM

Review of Systems

(+) Fatigue and frequent body aches with muscle weakness in major muscle groups; (+) pain in joints of hands, ankles, and knees; reports weight gain in her abdomen, face, and around her neck and shoulders; (+) acne and excess hair growth on her face and neck; (+) generalized depressed mood and insomnia; (+) thin, dry skin with occasional bruising; notes irregular light periods; (+) increased urination; (+) increased thirst

Physical Examination

▶ *General*

Cushingoid-appearing, obese, middle-aged Caucasian woman in slight distress

▶ *Vital Signs*

BP 144/86 mm Hg, P 80, RR 16, T 37°C

Weight 188.1 lb (85.5 kg)

Height 63 in. (160 cm)

Pain 7/10 in joints of hands, ankles, and knees

▶ *Skin*

Thin, dry-appearing skin with several small bruises; (−) rashes; pink and purple striae visible on abdomen and bilateral breasts

▶ *HEENT*

Round face; excess facial hair; PERRLA, EOMI; (−) sinus tenderness; TMs appear normal

▶ *Neck and Lymph Nodes*

(−) Lymphadenopathy; (−) carotid bruits, JVD, or thyromegaly

▶ *Chest*

Clear to auscultation bilaterally

▶ *Breasts*

Normal with some pink and purple striae bilaterally; (−) lumps

▶ *Cardiovascular*

RRR, normal S_1, S_2; (−) S_3 or S_4

▶ *Abdomen*

Soft; not tender; obese with pink and purple striae; (−) organomegaly

▶ *Neurology*

Grossly intact; DTRs normal

▶ *Genitourinary*

Examination deferred

▶ *Rectal*

Examination deferred

▶ *Musculoskeletal/Extremities*

Decreased muscle strength in upper and lower extremities bilaterally; bilateral symmetrical tenderness at metacarpophylangeal (MCP) and proximal interphalangeal (PIP) joints of the hands and joints of ankles

Laboratory Tests

Fasting

	Conventional Units	SI Units
Na	139 mEq/L	139 mmol/L
K	3.6 mEq/L	3.6 mmol/L
Cl	102 mEq/L	102 mmol/L
CO_2	24 mEq/L	24 mmol/L
BUN	13 mg/dL	4.6 mmol/L
SCr	0.8 mg/dL	71 μmol/L
Glu	133 mg/dL	7.4 mmol/L
Ca	9.6 mg/dL	2.40 mmol/L
Mg	1.9 mEq/L	0.95 mmol/L
Phosphate	3.7 mg/dL	1.20 mmol/L
Total cholesterol	228 mg/dL	5.90 mmol/L
LDL cholesterol	142 mg/dL	3.67 mmol/L
HDL cholesterol	48 mg/dL	1.24 mmol/L
Triglycerides	190 mg/dL	2.15 mmol/L
Hgb	13.5 g/dL	135 g/L; 8.37 mmol/L
Hct	38.7%	0.387
MCV	86 μm³	86 fL
WBC	$6.6 \times 10^3/mm^3$	$6.6 \times 10^9/L$
Platelets	$280 \times 10^3/mm^3$	$280 \times 10^9/L$
Albumin	3.8 g/dL	38 g/L
Total bilirubin	0.5 mg/dL	8.6 μmol/L
Direct bilirubin	0.1 mg/dL	1.7 μmol/L
AST	32 IU/L	0.53 μkat/L
ALT	26 IU/L	0.43 μkat/L
Alkaline phosphatase	112 IU/L	1.87 μkat/L
Rheumatoid factor (+)		
ACTH	9 pg/mL (9 ng/L)	2.0 pmol/L
Cortisol (24-h free urinary via HPLC)	296 mcg/d	817 nmol/d
Serum cortisol for 1-mg overnight dexamethasone suppression test	15 mcg/dL	414 nmol/L

Assessment

Forty-five-year-old woman with clinical presentation consistent with Cushing syndrome

Student Workup

Missing Information?

Evaluate: Patient Database

Drug Therapy Problems

Care Plan (by Problem)

TARGETED QUESTIONS

1. What signs and symptoms of Cushing syndrome does the patient exhibit?

   Hint: See p. 794 in PPP

2. What is the likely etiology of Cushing syndrome in the patient?

   Hint: See pp. 791 and 792 and Table 45-4 in PPP

3. How would you treat Cushing syndrome in the patient?

   Hint: See pp. 792, 793, and 795 and Table 45-7 in PPP

4. What are the potential risks of therapy that need to be discussed with the patient?

   Hint: See pp. 790 and 791 and Table 45-8 in PPP

5. Should the patient receive drug treatment for her hyperglycemia?

   Hint: Does she have a diagnosis of DM? See p. 792 in PPP

FOLLOW-UP

6. JT was tapered off the prednisone and started on methotrexate 10 mg once a week, along with folic acid 1 mg once daily to prophylax against methotrexate's side effects. She will follow-up with her rheumatologist in 2 weeks for further assessment of her therapy for RA. Four weeks after her initial PCP visit, JT returns for a follow-up with the PCP. She has more energy, can sleep better, and has less depressed feelings. Her early morning cortisol level at this visit is 18 mcg/dL (497 nmol/L). What could be the reason why her cortisol level is slightly low? What are the risks associated with a suppressed cortisol level? What actions, if any, would you take?

   Hint: See pp. 790 and 791 and Table 45-8 in PPP

⊙ GLOBAL PERSPECTIVE

Cushing syndrome is most commonly caused by chronic administration of exogenous glucocorticoids. Endogenous Cushing syndrome is an uncommon disorder. According to European population-based studies, the incidence of endogenous Cushing syndrome is two to three cases per 1 million inhabitants per year.[1] A study conducted in Spain reports that Cushing disease due to a pituitary adenoma is the most frequent cause of endogenous Cushing syndrome, which is five to six times more frequent than adrenal Cushing syndrome, with an incidence of 1.2 to 2.4 cases per 1 million inhabitants per year.[2] Treatment options for various types of endogenous Cushing syndrome include surgery and pharmacotherapeutic options, which are discussed in the PPP Chapter 45.

REFERENCES

1. Nieman LK, Biller BM, Findling JW, et al. The diagnosis of Cushing's syndrome: An Endocrine Society Clinical Practice Guideline. J Clin Endocrinol Metab 2008 93:1526–1540.

2. Lindholm J, Juul S, Jorgensen AO, et al. Incidence and late prognosis of Cushing's Syndrome: A population-based study. J Clin Endocrinol Metab 2001 86:117–123.

CASE SUMMARY

- The patient's current clinical presentation is consistent with steroid-induced Cushing syndrome. Gradual tapering and discontinuation of prednisone therapy should be initiated. Her Cushing symptoms should resolve on discontinuation of prednisone therapy.

- Morning cortisol level can be rechecked 4 weeks after start of taper to assess the need for continued slow taper or whether prednisone can be discontinued at this time.

- The patient should be educated about the possibility of adrenal insufficiency and symptoms of an acute adrenal crisis.

- Alternative treatment for RA should be initiated while prednisone is being tapered.

For more information on the care plan and facilitator's guide please visit http://www.mhpharmacotherapy.com.

50 Pregnancy

Ema Ferreira   Caroline Morin

Évelyne Rey

CASE LEARNING OBJECTIVES

- Develop an appropriate treatment plan during pregnancy
- Properly educate a patient taking drugs during pregnancy
- Identify the risks of epilepsy during pregnancy
- Identify the risks of anticonvulsants during pregnancy and lactation

PATIENT PRESENTATION

Chief Complaint

"I think I am pregnant."

History of Present Illness

Loretta Baldwin is a 26-year-old woman who presents to her primary care physician after completing a pharmacy pregnancy test that was positive 2 days ago. Her period is 3 weeks late. Her menstrual cycle is usually 28 to 32 days. She stopped her medications yesterday because she has been told that they may cause fetal malformations. She has never been pregnant before.

Past Medical History

Epilepsy (generalized tonic–clonic seizures) for 13 years following viral encephalitis. No seizures since one episode last year. Last visit to her neurologist 6 months ago.

Overweight since childhood

Chronic HAs

Occasional constipation

Family History

Mother is alive at age 51 with DM, obesity, and HTN. She had two inconsecutive miscarriages. Father is alive at age 53 with hypothyroidism. She has one brother who is healthy and two sisters who had normal pregnancies. There have been no multiple pregnancies in the family.

Social History

Born in the United States. Married and lives with her husband. Works full time as a clerk. Dislikes fruit and vegetables, eats two meals a day, often in fast-food restaurants. (−) Exercise. No pets.

Tobacco/Alcohol/Substance Use

Social drinker; (−) tobacco or illicit drug use

Allergies/Intolerances/Adverse Drug Events

Phenytoin (unknown reaction at age 13)

Medications (Current)

Lamotrigine 200 mg PO twice daily, stopped yesterday

Carbamazepine CR 400 mg PO twice daily, stopped yesterday

MOM 30 mL PO once daily as needed for constipation

Feverfew herbal tea two to five times a week

Ibuprofen 400 mg PO as needed for HA, twice weekly in the last month

Review of Systems

No seizure; occasional HA relieved with ibuprofen; increased urinary frequency and constipation in the past 2 weeks; occasionally SOB; tiredness and mild nausea.

Physical Examination

▶ *General*

Overweight young Caucasian woman in no acute distress

▶ *Vital Signs*

BP 112/76 mm Hg, P 89, RR 12, T 36.2°C

Weight 207.2 lb (94.2 kg)

Height 67 in. (170 cm)

Denies pain

▶ **Skin**

Normal

▶ **HEENT**

PERRLA, EOMI; TMs normal

▶ **Neck and Lymph Nodes**

Thyroid gland not palpable

▶ **Chest**

Clear to auscultation

▶ **Breasts**

Slight tenderness; no nodule, discharge, or skin deformation

▶ **Cardiovascular**

RRR, normal S_1, S_2; (−) S_3 or S_4; systolic ejection murmur at the left second intercostal space without irradiation

▶ **Abdomen**

Not tender/not distended; (−) organomegaly

▶ **Neurology**

Grossly intact; DTRs normal

▶ **Genitourinary**

(−) discharge or lesions; cervix closed; bimanual examination normal

▶ **Rectal**

Examination deferred

Laboratory Tests

Nonfasting, obtained the same day

	Conventional Units	SI Units
Urine pregnancy test	(+)	
Hgb	12.3 g/dL	123 g/L; 7.63 mmol/L
Hct	37.8%	0.378
WBC	$5.4 \times 10^3/mm^3$	$5.4 \times 10^9/L$
MCV	82 μm³	82 fL
Platelets	$203 \times 10^3/mm^3$	$203 \times 10^9/L$
SCr	0.63 mg/dL	56 μmol/L
Glu	101 mg/dL	5.6 mmol/L
Lamotrigine level	Not done	
Urinalysis	Normal	
Urine culture	(−)	
Blood group/rhesus type	O⁺	

Rubella antibody	(+)	
Hepatitis B surface antigen	(−)	
HIV antibody	(−)	
Vaginal culture	(−)	
Carbamazepine level	4.2 mcg/mL	18 μmol/L

Assessment

Twenty-six-year-old woman, 7 weeks pregnant, wanting to stop her antiepileptic therapy

Student Workup

Missing Information?

Evaluate: Patient Database
Drug Therapy Problems
Care Plan (by Problem)

TARGETED QUESTIONS

1. What risks and adverse effects of epilepsy/therapy would you discuss with the patient?

   Hint: See Tables 47-1 and 47-3 and p. 827 in PPP

2. How should headaches be treated?

   Hint: See Table 47-3 in PPP

3. Should other medication be added?

   Hint: See Table 47-8 and p. 827 in PPP

4. How could nausea affect the actual therapy? What is the approach of nausea?

   Hint: See Table 47-8 and p. 829 in PPP

FOLLOW-UP

Two weeks later, the patient returns for follow-up. She is taking her usual anticonvulsants and folic acid as recommended by a fetomaternal obstetrician who asked for fetal ultrasounds at 12 and 20 weeks and carbamazepine blood levels every month. Despite a diet rich in fiber and psyllium supplement, she complains of constipation.

5. Why are carbamazepine and lamotrigine levels assessed and how should the results be interpreted?

   Hint: See Table 47-6 in PPP

6. What do you suggest for persistent constipation?

   Hint: See Table 47-8 and p. 829 in PPP

⟳ GLOBAL PERSPECTIVE

Anticonvulsants should not be stopped during pregnancy because it puts the woman at risk of seizures. Triggers of seizures, such as tiredness and vomiting, should be avoided.

Anticonvulsants increase the risk of fetal malformations, a topic that should be discussed with the woman. In general, pregnant women overestimate the teratogenic risk of drugs. Lifestyle modifications should be discussed, and folic acid 4 mg should be prescribed at the first prenatal visit (if not already taken). Planning a pregnancy is especially important in women with epilepsy because folic acid is more efficient in preventing fetal malformations when started 3 months before pregnancy (general population). Multivitamins, containing vitamin D, calcium, and iron, should be considered in women with a poor diet or lack of sun exposure. Other drugs, for which proven safe alternatives are available or that have no proven efficacy, should be stopped.

CASE SUMMARY

- The current clinical picture is consistent with pregnancy.
- The risks and benefits of anticonvulsants were not well understood before pregnancy.

- The anticonvulsants should not be stopped.
- Pregnancy causes a decrease in total anticonvulsant blood levels.
- Folic acid 4 mg should be added to current medications.
- Ibuprofen and NSAIDs should not be used regularly during pregnancy, and should be stopped at 26 weeks of pregnancy. Acetaminophen is the first-line drug for aches.
- Herbal medications should not be used in pregnancy unless their safety has been proved.
- N/V can affect drug absorption and efficacy.
- Constipation and nausea of pregnancy could be relieved by diet modifications. Psyllium preparations are the first-line drugs for constipation.

For more information on the care plan and facilitator's guide please visit http://www.mhpharmacotherapy.com.

51 Contraception

Shareen Y. El-Ibiary

CASE LEARNING OBJECTIVES

- Assess patient needs for hormonal contraceptives
- Manage and minimize side effects associated with hormonal contraceptives on the basis of patient needs
- Identify drug interactions and contraindications associated with hormonal contraceptives
- Recommend an appropriate contraceptive method on the basis of patient characteristics and needs
- Properly educate a patient using a recommended contraceptive method

PATIENT PRESENTATION

Chief Complaint

"I'm getting married soon, and I need to start birth control."

History of Present Illness

Carrie Anderson is a 36-year-old woman who presents to her primary care physician (PCP) for a routine follow-up appointment and excitedly states that she is getting married in 4 months and "needs to start birth control." She has been seeing her PCP regularly for the management of HTN and depression. She and her fiancé are currently using condoms for pregnancy prevention, but states that she wants "something easier" since she will be married. She would like to have children "in a year or so." She was treated for depression 1 year ago with sertraline 50 mg PO daily for 6 months and her BP is controlled with HCTZ 25 mg PO daily and recent addition of ramipril 5 mg PO 6 weeks ago. Overall, she is feeling well and very happy. She admits to a nagging cough that started about 2 weeks ago, but otherwise, she is seeking to start on a hormonal contraceptive.

Past Medical History

HTN diagnosed 2 years ago

Depression treated successfully 1 year ago (6-month treatment course)

Family History

Father is alive at age 67 with HTN. Mother is alive at age 65 with osteoporosis and HTN. She has one brother and one sister who are healthy.

Social History

Single, planning to get married for the first time in 4 months, no children, but plans to have children in 1 year. Caucasian, English speaking, United States born.

Tobacco/Alcohol/Substance Use

Social drinker; admits to smoking ½ ppd, but would like to quit

Allergies/Intolerances/Adverse Drug Events

NKDA

Medications (Current)

HCTZ 25 mg PO daily

Ramipril 5 mg PO daily

Ibuprofen 200 mg PO PRN menstrual cramps

Dextromethorphan/guaifenesin 5 mL PO q 6 h PRN cough

Review of Systems

Noticed dry cough, attributes it to possibly new allergies; (−) fever, chills, sore throat; otherwise feeling well

Physical Examination

▶ *General*

Obese, well-appearing, Caucasian woman in no acute distress

▶ *Vital Signs*

BP 137/82 mm Hg, P 84, RR 12, T 36.2°C

Weight 202.4 lb (92 kg)

Height 67 in. (170.2 cm)

► **Skin**

Supple, normal appearance

► **HEENT**

PERRLA, EOMI; (−) sinus tenderness; TMs appear normal

► **Neck and Lymph Nodes**

Thyroid gland smooth, slightly enlarged symmetrically; (−) thyroid nodules; (−) lymphadenopathy; (−) carotid bruits

► **Chest**

Clear to auscultation

► **Breasts**

Examination deferred

► **Cardiovascular**

RRR, normal S_1, S_2; (−) S_3 or S_4

► **Abdomen**

Not tender/not distended; (−) organomegaly

► **Neurology**

Grossly intact; DTRs normal

► **Genitourinary**

Examination deferred

► **Rectal**

Examination deferred

Laboratory Tests

Fasting, obtained this morning

	Conventional Units	SI Units
Na	139 mEq/L	139 mmol/L
K	4.3 mEq/L	4.3 mmol/L
Cl	101 mEq/L	101 mmol/L
HCO$_3$	25 mEq/L	25 mmol/L
BUN	10 mg/dL	3.6 mmol/L
SCr	0.62 mg/dL	55 μmol/L
Glu	104 mg/dL	5.8 mmol/L
Ca	9.1 mg/dL	2.28 mmol/L
Hgb	13.5 g/dL	135 g/L; 8.38 mmol/L
Hct	39.7%	0.397
WBC	5.1×10^3/mm^3	5.1×10^9/L
Albumin	4.1 g/dL	41 g/L

AST	29 U/L	0.48 μkat/L
ALT	30 U/L	0.50 μkat/L
Alk phos	63 U/L	1.05 μkat/L

Assessment

Thirty-six-year-old woman with history of depression, HTN, obesity, smoking, and mild cough requesting a hormonal contraceptive

Student Workup

Missing Information?

Evaluate: Patient Database

Drug Therapy Problems

Care Plan (by Problem)

TARGETED QUESTIONS

1. What hormonal contraceptives should be avoided in this patient and why?

   Hint: See Table 48-3 in PPP

2. Why is smoking in women older than 35 years and uncontrolled HTN contraindicated with combined hormonal contraceptives?

   Hint: See p. 846 in PPP

3. What medications interact with hormonal contraceptives based on this patient's medication regimen?

   Hint: See pp. 849 and Table 48-4 in PPP

4. What risks and adverse effects of hormonal contraceptives would you discuss with this patient?

   Hint: See pp. 845–846 in PPP

5. How do this patient's needs influence the choice of hormonal contraceptive agents?

   Hint: Important to consider this patient's desire to have children in the near future and her age of 36 years. Consider the return to fertility of different contraceptive agents in this patient. The patient is also obese and contraceptive agents that heavily contribute to weight gain should also be avoided. See pp. 848 and 851 in PPP

FOLLOW-UP

6. Eight weeks later, the patient returns for follow-up. Her cough has resolved after discontinuing ramipril and starting losartan 50 mg PO daily. She has been taking her progestin-only pills every morning right after brushing her teeth, but missed a dose when she went out of town for a night. What are some reasons her cough went away after discontinuing ramipril? What counseling would you provide the patient with regard to missing a progestin-only pill?

⊙ GLOBAL PERSPECTIVE

Hormonal contraception is mainly used for pregnancy prevention, but has other uses as well, such as treating acne, hirsutism, dysmenorrhea, menorrhagia, polycystic ovary syndrome, iron-deficiency anemia, premenstrual dysphoric disorder, and premenstrual syndrome. In the developing world, however, hormonal contraceptives are mainly desired for pregnancy prevention. Survey information provided by the Guttmacher institute (www.guttmacher.org, May 2007) states that 15% of married women aged 15 to 49 years in 53 developing countries have an unmet need for contraception, with the highest percent reported in sub-Saharan Africa of 24%. Reports also state that almost 71 million married women in 53 countries and 4.2 million unmarried women in a survey of 36 countries are at risk of an unplanned pregnancy and not using a family planning method. Contraception in developing countries may be particularly important in preventing abortions of unplanned babies, decreasing the spread of diseases such as HIV from partner to partner and mother to infant, preventing pregnancy in areas where risks of nonconsensual intercourse is high, and preventing pregnancy in women who have multiple children and cannot afford to have another. Improving access to contraception whether barrier, hormonal, or surgical in developing countries and in the United States may help to decrease unplanned pregnancies and prevent the associated consequences.

CASE SUMMARY

- The patient's contraceptive needs include an easier birth control method than condoms. Ideally, this method could be a hormonal contraceptive that includes the following characteristics: effective with her current weight, does not increase her weight significantly, does not increase her risk of stroke and CV risk because of her HTN and smoker status, does not increase her potassium level, and has a quick return to fertility.

- A progestin-only pill or IUD would be appropriate in this patient with monitoring of mood symptoms in case the progestin induces depression symptoms.

For more information on the care plan and facilitator's guide please visit http://www.mhpharmacotherapy.com.

52 Dysmenorrhea/ Menorrhagia

Jacqueline M. Klootwyk   Elena Umland

CASE LEARNING OBJECTIVES

- Describe the clinical presentation of dysmenorrhea and menorrhagia
- Recommend appropriate nonpharmacologic and pharmacologic interventions for patients with dysmenorrhea and menorrhagia
- Develop a monitoring plan to assess the effectiveness and safety of pharmacologic therapies for dysmenorrhea and menorrhagia
- Identify the goals of therapy for dysmenorrhea and menorrhagia

PATIENT PRESENTATION

Chief Complaint

"My cramps are unbearable!"

History of Present Illness

Anita Jacob is a 21-year-old Caucasian woman who presents to the clinic complaining of painful menses for the past few months. Her menses last between 6 and 8 days on average and have become increasingly painful. The pain begins 1 day prior to the onset of menses and lasts 2 to 3 days. The pain is "crampy" in nature. She has heavy menses for 2 days that require her to change feminine hygiene products every 2 to 3 hours. She has a history of iron-deficiency anemia secondary to menorrhagia that has been successfully treated with iron supplementation. She has tried an OTC product (Midol Menstrual Complete) and ibuprofen without success. Today, she is also complaining of abdominal pain, but denies vaginal discharge.

Past Medical History

Iron-deficiency anemia × 6 months

Menorrhagia × 6 months

Seasonal allergic rhinitis × 2 years

Family History

Father is alive at age 56 with CHD, H/O MI at age 55, dyslipidemia, HTN, and osteoarthritis. Mother is alive at age 54 with osteopenia, HTN, and H/O ovarian cancer. She has one older brother (age 30) and one older sister (age 27) who are both alive and well.

Social History

The patient is a single, heterosexual, sexually active female. She has been sexually active since age 15. She does not desire pregnancy at this time. She has had vaginal intercourse with multiple partners (approximately 10–12 men). Her partners use condoms only occasionally. She has been in a monogamous relationship for the past 8 months. She is a student at the local university.

Tobacco/Alcohol/Substance Use

Social drinker (3–5 drinks per weekend); (+) tobacco use (1 ppd); (−) illicit drug use. The patient is not ready to quit smoking at this time.

Allergies/Intolerances/Adverse Drug Events

Penicillin (rash)

Medications (Current)

Fexofenadine 180 mg PO once daily

Ferrous sulfate 325 mg PO twice daily

Ibuprofen 200 mg two tablets PO PRN headache and menstrual cramps

Midol Menstrual Complete two tablets PO PRN menstrual cramps

Medications (Past)

Kava kava root capsules 500 mg PO two to three times daily PRN menstrual cramps

Review of Systems

Occasional HA relieved with NSAID medication; seasonal allergies relieved with antihistamine; (−) GI upset, heartburn, or constipation, but (+) abdominal pain; (−) change in urinary frequency; (−) dysuria; (−) vaginal discharge; (+) menorrhagia, (+) dysmenorrhea; LMP 27 days ago; age at menarche 14 years.

Physical Examination

▶ *General*

Overweight-appearing, young, Caucasian woman in no apparent distress

▶ *Vital Signs*

BP 114/72 mm Hg, P 76, RR 12, T 37.0°C

Weight 170 lb (77.3 kg)

Height 65 in. (165.1 cm)

Pain score 2/10

▶ *Skin*

Normal-appearing skin and nails; (−) rashes or lesions

▶ *HEENT*

PERRLA, EOMI; TMs appear normal

▶ *Neck and Lymph Nodes*

No nodules

▶ *Chest*

Clear to auscultation bilaterally; (−) chest pain

▶ *Breasts*

Nontender; (−) masses

▶ *Cardiovascular*

RRR, normal S_1, S_2; (−) S_3 or S_4

▶ *Abdomen*

Soft, tender, nondistended; (−) hepatosplenomegaly

▶ *Neurology*

Grossly intact; DTRs normal

▶ *Genitourinary*

Normal external appearance of labia; (−) lesions on cervix; (−) cervical motion tenderness; (−) vaginal discharge

▶ *Rectal*

Examination deferred

Laboratory and Other Diagnostic Tests

Today

- Urine pregnancy test: Negative
- Urine gonorrhea/chlamydia screening: Pending

Fasting, obtained 3 months ago

	Conventional Units	SI Units
Na	138 mEq/L	138 mmol/L
K	4.8 mEq/L	4.8 mmol/L
Cl	104 mEq/L	104 mmol/L
CO_2	25 mEq/L	25 mmol/L
BUN	12 mg/dL	4.3 mmol/L
SCr	0.9 mg/dL	80 μmol/L
Glu	85 mg/dL	4.7 mmol/L
Hgb	12.8 g/dL	128 g/L; 7.94 mmol/L
Hct	37.2%	0.372
MCV	84 μm³	84 fL
WBC	6.9×10^3/mm³	6.9×10^9/L
Platelet	255×10^3/mm³	255×10^9/L
Iron	54 mcg/dL	9.7 μmol/L
Ferritin	45 ng/mL	45 mcg/L
TIBC	382 mcg/dL	68.4 μmol/L
Transferrin saturation	26%	0.26

Fasting, obtained 6 months ago

	Conventional Units	SI Units
Na	140 mEq/L	140 mmol/L
K	4.5 mEq/L	4.5 mmol/L
Cl	102 mEq/L	102 mmol/L
CO_2	24 mEq/L	24 mmol/L
BUN	11 mg/dL	3.9 mmol/L
SCr	0.8 mg/dL	71 μmol/L
Glu	78 mg/dL	4.3 mmol/L
AST	23 IU/L	0.38 μkat/L
ALT	17 IU/L	0.28 μkat/L
Hgb	9.8 g/dL	98 g/L; 6.08 mmol/L
Hct	30.9%	0.309
MCV	72 μm³	72 fL
WBC	5.5×10^3/mm³	5.5×10^9/L
Platelet	220×10^3/mm³	220×10^9/L
Iron	20 mcg/dL	3.6 μmol/L
Ferritin	6 ng/mL	6 mcg/L
TIBC	465 mcg/dL	83.2 μmol/L
Transferrin saturation	12%	0.12

Diagnostic tests, 6 months ago
   Pap smear: (−) cervical changes
   Pelvic ultrasound: (−) masses or lesions, (−) ovarian cysts or endometriomas

Assessment

Twenty-one-year-old woman with signs and symptoms consistent with dysmenorrhea secondary to menorrhagia proposed that some of these variations can be explained by the cultural perceptions of menstruation. Those cultures that have a more negative view of menstruation appear to report higher levels of dysmenorrhea.[5] Further, these negative expectations also seem to impact and be associated with higher levels of absenteeism.[2] Knowledge of such cultural differences may be of benefit in the assessment and treatment of women presenting with complaints consistent with dysmenorrhea.

REFERENCES

1. Ohde S, Tokuda Y, Takahashi O, Yanai H, Hinohara S, Fukui T. Dysmenorrhea among Japanese women. Int J Gynecol Obstet 2008 100:13–17.
2. Houston AM, Abraham A, Huang Z, D'Angelo LJ. Knowledge, attitudes, and consequences of menstrual health in urban adolescents. J Pediatr Adolesc Gynecol 2006 19:271–275.
3. Ortiz MI, Rangel-Flores E, Carrillo-Alarcon LC, Veras-Godoy HA. Prevalence and impact of primary dysmenorrhea among Mexican high school students. Int J Gynecol Obstet 2009 107(3):240–243.
4. Banikarim C, Chacko MR, Kelder SH. Prevalence and impact of dysmenorrhea on Hispanic female adolescents. Arch Pediatr Adolesc Med 2000 154:1226–1229.
5. Bettendorf B, Shay S, Tu F. Dysmenorrhea: Contemporary perspectives. Obstet Gynecol Surv 2008 63:597–603.

Student Workup

Missing Information?

Evaluate: Patient Database

Drug Therapy Problems

Care Plan (by Problem)

TARGETED QUESTIONS

1. What signs and symptoms of dysmenorrhea does the patient have?

   Hint: See p. 858 in PPP

2. Why are NSAIDs the treatment of choice for most patients with dysmenorrhea?

   Hint: See p. 861 in PPP

3. What nonpharmacologic therapies have been shown to be beneficial in the treatment of dysmenorrhea?

   Hint: See p. 861 in PPP

4. What risks and adverse effects of therapy would you discuss with the patient?

   Hint: See Table 49-2 in PPP

FOLLOW-UP

5. Three months later, the patient returns for follow-up. Her symptoms have improved dramatically with a reduction in menstrual flow and pain. Her iron studies, drawn last week, are iron 85 mcg/dL (15.2 μmol/L), ferritin 70 ng/mL (70 mcg/L), TIBC 325 mcg/dL (58.2 μmol/L), and transferrin saturation 32% (0.32). Would you recommend discontinuing the iron supplementation?

   Hint: See pp. 1113–1116 in PPP

☿ GLOBAL PERSPECTIVE

Reports of primary dysmenorrhea have been shown to vary among different cultures. It has been reported by 15.8% of Japanese women,[1] 65% of African American adolescents,[2] 48% of Mexican adolescents,[3] 85% of Hispanic adolescents,[4] and more than 80% of Caucasian women.[5] It has been

CASE SUMMARY

- The patient's current clinical picture is consistent with dysmenorrhea and menorrhagia, and an oral contraceptive should be initiated.
- Given the patient's family history of ovarian cancer and her occasional use of a barrier contraceptive, a combination oral contraceptive would be a good alternative to NSAIDs.
- Resolution of symptoms (both dysmenorrhea and menorrhagia) should occur within one to three menstrual cycles.

For more information on the care plan and facilitator's guide please visit http://www.mhpharmacotherapy.com.

53 Menopause

Leigh V. Maine

CASE LEARNING OBJECTIVES

- Identify the signs and symptoms associated with menopause
- Explain how to evaluate a patient for the appropriate use of hormone replacement therapy
- Recommend nonpharmacologic therapy for menopausal symptoms
- Differentiate between topical and systemic forms of hormone replacement therapy
- Educate a patient regarding the proper use and potential adverse effects of hormone replacement therapy

PATIENT PRESENTATION

Chief Complaint

"It has been very painful to have intercourse recently; nothing I've tried from the drugstore seems to help."

History of Present Illness

Shirley Davis is a 52-year-old Caucasian woman who presents to her primary care physician complaining of dyspareunia for the last 2 months. Due to her embarrassment over the issue, she has tried several OTC lubricants in order to relieve her problem rather than seek medical attention. Within the last year, she has informed her physician that her menstrual cycle has stopped. She denied having hot flashes or mood changes approximately a year ago. Currently, she admits to interruptions in her day several times per week due to profuse sweating and mood swings. She states it usually happens after having hot tea or soup for lunch.

Past Medical History

Amenorrhea × 1 year

HTN × 3 years

Hyperlipidemia × 4 years

Past Surgical History

Hysterectomy 1 year ago

Oophorectomy (left ovary) 32 years ago

Tonsillectomy 44 years ago

Family History

Father is 78 and has CHD and DM. Mother is 76 and is in overall good health, is a survivor of breast cancer, and had a double mastectomy 20 years ago. SD has no siblings.

Social History

SD is a married mother of three children, ages 27, 25, and 23. She has been married for 27 years. She works as a librarian.

Tobacco/Alcohol/Substance Use

Three to five alcoholic drinks/wk; states she drinks wine to help her cholesterol; (−) tobacco or illicit drug use

Allergies/Intolerances/Adverse Drug Events

HCTZ (hypokalemia)

Medications (Current)

Amlodipine/benazepril 5 mg/10 mg PO q 24 h

Fenofibrate 145 mg PO q 24 h

Calcium with vitamin D 600 mg/400 IU PO bid

Multivitamin one tablet PO q 24 h

Ibuprofen 200 mg PO PRN joint pain after gardening

Review of Systems

Several incidences of painful intercourse; (+) dyspareunia; also episodes of increased body temperature and irritability; (+) vasomotor symptoms; (−) night sweats; (−) chest pain; (−) palpitations; (−) tachycardia

Physical Examination

▶ General

Fifty-two-year-old Caucasian woman in no acute distress

▶ Vital Signs

BP 104/70 mm Hg, P 70, RR 18, pulse O$_2$ 97% (0.97),
 T 96.7°F (35.9°C)

Weight 141.2 lb (64.2 kg)

Height 62.8 in. (159.5 cm)

Pain score 0/10

▶ Skin

Denies history of skin cancer. No rashes or new or unusual skin lesions

▶ HEENT

PERRLA, EOMI; intact without nystagmus, conjunctivas clear, sclera anicteric, canals clear, oropharynx clear without exudate

▶ Neck and Lymph Nodes

No masses or crepitance, symmetric, thyroid without nodularity, midline trachea

▶ Breasts

No discrete nodules

▶ Cardiovascular

Regular rate and rhythm, no murmurs, no jugular venous distention

▶ Lungs

Clear to auscultation

▶ Abdomen

No tenderness, organomegaly, or masses

▶ Neurology

No history of seizures, migraines, falls, or vertigo

▶ Genitourinary

No urinary problems, negative for renal stones

▶ External Genitalia

No unusual findings

▶ Vagina

Atrophic, erythematous mucosa

▶ Psychiatric

Mood swings, irritability

Laboratory Tests

Fasting, obtained this morning

	Conventional Units	SI Units
Na	137 mEq/L	137 mmol/L
K	5 mEq/L	5 mmol/L
Cl	106 mEq/L	106 mmol/L
CO$_2$	22 mEq/L	22 mmol/L
BUN	7 mg/dL	2.5 mmol/L
SCr	0.7 mg/dL	62 μmol/L
Glu	78 mg/dL	4.3 mmol/L
Ca	8 mg/dL	2 mmol/L
Mg	1.6 mEq/L	0.80 mmol/L
Phosphate	3.7 mg/dL	1.20 mmol/L
Hgb	12.8 g/dL	128 g/L; 7.93 mmol/L
Hct	37.5%	0.375
WBC	5 × 10^3/mm^3	5 × 10^9/L
MCV	87 μm^3	87 fL
Albumin	3.8 g/dL	38 g/L
TSH	3.5 μIU/mL	3.5 mIU/L
Free T$_4$	0.84 ng/dL	10.8 pmol/L
Total cholesterol	213 mg/dL	5.51 mmol/L
LDL cholesterol	114 mg/dL	2.95 mmol/L
HDL cholesterol	80 mg/dL	2.07 mmol/L
TG	94 mg/dL	1.06 mmol/L

Assessment

Fifty-two-year-old woman with s/s consistent with menopause

Student Workup

Missing Information?

Evaluate: Patient Database

 Drug Therapy Problems

 Care Plan (by Problem)

TARGETED QUESTIONS

1. What s/s of menopause does SD have?

 Hint: See p. 871 in PPP

2. What factors in SD's medical history must we consider when deciding medication therapy?

 Hint: See pp. 871 and 887 in PPP

3. What pharmacologic/nonpharmacologic therapy would be recommended in SD's case?

 Hint: See pp. 872, 874, 878, and 879 in PPP

4. What risks and adverse effects of therapy would you discuss with SD?

 Hint: See pp. 879 and 880 in PPP

FOLLOW-UP

5. Six weeks later, SD is back for a follow-up appointment. She denies dyspareunia and reports her vasomotor symptoms have improved. If started on hormone replacement therapy, when should discontinuation be considered?

   Hint: See p. 878 in PPP

◎ GLOBAL PERSPECTIVE

Menopause happens to every woman in the world when considering menopause as a physiologic change. However, when comparing how menopause manifests itself through signs and symptoms across cultures, the results differ greatly. Signs and symptoms of menopause can differ in quality and duration depending on the culture. Use of medication or alternative therapies can vary considerably as well.

CASE SUMMARY

- SD's clinical condition is consistent with menopause and therapy should be initiated.
- Use of topical estrogen and an SSRI are acceptable given her PMH of hysterectomy and risk factors for CHD and breast cancer.
- Close follow-up (4–6 weeks) may be desired initially to ensure success of medication therapy, and then 6-month follow-up would be acceptable.

For more information on the care plan and facilitator's guide please visit http://www.mhpharmacotherapy.com.

54 Erectile Dysfunction

Nicole Brandt   Allison Chilipko

CASE LEARNING OBJECTIVES

- Differentiate between organic and psychogenic erectile dysfunction (ED) with regard to etiology and pathophysiology
- Identify the drug classes most likely to contribute to ED
- Define the essential components of history, physical examination, and laboratory data needed to evaluate the patient presenting with ED
- Describe current nonpharmacologic and pharmacologic options for ED treatment to determine an appropriate first-line therapy for a specific patient
- Compare and contrast the benefits and risks for current phosphodiesterase inhibitors
- Recommend an appropriate treatment approach for patients with ED and significant cardiovascular risk factors

PATIENT PRESENTATION

Chief Complaint

"I am having trouble in the bedroom."

History of Present Illness

JM is a 67-year-old African American male who comes to your medication management clinic complaining about "not getting it up." He has a new girlfriend, and he is frustrated that they cannot be intimate. He has not been sexually active for at least 10 years, yet really wants to get back "on the horse," but needs help. He wants to know if he can get one of those pills he saw on television. In terms of his other medications, he admits to not taking his depression medication regularly as well as his cholesterol medication.

Past Medical History

HTN × 25 years

Angina × 10 years

Hyperlipidemia × 20 years

Depression × 5 years

Family History

Father died at age 75 from lung cancer. Mother died at age 70 from complications of diabetes. He has one brother who is healthy (age 61) and one sister who has diabetes and HTN (age 56). He has two sons (ages 42 and 27) who both have HTN and diabetes.

Social/Work History

The patient retired from the real estate business to take care of his wife about 10 years ago. For the last 3 years, he has been living in an apartment within a retirement community. Prior to this transition, he was living in his own home; however, he was lonely due to his wife's death 7 years ago from cancer. He has completed a few years of college but was unable to graduate. Now, he has a new girlfriend in his building.

Tobacco/Alcohol/Substance Use

He has a history of smoking about ½ to 1 ppd for the last 50 years. He admits he is trying to cut back. Currently, he regularly drinks about two cans of beer per night and occasionally more during "Happy Hours" at the facility on Friday.

Allergy/Intolerance/Adverse Event History

No known drug allergies

Medications (Current)

HCTZ 25 mg PO q 24 h (for the past 6 years)

Paroxetine 40 mg PO daily (for the past 3 years)

Isosorbide mononitrate 60 mg PO daily (for the past 10 years)

Atorvastatin 40 mg once daily (for the past 10 years)

Clonidine 0.2 mg PO twice daily (for the past 10 years)

Multivitamin one tablet PO daily

Enteric-coated aspirin 81 mg PO daily

Current Insurance Plan

Rx payment: Medicare Part D plan

Review of Systems

The patient has occasional dry mouth and stuffy nose with occasional cough. He denies any chest pain or tightness, but admits to occasional DOE when walking up a hill and with exercise. The patient denies any urinary hesitancy, but some issues with urgency due to the water pill. He notes it is hard for him to get and maintain an erection. He describes suffering from depressive episodes since his wife died. Now, though, the patient is happy to have made a new friend, but he is anxious about intimacy. He notes history of pain and tingling in both feet.

Physical Examination

▶ **General**

Pleasant, well-groomed and dressed male in no apparent distress, accompanied by his "friend."

▶ **Vital Signs**

BP 126/76 mm Hg (left arm, sitting), P 62 (regular), RR 20 (unlabored), T 98.0°F (36.7 °C) (oral)

Weight 225 lb (102 kg)

Height 73 in. (185 cm)

Pain 0/10

▶ **HEENT**

PERRLA, EOMI

▶ **Chest**

Clear to auscultation bilaterally

▶ **Cardiovascular**

RRR, nl S_1, S_2; no murmurs, rubs, or gallops

▶ **Abdomen**

Nontender, nondistended, normal bowel sounds

▶ **Neurology**

Cranial nerves intact, normal reflexes, good strength throughout

▶ **Genitourinary**

Slightly enlarged prostate gland, smooth, no nodules, tenderness, or warmth

▶ **Extremities**

Good muscle strength and tone throughout, with no decrease in range of motion noted

Laboratory Tests

Measured today after 12-hour fasting

	Conventional Units	SI Units
Na	135 mEq/L	135 mmol/L
K	4 mEq/L	4 mmol/L
Cl	100 mEq/L	100 mmol/L
CO_2	22 mEq/L	22 mmol/L
BUN	38 mg/dL	13.6 mmol/L
SCr	1.1 mg/dL	97 μmol/L
Glu	92 mg/dL	5.1 mmol/L
Urinalysis	(−)	
TSH	2.8 μIU/mL	2.8 mIU/L
Hgb	13.5 g/dL	135 g/L; 8.38 mmol/L
Hct	39.7%	0.397
WBC	$7.6 \times 10^3/mm^3$	$7.6 \times 10^9/L$
Albumin	3.8 g/dL	38 g/L
PSA	3.6 ng/mL	3.6 mcg/L
Free testosterone	10 ng/dL	0.35 nmol/L
Total cholesterol	185 mg/dL	4.78 mmol/L
LDL cholesterol	98 mg/dL	2.53 mmol/L
HDL cholesterol	45 mg/dL	1.16 mmol/L
Triglycerides	128 mg/dL	1.45 mmol/L

Assessment

This is a 67-year-old African American man with ED, who is not currently receiving treatment.

Student Workup

Missing Information?

Evaluate: Patient Database

Drug Therapy Problems

Care Plan (by Problem)

TARGETED QUESTIONS

1. What potential etiologies may be responsible for this patient's ED?

   Hint: See pp. 884 and 885, and Table 51-1 in PPP

2. What medications may be causing or contributing to this patient's ED?

   Hint: See Table 51-2 in PPP

3. Why are phosphodiesterase inhibitors not a treatment consideration for this patient?

   Hint: See pp. 888 and 889, and Table 51-5 in PPP

4. Why should a vacuum erection device, representative of nonpharmacologic means, be considered with drug therapy in this patient?

   Hint: See pp. 887–888 in PPP

5. What risks and adverse effects of therapy would you discuss with this patient?

   Hint: See pp. 887–888 in PPP

FOLLOW-UP

6. One year later, JM comes back to your clinic to follow-up with you. Over the last year, he underwent a three-vessel CABG for his heart disease and since his angina has resolved. He underwent extensive cardiac rehab, and his cardiologist notes that he is stable off of his isosorbide mononitrate. He wants to know if he can now take "Viagra" because he was not satisfied with the results from the previous recommendation. On the basis of the changes in his comorbid conditions and medications, how would you change your treatment recommendations?

   Hint: See Table 51-4 in PPP

⊙ GLOBAL PERSPECTIVE

ED may not be incorporated into conventional screening measures for older men despite its prevalence of occurrence.

This omission may be due to the health care providers' level of comfort with the topic or lack of time to properly evaluate the patient given the potential for multiple etiologies. The increasing prevalence of ED could be due to physiologic changes that occur with aging, the onset of chronic disease states associated with ED (e.g., HTN, DM), increased medication use (e.g., antihypertensives, antidepressants), lifestyle factors (e.g., smoking, drinking, obesity), or a combination of the above influences. Although there appears to be a difference in reporting among certain cultures (e.g., Hispanic men), overall, it seems that the prevalence may be more attributable to the interplay of above-mentioned risk factors.

CASE SUMMARY

- ED is very common in older adults but is often not discussed or treated appropriately.
- *All* potential etiologies (e.g., vasculogenic, psychogenic medications) need to be considered and investigated before starting treatments with unrealistic expectations for symptomatic improvement.
- Monitoring patients over time is essential to assess the efficacy, toxicity, and need for alternative treatment options.

For more information on the care plan and facilitator's guide please visit http://www.mhpharmacotherapy.com.

55 Benign Prostatic Hyperplasia

Mary Lee   Roohollah Sharifi

CASE LEARNING OBJECTIVES

- Recognize the symptoms and signs of benign prostatic hyperplasia (BPH) in individual patients
- List the desired treatment outcomes for a patient with BPH
- Identify the factors that guide selection of a particular α-adrenergic antagonist for an individual patient
- Compare and contrast the α-adrenergic antagonists versus 5-α-reductase inhibitors in terms of mechanism of action, treatment outcomes, adverse effects, and interactions when used for management of BPH
- Describe the indications for combination drug treatment of BPH
- Describe the indications for surgical treatment of BPH
- Formulate a monitoring plan for a patient on a given drug treatment regimen on the basis of patient-specific information and formulate appropriate counseling information for patients receiving drug treatment for BPH

PATIENT PRESENTATION

Chief Complaint

"I'm taking two drugs for my big prostate, but my urine flow is still too slow. I have urinary frequency day and night. I feel like I can't empty my bladder. Sometimes I can't get to the bathroom on time and I leak on myself."

History of Present Illness

George Gold is a 73-year-old male with long-standing lower urinary tract symptoms (LUTS) who is referred to the urology service after failing maximal medication therapy for BPH. He has been taking terazosin 20 mg orally daily and finasteride 5 mg orally daily for 9 months. His current complaints include urgency with urge incontinence, nocturia two to three times a night, a weak urinary stream, and small-volume voids. He denies hematuria, dysuria, suprapubic or flank pain. He has no fever, chills, nausea, or vomiting. His American Urological Association (AUA) symptom score is 30.

Past Medical History

Essential HTN × 10 years

Hyperlipidemia × 10 years

Obesity, BMI 35 kg/m²

OA with chronic lower back pain × 5 years

History of a bleeding ulcer secondary to aspirin overuse

S/p transurethral incision of the prostate (TUIP) in 1996

Family History

Father died of a stroke. Mother died of breast cancer. Sister, alive, has breast cancer.

Social History

Married for 45 years; has two children: a son and a daughter, both alive and healthy.

Tobacco/Alcohol/Substance Use

Negative for all

Allergies/Intolerances/Adverse Drug Events

Sulfonamides; develops hives and shortness of breath when exposed. Cannot use Bactrim or Septra (trimethoprim/sulfamethoxazole)

Medications (Current)

Docusate 100 mg PO daily

Finasteride 5 mg PO daily

Furosemide 40 mg PO daily

Lisinopril 40 mg PO daily

Metoprolol 50 mg PO twice a day

Nifedipine 60 mg extended release two tablets PO daily

Terazosin 20 mg PO at bedtime

Simvastatin 80 mg PO at bedtime

Hydrocodone 5 mg/acetaminophen 500 mg two tablets PO twice a day

Review of Systems

The patient has chronic moderately severe low back pain that is only slightly relieved with analgesic. He takes narcotic analgesic only as needed; he is worried about addiction. To prevent constipation, he takes docusate and eats a high-fiber diet. Medications for HTN make him dizzy, particularly when he kneels down or suddenly changes body positions. He is most bothered by urinary incontinence. He has had to curb some social activities because of it.

Physical Examination

▶ General

Well-developed, well-nourished male in no apparent distress

▶ Vital Signs

BP 132/64 mm Hg, P 62, RR 14, T 37°C

Weight 222 lb (101 kg)

Height 66.5 in. (168.9 cm)

▶ Skin

(−) Rashes or lesions

▶ HEENT

PERRLA, EOMI

▶ Neck and Lymph Nodes

Thyroid gland is smooth and symmetrical; (−) thyroid nodules; (−) lymphadenopathy; (−) carotid bruits

▶ Chest

Clear to auscultation and percussion

▶ Cardiovascular

RRR; no murmurs

▶ Abdomen

Soft, not tender, or distended; no masses or organomegaly

▶ Neurology

Grossly intact; deep tendon reflexes normal

▶ Extremities

Trace bilateral lower extremity edema; good range of motion; normal pedal pulses

▶ Genitourinary

Digital rectal examination shows a large (50 g), soft, symmetric nontender prostate, no nodules, and no areas of induration. Normal external genitalia. No costovertebral angle tenderness. No rectal pathology.

▶ Rectum

No hemorrhoids

Laboratory Tests

	Conventional Units	SI Units
Na	143 mEq/L	143 mmol/L
K	4.6 mEq/L	4.6 mmol/L
Cl	107 mEq/L	107 mmol/L
CO_2	27.1 mEq/L	27.1 mmol/L
BUN	30 mg/dL	10.7 mmol/L
SCr	1.6 mg/dL	141 μmol/L
Glu fasting	95 mg/dL	5.3 mmol/L
Ca	8.7 mg/dL	2.18 mg/dL
Urinalysis—yellow, clear		
pH	5	
Specific gravity	1.027	
WBC	2/lpf	
RBC	0/lpf	
Protein	Trace	
Glucose	(−)	
Ketones	(−)	
Blood	(−)	
Hyaline casts	6–10/lpf	
Hgb	13.8 g/dL	138 g/L; 8.57 mmol/L
Hct	40.7%	0.407
WBC	$6.7 \times 10^3/mm^3$	$6.7 \times 10^9/L$
Platelets	$167 \times 10^3/mm^3$	$167 \times 10^9/L$
Albumin	3.8 g/dL	38 g/L
Total cholesterol	123 mg/dL	3.18 mmol/L
LDL cholesterol	63 mg/dL	1.63 mmol/L
HDL cholesterol	32 mg/dL	0.83 mmol/L
PSA	1.6 ng/mL	1.6 mcg/L
PSA (1 yr ago)	3.0 ng/mL	3 mcg/L

Assessment

The patient has severe LUTS, s/p TUIP, and is not responding to maximum doses of terazosin and finasteride after 9 months. He has urinary incontinence and impaired renal function, and is at risk of additional complications of BPH on the basis of size of prostate and PSA. Patient to undergo preoperative testing for a prostatectomy, which will include uroflowmetry, postvoid residual volume, and transrectal ultrasound (TRUS) of the prostate.

Student Workup

Missing Information?

Evaluate: Patient Database

Drug Therapy Problems

Care Plan (by Problem)

TARGETED QUESTIONS

1. What symptoms and signs of BPH does this patient have?

    Hint: See pp. 897 and 898 in PPP

2. Explain the mechanism of terazosin and finasteride in the management of BPH. Contrast their onset of action, clinical benefits, and adverse effects.

    Hint: See pp. 896 and 897 and Table 52-2 in PPP

3. Was this patient given an adequate medication treatment trial? Explain your answer.

    Hint: See pp. 898 and 906 in PPP

4. Interpret the change in this patient's PSA over the past year.

    Hint: See p. 907 in PPP

5. In view of this patient's renal impairment, are the doses of terazosin and finasteride appropriate?

    Hint: See Tables 52-6 and 52-7 in PPP

FOLLOW-UP

Preoperative testing is done. Test results reveal the following: maximum urine flow rate 8 mL/s (normal, at least 10–14 mL/s) with a voided volume of 150 mL, postvoid residual urine volume 150 mL (normal, 0 mL), and TRUS shows a prostate size of 50 cm³. One week after this clinic visit, the patient is scheduled for an outpatient transurethral resection of the prostate (TURP). Surgery is uneventful. Three months after the TURP, the patient returns to the clinic. AUA symptom score is 9, maximum urine flow rate is 18 mL/s, and postvoid residual urine volume is 0 mL. The patient reports that he is able to sleep through the night without having to wake up to urinate. He has noticed no blood clots or red coloring of his urine. He has no incontinence, urinary frequency, or urgency.

6. Interpret the preoperative and postoperative laboratory tests performed on this patient. Are the postoperative tests consistent with improvement in the symptoms and signs of BPH?

    Hint: See Table 52-2 in PPP

⊙ GLOBAL PERSPECTIVE

Treatment of BPH may differ in countries outside the United States because of the use of herbals to control obstructive or irritative voiding symptoms. The American Urological Association and the Food and Drug Administration have concluded that clinical evidence is not sufficient to document the efficacy of any herbal product for this disorder, which should dissuade physicians from prescribing such agents. However, in other countries, widespread use of herbals including saw palmetto, pygeum (African plum), secale cereale (rye pollen), and hypoxis rooperi (South African star grass) is common. Such agents may be taken on their own, in combination with other herbals, or in common with prescription medications.

CASE SUMMARY

- First-line drug treatment for moderate-to-severe BPH is an α-adrenergic antagonist. A uroselective α-adrenergic antagonist or an extended-release α-adrenergic antagonist is preferred in patients who cannot tolerate the cardiovascular side effects of immediate-release terazosin or doxazosin. All α-adrenergic antagonists quickly relieve voiding symptoms and have comparable efficacy in relieving voiding symptoms.

- For a patient with a moderately enlarged prostate, 40 g or more, a 5-α-reductase inhibitor may be considered. However, these agents require a clinical trial of 6 months minimum. Onset is delayed as the prostate gland must shrink in size and this takes time.

- Combination drug therapy with an α-adrenergic antagonist and a 5-α-reductase inhibitor is considered in those patients with moderate-to-severe disease who also have an enlarged prostate gland of at least 30 to 40 g and a PSA greater than 1.5 ng/mL (1.5 mcg/L). In such patients, combination therapy may relieve LUTS, slow disease progression, and reduce the need for prostatectomy.

- For patients who fail drug therapy or for those with complications of BPH, surgery is the treatment of choice.

For more information on the care plan and facilitator's guide please visit http://www.mhpharmacotherapy.com.

56 Urinary Incontinence: Overactive Bladder

Thomas E. Lackner

CASE LEARNING OBJECTIVES

- Contrast the pathophysiology of overactive bladder with other major types of urinary incontinence (i.e., stress, overflow, and functional)
- Recognize the signs and symptoms of overactive bladder
- List the treatment goals for a patient with urinary incontinence, including overactive bladder
- Compare and contrast anticholinergics/antispasmodics, vaginal estrogens, tricyclic antidepressants, and α-adrenoceptor antagonists in terms of mechanism of action, treatment outcomes, adverse effects, and drug–drug interaction potential when used to manage overactive bladder
- Identify the factors that guide drug selection for an individual patient
- Formulate a monitoring plan for a patient on a given treatment regimen using patient-specific information
- Describe the indicators for combination drug therapy of urinary incontinence
- Describe the nonpharmacologic treatment approaches (including surgery) for overactive bladder
- Formulate appropriate patient-counseling information for patients undergoing drug therapy for overactive bladder

Chief Complaint

"I tried bladder medicine but it didn't help my overactive bladder very much. Do you have any better pads than these to protect me when I need it?"

History of Present Illness

Phoebe J. Engling, a 72-year-old woman, comes to the pharmacy for a refill of her pain medicine. She was recently hospitalized for dehydration and possible head injury after falling. Despite behavioral therapy and regular use of absorbent pads and undergarments, she is embarrassed and bothered by uncontrollable wetting of her clothing for at least a couple of years. She was initially told by her physician not to worry about urine leakage, that this can be expected with aging. With trepidation, she revealed she may have become dehydrated while trying to relieve her wetting accidents by limiting her fluid consumption and doubling the dose of her prescribed diuretic. This led to being hospitalized last month for severe dehydration with a fall without hitting head or bone fracture. At hospital discharge, she was given a prescription for oxybutynin. In a hurry to get home before she had another "accident" she declined medication counseling from the pharmacist. She stopped taking oxubutynin after a few days' use due to the lack of substantial improvement in her urinary symptoms.

Past Medical History

Overactive bladder (06/08/2009)

Type 2 DM (diagnosed 4 years ago)

HTN (for over 10 years)

OA (diagnosed last year)

Dehydration (06/08/2009) (resolved)

Fall (06/08/2009, and twice more the past year)

Depression diagnosed 6 months ago

Insomnia diagnosed 6 months ago

Cerebrovascular disease (stroke 2003)

Glaucoma for more than 20 years

Chronic constipation (late 2007)

Family History
No details

Social History
Widowed, three children, worked as a hospital laboratory phlebotomist for 40 years

Tobacco/Ethanol/Substance Use
Denies tobacco; drinks one glass of wine at bedtime to help sleep and three to five cups of caffeinated coffee daily

Allergies/Intolerances/Adverse Drug Events
Amoxicillin (rash), tetracycline (GI discomfort)

Medications (Current)
Immediate-release oxybutynin 5 mg PO bid

Propoxyphene 100 mg/acetaminophen 650 mg PO q 6 h

Propoxyphene 100 mg/acetaminophen 650 mg PO q 4–6 h PRN knee pain

Senna 8.6 mg PO hs

HCTZ 25 mg PO q 24 h

Metformin 500 mg PO bid

Enteric-coated aspirin 81 mg PO q 24 h

Lisinopril 10 mg PO q 24 h

Citalopram 20 mg PO q 24 h

Simvastatin 40 mg PO every evening

Acetaminophen 500 mg/diphenhydramine 25 mg PO hs PRN insomnia

Bimatoprost ophthalmic solution 0.03% one drop both eyes every night

Timolol maleate ophthalmic solution 0.5% one drop in the right eye every morning

Review of Systems
Overall, the patient's appetite is adequate. Her cataracts are stable, but she is hard of hearing. She has had insomnia for a couple of years; she has recently started taking a glass of wine nightly to help her relax, and believes that can prevent urinary urgency that awakens her during the night. The patient uses an absorbent pad. She has chronic urinary incontinence (incontinent several times per week). She needs to void within a couple of minutes or large urine loss. She urinates as frequently as every 1 to 2 hours during the day. She wakes up as many as five times nightly with a strong urge to void. The patient also has pain in knees and hips; balance is fine with walker (uses all the time), but unsteady gait. She has right-hand weakness.

Physical Examination

▶ **General**

Obese white female in no acute distress. Decreased normal fluid intake

▶ **Vital Signs**

BP 129/78 mm Hg, P 72, RR 18, T 36.3°C

Weight 182 lb (82.7 kg)

Height 62 in. (157 cm)

▶ **Skin**

Dry-appearing skin

▶ **HEENT**

Dry oral mucosal membranes

PER, EMI

▶ **Neck and Lymph Nodes**

No masses

▶ **Chest**

Clear lung fields

▶ **Breasts**

No masses

▶ **Cardiovascular**

RRR; no murmurs heard

▶ **Abdomen**

Obese; bowel sounds

▶ **Neurology**

Slight EOMI, motor strength 5/5 symmetrical

▶ **Genitourinary**

Incontinence

▶ **Rectal**

Examination deferred

Laboratory Tests
Two days ago (7/7/2009)

	Conventional Units	SI Units
Na	137 mEq/L	137 mmol/L
K	4.5 mEq/L	4.5 mmol/L
Cl	100 mEq/L	100 mmol/L

CO_2	24 mEq/L	24 mmol/L
BUN	17 mg/dL	6.1 mmol/L
SCr	0.52 mg/dL	46 mmol/L
Glucose (fasting)	162 mg/dL	9 mmol/L
Ca	8.8 mg/dL	2.20 mmol/L
Hgb	13.9 g/dL	139 g/L; 8.63 mmol/L
HCT	39.7%	0.397
MCV	93 um^3	93 fL
WBC	$7.2 \times 10^3/mm^3$	$7.2 \times 10^9/L$
Platelets	$156 \times 10^3/mm^3$	$156 \times 10^9/L$
Albumin	3.8 g/dL	38 g/L
A_{1C}	8.8%	0.088
TSH	2.25 mIU/mL	2.25 mIU/L

Postvoid residual urine volume 89 mL

Assessment

Seventy-two-year-old woman with signs and symptoms consistent with overactive bladder along with numerous other comorbid conditions

Student Workup

Missing Information?

Evaluate: Patient Database

               Drug Therapy Problems

               Care Plan (by Problem)

TARGETED QUESTIONS

1. What signs and symptoms of overactive bladder does the patient have?

   Hint: See pp. 910 and 911 in PPP

2. Why is antimuscarinic medication the pharmacologic treatment of choice for patients with overactive bladder?

   Hint: See p. 915 in PPP

3. What medications can cause overactive bladder?

   Hint: See Table 52-1 in PPP

4. What risks and adverse effects of pharmacotherapy would you discuss with the patient?

   Hint: See p. 915 in PPP

5. Should the patient receive specific (other) pharmacotherapy that could indirectly improve overactive bladder symptoms?

   Hint: See pp. 914 and 915 in PPP

Student Workup

Missing Information?

Evaluate: Patient Database

               Drug Therapy Problems

               Care Plan (by Problem)

FOLLOW-UP

6. One month later, the patient returns for a refill of oxybutynin. She reports moderate improvement in her overactive bladder symptoms, with this documented in a bladder diary. However, she complains of dry mouth and worsened constipation. What actions, if any, would you take?

   Hint: See p. 915 in PPP

⊙ GLOBAL PERSPECTIVE

It is estimated by the World Health Organization that more than 200 million people worldwide have some type of bladder-control issue. Considering pathophysiology, it is not surprising that there is no evidence of significant international differences in the prevalence of overactive bladder or other types of urinary incontinence and their symptoms and drug response. The female sex and older age are associated with a higher risk of development of bladder-control issues, likely due to the stress of childbirth and menopause. Differences in continence services for managing urinary incontinence outside of North America are attributed to government policies.

CASE SUMMARY

- Her current clinical presentation is consistent with overactive bladder with urge urinary incontinence.

- The patient's glaucoma is a contraindication for use of an antimuscarinic agent, therefore, requires clarification regarding its type and whether her intraocular pressures are controlled by her current ophthalmic medicine. Because the use of an antimuscarinic agent with uncontrolled narrow-angle glaucoma could potentially cause serious damage to the optic nerve, this therapy should be confirmed with her ophthalmologist before starting therapy.

- If the antimuscarinic medication cannot be used, transient factors and elements of functional incontinence should be managed.

- Antimuscarinic therapy should be started at the lowest recommended dose during or after amelioration of transient factors and potential functional incontinence in the patient, especially with her advanced age. If bothersome adverse effects occur, if possible, the dose should be reduced or the current antimuscarinic agent replaced with the lowest dose of a different antimuscarinic agent, preferably an extended-release or transdermal formulation.

- An excessive dose of the antimuscarinic agent should be avoided, especially with her advanced age, history of constipation, diuretic use that predisposes to dry mouth and constipation, and glaucoma that predisposes to vision disturbances.

For more information on the care plan and facilitator's guide please visit http://www.mhpharmacotherapy.com.

57 Drug Allergy

Lauren S. Schlesselman

CASE LEARNING OBJECTIVES

- Recognize the signs and symptoms of anaphylaxis
- Identify the goals of therapy for anaphylaxis
- Develop an appropriate treatment and monitoring plan for anaphylaxis based on individual patient characteristics
- Select an appropriate product for treating the underlying condition on the basis of patient's allergic history
- Properly educate a patient with a history of drug allergies

PATIENT PRESENTATION

Chief Complaint

"I was walking back from the mailbox when I heard a rustling sound in the woods. A raccoon came charging out of the woods at me. I tried to run but he caught up to me and bit my leg."

History of Present Illness

Faith Stevens is a 19-year-old woman who presents to the emergency department with a raccoon bite to her left leg. While walking in her yard during daylight hours, a raccoon (whose whereabouts are currently unknown) raced across the lawn to bite her. The patient describes attempting to shake the raccoon from her leg. Damage to the leg confirms raccoon-inflicted significant damage to the skin and muscles on the left calf.

On arrival at the hospital, cleaning of the wound began with soap and water, followed by povidine–iodine. During this time, a single dose of amoxicillin/clavulanate 875/125 mg was orally administered. Within 30 minutes of the dose, the patient began complaining of SOB, abdominal pain, itchiness, nausea, and rapid heart rate. Nurse noted audible wheezing and pruritis on trunk and arms.

Past Medical History

History of Stevens–Johnson syndrome with sulfa

Family History

Father is alive with no significant medical history at age 44. Mother is alive with no significant medical history at age 42. She has two young sisters who are healthy.

Social History

College student pursuing degree in psychology. Single, lives with her parents and sisters; has no children. Works part-time at a local library

Tobacco/Alcohol/Substance Use

Social drinker; (−) tobacco or illicit drug use

Allergies/Intolerances/Adverse Drug Events

Sulfa-induced Stevens–Johnson syndrome

Codeine-induced nausea

Ibuprofen (GI upset and abdominal pain)

Meperidine (hallucinations)

Medications (Current)

No outpatient medications

Physical Examination

▶ *General*

Teenaged, Caucasian woman in acute distress

▶ *Vital Signs*

BP 90/45 mm Hg, P 98, RR 16, T 37.2°C

Weight 134.2 lb (61 kg)

Height 68 in. (172.7 cm)

Pain 7 (scale 0–10)

231

▶ **Skin**

Clammy skin

Laceration of left calf 4 inch (10 cm) in diameter with underlying tissue and muscle damage; significant bleeding at site; (+) urticaria on trunk and arms

▶ **HEENT**

PERRLA, EOMI; (−) trace periorbital edema; (−) sinus tenderness

▶ **Neck and Lymph Nodes**

(−) Lymphadenopathy; (−) carotid bruits

▶ **Chest**

Audible wheezing

▶ **Breasts**

Examination deferred

▶ **Cardiovascular**

Normal rhythm; tachycardia; normal S_1, S_2; (−) S_3 or S_4

▶ **Abdomen**

Not tender/not distended; (−) organomegaly

▶ **Neurology**

Grossly intact; deep tendon reflexes normal

▶ **Genitourinary**

Examination deferred

▶ **Rectal**

Examination deferred

Laboratory Tests

Nonfasting

	Conventional Units	SI Units
Na	140 mEq/L	140 mmol/L
K	4 mEq/L	4 mmol/L
Cl	100 mEq/L	100 mmol/L
CO_2	24 mEq/L	24 mmol/L
BUN	8 mg/dL	2.9 mmol/L
SCr	0.7 mg/dL	62 μmol/L
Glu	105 mg/dL	5.8 mmol/L
Ca	9.4 mg/dL	2.35 mmol/L
Mg	1.8 mEq/L	0.90 mmol/L
Phosphate	3.8 mg/dL	1.23 mmol/L
Hgb	13.5 g/dL	135 g/L; 8.38 mmol/L
Hct	39.7%	0.397
WBC	$9.2 \times 10^3/mm^3$	$9.2 \times 10^9/L$
MCV	$83\ \mu m^3$	83 fL
Albumin	4.3 g/dL	43 g/L

Assessment

Nineteen-year-old woman with signs and symptoms consistent with anaphylaxis following antibiotic administration; also with signs consistent for animal bite

---

Student Workup

Missing Information?

Evaluate: Patient Database
Drug Therapy Problems
Care Plan (by Problem)

TARGETED QUESTIONS

1. What signs and symptoms of anaphylaxis does the patient have?

   Hint: See p. 930 and Table 54-1 in PPP

2. Why are epinephrine and fluids the treatment of choice for patients with anaphylaxis?

   Hint: See p. 928 and Table 64-3 in PPP

3. How long should patients who have experienced an anaphylactic reaction be observed and why?

   Hint: See p. 930 in PPP

4. What classes of medications are frequently associated with anaphylaxis?

   Hint: See Table 54-1 in PPP

5. What steps can the patient and health care providers take to prevent exposure to medications to which she is allergic?

   Hint: See p. 936 in PPP

FOLLOW-UP

6. After administration of her five doses of rabies vaccine, the patient is seen by her primary care provider for follow-up. She feels much better with significant wound healing and limited discomfort. Is the patient a candidate for desensitization to penicillin or sulfa? If so, how would this be done?

   Hint: See pp. 933–935 in PPP

⊙ GLOBAL PERSPECTIVE

Drug allergy is an adverse immune response to a stimulus. Such responses, categorized utilizing the Gell and Coombs categories, can be type I, II, III, IV, or a combination of these. Classes of medications frequently associated with anaphylaxis include penicillins, sulfa, vaccines, NSAIDs, and radiocontrast media. Available medications commonly associated with allergies and skin tests vary by country. For example, penicillin minor-determinant skin tests are not available in the United States, but are used in Europe. Additionally, many medication-related allergic reactions have been associated with impurities in medication solutions, which depends on manufacturing procedures and regulations in different countries.

CASE SUMMARY

- Her current clinical picture is consistent with anaphylaxis and epinephrine and fluid replacement should be initiated.

- An initial epinephrine dose of 0.2 to 0.5 mg IM or SC, repeated every 5 minutes as needed, is appropriate. This should be accompanied by 1 to 2 L of normal saline at 5 to 10 mL/kg in the first 5 minutes followed by a slower infusion.

- Anaphylaxis can reoccur 6 to 8 hours after presentation, so patients should be monitored for at least 12 hours.

- Documentation of allergies in the patient's medical records in the hospital, physician's office, and pharmacy is a critical component in preventing exposure to these medications in the future. Differentiation between true allergies and adverse reactions is also essential.

For more information on the care plan and facilitator's guide please visit http://www.mhpharmacotherapy.com.

58 Solid Organ Transplantation

R. Carlin Walsh   Rita R. Alloway

CASE LEARNING OBJECTIVES

- Identify the signs and symptoms of renal transplant rejection
- Develop a comprehensive treatment plan for renal transplant rejection
- Determine a cytomegalovirus (CMV) therapeutic regimen and monitoring parameters for that regimen
- Formulate a medication-counseling plan for a renal transplant recipient

Chief Complaint

"I'm just here for my regular check up."

History of Present Illness

Robert Weaver is a 43-year-old African American gentleman with a history of end-stage renal disease (ESRD) secondary to hypertension and type 2 diabetes mellitus. He underwent a three-antigen mismatched deceased-donor kidney transplant 4 months previously. This was his second transplant. Prior to his second transplant, he was on hemodialysis three times a week for 2 years. He received blood transfusions due to anemia on two occasions while he was on dialysis. Pretransplant testing revealed a peak cytotoxic panel-reactive antibody (PRA) of 54% and current cytotoxic PRA of 18%. He received induction with rabbit antithymocyte globulin and a rapid steroid taper. Pretransplant viral serologies showed that Mr. Weaver was CMV IgG negative and the donor was CMV IgG positive. Maintenance immunosuppression includes tacrolimus and mycophenolate mofetil. Posttransplant, his serum creatinine nadir was 1.1 mg/dL (97 μmol/L) and has remained relatively constant. He was last seen in renal transplant clinic 3 weeks prior. He states that he is feeling fine, but thinks that he might be somewhat dehydrated. He has noticed a slight decrease in his urine output, which he attributes to not drinking enough water. He endorses that he has missed "a couple days" of immunosuppressive medications due to issues with insurance co-pays.

Past Medical History

ESRD status post (s/p) deceased-donor kidney transplant

HTN × 25 years

Diabetes mellitus type 2 × 19 years

Hyperlipidemia × 16 years

Past Surgical History

Four months s/p deceased-donor kidney transplant

Tonsillectomy at age 9

Family History

Mother is alive at 67 years with HTN and type 2 diabetes mellitus. Father had HTN and hyperlipidemia and he died last year due to MI at the age of 68.

Social History

He is married with three children (aged 16, 14, and 10), all of whom are alive and well. He worked as a retail store manager, but is currently on disability and is not working.

Tobacco/Alcohol/Substance Use

Previously, social drinker (last approximately 4 years ago); denies tobacco use and illicit drug use

Allergies

NKDA

Medications (Current)

Tacrolimus 6 mg PO twice daily

Mycophenolate mofetil 1,000 mg PO twice daily

Valganciclovir 450 mg PO daily until 6 months s/p transplant

Sulfamethoxazole/trimethoprim 400 mg/80 mg PO daily

Metoprolol 100 mg PO twice daily

Nifedipine ER 60 mg PO daily

Lisinopril 10 mg PO daily

Aspirin EC 81 mg PO daily

Metoclopromide 5 mg PO three times daily before meals

Omeprazole 20 mg PO daily

Simvastatin 20 mg PO at bedtime

Insulin glargine 24 units SC at bedtime

Multivitamin one tablet PO daily

Magnesium oxide 400 mg PO twice daily

Review of Systems

Denies dysuria; denies fever, nausea/vomiting, diarrhea, chest pain, or shortness of breath; endorses subjective decrease in urinary output

Physical Examination

▶ General

Well-nourished, middle-aged, African American male in no apparent distress

▶ Vital Signs

BP 138/86 mm Hg, P 74, RR 16, T 37.2°C

Weight 242 lb (110 kg)

Height 70 in. (178 cm)

Pain score 0/10

▶ HEENT

PERRLA; EOMI

▶ Chest

Clear to auscultation bilaterally

▶ Cardiovascular

RRR; (+) S1, S2; (−) murmurs

▶ Abdomen

Nontender; nondistended; (+) bowel sounds

▶ Neurology

Alert and oriented × 3; CN II–XII intact; no focal deficits

▶ Genitourinary/Rectal

Examination deferred

Laboratory Tests

Fasting

	Conventional Units	SI Units
Na	143 mEq/L	143 mmol/L
K	5.3 mEq/L	5.3 mmol/L
Cl	107 mEq/L	107 mmol/L
CO_2	20 mEq/L	20 mmol/L
BUN	38 mg/dL	13.6 mmol/L
SCr	1.9 mg/dL	168 µmol/L
Glu	112 mg/dL	6.2 mmol/L
Ca	8.6 mg/dL	2.15 mmol/L
Mg	1.7 mEq/L	0.85 mmol/L
Phos	3.8 mg/dL	1.23 mmol/L
Hgb	11.3 g/dL	113 g/L; 7.01 mmol/L
Hct	32.7%	0.327
WBC	$5.4 \times 10^3/mm^3$	$5.4 \times 10^9/L$
MCV	87 µm³	87 fL
Albumin	3.6 g/dL	36 g/L
Total cholesterol	172 mg/dL	4.45 mmol/L
LDL cholesterol	93 mg/dL	2.41 mmol/L
HDL cholesterol	51 mg/dL	1.32 mmol/L
Tacrolimus	3.6 ng/mL or mcg/L	4.5 nmol/L

Renal Biopsy Pathology

Acute cellular rejection—Banff grade IB

Assessment

Mr. Weaver is a 43-year-old gentleman who is 4 months s/p deceased-donor kidney transplant, and presents with clinical symptoms, laboratory tests, and pathology findings consistent with acute cellular rejection.

TARGETED QUESTIONS

1. What risk factors for acute cellular rejection does Mr. Weaver have?

   Hint: See p. 943 in PPP

2. What therapies could be used for the treatment of acute cellular rejection?

   Hint: See p. 953 and Figure 55-2 (p. 949) in PPP

3. What clinical parameters should be monitored for efficacy of rejection treatment and resolution of acute cellular rejection?

   Hint: See Table 55-2 (p. 944) and Figure 55-2 (p. 949) in PPP

4. Three months later, Mr. Weaver presents to the renal transplant clinic with complaints of gastrointestinal pain and diarrhea over the last week. Of note, he recently completed a 7-day course of ciprofloxacin for a UTI. Laboratory evaluation reveals a SCr 1.3 mg/dL (115 µmol/L), WBC $1.3 \times 10^3/mm^3$ ($1.3 \times 10^9/L$), and an ANC $1.078 \times 10^3/mm^3$ ($1.078 \times 10^9/L$). What are possible explanations for Mr. Weaver's clinical symptoms of gastrointestinal pain and diarrhea?

   Hint: See pp. 956–957 in PPP

5. Serum CMV PCR results were positive with 275,000 copies/mL. A colonoscopy was performed and there was no evidence of invasive CMV disease. What therapeutic options are there for the treatment of CVM viremia and how should treatment efficacy be monitored?

   Hint: See p. 957 and Table 55-7 (p. 956) in PPP

⟳ GLOBAL PERSPECTIVE

Immunosuppression practices vary widely from region to region and country to country. The one consistent tenet is that as risk for rejection increases, the level of baseline immunosuppression used increases. However, different immunosuppressive medications may be utilized to achieve this ultimate goal. Examples of this include the use of steroid-minimization or -avoidance protocols, choice of antiproliferative agent, or choice of calcineurin inhibitor.

CASE SUMMARY

- Initial clinical presentation is consistent with acute cellular rejection in a kidney transplant recipient due to subtherapeutic doses of immunosuppressive medications.

- There is a risk of opportunistic infection in patients with immunosuppression. Therefore, appropriate prophylaxis and surveillance should be employed to improve patient outcomes.

For more information on the care plan and facilitator's guide please visit http://www.mhpharmacotherapy.com.

59 Osteoporosis

Alexis Horace   Beth Bryles Phillips

PATIENT PRESENTATION

Chief Complaint

"I am here to see my new physician."

History of Present Illness

DS is a 72-year-old Caucasian woman who presents to the internal medicine clinic to establish care at the urging of her daughter. She had been followed for a number of years by her previous physician who recently retired. She reports she has been taking calcitonin nasal spray for the past 5 years when her physician ordered a bone density test. She remembers asking her physician if she should take Fosamax instead because she knew several women in her book club who took the medication. She reports they discussed it, but he felt calcitonin may be a better choice due to her loss of height and presence of heartburn. She tries to walk on a regular basis for exercise, but finds that her speed and distance are not what they used to be since her hip was replaced 6 months ago. She reports consuming milk on a daily basis with her cereal. She only rarely takes in other dairy products. She drinks five to six cups of coffee daily and has been a heavy coffee drinker all of her life. She has had problems with heartburn "on and off" over the years. She currently takes omeprazole for her heartburn and feels that her symptoms are well controlled.

Past Medical History

Osteoporosis status post (s/p) vertebral fractures and left hip fracture with hip replacement 6 months ago

Gastroesophageal reflux disease

Hypertension

Peripheral artery disease

Hypothyroidism

Nicotine dependence

Osteoarthritis s/p total knee replacement 10 years ago

s/p deep venous thrombosis after knee surgery

Family History

Father deceased at age 94 due to cancer (type unknown). Mother deceased at age 92, history of hip fracture. She has one brother and one sister, who both are healthy.

Social History

The patient is married and lives with her husband of 44 years, and has five children. She is a retired social worker.

Tobacco/Alcohol/Substance Use

Social drinker; (+) tobacco 1 ppd × 54 years; (−) illicit drug use

Allergies/Intolerances/Adverse Drug Events

No known drug allergies

Medications (Current)

Calcitonin nasal spray 200 IU alternating nostrils daily

Omeprazole 20 mg daily

Hydrochlorothiazide 25 mg daily

Aspirin 325 mg daily

Levothyroxine 125 mcg daily

Naproxen 500 mg bid

Calcium carbonate 500 mg daily AM PRN

Review of Systems

(+) For heartburn treated with omeprazole; denies difficulty swallowing or burning in her throat; denies back or hip pain, but reports 2½ inch decrease in height since young adulthood; (+) kyphosis; denies heat intolerance, weight loss, or changes in texture of hair or skin

Physical Examination

▶ **General**

Thin, elderly woman who looks older than her stated age; mild kyphosis present

▶ **Vital Signs**

BP 132/76 mm Hg, P 78, RR 16, T 36.2°C

Weight 117 lb (53 kg)

Height 69 in. (175.3 cm)

Denies pain

▶ **Skin**

Normal turgor and color; warm

▶ **HEENT**

PERRLA, EOMI; disks flat; fundi with no hemorrhages or exudates

▶ **Neck and Lymph Nodes**

No lymphadenopathy, thyromegaly, or carotid bruits

▶ **Chest**

Clear to auscultation bilaterally

▶ **Breasts**

Examination deferred

▶ **Cardiovascular**

RRR; normal S_1 and S_2; no S_3 or S_4; no m/r/g

▶ **Abdomen**

Not tender/not distended; (−) organomegaly

▶ **Neurology**

A&O × 3; CN II–XII intact; DTR 2+

▶ **Extremities**

Cool; normal color; dorsalis pedis pulse weak

▶ **Genitourinary**

Examination deferred

▶ **Rectal**

Examination deferred

Laboratory Tests

Fasting, obtained 2 days ago

	Conventional Units	SI Units
Na	139 mEq/L	139 mmol/L
K	4.7 mEq/L	4.7 mmol/L
Cl	101 mEq/L	101 mmol/L
CO_2	30 mEq/L	30 mmol/L
BUN	14 mg/dL	5 mmol/L
SCr	0.8 mg/dL	71 µmol/L
Glu	99 mg/dL	5.5 mmol/L
Ca	9.3 mg/dL	2.33 mmol/L
TSH	0.2 µIU/mL	0.2 mIU/L
Hgb	15.5 g/dL	155 g/L; 9.61 mmol/L
Hct	48%	0.48
WBC	$7.6 \times 10^3/mm^3$	$7.6 \times 10^9/L$
MCV	79 µm³	79 fL
Albumin	3.8 g/dL	38 g/L
Total cholesterol	184 mg/dL	4.76 mmol/L
LDL cholesterol	96 mg/dL	2.48 mmol/L
HDL cholesterol	48 mg/dL	1.24 mmol/L
Triglyceride	184 mg/dl	2.08 mmol/L

Other Test

Bone mineral density

   5 years ago

      Total hip   T-score: −1.8

      Lumbar spine   T-score: −2.1

   3 months ago

      Total hip   T-score: −2.3

      Lumbar spine   T-score: −2.95

Assessment

Seventy-two-year-old female with signs and bone densitometry consistent with osteoporosis; recurrent osteoporotic fracture on current therapy

Student Workup

Missing Information?

Evaluate: Patient Database

                 Drug Therapy Problems

                 Care Plan (by Problem)

TARGETED QUESTIONS

1. What signs and symptoms of osteoporosis does the patient have?

   Hint: See p. 968 in PPP

2. What risk factors does the patient have for osteoporosis?

   Hint: See pp. 968-969 in PPP

3. What nonpharmacologic recommendations are important for the patient's treatment plan?

   Hint: See pp. 969-970 in PPP

4. What are the patient's calcium and vitamin D requirements? Is she a candidate for calcium and/or vitamin D supplementation? If so, which one would you recommend and why?

   Hint: See pp. 971-973 in PPP

5. Is the patient's current osteoporosis treatment effective? What alternative medications would you recommend for her?

   Hint: See pp. 973-974 in PPP

FOLLOW-UP

6. What if a follow-up bone mineral density scan in 2 years shows no improvement in T-scores and the patient has not had any recurrent fractures? Should her therapy be changed at that time?

   Hint: See p. 977 in PPP

7. What if the patient develops adverse gastrointestinal effects on therapy in 6 months? What alternative therapies are appropriate?

   Hint: See p. 977 in PPP

8. What if the patient had a history of breast cancer? Would that influence your choice of agent to treat osteoporosis?

   Hint: See pp. 974-975 in PPP

☉ GLOBAL PERSPECTIVE

Osteoporosis is the most common skeletal disorder caused by an imbalance of bone remodeling, which results in overall bone loss. The development of bone loss can lead to painful and debilitating bone fractures. Although osteoporosis affects more than 10 million Americans, the World Health Organization reports that osteoporosis affects approximately 75 million people in America, Europe, and Japan combined. The lifetime risk for developing wrist, vertebral, and hip fractures is 30% to 40% for these combined populations. Osteoporosis primarily affects the Caucasian ethnicity; however, significant risk has been reported for all ethnic backgrounds. Asian and non-Hispanic Caucasian women aged 50 years or older diagnosed with osteoporosis approximately 20% of Americans. Approximately 5% of American non-Hispanic black women within the same age group have osteoporosis. An estimated 35% of women in all three of these ethnic groups are estimated to have low bone mass. The risk of osteoporosis is increasing more in American Hispanic women when compared to other ethnic/racial groups. Ten percent of American Hispanic women aged 50 years and older are diagnosed with osteoporosis with 23% of those women estimated to have low bone mass. To add to the significance of these statistics for American Hispanic women, experts predict an increase in cost related to osteoporotic fractures for from $754 million in 2005 to $2 billion in 2025. To help decrease the mortality associated with osteoporosis, it is important to educate all patient populations irrelevant of race/ethnicity on the importance of proper nutrition, pharmacotherapy, and yearly bone mineral density screenings.

CASE SUMMARY

- Current pharmacotherapy for the treatment of osteoporosis has been ineffective in preventing fractures. Alternative therapy should be considered.

- Adequate calcium and vitamin D supplementation is needed to optimize osteoporosis treatment. A calcium supplement whose absorption is not dependent on an acidic gastric environment is needed.

- Oversuppression of thyroid can promote bone loss and increase risk for osteoporotic fracture and should be avoided.

For more information on the care plan and facilitator's guide please visit http://www.mhpharmacotherapy.com.

60 Rheumatoid Arthritis

Susan P. Bruce   Elaine M. Greifenstein

CASE LEARNING OBJECTIVES

- Discuss the comorbidities associated with rheumatoid arthritis (RA)
- Recognize the typical clinical presentation of RA
- Create treatment goals for a patient with RA arthritis on the basis of disease activity
- Compare and contrast the available pharmacotherapeutic options, selecting the most appropriate regimen for a given patient
- Propose a patient education plan that includes nonpharmacologic and pharmacologic treatment measures
- Formulate an initial prescreening and a long-term monitoring plan to evaluate the safety and efficacy of a therapeutic regimen designed for an individual patient with RA

PATIENT PRESENTATION

Chief Complaint

"I'm stiff and my joints are swollen."

History of Present Illness

Ching Li is a 55-year-old postmenopausal woman presenting to the rheumatologist for evaluation and treatment of RA. Ching presented to her primary care physician 3 months ago with complaints of symmetrical joint pain in her hands and feet and morning stiffness lasting more than an hour. She trialed ibuprofen followed by naproxen for about 2 months with limited pain relief. During a follow-up visit with her primary care physician approximately 1 month ago, naproxen was discontinued and low-dose corticosteroids were initiated. The corticosteroids have helped joint discomfort partially, but have not had an impact on joint swelling. She reports significant difficulty with dressing (especially buttons, zippers, and tying her shoes) and meal preparation. She has experienced progressive morning stiffness, now lasting for 2 to 3 hours daily. She reports that she feels down, but does not understand why. Her husband passed away 3 years ago and, in her opinion, she dealt with her husband's passing immediately after his death.

Past Medical History

Peptic ulcer disease diagnosed 7 months ago

Hypertension × 3 years

Blood transfusion following C-section in China 30 years ago

Menopause at age 50

Family History

Father had CAD and died of MI at age 82. Mother died at age 70 from hepatocellular carcinoma. Her only brother has dyslipidemia and hypertension. Daughter is alive and well.

Social History

Ching, a homemaker, moved to the United States from China to live with her daughter 3 years ago after her husband died. She speaks Mandarin and English.

Tobacco/Alcohol/Substance Use

(+) Tobacco—1 ppd × 40 years; (−) alcohol or illicit drug use

Allergies/Intolerances/Adverse Drug Events

Trimethoprim/sulfamethoxazole—rash

Medications (Current)

Hydrochlorothiazide 12.5 mg PO daily

Prednisone 5 mg PO daily in the morning

Lansoprazole 30 mg PO daily

Red yeast rice 1,200 mg PO twice daily

Kava kava 500 mg PO at bedtime

Review of Systems

Generalized malaise and fatigue for 4 months; unintentional 10 lb (4.5 kg) weight loss over the past 3 months; (−) fevers, night sweats, adenopathy, dry eyes, oral ulcers, or skin rashes; morning cough productive of clear sputum, resolves 15 to 30 minutes after arising; (−) hemoptysis, chest pain, shortness of breath, exertional chest discomfort, abdominal pain, or diarrhea; initial difficulty falling asleep at night due to joint discomfort, but then awakens two to three times per night for unknown reasons; self-prescribed use of kava kava at bedtime decreases the nighttime awakening; (−) suicidal ideation

Physical Examination

► General

Thin, middle-aged, Asian woman in obvious discomfort on shaking hands and arising from sitting

► Vital Signs

BP 146/88 mm Hg, P 72, RR 15, T 36.8°C

Weight 112.5 lb (51.1 kg)

Height 60 in. (152.4 cm)

Pain rated as 6/10

► Skin

(−) Rashes, lesions or evidence of vasculitis

► HEENT

(−) Conjunctival or sclera injection; (−) oral or nasal ulcers; mucus membranes moist

► Neck and Lymph Nodes

(−) Adenopathy, thyromegaly, or masses

► Chest

Prolonged expiratory phase bilaterally; (−) rales, rhonchi, wheezes, or rubs

► Breasts

(−) Nodules, masses, skin changes, or nipple discharge

► Cardiovascular

RRR; S_4 gallop present; (−) S_3 gallop or rubs

► Abdomen

Scaphoid and nontender; (−) masses, hepatomegaly, or splenomegaly

► Extremities

Small olecranon nodules bilaterally; 1+ synovitis and tenderness of the bilateral dorsal wrists; 2+ synovitis of the right metacarpophalangeal (MCP) joints and 1+ synovitis of the left MCP joints; 1+ synovitis and tenderness of the bilateral proximal interphalangeal joints (PIP) joints; 2+ synovitis and tenderness of the right metatarsophalangeal (MTP) joints and 1+ synovitis of the left MTP joints; (−) joint effusions.

► Genitourinary

Examination deferred

► Rectal

Normal sphincter tone; (−) masses; stool brown and (−) guaiac

Laboratory Tests

Fasting, obtained 2 weeks ago

	Conventional Units	SI Units
Na	140 mEq/L	140 mmol/L
K	4.2 mEq/L	4.2 mmol/L
Cl	99 mEq/L	99 mmol/L
CO_2	24 mEq/L	24 mmol/L
BUN	12 mg/dL	4.3 mmol/L
SCr	0.8 mg/dL	71 μmol/L
Glu	106 mg/dL	5.9 mmol/L
Ca	9.2 mg/dL	2.3 mmol/L
Mg	1.8 mEq/L	0.74 mmol/L
Phosphate	3.6 mg/dL	1.16 mmol/L
RF	200 IU/mL	200 kIU/L
Anti-CCP	(+)	
C-reactive protein (CRP)	3.2 mg/dL	32 mg/L
Hgb	12.2 g/dL	122 g/L; 7.56 mmol/L
Hct	36.8%	0.368
Platelets	$500 \times 10^3/\mu L$	$500 \times 10^9/L$
MCV	90 μm³	90 fL
WBC	$5.2 \times 10^3/mm^3$	$5.2 \times 10^9/L$
Albumin	4 g/dL	40 g/L
AST	26 IU/L	0.43 μKat/L
ALT	32 IU/L	0.53 μKat/L
ESR	52 mm/h	14.5 μm/s
Total cholesterol	247 mg/dL	6.39 mmol/L
LDL cholesterol	162 mg/dL	4.19 mmol/L
HDL cholesterol	28 mg/dL	0.72 mmol/L
Triglycerides	282 mg/dL	3.19 mmol/L

Assessment

Fifty-five-year-old woman with signs, symptoms, and laboratory tests consistent with RA of moderate-to-high disease activity and poor prognostic factors

Student Workup

Missing Information?

Evaluate: Patient Database

Drug Therapy Problems

Care Plan (by Problem)

TARGETED QUESTIONS

1. On the basis of initial disease activity, which medications are appropriate for the treatment of RA in this patient?

   Hint: See p. 985 and Table 57-3 in PPP

2. What tests should be included in the prescreening workup prior to initiating therapy? What tests should be included in the long-term monitoring for the therapeutic regimen you are recommending?

   Hint: See p. 984 in PPP

3. Which comorbid conditions related to RA or its treatment must also be addressed for this patient?

   Hint: See p. 983 in PPP

4. What is the most appropriate treatment for each comorbid condition?

   Hint: See p. 994 in PPP

5. What pharmacologic and nonpharmacologic measures should your patient education plan include?

   Hint: See p. 994 in PPP

FOLLOW-UP

Ching returns to the rheumatologist 3 months after initiation of DMARD (disease-modifying antirheumatic drug) and indicates her pain is 4 on a 0 to 10 scale. She notes some improvement in completing activities of daily living (dressing and bathing), but is still too fatigued to complete meal preparation for her family. Physical examination reveals improvement in joint synovitis and swelling overall, but persistent 1+ synovitis of the right MCP joints. Bilateral dorsal wrists remain tender to palpation. Small bilateral olecranon nodules are unchanged. X-rays of her hands and feet reveal periarticular osteopenia at the MCP and MTP joints, with erosions noted at the right second and third MCP joints. Significant laboratory values include ESR 45 mm/h (12.5 μm/s), CRP 2.5 mg/dL (25 mg/L), AST 35 IU/L (0.58 μKat/L), ALT 40 IU/L (0.67 μKat/L), SCr 1.0 mg/dL (88 μmol/L), and glucose (fasting) 120 mg/dL (6.7 mmol/L).

6. On the basis of the disease activity at follow-up, which medications are appropriate for the treatment of RA in this patient?

   Hint: See p. 985 and Table 57-3 in PPP

7. What, if any, tests should be included in the prescreening workup prior to initiating additional therapy? What tests should be included in the long-term monitoring for the therapeutic regimen you are recommending?

   Hint: See p. 994 in PPP

⊙ GLOBAL PERSPECTIVE

RA is a common chronic systemic autoimmune inflammatory disease with a prevalence of 1% to 2% across all populations. Women are affected more commonly than men, with a peak incidence in the fourth and fifth decades of life. Synovium is the primary site of inflammation and the condition typically progresses to a chronic state with substantial morbidity and disability. Comorbid diseases are common due to the ongoing inflammatory response with cardiovascular disease and infections representing the most common causes of death. Treatment of RA requires early assessment of disease activity with selection of disease-modifying agents and combination therapy representing the gold standard of care.

CASE SUMMARY

- Her current clinical picture is consistent with RA of moderate-to-high disease activity, and disease-modifying therapy should be initiated.

- Initial treatment with methotrexate with concomitant prednisone while improving her overall joint swelling and tenderness did not significantly reduce the disease activity (persistent synovitis at MCP joints, periarticular osteopenia and erosions on x-rays, and elevated ESR and CRP). At follow-up, she required initiation of combination therapy, including a biologic agent.

- Initiation and ongoing treatment with immunosuppressive therapy requires continual clinical vigilance for medication side effects.

- RA is associated with a number of comorbid conditions, including cardiovascular disease, depression, and osteoporosis, all of which should be addressed.

For more information on the care plan and facilitator's guide please visit http://www.mhpharmacotherapy.com.

61 Osteoarthritis

Steven M. Smith   John G. Gums

PATIENT PRESENTATION

Chief Complaint

"My knees are starting to hurt more and more every time I climb stairs. I also fell last week at work because my right knee gave out."

History of Present Illness

Bryce Johnson is a 68-year-old white male who presents to his primary care physician complaining of increasing bilateral knee pain over the past 4 months with recent joint instability, most notably in the right knee. His knee pain is frequently associated with climbing stairs. He also reports knee stiffness on waking, which lasts approximately 15 to 20 minutes and abates with ambulation. He has not previously sought care for his knee pain. On "bad" days, he reports taking acetaminophen 1,000 mg two to three times daily. Although this dose is generally inadequate to fully alleviate his pain, he is concerned about taking larger doses because of the recent news coverage of acetaminophen-induced liver toxicity. He has also been trying to lose weight using an over-the-counter product called Alli. He reports poor compliance with this medication due to diarrhea on numerous occasions. Lastly, he requests your advice on taking a product that a family member recommended, called Cosamin DS. He has been told that it prevents joint breakdown and is safer than pain killers.

Past Medical History

Hypertension × 7 years
Hyperlipidemia × 5 years

Insomnia × 8 months
Diabetes mellitus type 2 × 4 years
Obesity

Family History

Father died of MI at age 49.

Social/Work History

Retired, former packaging plant floor manager for a mail-order company. Currently, a part-time volunteer for a local political campaign. Divorced; has two children, aged 35 and 37.

Tobacco/Alcohol/Substance Use

Social drinker; (–) tobacco; 10 pack-year history, quit 18 years ago; (–) illicit drug use

Allergy/Intolerance/Adverse Event History

NKDA

Medications (Current)

Indapamide 2.5 mg PO once daily
Lisinopril 20 mg PO twice daily
Metformin/sitagliptin 1,000/50 mg PO twice daily
Simvastatin 40 mg PO once daily
Orlistat 120 mg PO three times daily with meals
Zolpidem 10 mg PO once daily at bedtime

Acetaminophen 1,000 mg PO q 8 h PRN pain

Os-Cal 500+D (calcium carbonate 500 mg/vitamin D 400 IU) PO q 12 h

Aspirin 81 mg PO once daily

Pantoprazole 40 mg PO once daily

Review of Systems

Knee pain (right > left) and right knee instability, most noticeable on climbing stairs; decreased quadriceps and hamstring strength in right leg; impaired range of motion due to knee pain; (−) hip and right ankle pain; (−) joint swelling; (−) joint tenderness. Negative for fever. Self-monitored blood glucose averages in the 130s to 160s mg/dL (~7–9.5 mmol/L) on most days of the week; no visual disturbances. Five-pound (2.3 kg) weight loss in previous 4 weeks

Physical Examination

▸ General

Pleasant obese, elderly, white male in no acute distress

▸ Vital Signs

BP 122/83 mm Hg, P 76, RR 14, T 36.6°C (97.9°F)

Weight 268 lb (121.8 kg), BMI 37.4 kg/m², 5 lb (2.3 kg) weight loss in last 4 weeks

Height 71 in. (180.3 cm)

(+) Pain, 5/10

▸ Skin

Large bruise on lateral aspect of the right thigh; (−) lesions or rash

▸ HEENT

PERRL, EOMI; TMs normal appearing

▸ Chest

Clear to auscultation

▸ Cardiovascular

RRR, normal S_1, S_2; (−) S_3 or S_4; (−) shortness of breath

▸ Abdomen

Obese, soft, nontender, nondistended; (−) organomegaly; (+) bowel sounds

▸ Neurology

Grossly intact; deep tendon reflexes equal bilaterally; muscle strength 4/5 on extension and flexion of right and left knees, 5/5 for upper extremities; muscle tone normal; slight gait impairment secondary to knee pain; no focal deficits

▸ Extremities

Range of motion in left knee limited by pain; (−) hip, ankle pain; (−) swelling; (−) tenderness; (−) heat

Laboratory Tests

Fasting

	Conventional Units	SI Units
Na	144 mEq/L	144 mmol/L
K	5 mEq/L	5 mmol/L
Cl	105 mEq/L	105 mmol/L
CO_2	26 mEq/L	26 mmol/L
Ca	8.9 mg/dL	2.23 mmol/L
Mg	2.1 mEq/L	1.05 mmol/L
Phosphate	3.5 mg/dL	1.13 mmol/L
SCr	1.1 mg/dL	97 µmol/L
BUN	9 mg/dL	3.2 mmol/L
Glu	113 mg/dL	6.3 mmol/L
A1c	6.6%	0.066
CK	41.4 IU/L	0.69 µkat/L
Hgb	12.8 g/dL	128 g/L; 7.94 mmol/L
Hct	44.3%	0.443
WBC	$8.4 \times 10^3/mm^3$	$8.4 \times 10^9/L$
Albumin	3.4 g/dL	34 g/L
AST	34 IU/L	0.57 µkat/L
ALT	37 IU/L	0.62 µkat/L
Total cholesterol	184 mg/dL	4.76 mmol/L
LDL cholesterol	116 mg/dL	3.00 mmol/L
HDL cholesterol	39 mg/dL	1.01 mmol/L
Triglycerides	145 mg/dL	1.64 mmol/L
Uric acid	6.1 mg/dL	363 µmol/L

Assessment

Sixty-eight-year-old obese male with signs and symptoms consistent with OA of the knee

Student Workup

Missing Information?

Evaluate: Patient Database

Drug Therapy Problems

Care Plan (by Problem)

TARGETED QUESTIONS

1. What signs and symptoms of OA does this patient have?

    Hint: See p. 999 in PPP

2. What are the first-line treatment options for OA?

    Hint: See pp. 1000–1004 in PPP and Table 58-2

3. Would this patient be a candidate for a COX-2 selective NSAID?

   Hint: Consider current gastrointestinal and cardiovascular risk factors and concomitant medications when choosing between a nonselective NSAID and COX-2 selective agent. See pp. 1004–1005 in PPP and Table 58-3

4. Would you recommend the use of glucosamine/chondroitin for this patient?

   Hint: Additional information with regard to allergies may be required before making this recommendation. See p. 1005 in PPP

5. How would you counsel this patient on the expected benefits and risks of NSAID therapy?

   Hint: See pp. 1002–1004 in PPP

FOLLOW-UP

The patient returns to the clinic after 3 months for routine follow-up. He reports decreased pain, but persistent joint instability in the right knee.

6. What nonpharmacologic strategies would you recommend for this patient to improve joint stability and reduce the risk of further joint deterioration?

   Hint: See p. 1000 in PPP

⟳ GLOBAL PERSPECTIVE

OA is the most common rheumatic disease worldwide; however, the prevalence of OA varies widely across geographic regions. Prevalence rates in Europe approximate those in North America and generally do not exceed 10%. In contrast, the prevalence in developing regions can range from 3% to 20%. These differences are probably more closely associated with differences in populations than geographic location because the development of OA is not predicated solely on environmental factors. For example, when compared with North American Caucasians, Asians exhibit higher rates of symptomatic knee OA, but lower rates of hip and hand OA. This finding may be attributable to the higher proportion of rural farmers and hard laborers in many Asian regions than in North America. Thus, the prevalence of OA in any region reflects population differences in age, lifestyle, genetics, and occupational history.

CASE SUMMARY

- The overall clinical picture is consistent with OA of the right knee.
- Acetaminophen has been only marginally effective in treating his knee pain.
- Nonpharmacologic therapies should reduce further joint damage and improve joint stability.

For more information on the care plan and facilitator's guide please visit http://www.mhpharmacotherapy.com.

62 Gout and Hyperuricemia

William Joshua Guffey

CASE LEARNING OBJECTIVES

- Recognize the major risk factors for developing gout
- Identify the goals of therapy for gout
- Select an appropriate drug to provide acute pain relief and reduce serum uric acid levels in patients with gout, and outline a plan for monitoring efficacy and toxicity
- Properly educate a patient on appropriate lifestyle modifications to help prevent gouty arthritis attacks

PATIENT PRESENTATION

Chief Complaint

"My feet throb when I walk or stand and my big toe is swollen."

History of Present Illness

John Smith is a 62-year-old Caucasian male who presents to his primary care physician complaining of bilateral foot pain (L > R) and swelling of the first phalanx (hallux) of the left foot. The patient describes the pain as a constant throbbing sensation when standing or walking. Initially the patient thought the pain could have been from an ingrown toenail, but became concerned when his other foot started to hurt and his left big toe started swelling with redness and warmth present. The pain has been present for approximately 2 weeks but has worsened over the past few days. He has tried to alleviate the pain through soaking his feet in a warm bath with Epsom salts with minimal relief. He has no prior history of diabetes, and his fasting blood glucose level 3 months ago was 105 mg/dL (5.8 mmol/L).

Past Medical History

Atrial fibrillation

HTN

Hyperlipidemia

Depression

Dyspepsia

Family History

Father had diabetes mellitus type 2 and died from a stroke at age 72; mother is alive at age 82 with hypertension and osteoarthritis.

Social History

Married and lives with his wife of 40 years; has no children; works as a service mechanic at a local automobile dealership.

Tobacco/Alcohol/Substance Use

Drinks three to four beers weekly and may consume more in social situations; nonsmoker ×10 years; denies any illicit drug use

Allergies/Intolerances/Adverse Drug Events

No known drug allergies

Medications (Current)

Atenolol 50 mg PO daily for hypertension

Hydrochlorothiazide/lisinopril 12.5/20 mg PO daily for hypertension

Omeprazole 20 mg PO q AM

Sertraline 100 mg PO daily

Simvastatin 40 mg PO daily

Extended-release niacin 1,000 mg PO q hs

Warfarin 5 mg PO q PM

Ibuprofen 200 mg PO q 4–6 h PRN

Review of Systems

Frequent headaches relieved with over-the-counter pain reliever; denies any recent chest pain, shortness of breath, abdominal pain, unusual bruising or bleeding, or changes in bladder or bowel habits

Physical Examination

▶ General

Obese, middle-aged, Caucasian male in acute distress

▶ Vital Signs

BP 140/84 mm Hg, P 99, RR 20, T 37.1°C, SpO$_2$ 98% (0.98)

Weight 276 lb (125.5 kg)

Height 73 in. (185.4 cm)

Reports pain score of 8/10

▶ Skin

Warm and dry to touch; (+) erythema and swelling of left foot

▶ HEENT

PERRLA, EOMI; (−) sinus tenderness; TMs appear normal

▶ Neck and Lymph Nodes

Unremarkable

▶ Chest

Clear to auscultation

▶ Breasts

Examination deferred

▶ Cardiovascular

RRR, normal S$_1$, S$_2$; (−) S$_3$ or S$_4$

▶ Abdomen

Obese; soft, nontender/nondistended; (−) organomegaly

▶ Neurology

Alert and oriented × 3; cranial nerves II to XII grossly intact; deep tendon reflexes normal

▶ Genitourinary

Examination deferred

▶ Rectal

Examination deferred

Laboratory Tests

Fasting, obtained today

	Conventional Units	SI Units
Na	136 mEq/L	136 mmol/L
K	4.9 mEq/L	4.9 mmol/L
Cl	97 mEq/L	97 mmol/L
CO$_2$	27 mEq/L	27 mmol/L
BUN	15 mg/dL	5.4 mmol/L
SCr	1.1 mg/dL	97 µmol/L
Glu	109 mg/dL	6 mmol/L
Ca	9.7 mg/dL	2.43 mmol/L
Uric acid	10.9 mg/dL	648 µmol/L
Hgb	13.8 g/dL	138 g/L; 8.56 mmol/L
Hct	39.9%	0.399
RBC	4.17 × 10^6/µL	4.17 × 10^{12}/L
Platelets	277 × 10^3/µL	277 × 10^9/L
Westergren ESR	26 mm/h	7.2 µm/s
MCV	95 µm^3	95 fL
WBC	8.8 × 10^3/µL	8.8 × 10^9/L
Neutrophils	82%	0.82
Lymphocytes	6%	0.06
Monocytes	10%	0.10
Eosinophils	1%	0.01
Basophils	1%	0.01
Bands	0%	0
INR	2.8	
Total cholesterol	158 mg/dL	4.09 mmol/L
LDL cholesterol	66 mg/dL	1.71 mmol/L
HDL cholesterol	36 mg/dL	0.93 mmol/L
Triglycerides	280 mg/dL	3.16 mmol/L

Assessment

Sixty-two-year-old man with signs, symptoms, and laboratory tests consistent with gout

Student Workup

Missing Information?

Evaluate: Patient Database

Drug Therapy Problems

Care Plan (by Problem)

TARGETED QUESTIONS

1. What signs and symptoms of gout does the patient have?
   Hint: See p. 1012 in PPP

2. What risk factors for the development of gout are present in the patient?
   Hint: See p. 1012 in PPP

3. What are the possible treatment options in most patients suffering from an acute gout attack?

   Hint: See pp. 1013–1015 in PPP

4. What risks and adverse effects of therapy would you discuss with the patient?

   Hint: See pp. 1016–1017 in PPP

5. What lifestyle modification patient education points should be discussed with the patient regarding the prevention of future gout attacks?

   Hint: See p. 1017 in PPP

FOLLOW-UP

Six months later, the patient returns to the clinic with an elevated uric acid level and recurrent acute gout attack.

6. What risks would persistent hyperuricemia and recurrent gout attacks pose to the patient?

   Hint: See p. 1012 in PPP

7. What would be an appropriate maintenance regimen for the prophylaxis of future gout attacks?

   Hint: See pp. 1015–1016 in PPP

8. What risks and adverse effects of therapy would you discuss with the patient?

   Hint: See pp. 1016–1017 in PPP

9. What would be an appropriate monitoring plan for the selected maintenance regimen?

   Hint: See p. 1017 in PPP

⟳ GLOBAL PERSPECTIVE

Gout is the most common form of inflammatory arthritis in the United States and western Europe. It is a condition caused by an abnormality of uric acid metabolism, resulting in hyperuricemia. The findings from the Rochester Epidemiology Project have estimated the annual incidence of gout in the United States as 62 cases/100,000. Over the past decade, the prevalence of gout in the United States has significantly increased due to several factors, including changes in diet, increased use of medications associated with the development of gout, increased rates of hypertension, dyslipidemias, metabolic syndrome, diabetes, and renal impairment, and an increase in the overall population life expectancy. Despite the increase in rates of the development of gout, there have been few new developments in therapeutic options for the management of gout.[1] To help decrease the incidence of gout and hyperuricemia, it is important for health care professionals to educate patients at risk for developing gout on the signs and symptoms of gout, potential drug interactions, and therapeutic lifestyle changes, including weight reduction and avoidance of foods high in purine content.

REFERENCES

1. Weaver AL. Epidemiology of gout. Cleve Clin J Med 2008 75(suppl 5):S9–S12.
2. Terkeltaub RA, Furst DE, Bennett K, et al. High versus low dosing of oral colchicine for early acute gout flare: Twenty-four-hour outcome of the first multicenter, randomized, double-blind, placebo-controlled, parallel group, dose-comparison colchicine study. Arthritis Rheum 2010;62:1060–1068.

CASE SUMMARY

- His current clinical picture is consistent with an acute gout attack, and an appropriate pain management therapy should be initiated.

- Colchicine would be a reasonable initial therapy for this patient with a dose of 1.2 mg PO immediately followed by 0.6 mg PO one hour later (1.8 mg/day) and then 0.6 mg PO 1–2 times daily until 24 hours after gout attack has subsided.[2] The patient should be educated on appropriate use and potential gastrointestinal side effects.

- Lifestyle modifications, including weight reduction and avoidance of substances with high purine content, should also be implemented.

- Maintenance therapy may not be indicated at this time since this is not a recurrent attack and there is no evidence of joint destruction or tophi present.

For more information on the care plan and facilitator's guide please visit http://www.mhpharmacotherapy.com.

63 Glaucoma

Jon P. Wietholter

CASE LEARNING OBJECTIVES

- List the goals of treatment for patients with primary open-angle glaucoma
- Choose the most appropriate therapy using patient-specific data for open-angle glaucoma
- Develop a monitoring plan for patients on specific pharmacologic regimens
- Counsel patients about glaucoma, drug therapy options, ophthalmic administration techniques, and the importance of adherence to the prescribed regimen

PATIENT PRESENTATION

Chief Complaint

"My eyes are hurting and I feel like my vision is worsening. It has been worsening over the last few months and now that I'm in the hospital, I'd like to have my eyes examined."

History of Present Illness

Carrie Kindred is a 52-year-old female who was admitted to the hospital 6 days ago for suspected community-acquired pneumonia (CAP). She had complained of a progressively worsening cough with increased sputum production and a tough time catching her breath on admission. These symptoms have improved drastically and are no longer a concern for this patient. While doing the initial review of systems with the patient, the physician who admitted her to the hospital asked her about any other problems she was currently experiencing. The only other problem she described was a dull, aching pain in her eyes and a subjective feeling that she needs new glasses or contacts as her vision seems to be worsening and becoming blurrier every day. When asked about this vision loss, she claims to be less able to see things to her sides and that her peripheral vision seems to be the main aspect of her vision loss. Additionally, she has noticed that she seems to have blind spots in her visual field that were not there previously.

Past Medical History

HTN diagnosed at age 43
AF diagnosed at age 47
COPD diagnosed last year
Insomnia, for the last 15 years

Family History

Father is alive and well with only medical problem being CAD. Mother passed away from breast cancer at age 74. Her mother also had a history of glaucoma and type 2 DM. Three younger siblings have no medical issues, except for her brother who has type 2 DM and HTN.

Social History

Works as a receptionist at a local dentist's office. Married for 30 years and lives with her husband. Has four children, aged 17, 22, 24, and 28.

Tobacco/Alcohol/Substance Use

Has smoked 2 ppd cigarettes for 25 years. (−) Illicit drug use. Drinks three to five glasses of wine per week (usually a glass of wine with dinner).

Allergies/Intolerances/Adverse Drug Events

Allergic to sulfamethoxazole/trimethoprim (anaphylaxis) and codeine (hives)

Medications (Current)

Metoprolol tartrate 50 mg PO twice daily

Amlodipine 5 mg PO daily

Albuterol inhaler two puffs every 4 hours as needed

Tiotropium 18 mcg inhaled daily

Fluticasone/salmeterol 250/50 one inhalation twice daily

Amitriptyline 25 mg PO before bedtime

Warfarin 4 mg PO daily

Ceftriaxone 1,000 mg IV daily (day 6 of 7 for CAP)

Azithromycin 500 mg PO daily (day 6 of 7 for CAP)

Physical Examination

▶ General

Patient in no acute distress. Sitting in bed without complaints other than that she is having trouble reading anything on the television.

▶ Vital Signs

BP 125/79 mm Hg, HR 81, RR 17, T 36.9°C, O_2 sat: 98% (0.98) on room air

Weight 130 lb (59 kg)

Height 67 in. (170 cm)

▶ Skin

Nothing acute; no acute rashes or lesions

▶ HEENT

EOMI; open anterior chamber angles noted; optic disc cupping noted; paracentral scotoma noted; IOP 35 mm Hg (4.7 kPa) on examination; TMs appear normal; (−) sinus tenderness; remainder of examination (−)

▶ Neck and Lymph Nodes

(−) Examination; no thyroid nodules or lymphadenopathy present

▶ Chest

Minor wheezing and rhonchi present on auscultation

▶ Breasts

(−) Examination

▶ Cardiovascular

Rate irregularly irregular; no discernable regularity in rhythm but rate seems to be in the 80s

▶ Abdomen

Nontender; (−) organomegaly

▶ Neurology

Grossly intact; deep tendon reflexes normal

▶ Genitourinary

Deferred

▶ Rectal

Deferred

Laboratory Tests

Fasting, obtained with the morning laboratory draw at 5 AM this morning

	Conventional Units	SI Units
Sodium	138 mEq/L	138 mmol/L
Potassium	4.1 mEq/L	4.1 mmol/L
Chloride	105 mEq/L	105 mmol/L
CO_2	24 mEq/L	24 mmol/L
BUN	8 mg/dL	2.9 mmol/L
SCr	1 mg/dL	88 µmol/L
Glucose	101 mg/dL	5.6 mmol/L
Calcium	8.9 mg/dL	2.23 mmol/L
Magnesium	2.1 mEq/L	1.05 mmol/L
Phosphate	3 mg/dL	0.97 mmol/L
Albumin	4.1 g/dL	41 g/L
INR	2.4	
Hgb	14.1 g/dL	141 g/L; 8.75 mmol/L
Hct	42.4%	0.424
WBC	$8 \times 10^3/mm^3$	$8 \times 10^9/L$
Platelets	$230 \times 10^3/mm^3$	$230 \times 10^9/L$
MCV	83 µm³	83 fL
AST	25 IU/L	0.42 µkat/L
ALT	27 IU/L	0.45 µkat/L
Total bilirubin	0.4 mg/dL	6.8 µmol/L
Direct bilirubin	0.1 mg/dL	1.7 µmol/L
Alkaline phosphatase	71 IU/L	1.18 µkat/L
Prothrombin time	23.9 s	

▶ Pertinent Diagnostic Tests

Chest x-ray done this morning shows resolving pneumonia.

Assessment

This is a hospitalized 52-year-old female with signs, symptoms, and physical examination consistent with uncontrolled primary open-angle glaucoma.

Student Workup

Missing Information?

Evaluate: Patient Database

Drug Therapy Problems

Pharmacotherapy Care Plan (by Problem)

Patient Education Needed

TARGETED QUESTIONS

1. What signs and symptoms of open-angle glaucoma is this patient currently experiencing?

   Hint: See p. 1035 in PPP

2. What are the goal(s) of therapy in this patient?

   Hint: See pp. 1036 and 1037 in PPP

3. Does this patient have any concomitant disease states that could factor into the selection of a medication to treat her glaucoma and how could that alter your drug selection? Additionally, is this patient on any current medications that could worsen or exacerbate her glaucoma?

   Hint: Think about what side effects each class of medications used for glaucoma can cause (see pp. 1040–1043 in PPP) and evaluate whether any of those side effects could be detrimental in any of her concomitant disease states contained in her PMH above. Additionally, this patient is on amitriptyline for her insomnia. This medication will have some unwanted anticholinergic side effects that could worsen or exacerbate her glaucoma. See p. 1043 in PPP

4. What are appropriate first-line treatment options in this patient and what adverse effects should be monitored for with each possible treatment option?

   Hint: See pp. 1040–1043 and Figure 61-4 in PPP

5. If this patient was instead experiencing acute angle-closure glaucoma, how would the treatment plan differ from your original suggestions for this patient's primary open-angle glaucoma?

   Hint: See pp. 1037 and 1040 in PPP

FOLLOW-UP

Three weeks later, the patient reports to the outpatient clinic affiliated with your hospital for a follow-up appointment. She says that her vision seems to be improving (at least not worsening) since you started her on timolol 0.5% eye drops (one drop to each eye twice daily). Her complaints at this point in time do not have to do with her eyes, but she claims that she has been really down in the dumps lately and that some days she feels so depressed that she will not leave the house. She also has had more trouble with shortness of breath since the timolol has been started. She is convinced that the timolol has caused all these symptoms.

6. What should you tell the patient in regard to her complaint and what would your therapeutic recommendation be in this patient?

Hint: Review common adverse effects from ocular β-blocker therapy on p. 1040 in PPP. Additionally, think if there is a patient-counseling point that should be made regarding the administration of her timolol eye drops that could possibly improve her clinical picture and reduce side effects.

⟳ GLOBAL PERSPECTIVE

Glaucoma is a disease state that affects people of all races and nationalities. Although many different countries and cultures use medications and procedures similar to what are used in the United States, there are many practitioners around the world that will turn to acupuncture or Chinese herbal remedies to aid in the treatment of both primary open-angle glaucoma and primary angle-closure glaucoma. Traditional Chinese medicine teaches that glaucoma suggests that there is a liver–kidney yin deficiency with liver yang rising. Although this may seem complicated, the practice of traditional Chinese medicine has been around for centuries and can be used to appropriately place acupuncture needles or select the appropriate combination(s) of herbal remedies (e.g., Wen Dan Tang and You Gui Wan) for the clinical scenario.

CASE SUMMARY

- Patient presentation is consistent with the diagnosis of primary open-angle glaucoma and should be appropriately treated.

- Appropriate first-line treatment options include an ocular β-blocker, a prostaglandin analog (AKA ocular hypotensive lipid), or brimonidine. Selection should be based on numerous factors including cost, concomitant disease states, and the patient's likelihood of compliance.

- Initial follow-up monitoring should take place at 2 to 4 weeks and adjustment of therapy should be based on improvement in IOP (initial goal is 20% lower than baseline).

- Care should be taken to not miss the diagnosis of acute angle-closure glaucoma as this is a medical emergency and should be surgically treated as soon as possible.

For more information on the care plan and facilitator's guide please visit http://www.mhpharmacotherapy.com.

64 Allergic Rhinitis

David A. Apgar

CASE LEARNING OBJECTIVES

- List the typical symptoms of allergic rhinitis (AR) and identify the most troublesome one
- List the reasons for referral to an allergy specialist
- Discuss the categories of pharmacotherapy choices for treatment of AR
- Rank the pharmacotherapy choices for efficacy in treating nasal congestion
- Describe an approach for treatment of mild AR with OTC drugs
- Create a therapy plan for treatment of moderate-to-severe AR

PATIENT PRESENTATION

Chief Complaint

"What can you recommend for my itchy, stuffy nose and sneezing?"

History of Present Illness

Brenda Baresdale is a 27-year-old female who comes into your retail pharmacy seeking advice for the above complaints. Your history reveals the following information. She began having significant nasal allergy symptoms for the first time about 8 years ago after moving to the southwest (Phoenix, AZ) from the midwest (Zionsville, IN). Her nose is affected most, but there are some mouth, throat, chest, and even occasional eye symptoms. The congestion in the nasal passages is so bad that she can breathe only through her mouth. The nasal symptoms are characterized by watery discharge, sneezing, itch, and severe congestion. Sometimes she has "itchiness" in the roof of the mouth and back of the throat. Sometimes there is cough, which seems to be stimulated by nasal discharge "dripping down" the back of the throat. The cough is usually mild and nonproductive. When her other symptoms are at their worst, there is sometimes a sensation of "chest tightness." Also, sometimes both her eyes become itchy, red, and even have increased tearing. She cannot identify specific triggers for her symptoms other than seasons of the year. Her condition is the worst from about May through July. However, in most years, she also has problems during the period from mid-September until the holiday season. Actually, in the last few years, she even noticed symptoms at other times, although less frequently and less severely. When her symptoms start in May and mid-September, they occur only two to three times per week. However, after 2

to 3 weeks, they are almost every day. She has horses, and cares for them every weekend, but her symptoms are not worse at those times. Sometimes her symptoms are worse when she spends a lot of time outdoors. However, she also notices that being in her kitchen can sometimes start her sneezing. She has tried several medications, some of which have helped. She began treating herself 4 to 5 years ago, with loratadine (Claritin), but that hardly helped at all. Next, she tried diphenhydramine, which did help, and she has continued that medication. The first few days she takes it, she notices sleepiness, but that "wears off" if she continues it for several days. She has tried decongestant nose sprays, usually oxymetazoline (e.g., Afrin), in the past, especially when the stuffy nose was bad. It did help for a while. She continues to use it intermittently. She has tried a neti (or nettie) pot, but finds it messy, hard to use, and not particularly helpful. Because her father uses fluticasone propionate (Flonase), she tried that about 3 years ago. She thought it helped, so she got a prescription for it from her primary care physician (PCP) several years ago. She tries to start using it in early May and during the second week of September before her seasonal symptoms begin. She starts with one spray into each nostril twice a day. Although it still seems to help, she notices some vague "belly" pain and sometimes even loses her appetite. She has paid close attention to this, and thinks that these symptoms occur about an hour after using the spray. As a result, she usually uses the spray only once a day, most often at bedtime. With that regimen, the Flonase still helps some, and she hardly notices the stomach symptoms. On further questioning, she admits to skipping some doses of Flonase because she dislikes the bitter aftertaste. A large portion of the dose seems to run down the back of her throat. Also, it smells bad and even affects her ability to smell normally sometimes. The same PCP also had her try an albuterol inhaler for the sensation of chest tightness. She used this during one summer season a few years ago, but noticed only that it made her feel nervous and jittery, but did not really help the chest tightness. Subsequently, her PCP had her try montelukast (Singulair) for the chest tightness. This seemed to work better than the albuterol, and it even seemed to help some of the nasal symptoms. She continues to use montelukast, one tablet daily, during the times when her symptoms are very bothersome. Except for the allergy symptoms specified above and the stomach symptoms that she attributes to the Flonase, she denies having other symptoms. She thinks that she needs more medication or something that will work better to control her symptoms, especially when they get worse.

Past Medical History

AR × 8 years

UTI about 9 months ago

Acute sinusitis about 2½ years ago

No unusual childhood diseases, no other chronic illnesses, and no history of surgery

Family History

Mother is alive and well, perimenopausal, but with no other chronic diseases. Father is alive and well, with AR and asthma. She has no siblings. She knows nothing about the health status of other, more remote family.

Social History

She is married, has no children, and is currently a full-time university student. She claims to have a "normal" diet. She has no formal exercise program. She denies being victimized by any type of abuse.

Tobacco/Alcohol/Substance Use

Denies all tobacco use; drinks alcohol "socially, but not to excess"; denies illicit drug/substance use except for remote (9 years ago) and brief "experimentation" with marijuana.

Allergies/Intolerances/Adverse Drug Reactions

Albuterol inhaler caused her to feel nervous and jittery.

Amoxicillin (diffuse, itchy, maculopapular skin rash during last few days of a 10-day course when used for sinus infection about 2½ years ago).

Ciprofloxacin [moderate-to-severe myalgias (both arms and shoulders) starting the last day of a 3-day course and continuing for 3 more days, about 9 months ago when used for treatment of a urine infection].

Fluticasone propionate (Flonase) seems to cause abdominal discomfort, and it tastes and smells bad, as mentioned in the HPI.

Medications (Current)

Diphenhydramine (generic) 50 mg capsule PO up to three times a day PRN allergy symptoms

Montelukast (Singulair) 10 mg tablet PO once daily, but only PRN for sensation of chest tightness

Fluticasone propionate (Flonase) nasal solution—one spray into both nostrils once or sometimes twice daily, at least during the time of her worst seasonal symptoms

Oxymetazoline (Afrin) nasal spray PRN severe nasal congestion

Acetaminophen 500 mg tablets—one to two tablets PO up to four times daily, only PRN for aches, pains, or headache

Seasonal influenza vaccine (for 2008–2009) given about 10 months ago

Denies other medications, including vitamins, dietary supplements, herbs, or other complementary and alternative remedies.

Review of Systems

Admits to feeling quite tired some days, and has some trouble sleeping, mostly due to nasal congestion. The tiredness causes her to miss some social events associated with school. Although she rarely misses any classes, she often has trouble paying attention and taking notes during lectures.

Denies fever, facial pain, headache or purulent nasal discharge.

Denies change in hearing, pain in ears, or discharge from ears.

Denies cough, but admits to occasional SOB or wheezing, but only when she has the "tightness in the chest" sensation.

Denies eyelids stuck shut in the mornings, purulent discharge from the eyes, or changes in vision or light sensitivity.

Admits to some abdominal discomfort and even anorexia, especially shortly after using Flonase during the day. Also admits to some heartburn, especially after big meals and sometimes at bedtime.

Denies dysuria, urinary frequency or urgency, and denies, fever, lower abdominal, back/flank pain, or bloody urine.

Physical Examination

▶ *General*

Well-developed, well-nourished Caucasian female who appears her stated age. Responds appropriately to questions in well-phrased, full sentences without breathlessness.

▶ *Vital Signs*

BP (left arm standing) 110/68 mm Hg and (right arm sitting) 114/66 mm Hg; P 64 and regular; RR 14; T 37.4°C

Weight 134.2 lb (61 kg)

Height 65 in. (165.1 cm)

Denies and has no indication of pain at the present time

► Skin

No obvious lesions seen with the patient fully clothed.

► HEEN(SMT)T

Conjunctivas are slightly injected, but there is no discharge in the eyes, no corneal lesions, and no discharge or matting on the eyelids; PERRLA; EOMI; fundi not examined.

Nasal examination (without instrumentation, except a small flashlight) reveals a somewhat red and swollen-appearing mucosa with some watery nasal discharge.

Deep palpation and/or percussion of the maxillary, frontal, and ethmoid sinuses cause no pain.

Mouth examination reveals normal oral mucosa, good dental hygiene, no malodorous breath, but some evidence of postnasal drip and a mildly irritated posterior oropharynx.

► Neck and Lymph Nodes

Neck examination is within normal limits, except for one small (2-mm) nontender, easily movable lymph node in the left submandibular area.

► Chest

Patient evaluated while fully clothed; respiratory excursions grossly normal; auscultation through blouse reveals no crackles or wheezes in posterior, lateral, and upper anterior lung fields.

► Breasts

Deferred

► Cardiovascular

Deferred

► Abdomen/Gastrointestinal–Hepatic

Deferred

► Neurology

Normal gait; normal facial movements during conversation; normal and appropriate responses to questions; remaining detail deferred

► Extremities

No deformities evident; apparent full range of motion of all four limbs; no clubbing, cyanosis, or edema; radial and dorsalis pedis pulses normal bilaterally

► Genitourinary

Deferred

► Rectal

Deferred

Laboratory Tests

The patient has the following printout of *fasting* laboratory results from her last (and annual) visit with her PCP, about *2 months ago.*

	Conventional Units	*SI Units*
Na	145 mEq/L	145 mmol/L
K	4.3 mEq/L	4.3 mmol/L
Cl	102 mEq/L	102 mmol/L
CO_2	27 mEq/L	27 mmol/L
BUN	8 mg/dL	2.9 mmol/L
SCr	0.8 mg/dL	71 μmol/L
Glu	94 mg/dL	5.2 mmol/L
Ca	9.7 mg/dL	2.43 mmol/L
Mg	1.8 mEq/L	0.90 mmol/L
Phosphate	4.1 mg/dL	1.32 mmol/L
Urinalysis		
pH	5.0	
Specific gravity	1.015	
Protein	(−)	
Glucose	(−)	
Ketones	(−)	
RBC	None seen	
WBC	0–2/hpf	
Nitrite	(−)	
Hgb	13.2 g/dL	132 g/L; 8.19 mmol/L
Hct	40%	0.40
MCV	87 μm³	87 fL
Platelets	$230 \times 10^3/mm^3$	$230 \times 10^9/L$
WBC	$6.2 \times 10^3/mm^3$	$6.2 \times 10^9/L$
Total cholesterol	157 mg/dL	4.06 mmol/L
LDL cholesterol	95 mg/dL	2.46 mmol/L
HDL cholesterol	52 mg/dL	1.34 mmol/L
Albumin	4.1 g/dL	41 g/L
Alanine aminotransferase (ALT)	32 IU/L	0.53 μkat/L
Aspartate aminotransferase (AST)	37 IU/L	0.62 μkat/L
Alkaline phosphatase	73 IU/L	1.22 μkat/L
Bilirubin, total	0.8 mg/dL	13.7 μmol/L

Assessment

Twenty-seven-year-old female with AR, which is predominantly seasonal but probably has a perennial component (by traditional classification), and is moderate to severe and persistent by new ARIA (Allergic Rhinitis and its Impact on Asthma) classification, which is not optimally controlled on her current regimen. There may be complicating factors of inadequate adherence, asthma, and GERD. She has a history of UTI and sinusitis.

Student Workup

Missing Information?

Evaluate: Patient Database

Drug Therapy Problems

Care Plan (by Problem)

TARGETED QUESTIONS

1. What additional information do you want to optimize your recommendations?

   Hint: See Table 62-3 in PPP for allergen avoidance information

2. What categories of medications are available to improve the control of her AR?

   Hint: See Table 62-4 in PPP

3. What categories of medications are most effective for management of the nasal congestion that is associated with AR?

   Hint: See Table 62-10 in PPP

4. What specific recommendations can you suggest to optimize her allergic rhinitis?

   Hint: See Tables 62-5 through 62-9 and the associated text (section titled First-Line Agents on pp. 1051–1054 and a portion of the section titled Adjunctive or Secondary-Choice Agents on pp. 1055–1057 in PPP)

5. If your initial recommendations do not help, what alternatives remain?

   Hint: See the Considerations for Referral section of the Clinical Presentation & Diagnosis textbox and the text on pp. 1048–1049 in PPP that relates to concurrence of AR and asthma

FOLLOW-UP

The same patient returns 6 months later. She is currently on a new regimen consisting of (1) appropriate use (no more than 3 days in a row) of intranasal decongestant (oxymetazoline) with supplemental as-needed intranasal antihistamine (olopatadine); (2) oral cetirizine taken as needed (in place of diphenhydramine); (3) mometasone intranasal corticosteroid (in place of fluticasone propionate) taken every day; (4) oral montelukast taken daily during her bad seasons; (5) ketotifen eye drops used as needed only for

bloodshot, itchy, and watery eyes; and (6) implementation of several environmental control measures (weekly laundering of bedclothes, treatment for elimination of cockroaches in her kitchen, and removal of cloth drapes in her bedroom). Her AR is quite well controlled. However, now she asks for a home pregnancy-test kit.

6. How will pregnancy change her symptoms and how might it change her medication regimen?

   Hint: See text on p. 1059 in PPP

⊕ GLOBAL PERSPECTIVE

There are many similarities concerning AR when one compares the United States to other countries of the world, however, there are some differences. Although AR is most common in the United States and the rest of the westernized world, some developing countries have recently seen an increase. This increase is predominantly in the more urbanized regions of those developing countries. There is evidence that "westernization," especially urbanization, increases the risk and prevalence of AR (as well as some other chronic allergic diseases). This phenomenon is usually attributed to the increased air and environmental pollution that is often associated with westernization (and industrialization). There may also be some contribution to this by the increasingly crowded living conditions often associated with urbanization. It is also said that immigrants from a rural area of a developing country may have an increased incidence of AR if they settle in an urbanized, westernized area of a developed country. Again, this is attributable to their being exposed to an increased number and probably amount of new (to them) pollutants and allergens. Complicating an evaluation of this is the fact that there is almost certainly an element of underdiagnosis of AR in developing countries. The basic approach to the management of AR is similar around the world. The only differences appear to be variable availability of certain specific medications in some classes of agents.

CASE SUMMARY

- This patient's condition is mixed seasonal and perennial AR, or as classified by the alternative system, it is moderate-to-severe and persistent AR. By either classification system, her condition is inadequately controlled by her current regimen.

- She has the most common symptoms of AR [runny, itchy nose, sneezing, and nasal congestion (which is the most bothersome and difficult to treat)], as well as other symptoms [some eye symptoms (itchy, red, and watery eyes sometimes)], sleep disturbance, tiredness, "presenteeism" (difficulty taking notes during class lectures), and decreased quality of life (decreased socialization). She also has some chest tightness, sometimes accompanied by SOB and wheezing.

- Several unanswered questions need clarification before an optimal regimen can be suggested. First, the detail of oxymetazoline usage must be determined. Second, a search for other identifiable triggers is appropriate. Third, when caring for any woman of childbearing age, it is always important to get a complete contraception and menstrual history. This may help with decisions concerning therapeutic management of that patient's medical conditions. Although it may be difficult, an attempt should be made to determine whether or not the current diphenhydramine is causing cognitive or performance problems.

- Depending on what is found out about the intranasal decongestant use (above), an intranasal antihistamine may be appropriate.

- A second-generation oral antihistamine should probably replace her diphenhydramine, as she may be having cognitive and performance degradation from the diphenhydramine without being aware of it.

- A replacement intranasal corticosteroid product should be used to minimize side effects and thus optimize adherence and efficacy.

- Monitoring should consist of tracking the usual three components that apply to monitoring of any chronic medical problem that is treated with medications. First, monitoring should consist of keeping careful records of her symptoms (frequency, severity, duration) to establish the efficacy of the new regimen. Second, monitoring should include tracking of any adverse events from any component of her new regimen, including considerations of adherence. Third, the symptoms of any known complications (e.g., sinusitis, otitis media) or other problems known to be associated with AR (asthma) should be monitored.

- Failure of the new regimen should be a consideration for referral to her PCP and possibly to an allergist. Benefits of referral include ruling out asthma (and if present, also ruling out GERD), ruling out sinusitis (because of her history of having at least one episode), and identifying specific allergens to both optimize avoidance and possibly facilitate implementation of appropriate immunotherapy.

For more information on the care plan and facilitator's guide please visit http://www.mhpharmacotherapy.com.

65 Conjunctivitis

Michelle L. Hilaire Jaime R. Hornecker

CASE LEARNING OBJECTIVES

- Differentiate between the various ophthalmic disorders using patient-specific information
- Choose an appropriate treatment regimen for an ophthalmic disorder
- Discuss the product differences that direct the selection of ophthalmic medications
- Educate patients about ophthalmic disease states and appropriate drug and nondrug therapies

PATIENT PRESENTATION

Chief Complaint

"My eyes are so red and watery. It started 2 days ago in my right eye and now my left eye is just as bad. I want to wear sunglasses because the light is making them water more. I hate coming to the office so you know I think it's serious."

History of Present Illness

Lena Petz is a 53-year-old woman who comes to see her physician because currently both of her eyes are red and watering. Two days ago, she noticed that her right eye was irritated and looked a little red, but she just figured that it was because she had been up late the previous night grading projects. She tried a couple drops of Visine but did not notice much difference. Yesterday, she noticed that she had to wipe away a watery discharge from her eye several times during the day. Today when she woke up, her left eye looked the same as the right. She thinks they look redder than yesterday and are watering more and now she is light-sensitive. She mentions that a lot of the children in her classes have been coughing and sniffling and having watery eyes recently.

Past Medical History

Osteopenia diagnosed 1 year ago
Type 2 DM diagnosed 2 years ago
HTN diagnosed 7 years ago

Family History

Mother has osteoporosis and HTN, and is alive at age 78. Father had lung cancer and died at age 60. She has a brother and a sister, who both have HTN and hyperlipidemia.

Social History

Married and lives with her husband of 32 years; has no children. Works as an art teacher at a local elementary school. Walks with husband 1 mile 3 days a week for exercise.

Tobacco/Alcohol/Substance Use

Social drinker (one to two drinks per week)
(−) Tobacco or illicit drug use

Allergies/Intolerances/Adverse Drug Events

Penicillin (breaks out in hives)

Medications (Current)

Glucophage 500 mg PO q 12 h
Lisinopril 20 mg PO daily
Calcium carbonate 1,000 mg PO q 12 h
Alendronate 35 mg PO weekly
Vitamin D 400 international units PO daily
Aspirin 81 mg PO daily
Ibuprofen 200 mg PO PRN headache

Review of Systems

(+) Eye discharge and tearing in both eyes
(−) Double vision and blind spots
Occasional headaches relieved with nonaspirin pain reliever

Physical Examination

▶ *General*

Well-developed, well-nourished, middle-aged, Caucasian female in no acute distress. Speech is clear and affect is appropriate.

▶ *Vital Signs*

BP 128/82 mm Hg, P 72, RR 15 (easy and nonlabored), T 36.9°C

Weight 155 lb (70 kg)

Height 66 in. (167.6 cm)

Denies pain

▶ *Skin*

Dry-appearing skin and scalp

(−) Rashes or lesions

▶ *HEENT*

Vision 20/40 in each eye with glasses

Both eyes—conjunctiva red and slightly swollen

PERRLA

EOMI

Ear canals without erythema, swelling, discharge, or cerumen

▶ *Neck and Lymph Nodes*

Physical examination of neck is unremarkable; (−) thyroid nodules; (−) lymphadenopathy; (−) carotid bruits

▶ *Chest*

Clear to auscultation bilaterally with no wheezing, ronchi, or rales

▶ *Breasts*

Examination deferred

▶ *Cardiovascular*

RRR

Normal S_1, S_2

(−) S_3 or S_4

No murmurs, rubs, or gallops

▶ *Abdomen*

Nontender/nondistended

(−) Organomegaly

▶ *Neurology*

Cranial nerves II to XII intact

Deep tendon reflexes normal

No complaints of weakness, numbness, or loss of coordination

▶ *Genitourinary*

Examination deferred

▶ *Rectal*

Examination deferred

Laboratory Tests

Fasting, obtained 6 months ago

	Conventional Units	*SI Units*
Na	138 mEq/L	138 mmol/L
K	4.2 mEq/L	4.2 mmol/L
Cl	104 mEq/L	104 mmol/L
CO_2	26 mEq/L	26 mmol/L
BUN	15 mg/dL	5.4 mmol/L
SCr	0.68 mg/dL	60 μmol/L
Ca	9.4 mg/dL	2.35 mmol/L
Mg	1.6 mEq/L	0.80 mmol/L
Phosphate	3.1 mg/dL	1 mmol/L
Hgb	13.1 g/dL	131 g/L; 8.13 mmol/L
Hct	40.1%	0.401
WBC	$7.2 \times 10^3/mm^3$	$7.2 \times 10^9/L$
MCV	89 mm^3	89 fL
Albumin	4.0 g/dL	40 g/L
Hemoglobin A_{1C}	7.6%	0.076
Glucose	146 mg/dL	8.1 mmol/L
Total cholesterol	232 mg/dL	6.00 mmol/L
LDL cholesterol	119 mg/dL	3.08 mmol/L
HDL cholesterol	46 mg/dL	1.19 mmol/L

Assessment

Fifty-three-year-old woman with signs and symptoms consistent with viral conjunctivitis (pink eye)

Student Workup

Missing Information?

Evaluate: Patient Database

Drug Therapy Problems

Care Plan (by Problem)

TARGETED QUESTIONS

1. What types of conjunctivitis exist?

   Hint: See Figure 63-1 in PPP

2. What is the primary cause of viral conjunctivitis?

   Hint: See pp. 1066 and 1067 in PPP

3. What pharmacologic therapy should be used to treat viral conjunctivitis?

   Hint: See p. 1067 in PPP

4. When should the patient see significant improvement in the viral conjunctivitis?

   Hint: See p. 1068 in PPP

FOLLOW-UP

Three weeks later, the patient returns for follow-up. Her symptoms have resolved, but she notes that her husband is experiencing similar symptoms.

5. What actions, if any, would you take? What nonpharmacologic measures would you share with the patient?

   Hint: See p. 1067 in PPP

⊙ GLOBAL PERSPECTIVE

Conjunctivitis is a worldwide ophthalmic disorder and viral conjunctivitis is one of the most common forms. This condition is very contagious and poses a significant health problem in schools and workplaces where touch contamination is poorly controlled. Poor living conditions can contribute to continuous cases of viral conjunctivitis as household items such as towels and pillows are shared. If the etiology of the conjunctivitis is not clear, the patient should be referred to an eye care practitioner.

CASE SUMMARY

- Her current clinical picture is consistent with viral conjunctivitis. Although it is self-limiting, the patient needs to observe nonpharmacologic measures to avoid spreading conjunctivitis to others.
- Antibiotic medications should be avoided in viral infections.

For more information on the care plan and facilitator's guide please visit http://www.mhpharmacotherapy.com.

66 Psoriasis

Meghan K. Sullivan

PATIENT PRESENTATION

Chief Complaint

"I'm so itchy! This stuff just keeps on spreading! I don't know what to do!"

History of Present Illness

Kathryn Leahy is a 24-year-old female who presents to her primary care provider complaining of severe itching, redness, and a psoriatic flare-up. She was diagnosed with psoriasis 4 years ago, and has experienced sporadic flare-ups during this time, the most recent being 4 months ago. She has been able to control her flare-ups over the years with a variety of creams and lotions. Most recently, she has been using betamethasone 1% cream and calcipotriol 50 mcg/g cream. Although this combination has worked well for her in the past, she is concerned that she is not seeing improvement in her current condition as rapidly as she has previously. The patient is also complaining of being physically and emotionally drained, and having difficulties sleeping.

Past Medical History

Psoriasis diagnosed 4 years ago

Melanoma diagnosed 2 years ago

Depression × 2 years

Anxiety × 6 weeks

Prediabetes × 6 months

Family History

Mother is alive at the age of 52 with type 1 DM, had a psoriatic episode in her late forties but has since been in remission. Father is alive at age 53. He has had two melanoma removed over the past 15 years. She has one brother and one sister, both of whom are healthy.

Social History

The patient is a third-year law student, one semester from graduation, and an intern at a local law firm. She is engaged to be married shortly after graduation. She has no children at present, but would like to start a family in the next 2 to 3 years.

Tobacco/Alcohol/Substance Use

Social drinker; (−) tobacco or illicit drug use

Allergies/Intolerances/Adverse Drug Events

Sulfa antibiotics (rash as child)

Codeine (rash postop melanoma)

Medications (Current)

Alprazolam 1 mg PO PRN test anxiety

Betamethasone valerate 1% cream daily PRN treatment of psoriasis plaques

Calcipotriol 50 mcg/g cream daily PRN treatment of psoriasis plaques

Ibuprofen 200 mg and diphenhydramine 38 mg PO PRN sleep

NuvaRing insert vaginally for 3 weeks and remove for 1 week

Sertraline 50 mg PO once daily

Review of Systems

(+) Depression; (+) test anxiety; (+) difficulty sleeping, relieved with NSAID/antihistamine combination product; (+)

multiple skin lesions/plaques, increased in the past 3 weeks; (+) pruritis.

Physical Examination

▶ General

The patient appears to be distressed/depressed about lesions.

▶ Vital Signs

BP 104/70 mm Hg, P 72, RR 14, T 36.2°C

Weight 165 lb (75 kg)

Height 68 in. (173 cm)

Denies pain and complains of pruritis

▶ Skin

Lesions on scalp, chest, back, and elbows

▶ HEENT

TMs normal; PERRLA

▶ Neck and Lymph Nodes

Within normal limits

▶ Chest

Within normal limits

▶ Breasts

Within normal limits

▶ Cardiovascular

Within normal limits

▶ Abdomen

Within normal limits

▶ Neurology

Reflexes normal

▶ Genitourinary

Examination deferred

▶ Rectal

Examination deferred

Laboratory Tests

Fasting, obtained during appointment

	Conventional Units	SI Units
Na	138 mEq/L	138 mmol/L
K	3.5 mEq/L	3.5 mmol/L
Cl	100 mEq/L	100 mmol/L
HCO₃	24 mEq/L	24 mmol/L
BUN	18 mg/dL	6.4 mmol/L
SCr	0.9 mg/dL	80 μmol/L
Glu	115 mg/dL	6.4 mmol/L
Ca	9.4 mg/dL	2.35 mmol/L
Mg	1.4 mEq/L	0.70 mmol/L
Phosphate	3.5 mg/dL	1.13 mmol/L
Hgb	13.8 g/dL	138 g/L; 8.57 mmol/L
Hematocrit	40.1%	0.401
MCV	88.2 μm³	88.2 fL
WBC	6.4 × 10³/mm³	6.4 × 10⁹/L
Albumin	3.8 g/dL	38 g/L
AST	14 IU/L	0.23 μkat/L
ALT	10 IU/L	0.17 μkat/L
Total cholesterol	110 mg/dL	2.84 mmol/L
LDL cholesterol	80 mg/dL	2.07 mmol/L
HDL cholesterol	50 mg/dL	1.29 mmol/L

Assessment

Twenty-four-year-old female with signs/symptoms consistent with a moderate-to-severe psoriasis exacerbation

---

Student Workup

Missing Information?

Evaluate: Patient Database

Drug Therapy Problems

Care Plan (by Problem)

TARGETED QUESTIONS

1. What signs and symptoms of moderate-to-severe psoriasis does this patient possess?

   Hint: See p. 1081 and Table 64-1 in PPP

2. What risk factors are present that may have influenced the exacerbation of a flare-up?

   Hint: See p. 1080 in PPP

3. What nonpharmacologic treatment should be recommended to this patient?

   Hint: See p. 1083 in PPP

4. Why would the addition of systemic therapy be preferred in this patient rather than phototherapy?

   Hint: See p. 1085 in PPP

5. What risks and adverse events should be discussed with this patient in regard to the chosen therapy?

   Hint: See pp. 1085 and 1086 in PPP

FOLLOW-UP

Four weeks later, the patient returns for follow-up. Improvement in her lesions is seen.

6. What actions will you take, if any, to enhance the therapeutic effect of this patient's current therapy? What additional steps will you take to ensure that she enters remission and experiences minimal flare-ups? In the future, what steps will need to be taken if the patient becomes pregnant? What therapeutic options will be available to her should finances no longer be an issue after graduation?

   Hint: See p. 1086 in PPP

🌎 GLOBAL PERSPECTIVE

Psoriasis is a common chronic inflammatory disease of the skin that is seen in people throughout the world. Incidence and prevalence of psoriasis continues to be studied on an ongoing basis. It is thought that psoriasis dates back to Biblical times as a common disorder is made mention of in the Bible. Throughout the years, the diagnosis of psoriasis has changed as more is learned about the disease. Several patterns have been identified in studies that have been conducted in patients suffering from psoriasis. However, these findings cannot always be deemed conclusive for the fact that many patients do not seek medical attention for the treatment of psoriasis. Observations that have been made include a greater incidence of psoriasis seen in patients living in regions further from the equator. Studies conducted in Australia show that people residing in southern Australia are more likely to suffer from psoriasis than those residing in northern Australia. The opposite is true for a study conducted in Norway, helping to prove the theory that those residing close to the equator are less likely to suffer from the disease. In terms of race, Caucasians have been found to suffer from psoriasis more often than those of Asian or African descent. Lifestyle plays a large role in the incidence and prevalence of the disease as well. Individuals living in third-world countries are less likely to suffer from psoriasis in comparison to developed countries where smoking, stress, and obesity are more prominent and have been shown to increase a person's risk for developing the disease.

CASE SUMMARY

- The patient's current condition can be classified as moderate psoriasis.

- The current flare-up is most likely due to ongoing stress in the patient's life. Stress, depression, anxiety, and trouble sleeping are all culprits of this flare-up. Encouragement of nonpharmacologic stress-reducing activities should be recommended (i.e., hobbies, exercise, and relaxation techniques).

- Current treatment with topical therapy is subpar. The addition of oral therapy (methotrexate) will be beneficial in this patient. Oral therapy needs to be monitored closely for side effects; pregnancy is of concern in the future.

- Past medical history positive for melanoma is of concern in regard to therapeutic options; UV therapy should not be considered in this patient.

For more information on the care plan and facilitator's guide please visit http://www.mhpharmacotherapy.com.

67 Acne

Jean E. Cunningham

CASE LEARNING OBJECTIVES

- Recognize the signs and symptoms of common skin disorders, such as acne, in a presenting patient
- Identify the goals of therapy for acne
- Develop an appropriate treatment and monitoring plan for acne, including nonpharmacologic and pharmacologic agents, on the basis of individual patient characteristics
- Select an appropriate product for acne disorders
- Properly educate a patient using acne treatment options

PATIENT PRESENTATION

Chief Complaint

"My son's acne medication is not working!"

History of Present Illness

Jefferson Roberts is a shy 17-year-old male who is brought into your pharmacy by his mother, Luanne Roberts, complaining that the acne medication prescribed to him is just not working. On further questioning and examination, you find that the patient currently has several papules and pustules on his chin and cheeks, and you also notice a lot of small depressed pits in the same area along with some excessively dry patches of skin. He has more closed comedones on his cheeks and forehead than open, with the majority of open comedones on his nose. His mother informs you that she watches the patient wash his face three times a day with soap and water, and reminds him constantly that dirty skin leads to "blackheads." The patient's mother admits to buying an "extraction tool" in which she uses to help "clean out the dirt and puss" in the patient's "zits." After looking at the patient's prescription history, you see that he has prescriptions from a local dermatologist. When questioned, you find out from the patient's mother that when he first started "breaking out" he was 13 years old, and Retin-A seemed to help. But in the past year, his acne has only worsened and she was hopeful his skin would further improve once his dermatologist added minocycline. However, she feels that these measures are not enough and wants to know what else they can do to clear up his skin. You hear the patient mumble something about wasting money on the soap that was advertised on television and also sense that he is very uncomfortable talking about his skin disorder.

Past Medical History

Hospitalized 5 years ago due to a severe upper respiratory infection

Family History

The patient is the youngest of three and his mother reports no one else in the family having so much trouble with acne.

Social History

The patient is a varsity swimmer and wants to try out for the US Olympic Water Polo team. He lives at home with his mother and is currently a high school junior. Family recently returned from a skiing vacation in Colorado. He has always been positive and upbeat until a few months ago and has now become more withdrawn and distressed. He works during the summer for his uncle's landscaping company.

Tobacco/Alcohol/Substance Use

Denies any and all use of tobacco, alcohol, or other substances

Allergies/Intolerances/Adverse Drug Events

No known allergies

Medications (Current)

Minocycline 100 mg PO once daily PRN acne

Retin-A (tretinoin) 0.01% gel—apply small amount q hs to clean, dry skin

Neutrogena Men skin-clearing salicylic acid face wash—washes face with cleanser three times per day

GNC skin vitamin

Previously purchased Proactiv, but currently is not using

Review of Systems

Painful swelling and redness located on face and reports similar issues with upper back and chest; (+) papules, pustules, open and closed comedones, moderately painful lesions; (+) scarring; (+) dry skin; (+) hyperpigmentation; (−) nodules.

Physical Examination

▶ *General*

Defensive, shy, and emotionally distressed, Caucasian teenager obviously embarrassed by physical appearance and mother's concern.

▶ *Vital Signs*

Weight 162 lb (74 kg)

Height 75 in. (190.5 cm)

Admits that swelling and inflammation are bothersome, but mostly embarrassing

▶ *Skin*

Red, flaky, swollen, and irritated skin; (+) papules and pustules on cheeks, chin, back, and chest; (+) closed comedones on cheeks and forehead; (+) open comedones on nose; (+) scarring and lesions; (−) nodules and conglobata

▶ *HEENT*

Wears contacts; also has glasses that he will not wear in public

Assessment

Seventeen-year-old male with signs, symptoms, and physical examination consistent with moderate acne

Student Workup

Missing Information?

Evaluate:	Patient Database
	Drug Therapy Problems
	Care Plan (by Problem)

TARGETED QUESTIONS

1. What signs and symptoms of moderate acne does the patient have?

   Hint: See Table 65-1 in PPP

2. For what type of acne is benzoyl peroxide the treatment of choice and why?

   Hint: See pp. 1096–1097 in PPP

3. What risks and adverse effects of topical and oral therapy would you discuss with the patient?

   Hint: See Tables 65-2, 65-3, and 65-4 in PPP

4. What are additional acne therapy options for the patient?

   Hint: See Figure 65-3 in PPP

5. Should the patient receive medical treatment for his psychologic distress associated with his acne?

   Hint: The patient's moderate acne is generally a self-limiting condition that with proper care may reduce the appearance and severity of the acne. Since the patient has no other signs or symptoms of depression besides apparent discomfort and awkwardness, the risk of medications for depressed mood far outweigh the benefit for the time being. It would be reasonable to optimize current acne therapy and reassess the patient for signs of improvement before suggesting additional measures. See p. 1094 in PPP

FOLLOW-UP

6. How would your treatment recommendation change if the patient returned in a few weeks presenting with extensive papules, pustules, nodules, and further scarring?

   Hint: See Figure 65-3 in PPP

7. What if the patient returns in 8 months with improved skin and only has a few issues with the open and closed comedones?

   Hint: See Figure 65-3 in PPP

8. If the patient were to begin isotretinoin capsules 40 mg PO twice daily, what are some considerations/counseling tips you would want to review with him?

   Hint: See Table 65-4 in PPP

⟳ GLOBAL PERSPECTIVE

Acne affects races and skin types differently, and may present with different clinical manifestations depending on the affected patient. Although acne is considered the most common disease in the United States, it is also common in other countries, but in different forms. Cystic acne is commonly found in countries such as Spain, Italy, Iran, and other countries in the Mediterranean region. African Americans or people of other ethnicities can also develop a certain type of acne commonly associated with the use of oil or ointment-based hair pomades. Although the primary cause of acne depends on pathogenic factors, additional factors, whether culturally related or not, such as the use of occluding cosmetic and hair products, certain medications, disease states, and items worn directly against skin that obstruct skin pores can worsen acne and should be identified, discussed, and avoided if possible.

CASE SUMMARY

- His current clinical picture is consistent with moderate papular pustular acne not responding to first-choice therapy, and alternative treatments should be initiated.

- Alternative pharmacologic therapy for moderate papular pustular acne includes the option to switch the patient to tretinoin (Retin-A Micro) 0.1% gel—apply small amount once daily at bedtime as it may be a less drying option. A change in oral antibiotic can also be considered, depending on the current length of therapy of the minocycline.

- Also, a topical benzoyl peroxide lotion can be recommended over the counter for the patient, since it can further treat the acne and also provide a much-needed moisturizer to help decrease his skin redness and irritation.

For more information on the care plan and facilitator's guide please visit http://www.mhpharmacotherapy.com.

68 Atopic Dermatitis

Kim W. Benner

CASE LEARNING OBJECTIVES

- Assess the signs and symptoms of common skin disorders in a presenting patient
- List the goals of treatment for patients with common skin disorders
- Select appropriate nonpharmacologic and pharmacologic treatment regimens to patients presenting with common skin disorders
- Identify the adverse effects that may result from pharmacologic agents used in the treatment of common skin disorders
- Develop a monitoring plan that will assess the safety and efficacy of the overall disease management of common skin disorders

PATIENT PRESENTATION

Chief Complaint

"This rash seems to be getting worse and it itches so bad that I cannot sleep at night."

History of Present Illness

Emily Evan is a 17-year-old female who presents to the dermatologist complaining of a rash on her hands and face that is getting worse. In these areas, the rash appears as pruritic, thickened plaques. A similar rash has recently appeared in the folds of her arms and legs; however, these areas are pruritic, erythematous papules and vesicles. She was recommended to use a nonprescription topical steroid (hydrocortisone) by a family friend who is a nurse. The patient recalls having a similar rash as a child that responded to the hydrocortisone, so she has tried it sporadically over the last several months. In addition, in her childhood, she also suffered food allergies to peanuts, eggs, and milk, but eventually outgrew this allergy and can tolerate these foods now. The rash, however, seems to come and go with the seasons and her stress level. She is currently having trouble in school and with her boyfriend; she is also trying to find a college despite her lack of funds and poor grades. Like most teenagers of her age, she frequently wears tightfitting clothes and wears much makeup and perfume.

Past Medical History

Food allergies to peanuts, eggs, and milk as an infant, now resolved

Allergic rhinitis since age 6

Family History

Both parents are alive. Father currently has asthma and mother has a history of allergic rhinitis. She has two younger sisters, one of which has asthma.

Social/Work History

Currently, she is a "C" student in high school and is not involved in extracurricular activities. She claims to have a boyfriend in college who likes to "spend a lot of time with her." She was employed part-time at a local fast-food restaurant but quit due to decreasing grades and to spend more time with her boyfriend.

Tobacco/Alcohol/Substance Abuse

Denies any routine use, but does admit to occasional alcohol use when around her friends. Admits her boyfriend smokes constantly

Allergies/Intolerances/Adverse Drug Events

None known at this time; seems to tolerate peanuts, eggs, and milk, but seldom eats them due to her childhood allergy

Medications (Current)

Hydrocortisone acetate cream, applies to rash on arms, hands, face, and legs PRN rash/itch

Fluticasone nasal spray, one spray in each nare two times a day, admits noncompliance

Yasmin 1 PO each day, questionable compliance

Review of Systems

(+) Dry skin all over. Thick plaques on hands and face. Fossa of legs and arms have erythematous lesions. No complaints of muscle or joint pain. Complains of being tired due to stress of school and boyfriend, and that she is up all night scratching her rash.

Physical Examination

▶ General

Tired and stressed teenager who appears anxious and depressed, yet in no acute distress

▶ Vital Signs

BP 104/65 mm Hg, P 72, RR 13, T 36.3°C

Weight 115 lb (52.3 kg)

Height 64 in. (163 cm)

▶ Skin

Generally dry all over; (+) thick fibrotic plaques with lichenification on hands and face. Pruritic, erythematous papules and vesicles on antecubital and popliteal fossa of arms and legs. She also has markings on her skin due to tightfitting clothes.

▶ HEENT

PERRLA, EOMI, nares moist with mucus; Dennie-Morgan lines present

▶ Neck and Lymph Nodes

Not significant

▶ Chest

CTA bilaterally

▶ Breasts

Normally developed female teenage breasts; the patient denies performing monthly breast examination.

▶ Cardiovascular

RRR; no m/r/g

▶ Abdomen

Not tender, not distended; (+) BS; (−) organomegaly

▶ Neurology

Grossly intact; A&O × 3; CNs intact

▶ Genitourinary

Patient menstruating

▶ Rectal

Deferred

Laboratory Tests

	Conventional Units	SI Units
Na	141 mEq/L	141 mmol/L
K	3.8 mEq/L	3.8 mmol/L
Cl	102 mEq/L	102 mmol/L
CO_2	24 mEq/L	24 mmol/L
BUN	10 mg/dL	3.6 mmol/L
SCr	0.6 mg/dL	53 mmol/L
Glu	92 mg/dL	5.1 mmol/L
Ca	9.1 mg/dL	2.28 mmol/L
Mg	1.9 mEq/L	0.95 mmol/L
Phosphate	3.6 mg/dL	1.16 mmol/L
Hgb	11.9 g/dL	119 g/L; 7.39 mmol/L
Hct	36%	0.36
WBC	$10.9 \times 10^3/mm^3$	$10.9 \times 10^9/L$
Eosinophils	9%	0.09
MCV	81 μm³	81 fL
IgE	400 IU/mL	400 kIU/L

Assessment

Seventeen-year-old female with signs and symptoms consistent with atopic dermatitis (AD)

Student Workup

Missing Information?

Evaluate: Patient Database
Drug Therapy Problems
Care Plan (by Problem)

TARGETED QUESTIONS

1. What signs and symptoms of AD does the patient have? Can the lesions be described as acute, subacute, or chronic?

   Hint: See pp. 1100–1102 in PPP

2. What nonpharmacologic therapy can you recommend for AD?

   Hint: See pp. 1101 and 1102 and Table 65-5 in PPP

3. Is a topical corticosteroid the treatment of choice for her? If so, what potency of steroid should be utilized?

   Hint: See Table 65-6 in PPP

4. What are the second-line options available for the acute control of AD?

   Hint: See pp. 1101 and 1102 in PPP

5. What adjunct therapy is needed for the more erythematous lesions on her arms and legs?

   Hint: Skin in AD is often colonized with bacteria.

FOLLOW-UP

Three weeks later, the patient returns for a follow-up and states that after using the prescribed initial therapy, her lesions are only moderately improved. She had begun to notice some "skin thinning" and discoloration in the areas of steroid use. She is interested in trying something other than topical steroids.

6. What therapy is available for long-term maintenance therapy or refractory cases?

    Hint: See pp. 1101 and 1102 in PPP

7. What can you recommend to help decrease the itching and help her sleep?

    Hint: See p. 1102 and Table 65-5 in PPP

8. What relation might the occurrence of AD have to her history of food allergies?

    Hint: See p. 1101 in PPP

⊙ GLOBAL PERSPECTIVE

Atopic dermatitis is a common skin disorder that is often associated with triggers such as food allergies. The incidence of food allergies can differ around the world due to variations in diets. For example, rice allergies occur more often in Asia where rice is a major component of Asian diet, whereas corn allergies may be more prevalent outside the United States since corn derivatives are commonplace in the US (and Canadian) diet. The most common allergies in many countries include milk, eggs, peanuts, treenuts, fish, shellfish, soy, wheat, and sesame. Seed allergies, especially sesame, have been reported to be increasing in many countries. The United States has the FDA to mandate appropriate labeling for possible allergens in the food supply, third-world countries may not have safeguards in place for consumers to take note of possible triggers. Often exposure to extreme hot or cold temperature can be a cause of an exacerbation, so inhabitants of such environments worldwide may suffer exacerbations more (or less) often.

CASE SUMMARY

- Her current skin problem is consistent with AD on her hands and face. Since she is uncontrolled on low-potency corticosteroids (first-line therapy), a stronger steroid may be utilized on the arm and leg lesions. However, due to the patient experiencing intolerable side effects, alternative therapy includes topical calcineurin inhibitors.

- Often nonpharmacologic measures and avoidance of triggers can decrease the severity of AD.

- Bacterial colonization often occurs with chronic lesions and can be exacerbated by the constant scratching. Topical and/or oral antibiotics may be beneficial.

For more information on the care plan and facilitator's guide please visit http://www.mhpharmacotherapy.com.

69 Iron-Deficiency Anemia

Colleen Clark Dula   Teri West

CASE LEARNING OBJECTIVES

- Identify the common causes of anemia
- Describe the common signs and symptoms of anemia
- Discuss the appropriate diagnostic evaluation to determine the type of anemia and guide therapeutic decisions
- State the desired therapeutic outcomes for patients with anemia
- Compare and contrast the various oral and parenteral iron preparations
- Recommend a specific treatment regimen for anemia considering the underlying cause of anemia and patient-specific variables
- Develop a plan to monitor the outcomes of anemia pharmacotherapy

PATIENT PRESENTATION

Chief Complaint

"I'm tired all the time, I just feel exhausted."

History of Present Illness

Neeraja Singh is a 30-year-old woman who presents to her primary care physician (PCP) complaining of fatigue that has continued to worsen over the past several months. She began an exercise regimen a few months ago after she was told this would help her blood pressure, but has been unable to stick to her routine lately because she has just been too tired and weak. She states that she checks her blood pressure once or twice a week and it usually runs in the 120–130s/80s mm Hg. She follows a traditional Indian diet; vegetables and rice are a large part of her diet and she does not eat meat.

Past Medical History

GERD

HTN × 1 year

Family History

Mother deceased at age 52 of breast cancer and father alive at age 65 with HTN and type 2 DM. She has two older brothers with HTN, both alive and well.

Social History

She is married for 2 years and lives with her husband; they currently have no children but would like to begin trying soon. She works full time as a receptionist at a dental clinic.

Tobacco/Alcohol/Substance Use

Denies alcohol, tobacco, or illicit drug use

Allergies/Intolerances/Adverse Drug Events

Codeine (stomach upset)

Medications (Current)

Omeprazole 20 mg PO every morning

Lisinopril 10 mg PO once daily

Review of Systems

(+) Fatigue; HA around periods; no CP or SOB; 28-day cycles, menses approximately 5 to 6 days (5 pads/d), LMP 14 days ago; denies any recent episodes of bleeding, including no hematochezia, melena, epitaxis, or hematuria

Physical Examination

▶ *General*

WDWN Indian woman in NAD, who appears her stated age

▶ **Vital Signs**

BP 134/88 mm Hg, P 80, RR 14, T 37°C

Weight 152 lb (69.1 kg)

Height 61 in. (155 cm)

▶ **Skin**

Dry skin

▶ **HEENT**

PERRLA, EOMI; pale conjunctivas; normal fundoscopic examination; no retinopathy; TMs intact; oropharynx clear

▶ **Neck and Lymph Nodes**

No thyromegaly, lymphadenopathy, or JVD

▶ **Chest**

CTA bilaterally

▶ **Breasts**

No masses or discharge

▶ **Cardiovascular**

RRR; normal S_1, S_2; w/o S_3 and S_4

▶ **Abdomen**

Normal bowel sounds, soft, not tender/not distended, no masses

▶ **Neurology**

A&O × 3; deep tendon reflexes normal

▶ **Genitourinary**

Examination deferred

▶ **Rectal**

(−) Stool guaiac

Laboratory Tests

Obtained today

	Conventional Units	SI Units
Na	135 mEq/L	135 mmol/L
K	4.2 mEq/L	4.2 mmol/L
Cl	105 mEq/L	105 mmol/L
CO_2	23 mEq/L	23 mmol/L
BUN	8 mg/dL	2.9 mmol/L
SCr	0.75 mg/dL	66 µmol/L
Glu	90 mg/dL	5 mmol/L
Ca	9 mg/dL	2.25 mmol/L
AST	23 IU/L	0.38 µkat/L
ALT	20 IU/L	0.33 µkat/L
Albumin	4 g/dL	40 g/L
TSH	3.76 µIU/mL	3.76 mIU/L
Hgb	8 g/dL	80 g/L; 4.96 mmol/L
Hct	26.3%	0.263
WBC	$6.1 \times 10^3/mm^3$	$6.1 \times 10^9/L$
RBC	$3.95 \times 10^6/µL$	$3.95 \times 10^{12}/L$
MCV	$66 \ µm^3$	66 fL
MCHC	30.6 g/dL	306 g/L
RDW	21.7%	0.217
Iron	8 mcg/dL	1.4 µmol/L
TIBC	493 mcg/dL	88.2 µmol/L
TSAT	2%	0.02
Ferritin	1 ng/mL	1 mcg/L

▶ **Peripheral Blood Smear**

Microcytic, hypochromic RBCs

Assessment

Thirty-year-old woman with signs, symptoms, and laboratory tests consistent with iron-deficiency anemia

Student Workup

Missing Information?

Evaluate: Patient Database

Drug Therapy Problems

Care Plan (by Problem)

TARGETED QUESTIONS

1. What signs, symptoms, and laboratory values are consistent with iron-deficiency anemia in this patient?

    Hint: See p. 1112 and Table 66-1 in PPP

2. What are the potential causes of iron-deficiency anemia?

    Hint: See p. 1111 in PPP

3. What iron replacement treatment options are available for this patient?

    Hint: See pp. 1113–1116 and Table 66-3 in PPP

4. What risks and adverse effects of therapy would you discuss with this patient?

    Hint: See pp. 1113–1116 and 1118 in PPP

5. Would you recommend a transfusion in this patient? If so why or why not?

    Hint: See pp. 1112 and 1113 in PPP

FOLLOW-UP

The patient tolerates the therapy well, and her Hgb and Hct stabilized over the first few weeks of therapy. At her 6-month follow-up, her laboratory tests showed that her iron stores returned to normal, so her PCP stopped the iron supplement. She was also started on a prenatal vitamin by her OB-GYN as she and her husband were actively trying to conceive.

One year later, the patient returns to your clinic with persistent fatigue and weakness. Her OB-GYN restarted the oral iron supplements 2 months ago suspecting anemia, and laboratory tests confirmed iron-deficiency anemia at that time [Hgb 8.8 g/dL (88 g/L; 5.46 mmol/L), Hct 26.3% (0.263), MCV 77 μm^3 (77 fL), ferritin 4 ng/mL (4 mcg/L)]. She informs you today that she is expecting twins and is about 28 weeks along in her pregnancy. She has had significant morning sickness and frequent vomiting throughout her entire pregnancy. She has tried several oral iron supplements, including ferrous sulfate, ferrous gluconate, and Niferex. Today's laboratory test results include Hgb 9.1g/dL (91 g/L; 5.65 mmol/L) and Hct 29.7% (0.297).

6. What are the potential reasons that she is not responding to oral iron therapy? What suggestions or changes would you make today?

   Hint: See pp. 1114 and 1115 in PPP

🌐 GLOBAL PERSPECTIVE

Iron-deficiency anemia is one of the most prevalent micronutrient deficiencies in the world and contributes to the global burden of disease. It has been estimated to affect 2 billion people in the world and is associated with approximately one-fifth of perinatal deaths and approximately one-tenth of maternal deaths in developing countries. In children living with iron-deficiency anemia, the disease can lead to retarded physical and mental development. In adults, iron-deficiency anemia can reduce aerobic capacity and work productivity of entire populations, resulting in serious economic consequences to a developing nation.

Many people around the world are at a high risk for iron-deficiency anemia, including those individuals with blood loss from parasitic infections such as hookworms, ascaris, and schistosomiasis. Others at high risk are individuals with acute or chronic infections of malaria, cancers, tuberculosis, and HIV. Additional precipitators of iron-deficiency anemia may include reduced iron intake in the diet. Iron absorption can be further reduced as a result of diets high in nonheme sources, such as plants and supplementation, when combined with foods that inhibit absorption, such as phylates (bran), phenolics (coffee and tea), or calcium (dairy) compounds.

Women are at a high risk for iron-deficiency anemia, particularly those who have experienced a pregnancy with multiple babies or more than one pregnancy. Women who are pregnant have higher iron demands due to blood volume expansion and subsequent increases in RBCs and Hgb production, and growth of the fetus, placenta, and maternal tissues. During the second and third trimester, there is a threefold increase in the demand for iron. Unlike many countries in the world, iron-deficiency anemia in the United States has declined over the past decade because of the availability of iron-fortified foods, increased iron supplementation, increased vitamin C, and the use of contraception to decrease the incidence of pregnancy.

CASE SUMMARY

- Her current signs, symptoms, and laboratory values are consistent with iron-deficiency anemia, and iron replacement therapy should be initiated.

- Oral iron therapy should be initiated with a total daily dose of 200 mg of elemental iron in divided doses.

For more information on the care plan and facilitator's guide please visit http://www.mhpharmacotherapy.com.

70 Vitamin B$_{12}$ Deficiency Anemia

Janice L. Stumpf

CASE LEARNING OBJECTIVES

- Identify the common causes of anemia
- Describe the common signs and symptoms of anemia
- Discuss the appropriate diagnostic evaluation to determine the type of anemia and guide therapeutic decisions
- State the desired therapeutic outcomes for patients with anemia
- Explain the optimal use of vitamin B$_{12}$ in patients with macrocytic anemia
- Recommend a specific treatment regimen for anemia considering the underlying cause of anemia and patient-specific variables
- Develop a plan to monitor the outcomes of pharmacotherapy of anemia

PATIENT PRESENTATION

Chief Complaint

"I think I have another UTI. I've really been tired out recently. It's been busy at work."

History of Present Illness

Ellie Harbison is a 28-year-old white female who presents to her physician with complaints of increased frequency and pain on urination over the past 2 days. She also notes a lack of energy. For the past 1 to 2 months, she has begun taking naps in the early evening, after work. In addition, she used to run 5 to 6 miles each morning, but has stopped recently because her legs feel weak after just a few blocks.

Past Medical History

History of UTI × 10 years—last 2 years ago

Appendectomy 4 years ago

Gravida 1, para 1

Family History

Mother with breast cancer, otherwise healthy. Father with HTN. No siblings.

Social History

Vegan since age 13 years—no meat, poultry, fish, eggs, or dairy products eaten. Married with 18-month old daughter. Manager of a department store.

Tobacco/Alcohol/Substance Use

Occasional alcohol (one to two glasses of red wine two to three times monthly); no tobacco; no illicit drugs

Allergies/Intolerances/Adverse Drug Events

Penicillin—rash

Medications (Current)

Calcium carbonate 650 mg PO once daily, when she remembers

Ibuprofen 400 mg PO PRN menstrual cramps

Review of Systems

Fatigue; weakness during exercise; sore, tender tongue, making eating difficult; increased frequency and pain with urination × 2 days, but no flank pain or blood in the urine; menstrual cramps relieved with ibuprofen; dry skin; fingernails break easily

Physical Examination

► **General**

Petite, thin, white female who appears pale and somewhat uncomfortable

► **Vital Signs**

BP 110/65 mm Hg, P 90, RR 16, T 38.2°C (100.8°F)

Weight 103 lb (46.8 kg)

Height 63 in. (160.0 cm)

Acute genitourinary pain only

► **Skin**

Pale, dry skin noted

► **HEENT**

PERRLA; glossitis: tongue smooth and red

► **Neck and Lymph Nodes**

Thyroid normal size; no lymphadenopathy noted

► **Chest**

Clear to auscultation

► **Breasts**

Normal breast examination

► **Cardiovascular**

RRR; normal S_1, S_2; (−) S_3 or S_4

► **Abdomen**

Not tender; no distention; no rebound

► **Neurology**

Grossly intact; normal deep tendon reflexes and sensory examination; some muscle weakness noted

► **Extremities**

Cold extremities; fingernails short and brittle

► **Genitourinary**

Normal female genitalia; no vaginal discharge noted

► **Rectal**

Examination deferred

Laboratory and Diagnostic Tests

	Conventional Units	SI Units
Na	138 mEq/L	138 mmol/L
K	3.6 mEq/L	3.6 mmol/L
Cl	110 mEq/L	110 mmol/L
CO_2	22 mEq/L	22 mmol/L
BUN	9.8 mg/dL	3.5 mmol/L
SCr	0.6 mg/dL	53 μmol/L
Glu (non-fasting)	160 mg/dL	8.9 mmol/L
Ca	9.0 mg/dL	2.25 mmol/L
Phosphate	3.4 mg/dL	1.10 mmol/L
Albumin	3.5 g/dL	35 g/L
WBC	$12 \times 10^3/mm^3$	$12 \times 10^9/L$
Hgb	10.8 g/dL (108 g/L)	108 g/L; 6.70 mmol/L
Hct	31.4%	0.314
RBC	$3.04 \times 10^6/\mu L$	$3.04 \times 10^{12}/L$
MCV	102.2 μm³	102.2 fL
MCH	31.8 pg/cell	
MCHC	34.4 g/dL	344 g/L
RDW	14.5%	0.145
Plasma folate	10.6 ng/mL	24 nmol/L
Vitamin B_{12}	158 pg/mL	117 pmol/L

Urinalysis

Color	Normal	
Appearance	Cloudy	
pH	6.4	
Specific gravity	1.025	
Protein	100 mg/dL	1 g/L
RBC	250 erythrocytes/μL	
Leukocyte esterase	25 leukocytes/μL	
Nitrite	(+)	

Urine Gram Stain and Culture

$>10^5$ CFU/mL ($>10^8$ CFU/L) Gram-negative rods; identification and susceptibilities pending

Assessment

Pleasant, febrile 28-year-old vegan female with history of urinary tract infections, who presents with symptoms of urinary tract infection as well as complaints of recent fatigue, muscle weakness, and tongue tenderness, likely related to anemia

Student Workup

Missing Information?

Evaluate: Patient Database

Drug Therapy Problems

Care Plan (by Problem)

TARGETED QUESTIONS

1. With what signs and symptoms of anemia does the patient present?

   Hint: See p. 1116 and Table 66-1 in PPP

2. What is the likely etiology of the patient's anemia?

   Hint: See p. 1110, Table 66-2, and Figure 66-3 in PPP

3. How should the patient's anemia be treated?

   Hint: See pp. 1111–1112 in PPP

4. What parameters should be monitored after treatment is initiated?

   Hint: See pp. 1112 and 1118 (Patient Care and Monitoring) in PPP

FOLLOW-UP

The patient returns to the clinic 6 months later, happily reporting that she is now 18 weeks pregnant. She continues on a regimen of cyanocobalamin 1,000 mcg intramuscularly once monthly. Her Hgb and Hct levels are within the normal range and she has no symptoms of anemia; however, her serum cyanocobalamin concentration is again low.

5. What may account for the low serum cyanocobalamin concentration?

   Hint: The patient's pregnancy may be increasing her vitamin B$_{12}$ requirements, leading to early signs of deficiency. In addition, high doses of folic acid can correct the macrocytic anemia associated with vitamin B$_{12}$ deficiency, so she should be questioned regarding the use of folate supplements. However, in light of her adherence to parenteral cyanocobalamin maintenance therapy and lack of clinical symptoms and laboratory measures consistent with anemia, it is unlikely that the patient is again deficient in vitamin B$_{12}$. Instead, low serum vitamin B$_{12}$ concentrations unrelated to anemia have been described during pregnancy. In vitamin B$_{12}$–deficient states, serum methylmalonic acid and homocysteine concentrations will be increased. Results of these determinations may therefore allow differentiation between pregnancy-related decreases in serum cyanocobalamin concentrations and true deficiency. See p. 1111 in PPP

🌐 GLOBAL PERSPECTIVE

Macrocytic anemia caused by micronutrient deficiencies occurs worldwide in those suffering from malnutrition. Vitamin B$_{12}$ is available from a variety of animal sources, including meat, fish, poultry, eggs, and dairy products; however, populations without ready access to these foods and who instead rely on plant sources for the majority of their calorie intake may develop deficiencies. Malabsorption of vitamin B$_{12}$ is more often the cause of deficiency in advanced nations, in which dietary ingestion is generally sufficient. According to the 1999 to 2000

National Health and Nutrition Examination Survey (NHANES), the median intake of vitamin B$_{12}$ for the United States population is 3.4 mcg/d, which is well above the 2.4-mcg recommended daily allowance for adults. Yet vitamin B$_{12}$ deficiency affects between 1.5% and 15% of the United States population. Malabsorption of vitamin B$_{12}$ is especially common in older people due to atrophic gastritis and subsequent reduced levels of gastric acid secretion, but it is also noted following gastric surgical procedures, in those with GI disorders such as Crohn's and celiac disease, and in patients with pernicious anemia. In addition, prolonged acid suppression therapy has been recognized as a cause of decreased vitamin B$_{12}$ absorption, although the clinical significance of this finding is debated.

In addition to macrocytic anemia, permanent neurologic damage may result if vitamin B$_{12}$ deficiency is not corrected. Although cognitive decline has been reported in vitamin B$_{12}$–deficient patients, supplementation in nondeficient patients with dementia or Alzheimer's disease has not improved cognitive function. A link between low vitamin B$_{12}$ concentrations and cardiovascular disease has also been suggested due to the effects of the nutrient on homocysteine metabolism. Elevated homocysteine concentrations are associated with an increased risk of stroke and coronary heart disease and are noted in vitamin B$_{12}$–deficient states. Despite reductions in homocysteine levels following administration of vitamin and mineral supplements that included vitamin B$_{12}$, differences in cardiovascular outcomes following long-term use of vitamin B$_{12}$ have not been documented. To date, data from large clinical trials do not support the use of vitamin B$_{12}$ supplements to protect against cardiovascular events.

CASE SUMMARY

- The patient's clinical picture is consistent with vitamin B$_{12}$ deficiency anemia resulting from inadequate dietary intake.
- Therapy with vitamin B$_{12}$ should be initiated, with parenteral therapy more reliably correcting the deficiency than oral therapy.
- Clinical symptoms should improve within days of vitamin B$_{12}$ supplementation. A CBC and serum cyanocobalamin concentrations should be obtained in 1 month to evaluate the efficacy of therapy.

For more information on the care plan and facilitator's guide please visit http://www.mhpharmacotherapy.com.

71 Folic Acid Deficiency Anemia

Janice L. Stumpf

CASE LEARNING OBJECTIVES

- Identify the common causes of anemia
- Describe the common signs and symptoms of anemia
- Discuss the appropriate diagnostic evaluation to determine the type of anemia and guide therapeutic decisions
- State the desired therapeutic outcomes for patients with anemia
- Explain the optimal use of folic acid in patients with macrocytic anemia
- Recommend a specific treatment regimen for anemia considering the underlying cause of anemia and patient-specific variables
- Develop a plan to monitor the outcomes of anemia pharmacotherapy

PATIENT PRESENTATION

Chief Complaint

"Why am I here? I need to go home now. You can't keep me here."

History of Present Illness

Charles Logan is a 68-year-old thin, white male brought to the emergency department by paramedics after being found unconscious on the grounds of a local church. He is now awake, but somewhat confused. He appears to be mildly hypothermic and dehydrated. He is known to the emergency department medical staff as a homeless veteran with a history of schizophrenia and alcoholism.

Past Medical History

Alcoholism × 45 years
Schizophrenia
Nonadherent with drug therapy

Family History

Unknown

Social History

Vietnam veteran. Homeless (long-term). Well known to local social agencies. Sister lives in town; no other family members.

Tobacco/Alcohol/Substance Use

Currently smokes 1 to 2 ppd × 50 years. Alcohol—up to two-fifths Southern Comfort per day. No illicit drug use reported.

Allergies/Intolerances/Adverse Drug Events

Reports allergies to all antipsychotic medications—"make him lose control of his mind"

Medications (Current)

Risperidone 6 mg PO once daily (not adherent)
Tums PRN stomach pain

Review of Systems

Hears voices, usually of his mother. Complains of cold extremities and tingling in his hands and feet. Occasional stomach pains that he relieves with Tums.

Physical Examination

▶ **General**

Thin, pale white male exhibiting some confusion about whereabouts. A&O × 2, to person and time only

▶ **Vital Signs**

BP 126/76 mm Hg, P 86, RR 18, T 34.4°C (36.6°C after 1 hour)

Weight 135.6 lb (61.6 kg)

Height 70 in. (177.8 cm)

"Fingertips hurt"

▶ **Skin**

Pale, especially extremities. Dry and thickened, showing signs of exposure to winter temperatures. No obvious signs of frostbite

▶ **HEENT**

PERRLA

▶ **Neck and Lymph Nodes**

Normal

▶ **Chest**

Decreased breath sounds. Slight wheezing

▶ **Cardiovascular**

RRR; normal S_1, S_2; (−) S_3 or S_4

▶ **Abdomen**

Not tender; no distention; no rebound

▶ **Neurology**

Deep tendon reflexes intact. Decreased sharp touch sensation in feet and hands

▶ **Extremities**

Cold to touch; palpable pulses

▶ **Genitourinary/Rectal**

Prostate somewhat enlarged

Laboratory and Diagnostic Tests

	Conventional Units	SI Units
Na	145 mEq/L	145 mmol/L
K	3.9 mEq/L	3.9 mmol/L
Cl	102 mEq/L	102 mmol/L
CO_2	31 mEq/L	31 mmol/L
BUN	24 mg/dL	8.6 mmol/L
SCr	1.5 mg/dL	133 μmol/L
Glu	80 mg/dL	4.4 mmol/L
Ca	8.8 mg/dL	2.20 mmol/L
Phosphate	2.4 mg/dL	0.78 mmol/L
Albumin	2.8 g/dL	28 g/L
AST	40 IU/L	0.67 μkat/L
ALT	60 IU/L	1 μkat/L
Alk phos	70 IU/L	1.17 μkat/L
Bilirubin	1.2 mg/dL	20.5 μmol/L
WBC	$9 \times 10^3/mm^3$	$9 \times 10^9/L$
Hgb	10.5 g/dL	105 g/L; 6.51 mmol/L
Hct	30.2%	0.302
Plt	$154 \times 10^3/\mu L$	$154 \times 10^9/L$
RBC	$2.97 \times 10^6/\mu L$	$2.97 \times 10^{12}/L$
MCV	101.7 μm³	101.7 fL
MCH	28.2 pg/cell	
MCHC	34.7 g/dL	347 g/L
RDW	24%	0.240
Plasma folate	2.8 ng/mL	6.3 nmol/L
Vitamin B_{12}	280 pg/mL	207 pmol/L
Blood alcohol	120 mg/dL	26 mmol/L
Hemoccult	(−)	

Student Workup

Missing Information?

Evaluate: Patient Database

Drug Therapy Problems

Care Plan (by Problem)

Assessment

Confused 68-year-old male with history of schizophrenia and alcoholism, who now presents s/p loss of consciousness with mild hypothermia, dehydration, and anemia

TARGETED QUESTIONS

1. What signs and symptoms of anemia does the patient have?

   Hint: See p. 1112 and Table 66-1 in PPP

2. What is the likely cause of the patient's anemia?

   Hint: See p. 1112 and Figure 66-3 in PPP

3. How should the patient's anemia be managed?

   Hint: See p. 1116 and Table 66-2 in PPP

4. How soon after initiating the therapy should the anemia resolve?

   Hint: See p. 1116 in PPP

FOLLOW-UP

The patient is admitted to the hospital and a thorough workup performed to evaluate the cause of his loss of consciousness. A CT scan reveals a recent head injury, and abnormal results are documented on an EEG. The neurologist recommends initiation of phenytoin therapy to prevent seizures.

5. What impact may folic acid supplementation have on the patient's anticonvulsant therapy?

> *Hint: There is a drug interaction between folic acid and phenytoin. Although the mechanism is not well understood, folic acid may decrease serum phenytoin concentrations by 15% to 50% and may also reduce its therapeutic efficacy. Higher phenytoin doses may therefore be required to achieve therapeutic concentrations. Phenytoin concentrations should be monitored closely during folic acid therapy and after folate supplementation is discontinued and the phenytoin dose adjusted as appropriate. In addition, folic acid concentrations may be decreased following long-term phenytoin administration, perhaps due to effects on absorption. Use of an alternative anticonvulsant for the patient while folic acid supplementation is required should be considered.*

☼ GLOBAL PERSPECTIVE

Because folic acid deficiency develops in all populations in which malnutrition is apparent, macrocytic anemia is a global health concern. Anemia affects an estimated 1.62 billion individuals, nearly 25% of the world's population. The primary cause of anemia worldwide is iron deficiency, although mixed anemias resulting from concurrent deficiencies in folic acid and vitamin B_{12} may also be noted.

Because of the association between low folic acid levels during pregnancy and neural tube birth defects, in 1998, the FDA mandated addition of folic acid to many grain products, including bread, pasta, and cereals. Foods in several other countries, including Australia, Canada, and Chile, are also fortified with folic acid. The folate food fortification program as well as increased awareness regarding the need for prenatal folic acid supplementation has reduced the incidence of neural tube defects by 30% to 50%. Low folate diets have also been associated with an increased risk of breast, pancreatic, and colon cancer. However, folic acid supplementation is not known to prevent particular cancers. In fact, some recent data show that high serum folate concentrations may actually increase the risk of cancer. In addition, low dietary ingestion of folic acid has been associated with an increase in the risk of coronary events, perhaps due to increases in homocysteine concentrations. Homocysteine is an amino acid that, when increased, has been associated with CHD and strokes. Supplementation with folic acid appears to reduce homocysteine levels to normal. Studies are under way to determine if folic acid supplementation reduces the risk of CV events.

CASE SUMMARY

- The patient's clinical picture is consistent with macrocytic anemia due to folic acid deficiency.
- Therapy with folic acid 1 mg PO daily should be initiated.
- Clinical symptoms should improve within days of initiating folic acid supplementation. CBC and plasma folate concentrations should be obtained in 2 months to assess response to therapy.

For more information on the care plan and facilitator's guide please visit http://www.mhpharmacotherapy.com.

72 Bacterial Meningitis

April D. Miller   P. Brandon Bookstaver

CASE LEARNING OBJECTIVES

- Describe the signs, symptoms, and clinical presentation of CNS infections
- List the most common pathogens causing CNS infections, and identify risk factors for infection with each pathogen
- State the goals of therapy for CNS infections
- Design appropriate empiric antimicrobial regimens for patients suspected of having CNS infections caused by any of the following pathogens or in the following settings and analyze the impact of antimicrobial resistance on both empiric and definitive therapy: *Neisseria meningitidis*, *Hemophilus influenzae*, *Listeria* spp., group B *Streptococcus* spp., Gram-negative bacillary, postneurosurgical infection, CNS shunt infection, and herpes simplex encephalitis
- Identify the candidates for vaccines and other prophylactic therapies to prevent CNS infections

PATIENT PRESENTATION

Chief Complaint

The patient is currently unresponsive. Her history is from medical records and nursing staff at long-term care facility, who report somnolence and "talking out of her head."

History of Present Illness

Ruth Johnson is a 67-year-old female resident of a local assisted-living facility, who presents to the ED with a 3-day history of worsening confusion and somnolence. Prior to her delirium, she also complained of headache and stiff neck. None of her friends/contacts at the nursing home have reported any signs or symptoms of illness, but her 10-year-old grandson who visited last week was recently diagnosed with pneumonia. She has a history of seizure disorder and one of her friends reported that she may have had some seizure-like activity yesterday.

Past Medical History

Type 2 DM diagnosed 1 year ago

Stroke at age 60, no residual neurologic deficits

Seizure disorder following stroke

Depression diagnosed at age 62 following the death of her husband

Family History

Father had CAD, deceased from MI at age 72. Mother had diabetes and osteoporosis and died of "old age." She had one brother who was killed in an accident at age 16.

Social History

The patient moved to assisted-living facility with her husband following stroke at age 60. Staff reports that she is independent in her ADLs, including taking her medications, and is quite active. She has two children, aged 45 and 40, and five grandchildren. She is a retired homemaker.

Tobacco/Alcohol/Substance Abuse

Unable to assess due to the patient's mental status; no known tobacco or illicit drug use.

Allergies/Intolerances/Adverse Drug Events

Morphine (itching)

Medications

▶ *Inpatient*

Naloxone 2 mg IV × 1 administered on arrival (no response)

Flumazenil 0.2 mg IV × 1 administered on arrival (no response)

0.9% sodium chloride IV at 125 mL/h

▸ *Home*

Aspirin 81 mg PO daily

Phenytoin ER 300 mg PO at bedtime

Sertraline 50 mg PO daily in the morning

Diphenhydramine 25 mg PO at bedtime

Review of Systems

Unable to attain secondary to the patient's condition

Physical Examination

▸ *General*

Unresponsive, ill-appearing elderly female in acute distress

▸ *Vital Signs*

BP 88/62 mm Hg, P 122, RR 20, T 38.8°C

Weight 140 lb (63.6 kg)

Height 65 in. (165.1 cm)

Unable to report pain

▸ *Skin*

Reduced skin turgor

▸ *HEENT*

PERRLA; TMs grossly normal

▸ *Neck and Lymph Nodes*

(+) Nuchal rigidity; (−) Kernig's sign; (−) Brudzinski's sign

▸ *Chest*

Clear to auscultation bilaterally

▸ *Breasts*

Examination deferred

▸ *Cardiovascular*

Sinus tachycardia

▸ *Abdomen*

Nontender; nondistended; no organomegaly

▸ *Neurology*

Normal DTRs; (+) corneal, gag, and cough reflexes

▸ *Genitourinary*

Examination deferred

▸ *Rectal*

Examination deferred

Laboratory Tests

Obtained in ED

	Conventional Units	SI Units
Na	140 mEq/L	140 mmol/L
K	3.9 mEq/L	3.9 mmol/L
Cl	100 mEq/L	100 mmol/L
CO_2	21 mEq/L	21 mmol/L
BUN	20 mg/dL	7.1 mmol/L
SCr	1.2 mg/dL	106 µmol/L
Glu	220 mg/dL	12.2 mmol/L
Ca	9.6 mg/dL	2.40 mmol/L
Mg	2 mEq/L	1 mmol/L
Phosphate	3.5 mg/dL	1.13 mmol/L
Hgb	12.5 g/dL	125 g/L; 7.75 mmol/L
Hct	37.5%	0.375
WBC	$15.7 \times 10^3/mm^3$	$15.7 \times 10^9/L$
Plt	$220 \times 10^3/mm^3$	$220 \times 10^9/L$
Albumin	3.8 g/dL	38 g/L
Phenytoin	6 mg/L	24 µmol/L
CSF Studies		
WBC	$6.3 \times 10^3/mm^3$	$6.3 \times 10^9/L$
WBC differential		
Monos	12%	0.12
PMNs	80%	0.80
Lymphs	8%	0.08
Protein	120 mg/dL	1,200 mg/L
Glu	66 mg/dL	3.7 mmol/L

▸ *Cultures*

Blood cultures × 2: Pending

CSF Gram stain: Gram-positive diplococci

Assessment

Sixty-seven-year-old female with signs, symptoms, and laboratory tests consistent with bacterial meningitis

Student Workup

Missing Information?

Evaluate: Patient Database

Drug Therapy Problems

Care Plan (by Problem)

TARGETED QUESTIONS

1. Which symptoms in this patient's history suggests the diagnosis of bacterial meningitis?

   Hint: See p. 1173 in PPP

2. What do this patient's CSF findings indicate?

   Hint: See Table 70-2 in PPP

3. What in this patient's history may indicate the causative organism of bacterial meningitis?

   Hint: See Table 70-1 in PPP

4. Why should empiric antibiotic therapy in bacterial meningitis include broad-spectrum coverage with more than one agent?

   Hint: See p. 1174 in PPP

5. What route(s) of antibiotic administration is(are) appropriate in bacterial meningitis?

   Hint: See Tables 70-3 and 70-4 in PPP

6. What vaccination(s) should be administered to help prevent invasive *Streptococcus pneumoniae* meningitis?

   Hint: See p. 1181 in PPP

FOLLOW-UP

Twenty-four hours later, CSF cultures return and are positive for *S. pneumoniae*. The patient continues to receive empiric antibiotics (as recommended in your Care Plan).

7. Should your antibiotic regimen be altered? If so, how? Also, what (if any) prophylaxis would you recommend for this patient's contacts?

   Hint: See p. 1181 and Table 70-3 in PPP

⚙ GLOBAL PERSPECTIVE

Worldwide, approximately 1.2 million cases of bacterial meningitis occur annually and result in 135,000 deaths. Vaccination has changed the microbiology and predominant causative organisms in the United States. Both *Haemophilus influenzae* and pneumococcal vaccination have decreased the incidence of infections secondary to these organisms in the United States. Due to limited vaccine availability and cost in developing countries, the incidence of disease secondary to these organisms has not decreased significantly. Likewise, polio and mumps vaccination in the United States has virtually eliminated these organisms as a cause of viral encephalitis. However, these remain important causative agents to consider in developing countries.

CASE SUMMARY

- The patient's clinical picture is consistent with a severe case of bacterial meningitis. Prompt initiation of broad-spectrum antimicrobial therapy is essential to ensure optimal patient outcomes.

- Initial broad-spectrum therapy should include agents such as a third-generation cephalosporin (ceftriaxone 2 g IV q 12 h), vancomycin dosed to target trough concentrations of 15 to 20 mg/L (10–14 µmol/L), and ampicillin 2 g IV q 4 h.

- Using culture and sensitivity data, the regimen can be narrowed to target-specific pathogens.

For more information on the care plan and facilitator's guide please visit http://www.mhpharmacotherapy.com.

73 Pneumonia

Diane M. Cappelletty

CASE LEARNING OBJECTIVES

- Recognize the signs and symptoms of mild and moderate-to-severe pneumonia
- Identify the goals of therapy for pneumonia
- Develop an appropriate empiric treatment and monitoring plan for pneumonia on the basis of individual patient characteristics
- Properly educate patients taking their antibiotic therapy
- Discuss the role of vaccination in pneumonia

PATIENT PRESENTATION

Chief Complaint

"For the last 2 days I have been more and more short of breath, especially on exertion. I have also been coughing and the color of the secretions is now green."

History of Present Illness

Cindy Milner is a 41-year-old woman who presents to the emergency department complaining of increasing SOB and increasing coughing. She has had a fever for the last 24 hours. She has some mild-to-moderate chest discomfort, but denies any sharp pains or heaviness in her chest. She does not have nausea, vomiting, or diarrhea.

Past Medical History

Asthma × 15 years

DM × 32 years

HTN × 10 years

Family History

Father died in a car accident at age 50. Mother had diabetes, HTN, and CRF, and died at age 56. She has one sister who has diabetes and HTN.

Social History

She lives with her husband and has no children. She works as a legal secretary.

Tobacco/Alcohol/Substance Use

Social drinker; (−) tobacco or illicit drug use

Allergies/Intolerances/Adverse Drug Events

Penicillin (sulfa)

Medications (Current)

Olmesartan (Benicar) 40 mg PO once daily

Insulin pump

Fluticasone/Salmeterol DPI (Advair) 100 mcg/50 mcg one inhalation twice daily

Acetaminophen 650 mg PO PRN headache

Review of Systems

Occasional headaches relieved with acetaminophen; occasional tinnitus; (−) vertigo; (−) history of seizures, syncope, or loss of consciousness; mild pain/discomfort in her chest/abdomen; SOB; (−) nausea, vomiting, or diarrhea.

Physical Examination

▶ *General*

Well-appearing, middle-aged woman breathing fast, appears in mild-to-moderate respiratory distress

▶ *Vital Signs*

BP 105/70 mm Hg, P 84, RR 22, T 38.8°C, pulse oximetry 89% (0.89) on room air

Weight 115 lb (52.3 kg)

Height 65 in. (165 cm)

▶ *Skin*

Normal; (−) rashes or lesions

▶ *HEENT*

PERRLA, EOMI; trace periorbital edema; (–) sinus tenderness; TMs appear normal

▶ *Neck and Lymph Nodes*

Negative for lymphadenopathy

▶ *Chest*

Wheezing bilaterally, worse on the left side; decreased breath sounds over the lower left lobe.

▶ *Cardiovascular*

RRR; normal S_1, S_2; (–) S_3 or S_4

▶ *Abdomen*

Not tender/not distended

▶ *Neurology*

Grossly intact; deep tendon reflexes normal

▶ *Radiologic Studies*

Chest x-ray: left lower lobe infiltrate

Laboratory Tests

	Conventional Units	SI Units
Na	142 mEq/L	142 mmol/L
K	4.1 mEq/L	4.1 mmol/L
Cl	100 mEq/L	100 mmol/L
CO_2	24 mEq/L	24 mmol/L
BUN	15 mg/dL	5.4 mmol/L
SCr	1.4 mg/dL	124 μmol/L
Glu	114 mg/dL	6.3 mmol/L
Ca	8.4 mg/dL	2.10 mmol/L
Mg	1.8 mEq/L	0.90 mmol/L
Phosphate	4.95 mg/dL	1.60 mmol/L
WBC	$13.4 \times 10^3/mm^3$	$13.4 \times 10^9/L$
WBC Differential		
Neutrophils	72%	0.72
Lymphocytes	20%	0.20
Monocytes	6%	0.06
Bands	2%	0.02
RBC	$3.6 \times 10^6/mm^3$	$3.6 \times 10^{12}/L$
Hgb	11.5 g/dL	115 g/L; 7.14 mmol/L
Hct	33.9%	0.339
MCV	87 μm³	87 fL
MCH	28 pg	
Platelets	$380 \times 10^3/mm^3$	$380 \times 10^9/L$

▶ *Sputum Culture*

Pending; Gram stain: moderate WBCs, rare squamous epithelial cells, no organisms seen

▶ *Blood Culture*

Pending

Assessment

Forty-one-year-old woman with signs, symptoms, and laboratory tests consistent with community-acquired pneumonia

Student Workup

Missing Information?

Evaluate: Patient Database

Drug Therapy Problems

Care Plan (by Problem)

TARGETED QUESTIONS

1. What signs, symptoms, and diagnostic tests support the diagnosis of pneumonia in the patient?

   Hint: See Chapter 71, pp. 1192 and 1193, in PPP

2. What are the top three organisms most likely causing pneumonia and what resistance issues are associated with these organisms?

   Hint: See pp. 1190, 1193, and 1194 in PPP

3. What patient factors need to be considered prior to selecting an empiric treatment regimen?

   Hint: See pp. 1193–1195 in PPP

4. What therapeutic regimen would you select (including the duration of therapy)?

   Hint: See pp. 1195–1197 and 1200 in PPP

5. How would you monitor the patient?

   Hint: See p. 1200 in PPP

6. What risks and adverse effects of therapy would you discuss with the patient?

   Hint: Focus on medication counseling. See p. 1200 in PPP

7. Should the patient be vaccinated, and if so, what vaccinations should she receive?

   Hint: See p. 1201 in PPP

FOLLOW-UP

8. What would happen to the therapeutic regimen or monitoring for each of the following situations:

   (a) What if the patient was pregnant?

   Hint: See pp. 1196 and 1201 in PPP

(b) What if the patient had a severe β-lactam allergy?

Hint: See p. 1196 for alternative therapy in PPP

(c) What if the patient had a condition that required warfarin therapy?

Hint: See p. 1196 for alternative therapy in PPP

◌ GLOBAL PERSPECTIVE

Viral pneumonia (specifically influenza) is of much greater concern for global spread causing pandemics than is bacterial pneumonia. Not all patients infected with influenza develop pneumonia, but those that do have a greater mortality risk than those without pneumonia. Vaccination against influenza can prevent the disease or minimize symptomology if the disease is contracted. The polysaccharide vaccine against *Streptococcus pneumoniae* covers 85% to 90% of the isolates responsible for causing disease in human beings.

CASE SUMMARY

- Her clinical picture is consistent with mild-to-moderate community-acquired pneumonia, and antimicrobial and oxygen therapy should be initiated.

- She is allergic to penicillin (rash) and sulfa drugs (rash). A third-generation cephalosporin could still be used in this patient since the risk of cross-reaction is low.

- Diabetes puts her at increased risk of infection; she should receive the pneumococcal vaccine once and the influenza vaccine yearly.

For more information on the care plan and facilitator's guide please visit http://www.mhpharmacotherapy.com.

74 Influenza

Heather L. VandenBussche

CASE LEARNING OBJECTIVES

- Identify the clinical signs and symptoms associated with influenza
- Develop an appropriate treatment plan for influenza using patient-specific information
- Create a monitoring plan for a patient with influenza using patient-specific information
- Educate patients about influenza and vaccination

PATIENT PRESENTATION

Chief Complaint

"My son has a fever, headache, and a cough. I'm worried he might need antibiotics."

History of Present Illness

Matthew Jackson is a 9-year-old boy who presents with his father to the pediatrician with complaints of fever, headache, and cough for 3 days. He began feeling ill 3 days ago when he developed a fever of 102.6°F (39.2°C) and chills. He has had an intermittent headache for 2 days that is worse when he coughs. His cough is nonproductive and dry. He is more tired than usual and he has not been eating or drinking as much as usual. His fever has been constant over the past 3 days, spiking to 103.5°F (39.7°C) yesterday, but it is responsive to "cold medicine." He also complains of achy muscles in his legs and wants to remain in bed most of the time. His father wants to know if his son needs antibiotic treatment and why Echinacea is not working.

Past Medical History

Exercise-induced asthma diagnosed 2 years ago
Sinusitis at age 4 and 6 years
Febrile seizure at age 2 years

Family History

Father's family has strong history of diabetes, heart disease, and lung cancer. Father has HTN and seasonal allergic rhinitis. Mother is deceased, but was healthy.

Social History

The patient lives with father and a 3-year-old sister. Father smokes cigarettes in the house and car. Sister is healthy. The patient is in third grade at private elementary school. No pets at home.

Allergies/Intolerances/Adverse Drug Events

Amoxicillin—(rash)

Medications (Current)

Children's Motrin Cold (ibuprofen 100 mg/5 mL; pseudoephedrine 15 mg/5 mL) 10 mL q 6 h as needed
Echinacea purpurea 180 mg daily
Albuterol MDI one puff as needed

Review of Systems

(+) Fatigue, fever, headache, chills; (−) rhinorrhea, nasal congestion, sneezing, neck stiffness, or ear pain; (+) intermittent dry cough; (−) difficulty breathing or wheezing; (+) reduced appetite; (−) abdominal pain, vomiting, constipation, or diarrhea; (+) reduction in urinary frequency

Physical Examination

▶ *General*

Generally well-appearing, mixed-race boy in no acute distress

▶ *Vital Signs*

BP 84/58 mm Hg, P 116, RR 18, T 101.1°F (38.4°C)
Weight 87.8 lb (39.9 kg)
Height 56.7 in. (144 cm)
Pain: 4/10 on numeric scale

▶ *Skin*

No rashes or bruises; 1-cm-long abrasion on left forearm

▶ *HEENT*

(−) Sinus or facial tenderness; PERRLA, EOMI; (−) conjunctivitis; left TM slightly erythematous, but with landmarks present and no effusion noted; right TM obscured with cerumen; nares patent with moist nasal mucosa; oral mucus membranes moist

▶ *Neck and Lymph Nodes*

(−) Neck stiffness or pain; neck supple; bilateral shotty anterior cervical lymphadenopathy

▶ *Chest*

Good air entry bilaterally; (−) crackles or wheezes heard

▶ *Cardiovascular*

Slightly tachycardic, but regular rhythm, normal S_1, S_2; (−) S_3 or S_4

▶ *Abdomen*

Positive bowel sounds; not tender or distended; (−) organomegaly or masses

▶ *Neurology*

Grossly intact; deep tendon reflexes normal; no focal deficits noted

▶ *Extremities*

No swelling or edema noted

▶ *Genitourinary*

Examination deferred

▶ *Rectal*

Examination deferred

Laboratory Tests

Nasopharyngeal swab positive for influenza A virus

Assessment

Nine-year-old boy with signs and symptoms consistent with influenza

Student Workup

Missing Information?

Evaluate: Patient Database

Drug Therapy Problems

Care Plan (by Problem)

TARGETED QUESTIONS

1. What signs and symptoms of influenza does this patient have?

   Hint: Symptoms of influenza are similar to those of the common cold (fatigue, headache, cough, fever), but it is typical to have higher fevers and muscle aches with influenza. See p. 1217 in PPP

2. What treatments could be considered for this patient?

   Hint: Symptomatic therapy is recommended. Antiviral therapy is not likely to affect the course of influenza after more than 48 hours of the onset of illness. See p. 1217 and Table 72-6 in PPP

3. What counseling points would you discuss with this patient's father?

   Hint: Many of the same principles that pertain to the common cold also apply to influenza. See pp. 1217–1219 in PPP

4. Is this patient a candidate for influenza vaccine?

   Hint: See p. 1410 and Table 86-1 in PPP

FOLLOW-UP

5. What if this patient was 6 years old instead of 9 years old?

   Hint: See p. 1217 in PPP

6. What if this patient had evidence of pneumonia at the time of presentation?

   Hint: See p. 1197 in PPP

7. What if this patient had a severe egg allergy?

   Hint: See p. 1410 and Table 86-1 in PPP

⟳ GLOBAL PERSPECTIVE

The global impact of influenza on morbidity and mortality is notable with more than 1 million deaths occurring annually. Influenza infection rates peak in cold winter months in temperate climates, but there is a high background rate of infection in tropical climates where epidemics also occur at certain times of the year. Poor outcome is associated with secondary bacterial infections or infection with certain strains of influenza (e.g., the recent H5N1 or avian influenza). Similar to the United States, morbidity and mortality is higher in the age extremes and those with certain chronic illnesses. Vaccination can limit the spread of infection, but is not as effective in preventing illness in the elderly. Limited resources in developing countries limit the impact of vaccination on the spread of influenza. Educational efforts should focus on hand hygiene, isolation of those who are ill, and other infection control measures where possible.

CASE SUMMARY

- His current clinical picture is consistent with influenza infection.
- Supportive treatment is recommended for fever or pain; single-ingredient acetaminophen or ibuprofen are appropriate choices. Other medications are not indicated at this time.

- He is a candidate for influenza vaccination once the acute stage of his illness is over, if he has not had one this year, and it is still influenza season. He should receive injectable influenza vaccine before each influenza season because of his underlying asthma; influenza vaccine is also indicated annually because of his age.

For more information on the care plan and facilitator's guide please visit http://www.mhpharmacotherapy.com.

75 Upper Respiratory Infection with Pharyngitis and Otitis Media

Heather L. VandenBussche

CASE LEARNING OBJECTIVES

- Identify the clinical signs and symptoms associated with streptococcal pharyngitis and acute otitis media (AOM)
- List the treatment goals for streptococcal pharyngitis and AOM
- Develop an appropriate treatment plan using patient-specific data
- Create a monitoring plan for a patient with streptococcal pharyngitis and AOM using patient-specific data
- Educate patients about upper respiratory tract infections and proper use of antibiotic therapy

PATIENT PRESENTATION

Chief Complaint

"My daughter has a head cold and fever. She needs antibiotics so she can go back to school tomorrow."

History of Present Illness

Jasmine Henderson is a 5-year-old girl who presents with her mother to the pediatrician with complaints of fatigue, nasal congestion, reduced appetite, fever, and ear and throat pain on swallowing. The patient began feeling tired 4 days ago and developed mild nasal congestion 1 day later. Her mother reports that the patient's appetite has diminished over the past couple of days. She complained of ear and throat pain on swallowing water this morning and she was sent home from school this morning with a fever of 102.4°F (39.1°C). Her mother has been giving her a nonprescription cold medication for the past 2 days, but it has not helped alleviate her symptoms. She is requesting antibiotics so that the patient can return to school tomorrow, and she wants to know what other nonprescription medicines she can give to her to relieve her symptoms.

Past Medical History

Perennial allergic rhinitis (cat dander, dust mites) diagnosed last year

Mild intermittent asthma diagnosed 2 years ago

Atopic dermatitis diagnosed 6 months ago

Iron-deficiency anemia diagnosed 6 months ago

Prior episodes of otitis media (age 14 months and 3 years)

Upper respiratory tract infections three to five times each year

Family History

Father has atopic dermatitis, hypercholesterolemia, and seasonal allergies. Mother has perennial allergic rhinitis and exercise-induced asthma. She has a 7-year-old sister and a 2-year-old brother, who are healthy.

Social History

Lives with mother, father, sister, and brother. Both parents work outside of the home. Has two pets (cat, goldfish). Attends kindergarten at public elementary school. No recent travel.

Allergies/Intolerances/Adverse Drug Events

Erythromycin—abdominal pain and diarrhea

Medications (Current)

Loratadine 5 mg PO q 24 h PRN allergy symptoms

Albuterol 2.5 mg solution for nebulization twice daily and q 6 h PRN wheezing

Hydrocortisone 1% ointment once daily to affected area(s)

Children's Tylenol Plus Cold (acetaminophen 160 mg/5 mL; chlorpheniramine 1 mg/5 mL; phenylephrine 2.5 mg/5 mL) 5 mL PO q 6 h PRN

Ferrous sulfate 150 mg/1.2 mL PO q 12 h

Review of Systems

(+) Fatigue, fever, headache, nasal congestion, throat and left ear pain; (+) hearing difficulty on left side; (−) conjunctivitis, rhinorrhea, sneezing, neck stiffness, or dizziness; (+) intermittent dry cough; (−) wheezing; (+) abdominal pain and reduced appetite; (−) nausea, vomiting, constipation, or diarrhea; (−) change in urinary frequency; (+) scaly itchy skin on left ankle.

Physical Examination

▸ General

Ill-appearing and slightly irritable young Caucasian female in no acute distress

▸ Vital Signs

BP 90/60 mm Hg, P 120, RR 24, T 101.8°F (38.8°C)

Weight 41.5 lb (18.9 kg)

Height 44.5 in. (113 cm)

Pain score: 6/10 on Faces scale

▸ Skin

Slightly pale skin; scaly patch (2 × 2 cm) on left medial ankle; no skin breakdown or discharge

▸ HEENT

(−) Sinus or facial tenderness; PERRLA, EOMI; (−) conjunctivitis; (+) erythematous left TM with bulging and limited mobility; (+) fluid behind right TM, but no erythema and normal mobility; (−) otorrhea; (+) inflamed nasal mucosa with no discharge; bilateral tonsillar hypertrophy with erythema and white exudates; foul-smelling breath; mucus membranes moist

▸ Neck and Lymph Nodes

(+) Bilateral tender cervical lymphadenopathy; (−) neck stiffness or pain

▸ Chest

Mild bilateral expiratory wheezes heard intermittently

▸ Cardiovascular

RRR, normal S_1, S_2; (−) S_3 or S_4

▸ Abdomen

Not tender or distended; (−) organomegaly

▸ Neurology

Grossly intact; deep tendon reflexes normal

▸ Extremities

No swelling or edema noted

▸ Genitourinary

Examination deferred

▸ Rectal

Examination deferred

Laboratory Tests

(+) Rapid streptococcal antigen from throat swab

Assessment

Five-year-old girl with signs, symptoms, and laboratory tests consistent with streptococcal pharyngitis and AOM

Student Workup

Missing Information?

Evaluate: Patient Database

Drug Therapy Problems

Care Plan (by Problem)

TARGETED QUESTIONS

1. What signs and symptoms of streptococcal pharyngitis does this patient have?

   Hint: See p. 1214 in PPP

2. What signs and symptoms of AOM does this patient have?

   Hint: See p. 1205 in PPP

3. Why is amoxicillin the treatment of choice for this patient?

   Hint: See pp. 1206 and 1215, Figures 72-1, 72-2, and 72-5, and Tables 72-2 and 72-5 in PPP

4. What counseling points regarding antibiotic treatment would you discuss with this patient's mother?

   Hint: See pp. 1206, 1209, and 1216, and Table 72-2 in PPP

5. What adjunctive treatments could be considered for this patient?

> *Hint: A viral upper respiratory tract infection may have preceded AOM and streptococcal pharyngitis in this patient. Nonprescription medication use should be limited in young children with viral upper respiratory tract infections. See pp. 1207 and 1216, and Figure 72-5 in PPP*

FOLLOW-UP

Three days later, the patient and her mother return to the pediatrician because the patient developed a rash. It is a pruritic, maculopapular rash on her trunk that is spreading to her groin and upper legs. Reported medication adherence is 100% and her last reported dose of amoxicillin was at 8 AM today. Her throat and ear pain have resolved and she has been afebrile for about 36 hours. However, she has bilateral middle ear effusions present at this time.

6. What actions, if any, would you take?

> *Hint: See pp. 1207 and 1216, Figure 72-2, and Tables 72-2 and 72-5 in PPP*

⟳ GLOBAL PERSPECTIVE

Group A streptococcus is a common contributor to global morbidity and mortality. Developing countries have significantly higher rates of streptococcal pharyngitis, rheumatic fever, heart disease, and poststreptococcal glomerulonephritis that lead to chronic cardiac and renal disease and their associated mortality in children and young adults. Antibiotics may not be readily available in less developed countries to treat infected patients in order to minimize the spread of infection and complications. Educational efforts should focus on reducing transmission of infection and use of secondary prophylaxis for rheumatic fever and heart disease.

AOM is a common childhood infection worldwide with an increased incidence in high-risk populations, such as American and Canadian Indians, Inuit, and aboriginal Australians. Complications such as mastoiditis and hearing impairment are more common in these high-risk groups, in children with lower socioeconomic status or who live in crowded conditions, and in developing countries. Geographic differences in bacterial causes of AOM, microbial resistance patterns, and access to pneumococcal conjugate vaccines can affect treatment choices that are based on likely etiologies of middle ear infections. Watchful waiting may be an appropriate option for most children in the developed world, but requires access to medical follow-up care. Risk factor reduction is an important educational target for developing countries and other high-risk groups that may lack access to modern medical care.

CASE SUMMARY

- Her current clinical picture is consistent with streptococcal pharyngitis and AOM, and antibiotic therapy with amoxicillin should be initiated. Amoxicillin is active against *Streptococcus pyogenes*, *Streptococcus pneumoniae*, and *Haemophilus influenzae*.

- An amoxicillin dose of 800 mg twice daily is reasonable (85 mg/kg/d) for treating AOM potentially caused by penicillin-resistant *S. pneumoniae*.

- Nonprescription medications such as single-ingredient acetaminophen or ibuprofen could be considered for pain and fever control; other nonprescription medications should be discouraged because of a lack of data supporting their safety and efficacy in young children.

For more information on the care plan and facilitator's guide please visit http://www.mhpharmacotherapy.com.

76 Cellulitis

Christy M. Weiland

CASE LEARNING OBJECTIVES

- Recognize the signs and symptoms of skin and skin-structure infections
- Understand the significant laboratory and imaging tests that should be performed to assist in the diagnosis and treatment of cellulitis
- Develop an appropriate treatment regimen for cellulitis
- Determine the appropriate monitoring parameters to evaluate therapeutic response to treatment of cellulitis

PATIENT PRESENTATION

Chief Complaint

"My leg has been hurting for the last few days and now it is red."

History of Present Illness

Richard Rogers is a 54-year-old male who presents to his primary care provider complaining of a painful leg that has become red within the last day. Last week, he was hiking with his son and they both ended up with multiple lower and upper extremity abrasions secondary to tree brush. The abrasions have mostly healed, but he noticed his left calf became painful 2 days ago and now today it has become erythematous. He is worried that it may be related to a tick since he removed one from his dog the day of the hike. He denies any fever, chills, nausea, or vomiting.

Past Medical History

Peripheral artery disease (diagnosed 2 years ago)

s/p lower extremity stent (6.5 months ago)

Diastolic heart failure [ejection fraction 60% (0.60) measured 10 months ago]

Hyperlipidemia (diagnosed 10 years ago, last lipid panel 3 years ago)

HTN (diagnosed 13 years ago, controlled on medications)

Family History

Father deceased at the age of 70 years secondary to an MI. Mother is alive at the age of 82 years with hypothyroidism, HTN, and history of breast cancer. The patient is negative for thrombolic disorders.

Social/Work History

The patient lives with his wife of 34 years. He has three adult children. He works as a lawyer.

Tobacco/Alcohol/Substance Use

The patient has a "few beers on the weekends." He smokes ½ ppd × 35 years. He denies illicit drug use.

Allergy/Intolerance/Adverse Event History

Codeine (unknown reaction)

Medication History

Clopidogrel 75 mg PO daily

Simvastatin 20 mg PO daily

Lisinopril/HCTZ 20/12.5 mg PO daily

Aspirin 81 mg PO daily

Naproxen 550 mg PO every 12 hours PRN pain

Review of Systems

(−) Fever, chills, nausea, or vomiting. Left calf has reproducible pain and erythema; pain and symptoms have been present for 2 days and lesions occurred last week; decreased perfusion to lower extremities secondary to peripheral artery disease and current smoking.

Physical Examination

▶ *General*

Well-nourished, middle-aged, white male who appears in no acute distress

► **Vital Signs**

BP 134/86 mm Hg, P 71 bpm, RR 18, T 38.7°C

Weight 240 lb (109 kg)

Height 72 in. (183 cm)

► **Skin**

Intact with healed abrasions noted under extremities; moist

► **HEENT**

Moist mucus membranes. Oropharynx is pink and moist. Pupils are equal, round, and reactive to light.

► **Chest**

Dull to auscultation at the base bilaterally

► **Cardiovascular**

RRR; no murmurs, rubs, or gallops

► **Abdomen**

Soft, nontender, not distended

► **Neurology**

CNs grossly intact; moves all extremities well × 4

► **Extremities**

Left calf has some erythema that is slightly tender with touch consistent with a previous lesion. It is slightly warmer than the right calf. He does have a full range of motion. No crepitations, no bulla, no petechia or purpura. Localized to the left leg. Multiple healed abrasions on lower extremities.

► **Genitourinary**

Not noted

Laboratory and Other Diagnostic Tests

	Conventional Units	SI Units
Na	136 mEq/L	136 mmol/L
K	4.1 mEq/L	4.1 mmol/L
Cl	103 mEq/L	103 mmol/L
CO_2	24 mEq/L	24 mmol/L
BUN	9 mg/dL	3.2 mmol/L
SCr	0.91 mg/dL	80 μmol/L
Glu	161 mg/dL	8.9 mmol/L
Hgb	14.5 g/dL	145 g/L; 9.00 mmol/L
Hct	43.5%	0.435
WBC	$13 \times 10^3/mm^3$	$13 \times 10^9/L$
Bands	12%	0.12
Eosinophils	0%	0.00
Albumin	4 g/dL	40 g/L

D-dimer	175 ng/mL	175 mcg/L
CRP	26 mg/dL	260 mg/L
Total cholesterol	180 mg/dL	4.65 mmol/L
LDL	93 mg/dL	2.40 mmol/L
HDL	19 mg/dL	0.49 mmol/L
Triglycerides	130 mg/dL	1.47 mmol/L

► **Blood Culture**

Pending

Assessment

Fifty-four-year-old male with left lower extremity cellulitis

Student Workup

Missing Information?

Evaluate: Patient Database

Drug Therapy Problems

Care Plan (by Problem)

TARGETED QUESTIONS

1. What signs, symptoms, and laboratory data support that this patient has an infection?

   Hint: Infections normally present with a source where organisms can enter the area such as broken skin barriers. Symptoms can present as both localized to the area of infection and systemic, so you would want to consider both. A CRP can be useful in this setting as it is a marker of acute inflammatory changes. CRP will show a rise within 4 to 6 hours of the onset of inflammation. CRP is very sensitive to inflammation, but has very low specificity. See p. 1224 in PPP

2. What laboratory data rule out other possible cause of this patient's symptoms?

   Hint: With pain specifically in a leg with a patient who is predisposed to a thrombosis process (peripheral artery disease), a DVT should be considered. A plasma D-dimer is a fibrin product generated by the action of plasmin on cross-linked fibrin molecules indicating that a clot has formed. It has a high sensitivity, but low specificity, leading to a significant amount of false positives. The negative D-dimer rules out a DVT. See pp. 1223 and 1224 in PPP

3. What disease states does this patient have that predispose and complicate the cellulitis?

   Hint: Peripheral artery disease leads to a decrease in the blood flow and perfusion to the extremities including arms and legs. With decreased blood flow the patient becomes predisposed to infection. Once a patient does have an infection, it makes it more difficult to treat since drug concentrations will be lower due to the decreased blood supply. In addition, smoking delays wound healing, leading to an increase in infection where the skin loses its integrity.

4. How would you classify this patient's cellulitis?

   Hint: See p. 1224 in PPP

5. How would this patient benefit from smoking cessation?

   Hint: Smoking decreases the blood flow by constricting arteries. Smoking cessation would not help this infection, but would provide benefit if he has a future infection which he is at a high risk for secondary to peripheral artery disease. Smoking cessation would also benefit his hyperlipidemia, HTN, and diastolic heart failure. These effects can start to reverse in just 2 months of cessation.

FOLLOW-UP

After starting the patient on amoxicillin/clavulanate 875 mg PO every 12 hours for 10 days, 3 days later, the sensitivities from the culture are received and are as follows:

Blood culture final—MRSA recovered from two of two bottles.

Drug		MIC (mcg/mL or mg/L)
Cefazolin	Resistant	>8
Levofloxacin	Sensitive	≤2
Linezolid	Sensitive	2
Vancomycin	Sensitive	1
Trimethoprim/ sulfamethoxazole	Sensitive	<0.5/9.5
Amoxicillin/clavulanate	Resistant	>4/2

After talking with the patient, his left leg has not improved, although it does not seem to be getting worse per the patient: the inflammation, temperature, and pain are the same.

6. Is this patient's infection being treated appropriately? Please explain your answer. If this patient is being treated inappropriately, what medication would you recommend on the basis of the new information? How long would the medication be continued for?

   Hint: See p. 1225 in PPP. When organisms are sensitive to many drug therapies, other factors should be taken into consideration, including allergies, simplicity of regimen (i.e., once-a-day vs. four-times-a-day medication), route of administration, side-effect profile of medication, and lastly cost. If an organism is resistant to an antibiotic, the patient should receive the full-recommended duration of therapy with the appropriate antibiotic since the patient was not on the appropriate therapy previously.

GLOBAL PERSPECTIVE

The organisms associated with cellulitis are consistent across the world, with *S. aureus* being the most common; however, the frequency of cellulitis and the type of *S. aureus* varies for travelers abroad. It has been noted that the second most common diagnosis in returned travels from international travel with skin problems is soft-tissue bacterial infections including cellulitis.[1] Bacterial skin infections are more common in those returning from sub-Saharan Africa or Southeast Asia, and hot spots identified by the GeoSentinel Network including Madagascar, Kenya, Philippines, Sri Lanka, South Africa, and Thailand. The tropical conditions including heat and humidity make organisms such as MRSA and PantoneValentine leukocidin toxin–associated *S. aureus* much more common. Travelers are at increased risk of PantoneValentine leukocidin strains of *S. aureus* infections, which are correlated with more severe tissue destruction. It is thought that the increased risk is due to the use of doxycycline that may select for it as well as reduced hygiene.

REFERENCE

1. O'Brian BM. A practical approach to common skin problems in returning travelers. Travel Med Infect Dis 2009 7:125–146.

CASE SUMMARY

- The patient's clinical presentation is typical for cellulitis with a recent wound, pain at site, and erythema.

- The majority of cellulitis infections are linked to Gram-positive organisms; however, due to comorbidities such as peripheral artery disease and smoking, the infection is at risk for containing Gram-positive and/or Gram-negative organisms.

- Both peripheral artery disease and smoking will delay the healing of lesions by decreasing the blood flow.

For more information on the care plan and facilitator's guide please visit http://www.mhpharmacotherapy.com.

77 Diabetic Foot Infections

Christy M. Weiland

CASE LEARNING OBJECTIVES

- Assess the signs and symptoms of diabetic foot infections
- List the goals of treatment for patients with diabetic foot infections
- Select appropriate nonpharmacologic and pharmacologic treatment regimens for patients presenting with diabetic foot infections
- Identify adverse effects that may result from pharmacologic agents used in the treatment of diabetic foot infections
- Develop a monitoring plan that will assess the safety and efficacy of the overall disease management of diabetic foot infections

PATIENT PRESENTATION

Chief Complaint

"I cannot handle the pain in my foot anymore, I need pain medication."

History of Present Illness

Ted Read is a 34-year-old male with type 1 DM who presents to the emergency department complaining of pain from an ulcer on the sole of his right foot. He reports having an ulcer in the past, but it healed after he borrowed a cream (unknown by the patient) from his friend. He has been using the same cream on this ulcer for the past week with no relief. He works in construction, so he needs to be on his feet all day, and today he could not take the pain anymore. The ulcer started about 2 weeks ago. He thinks there was a rock in his shoe for an entire work day that started it. The pain has continuously worsened. He reports not regularly checking his feet. He is worried that this will affect his job since he is concerned about getting laid off.

Past Medical History

Type 1 DM diagnosed at the age 6
History of one foot ulcer reported by the patient

Family History

Father is alive at age 56 with a history of suicide ideation. Mother is alive at age 54 with a history of hypothyroidism, HTN, and Addison's disease. He has two siblings who live locally. Medical history unknown.

Social/Work History

Single; has a child of age 4; works in construction; lately, reports an increase in stress due to concerns of getting laid off.

Tobacco/Alcohol/Substance Use

He admits to a few beers a night and maybe a little more on the weekends; no illicit drug use; he smokes cigarettes socially.

Allergy/Intolerance/Adverse Event History

Sulfa: Rash

Medication History

Insulin glargine injects 32 units subcutaneously at bedtime

Insulin lispro injects insulin according to carbohydrate intake and as needed prior to meals

Acetaminophen as needed

Ibuprofen 400 mg PO as needed for aches and pains

Hydrocodone/acetaminophen 5/500 mg PO as needed (he borrows from a friend occasionally; recently, due to the pain he has borrowed quite a bit)

Cream unknown, borrowed from a friend

Review of Systems

(+) Occasional pain mostly aches which he takes ibuprofen and acetaminophen for unknown doses. He also borrows hydrocodone/acetaminophen occasionally. Frequency of use has increased as pain has increased. (+) Right foot secondary to ulcer; (+) fever, (−) nausea, vomiting, chills, or SOB.

Physical Examination

▶ General

The patient is a well-nourished individual, who is A&O × 4 and in minimal distress.

▶ Vital Signs

BP 132/92 mm Hg, P 84 bpm, RR 16, T 38.9°C

Weight 180 lb (82 kg)

Height 72 in. (183 cm)

Pain 7/10

▶ Skin

Moist, cold to touch, intact except right foot as noted below

▶ HEENT

Pupils rounds and reactive to light; extraocular muscles intact; no pharyngeal erythema or edema

▶ Chest

(−) Chest pain; lungs are clear to auscultation bilaterally without wheezes, rhonchi, or rales

▶ Cardiovascular

Regular rate and rhythm without S_3, S_4, or murmurs

▶ Abdomen

Positive bowel sounds, soft, nontender, and nondistended

▶ Neurology

CNs II to XII grossly intact; 5/5 muscle strength bilaterally

▶ Extremities

No lower extremity edema. Very extensive ulcer distal to the great toe on the plantar surface extending up the heal of the right foot. Flesh erythematous around the ulcer and spreading 5 to 6 cm. Drainage of foul-smelling fluid on pressure. Unable to visualize the bone. Mild decreased rotation of the left foot. Left foot normal.

Laboratory and Other Diagnostic Tests

	Conventional Units	SI Units
Na	132 mEq/L	132 mmol/L
K	3.3 mEq/L	3.3 mmol/L
Cl	100 mEq/L	100 mmol/L
CO_2	23 mEq/L	23 mmol/L
BUN	20 mg/dL	7.1 mmol/L
SCr	0.9 mg/dL	80 μmol/L
Glu	412 mg/dL	22.9 mmol/L
Hgb	14 g/dL	140 g/L; 8.69 mmol/L
Hct	42%	0.42
WBC	$17 \times 10^3/mm^3$	$17 \times 10^9/L$
Bands	11%	0.11
Platelets	$312 \times 10^3/mm^3$	$312 \times 10^9/L$
Albumin	3.5 g/dL (35 g/L)	
AST	45 IU/L	0.75 μkat/L
ALT	33 IU/L	0.55 μkat/L
CRP	12.1 mg/dL	121 mg/L
HbA_{1c}	10.2%	0.102

▶ Cultures

Tissue: Pending

Blood × 2: Pending

Foot x-ray: Ruled out osteomyelitis

Assessment

A 34-year-old male with uncontrolled type 1 DM with an infected foot ulcer

---

Student Workup

Missing Information?

Evaluate:	Patient Database
	Drug Therapy Problems
	Care Plan (by Problem)

TARGETED QUESTIONS

1. What signs, symptoms, and laboratory data support the patient's diagnosis of infection?

   Hint: See pp. 1228 and 1229 in PPP

2. What is the classification of the patient s diabetic foot infection? Please explain your answer.

   Hint: See p. 1228 and Table 73-5 in PPP

3. Once the patient is treated, what are the patient s goals to prevent this from reoccurring?

   Hint: See p. 1229 in PPP

4. What would be the most appropriate antimicrobial regimen for this patient? Please include dose, route, frequency, and duration. Please explain the rationale.

   Hint: Anaerobic organisms are commonly malodorous or foul smelling. See pp. 1229 and 1230, and Table 73-6 in PPP

FOLLOW-UP

The patient was initiated on piperacillin/tazobactam 3.375 g IV every 6 hours and linezolid 600 mg IV every 12 hours. The patient has been afebrile for 48 hours. The foot has decreased erythema. His WBC has decreased to $9 \times 10^3/mm^3$ $(9 \times 10^9/L)$ with 3% (0.03) band neutrophils. Two days later, the following culture and sensitivities were reported:

- **Blood culture:** Negative (pending)
- **Tissue culture:** *Pseudomonas aeruginosa* from two of two bottles

Drug		MIC (mcg/mL or mg/L)
Cefazolin	Resistant	≥16
Levofloxacin	Sensitive	≤2
Ceftazidime	Resistant	10
Amoxicillin/clavulanate	Resistant	≥6/3
Piperacillin/tazobactam	Sensitive	<16/4

5. On the basis of the above culture, sensitivities, and the patient's clinical picture, would changing antibiotic therapy be appropriate? Please explain. If yes, what would be an appropriate therapy, including drug, dose, route, frequency, and duration?

> *Hint: Once the patient is afebrile for 24 to 48 hours and hemodynamically stable, it is appropriate to change the therapy from intravenous to by mouth. In addition, when able, narrow the spectrum of antibiotic therapy on the basis of the culture and sensitivities to decrease the incidence of antibiotic resistance and side effects to the patient, including risk of Clostridium difficile.*

☌ GLOBAL PERSPECTIVE

Diabetic foot infections are a global burden, resulting in major debilitating complications with severe morbidity and possible amputations across the globe; developing countries as compared to developed countries have additional barriers to overcome. Peripheral neuropathy in populations with type 2 DM tends to be higher in developing countries, which leads to a higher incidence of foot ulcerations. It has been estimated in India to be as high as 27.5%, Tanzania 28.1%, and Sudan 37% of all patients with type 2 DM.[1] One of the most important factors leading to an increase in diabetic foot infections is the lack of proper footwear, which has been noted in most developing countries. Other contributing factors include lack of proper education on diabetes, lack of proper hygiene, lack of health insurance, and cultural beliefs to surgical interventions. In India and many parts of Africa, the sociocultural practice is to walk barefoot; in Africa, it has been estimated that 70% of patients with diabetes have inadequate glycemic control; and in Africa, patients are reluctant to participate in any minor surgical intervention due to cultural beliefs, which is thought to contribute to an increase in mortality of diabetic foot infections.

REFERENCE

1. Ramachandra A. Specific problems of the diabetic foot in developing countries. Diabetes Metab Res Rev 2004 20(suppl 1):S19–S22.

CASE SUMMARY

- The patient's clinical presentation was a typical diabetic foot infection consistent with inflamed foot ulceration and elevated blood sugars.
- Diabetic foot infections are generally polymicrobial and require empiric broad-spectrum antibiotics for adequate organism coverage.
- Foot care maintenance, including daily foot inspection, is an essential part of maintaining healthy diabetic feet.

For more information on the care plan and facilitator's guide please visit http://www.mhpharmacotherapy.com.

78 Infective Endocarditis

Ronda L. Akins

CASE LEARNING OBJECTIVES

- Recognize the signs and symptoms of infective endocarditis (IE)
- Understand the significant laboratory and imaging tests that should be performed to assist in the diagnosis, treatment, and monitoring of IE
- Identify the initial and long-term goals of therapy for IE
- Develop an appropriate treatment regimen, including length of treatment, for this particular patient on the basis of organism characteristics and treatment guidelines for IE
- Determine appropriate monitoring parameters to evaluate response of the IE therapy
- Understand which patients need prophylactic therapy and what therapy is appropriate for the prevention of IE

PATIENT PRESENTATION

Chief Complaint

"I've had a fever off and on for the past 2 weeks. My leg hurts and is swollen. I just don't feel very good, my body aches and I am tired all the time."

History of Present Illness

LB is a 38-year-old Caucasian man who presents to the emergency department with complaints of intermittent high fever [103–104°F (39.4–40.4°C)], chills, malaise, myalgias, and arthralgias for the past 2 weeks, as well as lower right leg erythema and edema for the past 3 to 4 weeks. He has been treated numerous times for recurrent cellulitis over the area of a previous gunshot wound (GSW) with evidence of injection drug use noted in the same area. Over the past year, he has been admitted to the hospital three times with right leg cellulitis (last admission was 2 months ago). He has been treated in the past with cefazolin, vancomycin, and trimethoprim/sulfamethoxazole. The area of cellulitis extends down from the groin to midthigh. The patient reports that the last intravenous drug abuse (IVDA) was 4 weeks ago. He has chronic leg pain due to the GSW and takes tramadol, Lortab, and Percocet for pain control. He states that the pain has increased over the past month, and he has been taking more medication to control the pain.

Past Medical History

GSW 8 years ago (right upper leg/groin area)

Recurrent cellulitis over the past 3 to 4 years (CA-MRSA + in the past)

HTN

Hyperlipidemia × 3 years

Hepatitis B

Family History

Father and mother are both alive. Father is 55 and has a history of COPD and hyperlipidemia. Mother is 52 and has no significant past medical history. He has two younger siblings: one sister aged 24 and one brother aged 21; both are healthy.

Social History

He was married but divorced after being incarcerated for selling illicit drugs. He has one child, aged 14 years, but does not have any contact. He was in prison for 6 years, but was released about 1½ years ago. He lives with his girlfriend at the present time and is unemployed.

Tobacco/Alcohol/Substance Use

Admits to a 10-year history of injective drug use (reports heroin and cocaine use). Denies any use of alcohol. Admits to tobacco use (1 ppd × 18 years)

Allergies/Intolerances/Adverse Drug Events

Penicillin—unknown reaction

Medications (Current)

Simvastatin 20 mg PO q hs

Atenolol 100 mg PO bid

Citalopram 40 mg PO q day

Gabapentin 300 mg PO tid

Tramadol 50 to 100 mg PO q 6 h

Lortab 10/500 mg PO q 4 to 6 h PRN pain

Percocet 7.5/325 mg PO q 6 h PRN severe pain

Acetaminophen PO PRN fever × 2 weeks

Review of Systems

Significant right leg pain due to previous GSW, some relief with pain medications (tramadol, Lortab, and Percocet); recurrent cellulitis in right leg/groin area; no other significant medical problems

Physical Examination

▶ General

Ill-appearing, Caucasian man in mild-to-moderate distress

▶ Vital Signs

BP 145/90 mm Hg, P 120, RR 22, T 39.6°C

Weight 148.2 lb (67.4 kg)

Height 71 in. (180 cm)

Complains of significant right leg pain extending up into the groin

▶ Skin

Pale appearing with numerous areas of scarred and leathery skin secondary to IVDA; (+) petechial rash on trunk, multiple lesions, and track marks on right leg and groin

▶ HEENT

PERRLA, EOMI; no scleral icterus, (+) petechia on palate, dry mucus membranes, no exudates noted in throat

▶ Neck and Lymph Nodes

Supple; (−) lymphadenopathy

▶ Chest

Clear to auscultation bilaterally

▶ Cardiovascular

RRR, (+) murmur noted (newly identified)

▶ Abdomen

Soft, nondistended, nontender; (+) bowel sounds; (−) organomegaly

▶ Neurology

AAO × 3; (−) focal or sensory deficit noted

▶ Extremities

Significant edema in right leg; pulses are 2+ and equal bilaterally. No clubbing or cyanosis noted. Splinter hemorrhages noted on left, middle, and ring fingers

Laboratory Tests

On admission

	Conventional Units	SI Units
Na	132 mEq/L	132 mmol/L
K	3.9 mEq/L	3.9 mmol/L
Cl	102 mEq/L	102 mmol/L
CO_2	26 mEq/L	26 mmol/L
BUN	34 mg/dL	12.1 mmol/L
SCr	1.6 mg/dL	141 µmol/L
Glu	122 mg/dL	6.8 mmol/L
Albumin	2.9 g/dL	29 g/L
RBC	$3.14 \times 10^6/mm^3$	$3.14 \times 10^{12}/L$
Hgb	8.8 g/dL	88 g/L; 5.46 mmol/L
Hct	27.8%	0.278
Platelets	$184 \times 10^3/mm^3$	$184 \times 10^9/L$
WBC	$19.6 \times 10^3/mm^3$	$19.6 \times 10^9/L$
Neutrophils	78%	0.78
Bands	14%	0.14
Lymphocytes	7%	0.07
Monocytes	1%	0.01
Eosinophils	0%	0.00
Basophils	0%	0.00

Cultures

Blood cultures taken on admission; results pending

Assessment

A 38-year-old man with signs, symptoms, and laboratory tests consistent with right leg cellulitis and suspected bacteremia/endocarditis

Plan

Admit the patient to a hospital, begin broad-spectrum antibiotics, and perform additional tests to evaluate for IE

AFTER HOSPITAL ADMISSION

Cultures

Day 2: Gram stain of blood cultures × 2 taken at admission show Gram-positive cocci in clusters.

Day 3: Blood cultures × 2 show *Staphylococcus aureus*; sensitivities pending.

Day 4: Right leg abscess aspirate grows *S. aureus*; sensitivities pending.

Day 5: Culture sensitivities (see Table 78-1).

Day 17: Gram stain of blood cultures × 2 show Gram-positive cocci in clusters.

Day 18: Blood cultures show *S. aureus*; sensitivities pending.

Day 19: Culture sensitivities (see Table 78-1).

Day 26: Blood cultures × 2 are negative.

Imaging

Day 3: CT of the right groin showed a 3 × 4 cm (1.2 × 1.6 in) abscess. Surgery drains abscess and sends aspirate for culture.

Day 4: TTE showed possible small vegetation; poor visualization of the valves; results inconclusive.

Day 20: TEE shows large vegetation [1.9 × 3.8 cm (0.75 × 1.5 inch)] on the posterior leaflet of the tricuspid valve.

Pertinent Labs

During hospitalization

	Conventional Units	SI Units
Day 7:		
SCr	1.8 mg/dL	159 μmol/L
WBC	$15.5 \times 10^3/mm^3$	$15.5 \times 10^9/L$
Day 12:		
SCr	2.4 mg/dL	212 μmol/L
WBC	$16.2 \times 10^3/mm^3$	$16.2 \times 10^9/L$
Day 22:		
SCr	1.9 mg/dL	168 μmol/L
WBC	$14.3 \times 10^3/mm^3$	$14.3 \times 10^9/L$
Day 30:		
SCr	1.3 mg/dL	115 μmol/L
WBC	$10.7 \times 10^3/mm^3$	$10.7 \times 10^3/mm^3$

TABLE 78-1.   CULTURE SENSITIVITIES

	Blood Culture—Aerobic and Anaerobic Bottles (Arm—Left) Specimen # B31126 09/05/2009 16:24	Blood Culture—Aerobic and Anaerobic Bottles (Right Internal Jugular Triple-Lumen Catheter) Specimen # B31278 09/05/2009 18:45	Abscess Fluid Right Groin—Aerobic and Anaerobic Bottles Note: Patient on Vancomycin Specimen # X48002 09/07/2009 10:18	Blood Culture—Aerobic and Anaerobic Bottles (Arm—Left Peripherally Inserted Center Catheter, PICC; Arm—Right) Note: Patient on Vancomycin Specimen # B42151; B42189 09/22/2009 21:52; 21:55
Gram stain	Gram-positive cocci in clusters	Gram-positive cocci in clusters	Gram-positive cocci in clusters	Gram-positive cocci in clusters
Organism	*S. aureus*	*S. aureus*	*S. aureus*	*S. aureus*
	MIC (mcg/mL; mg/L)	MIC (mcg/mL; mg/L)	MIC (mcg/mL; mg/L)	MIC (mcg/mL; mg/L)
Clindamycin	>4 (R)	>4 (R)	>4 (R)	>4 (R)
Daptomycin	0.5 (S)	0.5 (S)	0.5 (S)	1.0 (S)
Erythromycin	>4 (R)	>4 (R)	>4 (R)	>4 (R)
Gentamicin	>8 (R)	>8 (R)	>8 (R)	>8 (R)
Moxifloxacin	>4 (R)	>4 (R)	>4 (R)	>4 (R)
Linezolid	1 (S)	1 (S)	2 (S)	2 (S)
Oxacillin	>2 (R)	>2 (R)	>2 (R)	>2 (R)
Penicillin	>8 (R)	>8 (R)	>8 (R)	>8 (R)
Rifampin	≤1 (S)	≤1 (S)	≤1 (S)	≤1 (S)
Quinupristin/ dalfopristin	≤0.25 (S)	≤0.25 (S)	0.50 (S)	0.50 (S)
Tetracycline	≤1 (S)	≤1 (S)	≤1 (S)	≤1 (S)
Trimethoprim/ sulfamethoxazole	≤0.5/9.5 (S)	≤0.5/9.5 (S)	≤0.5/9.5 (S)	≤0.5/9.5 (S)
Vancomycin	1 (S)	1 (S)	2 (S)	2 (S)

Treatment in Hospital

The patient was placed on vancomycin 1,000 mg IV q 12 h and gentamicin 150 mg IV q 8 h for broad coverage of common organisms of IE and right upper leg cellulitis/abscess. He continues to have intermittent febrile episodes [spikes up to 38.8°C (101.8°F)] despite therapy. On hospital day 12, peaks and troughs were drawn for both vancomycin and gentamicin, and results were as follows: vancomycin, peak 41.6 mcg/mL (41.6 mg/L; 28.7 μmol/L) (11:40) and trough 15.3 mcg/mL (15.3 mg/L; 10.6 μmol/L) (08:15); gentamicin, peak 12.2 mcg/mL (12.2 mg/L; 25.5 μmol/L) (17:30) and trough 4.8 mcg/mL (4.8 mg/L; 10.0 μmol/L) (15:20). At this time, gentamicin was discontinued and vancomycin was held for one dose and then restarted at the same dose. On hospital day 16, the patient became SOB with complaints of a dry cough and chest pain. A chest x-ray revealed bilateral lower infiltrates, which were believed to be septic pulmonary emboli. He had repeat blood cultures on hospital day 17, which grew *S. aureus* (see Table 78-1). Antimicrobial therapy was reassessed on the basis of the patient's clinical deterioration (large vegetation on TEE), development of IE complications (septic emboli), and continued positive cultures showing increased MICs. At this time (day 20), vancomycin was discontinued and daptomycin 300 mg q 24 h was started.

Student Workup

Missing Information?

Evaluate:	Patient Database
	Drug Therapy Problems/Monitoring Issues
	Care Plan (by Problem)

TARGETED QUESTIONS

1. What signs and symptoms of IE does this patient have? Categorize by Duke classifications as major or minor criteria and specify what "type" of clinical diagnosis is appropriate for this patient.

   Hint: See p. 1237 and Table 74-2 in PPP

2. Is it appropriate to start vancomycin as empiric therapy in this patient?

   Hint: See pp. 1238, 1241, and 1242 in PPP

3. Is synergistic therapy with gentamicin appropriate in this patient?

   Hint: See pp. 1241–1243 in PPP

4. What should you recommend after reviewing this patient's vancomycin and gentamicin levels?

   Hint: See Tables 74-4 and 74-6 (footnotes) in PPP, and see the following article:

Rybak MJ, Lomaestro BM, Rotschafer JC, Moellering RC, Craig WA, Billeter M, Dalovisio JR, Levine DP. Therapeutic monitoring of vancomycin in adults—summary of consensus recommendations from the American Society of Health-System Pharmacists, the Infectious Diseases Society of America, and the Society of Infectious Diseases Pharmacists. Pharmacotherapy 2009 29(11):1275–1279.

5. What concerns develop with the empiric therapy during the initial hospital course of this patient?

   Hint: See pp. 1242 and 1243, and Tables 74-5 and 74-7 in PPP

6. Is it appropriate to change therapy?

   Hint: See the following articles:

   Hidayat LK, Hsu DI, Quist R, Shriner KA, Wong-Beringer A. High-dose vancomycin therapy for methicillin-resistant *Staphylococcus aureus* infections. Arch Intern Med 2006 166:2138–2214.

   Rybak MJ, Lomaestro BM, Rotschafer JC, Moellering RC, Craig WA, Billeter M, Dalovisio JR, Levine DP. Therapeutic monitoring of vancomycin in adults—summary of consensus recommendations from the American Society of Health-System Pharmacists, the Infectious Diseases Society of America, and the Society of Infectious Diseases Pharmacists. Pharmacotherapy 2009 29(11):1275–1279.

7. Is daptomycin an appropriate alternative therapy?

   Hint: See pp. 1243 and 1246 in PPP, and see the following article:

   Fowler V, Boucher HW, Corey GR, et al. Daptomycin versus standard therapy for bacteremia and IE caused by *Staphylococcus aureus*. N Engl J Med 2006 355:653–665.

8. Are there any concerns with concurrent drug therapy and daptomycin?

   Hint: See p. 1243 and Table 74-7 in PPP, and the Cubicin package insert pp. 11 and 13 (http://www.cubicin.com/pdf/PrescribingInformation.pdf), and see the following article:

   Fowler V, Boucher HW, Corey GR, et al. Daptomycin versus standard therapy for bacteremia and IE caused by *Staphylococcus aureus*. N Engl J Med 2006 355:653–665.

9. How long this patient should be treated?

   Hint: See Table 74-4 in PPP. In addition, take into account that the patient had a positive culture on day 18 with worsening symptoms when therapy was changed.

10. How should this patient be monitored for resolution of infection/adverse drug effects? Include additional tests, procedures, etc.

    Hint: See pp. 1248, 1250, and 1251, and Table 74-7 in PPP

11. Should this patient receive IE prophylactic therapy for future invasive dental procedures? Include reason and regimen as appropriate.

    Hint: See pp. 1249–1251 in PPP

CLINICAL COURSE

During the first 2 weeks of therapy, the patient showed some initial improvement. The WBC decreased but then began to show an increase and the patient continued to have intermittent febrile episodes. Over these 2 weeks, the right upper leg cellulitis resolved but not cured. The right groin abscess remained visible on repeat CT, but was smaller in size. During week 3, the patient's renal function declined and drug levels for vancomycin and gentamicin were drawn, showing abnormal levels. Dosage recommendations were made by the pharmacokinetic pharmacy service. After the patient deteriorated clinically, experienced a complication of IE (pulmonary septic emboli), and had positive repeat blood cultures with increased MICs, therapy was changed to daptomycin. Over the next week, the patient's bacteremia resolved, right upper leg cellulitis resolved, and the right groin abscess was healing. The patient reported that he was feeling much better and had no complaints. The medicine team recommended continuing therapy for the appropriate length of treatment for his IE.

⚙ GLOBAL PERSPECTIVE

IE is an infection typically involving the heart valves and nearby endocardial tissue. This disease state often has an aggressive clinical course with numerous complications and high mortality rates. Incidence of IE appears to be similar throughout developed countries. Patients have various clinical presentations, ranging from subtle illness to severe sepsis with multiple complications. Certain patients (IVDA, diabetics, elderly) have an increased risk of having less common organisms and/or resistant organisms. Regardless of patient type, IE can be difficult to diagnose and treat. The patient must be carefully monitored throughout treatment for disease complications, therapeutic or toxic drug levels (as appropriate), drug interactions, and clinical improvement (both laboratory results and patient response). Patient follow-up is critical in ensuring that a cure has been achieved and that no adverse events have occurred.

CASE SUMMARY

- His clinical presentation is consistent with IE requiring appropriate antibiotic therapy.
- Vancomycin therapy on the basis of organism and susceptibilities is appropriate per IE treatment guidelines.
- Worsening clinical picture and susceptibilities require reassessment of therapy.

For more information on the care plan and facilitator's guide please visit http://www.mhpharmacotherapy.com.

79 Tuberculosis

Rocsanna Namdar

CASE LEARNING OBJECTIVES

- Identify the risk factors for active tuberculosis (TB) disease
- Design a therapeutic plan for active TB disease in immunocompetent and immunocompromised patients
- Assess the effectiveness of therapy in patients with TB
- Design appropriate regimens for the treatment of latent TB infection

PATIENT PRESENTATION

Chief Complaint

"I have had a cough for a month. Two nights ago I woke up with a sharp pain and I coughed up some blood."

History of Present Illness

HS is a 52 year-old Hispanic female who presents to the emergency department with complaints of cough, productive of small amounts of yellow sputum within the last month. She has experienced increasing fatigue, occasional SOB on exertion, and mild, nonpleuritic, substernal chest discomfort. She has had periodic night sweats; last night her temperature was 102°F (38.9°C). Two nights ago, she noticed streaks of bright-red blood in her sputum without any particular odor or taste. The only medication she has taken is an over-the-counter cough preparation (Robitussin). Three months ago, the patient presented to a free clinic with fatigue, increased urinary frequency, and headaches. Evaluation revealed a diagnosis of diabetes and stage 1 HTN. A purified protein derivative (ppd) test, required for work clearance, was placed. She was noted to have a positive ppd test, but because her CXR showed no active disease, she was cleared to work.

Past Medical History

HTN diagnosed 3 months ago
Type 2 DM diagnosed 3 months ago
Depression diagnosed 3 months ago
Immunized with BCG

Family History

Mother (age 77) is in good health. Sisters (age 49 and 56) have HTN. Her father in Mexico died of lung disease 4 years ago at age 72. Her husband died of colon cancer 2 years ago.

Social History

The patient immigrated to the United States from Mexico 1 year ago. She lives with her son and his family. She has two daughters that still live in Mexico and has visited them on several occasions during the past year. She has recently started working at a day care.

Tobacco/Alcohol/Substance Use

Social drinker; (−) tobacco or illicit drug use

Allergies/Intolerances/Adverse Drug Events

Penicillin (rash)

Medications (Current)

Lisinopril 20 mg PO daily
Metformin 500 mg PO twice daily
Sertraline 50 mg PO daily
Calcium carbonate 1,000 mg PO daily
Motrin PRN pain

Review of Systems

The patient reports a more-than-9 lb (4-kg) weight loss over the past 2 months. She also complains of fever, body aches, intermittent chest pain associated with cough, SOB, and intermittent cough productive of sputum and blood. She states that she has had improvement in urinary frequency since starting metformin.

Physical Examination

▶ General

Pleasant, slightly overweight Hispanic female in no acute distress

▶ Vital Signs

BP 135/85 mm Hg, P 82, RR 18, T 37.9°C (100.2°F)

Weight 140 lb (63.6 kg)

Height 61 in. (154.9 cm)

▶ HEENT

PERRLA, EOMI; pharynx: slightly inflamed, no exudate

▶ Neck and Lymph Nodes

Few small 2- to 3-mm nontender, freely movable lymph nodes in left anterior cervical and axial area

▶ Chest

Configuration and expansion symmetrical. Tactile fremitus, percussion symmetrical bilaterally. Breath sounds and vocal fremitus are normal. A few posttussive rales are noted at the left apex posteriorly.

▶ Cardiovascular

RRR, normal S_1, S_2

▶ Abdomen

Not tender/not distended; (−) organomegaly

▶ Neurology

Grossly intact; deep tendon reflexes normal

▶ Genitourinary

Examination deferred

▶ Rectal

Examination deferred

Laboratory Tests

On admission

	Conventional Units	SI Units
Na	139 mEq/L	139 mmol/L
K	3.9 mEq/L	3.9 mmol/L
Cl	98 mEq/L	98 mmol/L
CO_2	26 mEq/L	26 mmol/L
BUN	20 mg/dL	7.1 mmol/L
SCr	0.7 mg/dL	62 μmol/L
Glu	153 mg/dL	8.5 mmol/L
AST	55 IU/L	0.92 μkat/L
ALT	61 IU/L	1.02 μkat/L
Total bilirubin	1 mg/dL	17.1 μmol/L

HbA_{1c}	8%	0.08
Urinalysis		
Protein	Trace	
Microalbumin	<30 mg/24 h	
Glucose	(−)	
Ketone	(−)	
Sputum culture	Normal respiratory flora	
Acid-fast bacilli smear	(+)	
Hgb	13.5 g/dL	135 g/L; 8.38 mmol/L
Hct	40%	0.40
WBC	$10.6 \times 10^3/mm^3$	$10.6 \times 10^9/L$
PMN	62%	0.62
Lymphocytes	34%	0.34
Monocytes	5%	0.05
RBC	$4.6 \times 10^6/mm^3$	$4.6 \times 10^{12}/L$

▶ Skin Test Results

PPD (tuberculin) 16 mm (0.63 inch) at 48 hours

▶ Chest X-Ray

Bilateral upper lobe infiltrates with well-defined cavitating lesion of the left apex

Assessment

A 52-year-old woman with signs, symptoms, and laboratory tests consistent with active TB

Student Workup

Missing Information?

Evaluate: Patient Database

Drug Therapy Problems

Care Plan (by Problem)

TARGETED QUESTIONS

1. What groups are at high risk for developing TB? What are the most common risk factors for development of TB?
   Hint: See pp. 1254 and 1255 in PPP

2. How does vaccination with BCG affect ppd test results?
   Hint: See p. 1256 in PPP

3. In patients with laboratory-confirmed drug-susceptible active pulmonary *Mycobacterium tuberculosis* (MTB), what are the standard medication(s) and duration of

treatment? How would this differ if the patient were HIV positive?

Hint: See Table 75-3 in PPP

4. The patient's liver function tests are slightly elevated. Why is this important and does it change the management of her TB infection?

Hint: See p. 1262 in PPP

5. How is the efficacy of therapy assessed in the treatment of TB?

Hint: See pp. 1262 and 1263 in PPP

FOLLOW-UP

Four weeks later, the patient returns for follow-up. Her sputum cultures are positive for AFB and the organism is identified as *Mycobacterium tuberculosis* resistant to isoniazid (INH).

6. How does this information change your recommended drug combination and duration of drug therapy?

Hint: See pp. 1258 and 1259 in PPP

7. How should the close contacts of this patient be treated?

Hint: See Table 75-2 in PPP

🌐 GLOBAL PERSPECTIVE

TB remains a leading infectious killer globally. Approximately 2 billion people are infected by *M. tuberculosis*, and roughly 2 million people die from active TB each year despite the fact that it is curable.[1] India, China, Indonesia, Nigeria, and South Africa have the highest number of reported incident cases worldwide. Africa accounts for approximately 80% of the HIV-positive TB cases. HIV is the most important risk factor for active TB, especially among people 25 to 44 years of age. The countries with the highest incidence of multi drug-resistant TB (MDR-TB) are India, China, and Russian Federation.

MDR-TB is defined as resistance to at least INH and rifampin (RIF). Extremely MDRTB (XDR-TB) is MDR-TB that is also resistant to any fluoroquinolone, and at least one of three injectable second-line drugs. MDR- and XDR-TB pose a serious threat to TB control. Other challenges in TB treatment worldwide include lack of qualified human resources, poor infection control, development of new drugs, limitations of available treatment options, insufficient laboratory capacity, and weak surveillance systems.[2] Directly observed therapy (DOT) and therapeutic drug monitoring are ways to optimize therapy. DOT programs have been expanded across the world to ensure that patients with TB can have access to optimal care.

REFERENCES

1. WHO. Global Tuberculosis Control: Epidemiology, Strategy, Financing. WHO Report 2009.
2. The Global Plan to Stop TB 2006-2015: Progress Report 2006-2008. Stop TB Partnership 2009.

CASE SUMMARY

- This patient's current clinical picture is consistent with pulmonary TB, and therapy should be initiated.
- Initial treatment with INH, RIF, PZA, and EMB is recommended. However, after susceptibility test results, the treatment regimen must be revised.
- Liver function tests should be monitored due to drug toxicity and preexisting enzyme elevations.
- Close contacts should be treated with RIF because of INH-resistant strain in the patient.

For more information on the care plan and facilitator's guide please visit http://www.mhpharmacotherapy.com.

80 *Clostridium difficile*— Associated Diarrhea

Jeremiah J. Duby   Brett H. Heintz

CASE LEARNING OBJECTIVES

- Identify the signs and symptoms of *Clostridium difficile*–associated diarrhea (CDAD)
- List the risk factors for CDAD
- Select an appropriate treatment and monitoring plan for antimicrobial therapy
- Consider the role of adjunctive agents and supportive care

PATIENT PRESENTATION

Chief Complaint

"Please give me something for this cramping, diarrhea, and nausea."

History of Present Illness

Shannon Rasmussen is a 69-year-old woman who is brought to the emergency department for a 3-day history of diffuse abdominal pain, fever/chills, frequent, voluminous, foul-smelling stools, and lethargy. Her husband reports that "she has not been able to keep anything down" since her recent discharge and has had 5 to 10 profuse, watery bowel movements per day. The patient was in her usual state of health until a week ago when she developed severe, acute abdominal pain. She was admitted at that time with a small bowel obstruction and received an urgent exploratory laparotomy with resection. Her postoperative course was complicated by a polymicrobial intra-abdominal abscess. She was empirically treated with cefepime and clindamycin, which was changed to ampicillin–sulbactam on the basis of the culture/susceptibility results. She was discharged on amoxicillin–clavulanate to complete a 14-day course.

Past Medical History

Type 2 DM

HTN

OA

Family History

Father died of bone cancer at age 66. Mother died of MI at age 72.

Social History

Married and lives with her husband, aged 45 years.

Tobacco/Alcohol/Substance Use

Social drinker (one to two glasses of wine daily); (−) tobacco or illicit drug use

Allergies/Intolerances/Adverse Drug Events

"Sulfa drugs" cause a rash.

Medications (Current)

Metformin 500 mg PO twice daily

Metoprolol 50 mg PO twice daily

Lisinopril 40 mg PO at bedtime

Ibuprofen 200 to 400 mg PO q 3–4 h as needed

Amoxicillin–clavulanate 875/125 mg PO twice daily (day 13/14)

REVIEW OF SYSTEMS

In addition to her symptoms (as noted in "history of present illness"), the patient reports that her husband gave her some of his prescription-strength esomeprazole for her abdominal pain; however, it did not help. Also, the patient states that she thinks she has lost several pounds over the last month, "since this all began."

Physical Examination

▶ *General*

Elderly woman in acute distress

▶ *Vital Signs*

BP 85/40 mm Hg, HR 120, RR 22, T 38.4°C

Weight 150 lb (68.2 kg)

Height 66 in. (167.6 cm)

Abdominal pain 6/10

▶ *Skin*

Dry and warm with poor turgor

▶ *HEENT*

PERRLA, EOMI; trace of periorbital edema; (−) sinus tenderness; TMs appear normal

▶ *Neck and Lymph Nodes*

Supple. No JVD or palpable lymph nodes

▶ *Chest*

Clear to auscultation. Shallow/rapid breathing

▶ *Breasts*

Examination deferred

▶ *Cardiovascular*

Sinus tachycardia, normal S_1, S_2; (−) S_3 or S_4

▶ *Abdomen*

Abdomen is positive for guarding, tender, and distended. Pain is sharp but diffuse, and it is exacerbated by pressure and movement. Diminished bowel sounds. Recent midline incision is noted.

▶ *Neurology*

Oriented times 2/4. Grossly apathetic and lethargic. Deep tendon reflexes normal

▶ *Genitourinary*

Examination deferred

▶ *Rectal*

Negative guaiac

Laboratory Tests

On admission

	Conventional Units	SI Units
Na	160 mEq/L	160 mmol/L
K	5.2 mEq/L	5.2 mmol/L
Cl	100 mEq/L	100 mmol/L
CO_2	16 mEq/L	16 mmol/L
BUN	42 mg/dL	15 mmol/L
SCr	1.7 mg/dL	150 μmol/L
Glu	180 mg/dL	10 mmol/L
Ca	8 mg/dL	2 mmol/L
Mg	2 mEq/L	1 mmol/L
Phosphate	4.6 mg/dL	1.5 mmol/L
Hgb	9.7 g/dL	97 g/L; 6 mmol/L
Hct	29%	0.29
WBC	$52 \times 10^3/mm^3$	$52 \times 10^9/L$
MCV	$80 \ \mu m^3$	80 fL
Albumin	3 g/dL	30 g/L
Stool sample	Positive for *C. difficile* toxins A/B	

ABG

pH	7.31	
PaO_2	32 mm Hg	4.3 kPa
$PaCO_2$	94 mm Hg	12.5 kPa

Procedures

CT of the abdomen indicates postoperative changes, including a profound ileus and acute dilation of the colon suggestive of toxic megacolon, but reveals complete resolution of the previous abscess.

Sigmoidoscopic examination indicates diffuse erythematous colitis characterized by yellow plaques in distal colon.

Assessment

A 69-year-old woman with signs, symptoms, and laboratory tests consistent with severe CDAD and complications that require direct transfer to the ICU.

Student Workup

Missing Information?

Evaluate: Patient Database

Drug Therapy Problems

Care Plan (by Problem)

TARGETED QUESTIONS

1. What signs and symptoms of CDAD does the patient have?

   Hint: See p. 1275 in PPP

2. What are the patient's risk factors for CDAD?

   Hint: See p. 1274 in PPP

3. What antimicrobial agents are active against *C. difficile*?

   Hint: See pp. 1274 and 1276 in PPP

4. What antimicrobial agent(s) are most appropriate for the patient? (Please include dose, route, frequency, and duration of therapy.)

   Hint: See pp. 1274 and 1276 in PPP

5. List other pharmacologic and nonpharmacologic changes to the patient's therapy that may improve her outcome?

   Hint: See pp. 1274 and 1276 in PPP

6. What clinical and laboratory endpoints should be used to monitor the patient's progress?

   Hint: See p. 1276 in PPP

FOLLOW-UP

The patient presents to the outpatient surgery clinic 8 weeks after successful treatment and discharge with symptoms that she describes as "exactly the same but much milder" compared to those from her previous presentation.

7. How would you characterize another episode of CDAD in the patient? What is the most appropriate antimicrobial therapy at this time? What recommendations can you provide the patient to prevent future episodes?

   Hint: See p. 1276 in PPP

⊙ GLOBAL FOLLOW-UP

Several outbreaks of *C. difficile* have been associated with highly virulent strain (NAP1/027) across the world, specifically first recognized in Canada and United Kingdom in 2003.[1] Since this time, several other outbreaks have been associated with this strain of *C. difficile* with high

toxin production. Oral vancomycin therapy is currently recommended for severe *C. difficile* infection, but many patients may require surgical intervention. The availability of oral vancomycin therapy is limited in certain countries and the IV formulation of vancomycin administered orally is prescribed.

REFERENCE

1. Cohen SH, Gerding DN, Johnson S, et al. Clinical practice guidelines for *Clostridium difficile* infection in adults: 2010 update by the Society of Healthcare Epidemiology of America (SHEA) and the Infectious Diseases Society of America (IDSA). Infect Control Hosp Epidemiol 2010 31(5):431–455.

CASE SUMMARY

- Her current clinical picture is consistent with a *C. difficile* infection, and appropriate antimicrobial therapy should be initiated.

- Oral vancomycin therapy would be a reasonable initial therapy for this patient with a dose of 125 mg PO q 6 h. The patient should be educated on appropriate use and potential GI side effects.

- Since the patient has evidence of toxic megacolon, she may require surgical intervention to remove the affected bowel.

For more information on the care plan and facilitator's guide please visit http://www.mhpharmacotherapy.com.

81 Intra-Abdominal Infection

Sarah M. Adriance   Brian L. Erstad

CASE LEARNING OBJECTIVES

- Recognize the clinical presentation of a secondary intra-abdominal infection involving abscess
- Identify the microorganisms typically involved in secondary intra-abdominal infections
- Develop an appropriate treatment and monitoring plan for a secondary intra-abdominal infection on the basis of specific patient characteristics
- Recommend the most appropriate drug and nondrug interventions to treat a secondary intra-abdominal infection

PATIENT PRESENTATION

Chief Complaint

"I feel sick. My stomach hurts, especially right by my belly button. I have been running a fever for two days."

History of Present Illness

Donny Westling is a 34-year-old male who presents to the emergency department complaining of acute onset of severe abdominal pain, localized in the periumbilical region. Crohn's disease was diagnosed 15 years ago. The patient states that his persistent fever and a localized region of pain in his abdomen are new symptoms for him. His oral intake has decreased over the past week due to the pain. Currently, he receives infliximab infusions for Crohn's disease. Methotrexate was prescribed in the past, but was not tolerated. In the past, intermittent high-dose corticosteroid tapers had been used for disease exacerbations with success. His last flare was 1 month ago. Past medical history also includes a colostomy performed 12 years ago with no subsequent complications.

Past Medical History

Crohn's disease (ileocolonic) diagnosed 15 years ago

Colostomy placement 12 years ago

Family History

Father died at age 36 from colon cancer. Paternal grandmother suffers from osteoporosis.

Social History

Works for a local nonprofit organization. No recent travel history outside the United States.

Tobacco/Alcohol/Substance Use

(−) Alcohol; (−) tobacco or illicit drug use

Allergies/Intolerances/Adverse Drug Events

No known medication allergies

Medications (Current)

Infliximab 760 mg IV q 8 wk

Review of Systems

Malaise and fever for a couple of days despite use of acetaminophen; abdomen tender right of umbilicus with palpable mass that has developed over past few days; abdomen pain increases with eating; (−) significant weight loss, but states that he has lost a couple of pounds this past week; (−) hematochezia; patient reports increase in colostomy output during last week; no history of fistula or abscess formation.

Physical Examination

▶ *General*

Ill-appearing, diaphoretic Caucasian male in moderate acute distress

▶ *Vital Signs*

BP 108/43 mm Hg, P 101, RR 22, T 39.1°C

Weight 145 lb (66 kg)

Height 70 in. (177.8 cm)

Abdominal pain 8/10

▶ *Skin*

(−) Rash, ulcerations, or other skin lesions

▶ *HEENT*

PERRLA, EOMI

▶ *Neck and Lymph Nodes*

Supple; (−) lymphadenopathy

▶ *Chest*

Clear to auscultation

▶ *Cardiovascular*

RRR, normal S_1, S_2; (−) S_3 or S_4

▶ *Abdomen*

Tender with mild guarding to palpitation, small palpable mass present just right of umbilicus; (−) distension

▶ *Neurology*

Grossly intact; deep tendon reflexes normal

▶ *Colorectal*

(+) Colostomy; stoma appears normal

Laboratory Tests

On admission

	Conventional Units	SI Units
Na	140 mEq/L	140 mmol/L
K	3.9 mEq/L	3.9 mmol/L
Cl	101 mEq/L	101 mmol/L
CO_2	22 mEq/L	22 mmol/L
BUN	10 mg/dL	3.6 mmol/L
SCr	0.9 mg/dL	80 µmol/L
Glu	102 mg/dL	5.7 mmol/L
Ca	9.2 mg/dL	2.30 mmol/L
Mg	1.8 mEq/L	0.90 mmol/L
Phosphate	4.2 mg/dL	1.36 mmol/L
Hgb	14.2 g/dL	142 g/L; 8.81 mmol/L
Hct	39.3%	0.393
WBC	$15 \times 10^3/mm^3$	$15 \times 10^9/L$
Albumin	3.1 g/dL	31 g/L
Prealbumin	10 mg/dL	100 mg/L

▶ *Microbiologic Data*

Blood cultures pending

▶ *Imaging*

Abdominal CT shows evidence of abdominal wall abscess arising from terminal ileum.

Assessment

A 34-year-old male with signs, symptoms, and clinical evidence of an intra-abdominal infection secondary to an anterior abdominal wall abscess attributable to the underlying Crohn's disease

Student Workup

Missing Information?

Evaluate: Patient Database
Drug Therapy Problems
Care Plan (by Problem)

TARGETED QUESTIONS

1. What characteristics of the patient's case are consistent with a secondary intra-abdominal infection?

   Hint: See pp. 1283 and 1284 in PPP

2. On the basis of the patient's history and presentation, should empiric antibiotic treatment cover for a monomicrobial or polymicrobial infection?

   Hint: See pp. 1283 and 1286 in PPP

3. What are the likely pathogens on the basis of the patient's site of infection and underlying disease process?

   Hint: See Table 77-1 in PPP

4. What intervention is foremost in the management of an intra-abdominal abscess?

   Hint: See p. 1284 in PPP

FOLLOW-UP

Abdominal wall abscess was accessible via percutaneous CT-guided drainage, which was carried out on day 2 of admission. On discharge, IV antimicrobial therapy was continued and radiologic-evaluation follow-up was scheduled at the end of therapy.

5. For how long should the patient be treated? What are some other aspects of care that should be addressed in the patient?

   Hint: See pp. 1289 and 1290 in PPP

⟳ GLOBAL PERSPECTIVE

Crohn's disease is becoming increasingly common across the world, but there is a higher incidence in industrialized, northern countries potentially due to environmental factors. Additionally, a bimodal age distribution has been shown in certain European countries and the United States. Of these patients with Crohn's disease, up to 30% may experience an intra-abdominal or pelvic abscess during the course of their illness. Abscess formation in Crohn's disease arises from deep fissuring ulceration associated with the transmural nature of the inflammatory process of Crohn's disease. Surgical drainage followed by resection of the bowel disease was once conventional therapy in these patients; however, current management involves percutaneous drainage with interventional radiologic techniques if the abscess is accessible. Appropriate nutrition and consideration of potential complications such as osteoporosis, which can occur due to malabsorption or long-term corticosteroid therapy, are also important aspects of care.

CASE SUMMARY

- The patient's current clinical picture is consistent with a secondary intra-abdominal infection in which management should focus primarily on infection source control with abscess drainage.

- Appropriate empiric antibiotic therapy should cover typical organisms inhabiting area, including enteric Gram-negative bacilli and anaerobic pathogens.

- De-escalation of antibiotic therapy should be initiated when a pathogen(s) is identified to avoid overuse of broad-spectrum antibiotics, although anaerobic coverage should be continued regardless of growth on cultures.

For more information on the care plan and facilitator's guide please visit http://www.mhpharmacotherapy.com.

82 Uncomplicated Urinary Tract Infection

Kathryn R. Matthias

CASE LEARNING OBJECTIVES

- Recognize the common signs and symptoms of uncomplicated urinary tract infections
- Describe factors that may affect empiric therapy for uncomplicated urinary tract infections
- Develop an appropriate plan for treatment of an uncomplicated urinary tract infection
- Evaluate factors that may decrease risk of recurrent urinary tract infections

PATIENT PRESENTATION

Chief Complaint

"I have to go to the bathroom more often and it is getting really annoying."

History of Present Illness

Elizabeth Wilson is a 26-year-old woman who presents to the emergency department with complaints of increased urinary urgency over the past 4 days. The patient reports that she had been diagnosed with a urinary tract infection at the age of 14 years but has had no other urinary tract issues since that time. The patient states that she heard cranberry juice may help with urinary tract infections (UTI) and has drank about 10 cups of cranberry juice over the past couple days but her urinary urgency symptoms seem to be getting worse.

Past Medical History

UTI at age 14 years (treated with trimethoprim–
　　sulfamethoxazole)

History of generalized tonic–clonic seizures (last reported
　　seizure 3.5 years ago)

Hypothyroidism

Seasonal allergies

Family History

Mother and father are both alive. Father is 49 and has a history of HTN. Mother is also 49 and has a history of hypothyroidism.

Social History

Patient works currently as a waitress at a local sandwich cafe but does not have health insurance. She is currently single and broke up with her previous boyfriend 2 weeks ago. She denies smoking, alcohol, and intravenous drug abuse.

Allergies/Intolerances/Adverse Drug Events

Penicillin (unknown reaction)

Valproic acid (rash)

Medications

Cetirizine 10 mg PO daily PRN seasonal allergies

Levothyroxine 50 mcg PO daily

Phenytoin extended-release 300 mg PO daily

Review of Systems

Denies chest pain, SOB, abdominal pain; (+) Dysuria; (+) increase in urinary frequency or urgency (every 1–3 hours during the past 2 days)

Physical Examination

▶ *General*

Well appearing, obese 26-year-old Caucasian woman in no acute distress

▶ *Vital Signs*

BP 122/78 mm Hg, P 72, RR 16, T 38.5°C

Weight 175 lb (80 kg)

Height 61 in. (155 cm)

▶ **Skin**

Dry appearing skin; (−) rashes or lesions

▶ **HEENT**

PERRLA, EOMI; (−) sinus tenderness; TMs appear normal

▶ **Neck and Lymph Nodes**

Thyroid gland symmetrical; (−) nodules; (−) lymphadenopathy

▶ **Chest**

Clear to auscultation

▶ **Cardiovascular**

RRR, normal S_1, S_2; (−) S_3 or S_4

▶ **Abdomen**

Not tender; not distended; (−) organomegaly

▶ **Neurology**

Grossly intact; DTRs normal

▶ **Genitourinary**

Normal external genitalia; (−) vaginal discharge

▶ **Rectal**

No hemorrhoids

Laboratory Tests

	Conventional Units	SI Units
Na	138 mEq/L	138 mmol/L
K	4.5 mEq/L	4.5 mmol/L
Cl	104 mEq/L	104 mmol/L
CO_2	22 mEq/L	22 mmol/L
BUN	5 mg/dL	1.8 mmol/L
SCr	0.6 mg/dL	54 μmol/L
Glu	70 mg/dL	3.9 mmol/L
WBC	13.5×10^3/mm³	13.5×10^9/L
TSH	1.3 μIU/mL	1.3 mIU/L
Phenytoin	12.1 mg/L	47.9 μmol/L
Urinalysis	Urine is yellow, cloudy	
Ph	5.2	

Specific gravity	1.023	
WBC	28 cells/mm³	28×10^6/L
RBC	3 cells/mm³	3×10^6/L
Protein	Trace	
Glucose	(−)	
Ketones	(−)	
Blood	(−)	

▶ **Urine Cultures**

(+) Gram-negative rods—final results pending

Assessment

Twenty-six-year-old woman with s/s, and laboratory tests consistent with an uncomplicated UTI

Student Workup

Missing Information?

Evaluate: Patient Database

Drug Therapy Problems

Care Plan (by Problem)

TARGETED QUESTIONS

1. What signs and symptoms of an uncomplicated UTI does the patient have?

   Hint: See pp. 1307 and 1309 in PPP

2. What risk factors does the patient have for uncomplicated UTIs?

   Hint: See p. 1309 in PPP

3. What treatment options including duration of therapy should be considered in this patient?

   Hint: See p. 1310 and Tables 79-2 and 79-3 in PPP

4. What risks and adverse effects of therapy should be discussed with the patient?

   Hint: Remember to evaluate potential drug–drug interactions with patient's current medication and treatment options. Remember to consider any missing laboratory tests that should be potentially performed prior to start of therapy. See p. 1313 and Table 79-4 in PPP

5. How would you counsel this patient on the expected benefits of "cranberry juice"?

   Hint: Is there any proven benefit of cranberry juice for treatment of UTIs. See p. 1310 in PPP

FOLLOW-UP

One day later, the patient's urine culture and sensitivity results are reported:

Urine culture: *Escherichia coli*

Drug		MIC (mcg/mL or mg/L)
Ampicillin	Sensitive	4
Ampicillin-sulbactam	Sensitive	≤8/4
Amoxicillin-clavulanic acid	Sensitive	≤8/4
Cefazolin	Sensitive	≤8
Ciprofloxacin	Sensitive	0.5
Gentamicin	Resistant	>8
Imipenem	Sensitive	≤0.25
Levofloxacin	Sensitive	≤2
Nitrofurantoin	Sensitive	≤32
Tetracycline	Sensitive	≤4
Trimethoprim–sulfamethoxazole	Resistant	≥8/152

6. Based on the above culture and sensitivity results along with the patient's clinical status, how would you change the patient's UTI therapy?

   Hint: See p. 1314 in Patient Care and Monitoring section in PPP

☽ GLOBAL PERSPECTIVE

Approximately 130 to 175 million cases of uncomplicated cystitis due to *E. coli* occur in premenopausal women worldwide every year. In the United States, these infections have been associated with over $1 billion direct (2003 dollars) in health-care costs per year plus indirect costs due to an average of two restricted-activity days. Although *E. coli* urinary isolate resistance rates to ampicillin and trimethoprim–sulfamethoxazole have increased over the past couple of decades worldwide based on surveillance reports, fluoroquinolone resistance rates (specifically ciprofloxacin and levofloxacin) have also increased significantly in Europe and Canada in the past decade. Development of such resistance has limited empiric treatment options in certain patient populations.[2,3]

REFERENCE

1. Russo TA, Johnson JR. Medical and economic impact of extraintestinal infections due to *Escherichia coli*: Focus on an increasingly important endemic problem. Microbes Infect 2003 5:449–456.
2. Oteo J, Pérez-Vázquez M, Campos J. Extended-spectrum beta-lactamase producing *Escherichia coli*: changing epidemiology and clinical impact. Curr Opin Infect Dis 2010 23:320–326.
3. Johnson JR, Johnston B, Calbots C, et al. *Escherichia coli* sequence type ST131 as the major cause of serious multidrug-resistant *E. coli* infections in the United States. Clin Infect Dis 2010 51:286–294.

CASE SUMMARY

- The patient's signs and symptoms are consistent with an uncomplicated urinary tract infection.
- Although there are several options for empiric uncomplicated urinary tract infection therapy, patient-specific factors including drug allergies, renal function, potential drug–drug interactions, and teratogenicity potential should be evaluated prior to antibiotic selection.
- The patient should be counseled on potential adverse effects of antibiotic therapy.

For more information on the care plan and facilitator's guide please visit http://www.mhpharmacotherapy.com.

83 Complicated Urinary Tract Infection

Kathryn R. Matthias

CASE LEARNING OBJECTIVES

- Recognize the common signs and symptoms of complicated urinary tract infections
- Describe factors that may affect empiric therapy for complicated urinary tract infections
- Develop an appropriate plan for treatment of an complicated urinary tract infection
- Evaluate factors that may decrease risk of recurrent complicated urinary tract infections

PATIENT PRESENTATION

Chief Complaint (from Patient's Wife)

"He is not acting like himself … he seems really confused."

History of Present Illness

Joseph Jones is a 74-year-old man, assisted-living facility resident, who is transferred to ABC Medical Center due to altered mental status. Initial differential diagnosis includes bacteremia, sepsis from a urinary source, UTI, or meningitis. On the basis of diagnostic studies including a chest x-ray and CT scan along with laboratory data, it is determined that the patient's altered mental status is due to a complicated UTI and dehydration from acute N/V. The patient is started on ciprofloxacin 200 mg IV q 12.

Past Medical History

History of acute kidney injury, resolved 6 months ago
HTN

Past Surgical History

Kidney abscess, s/p drainage with pigtail catheter
    6 months ago
Right knee surgery in 1974

Family History

Mother died at the age of 68 and had a past medical history significant for HTN and type 2 diabetes mellitus. Father died at the age of 72 and had a past medical history significant for COPD. Patient has two children and five grandchildren, none with any significant medical history.

Social History

Patient and his wife are currently residents of an assisted-living facility. They moved to this facility 4 years ago after his wife's hip replacement. As per the patient's wife, he does not smoke or drink alcohol.

Allergies/Intolerances/Adverse Drug Events

NKDA

Medications

Fluoxetine 10 mg PO daily
Esomeprazole 40 mg PO daily

Review of Systems

(+) Fever; (+) vomiting; (−) eye changes; (−) complaints of chest pain or shortness of breath

Physical Examination

▶ *General*

Acutely ill male with decreased level of consciousness who is sleepy but arousable and able to answer yes and no questions

▶ **Vital Signs**

BP 102/56 mm Hg, P 108, RR 24, T 38.3°C, saturation 100% on a nonrebreather mask

Weight 154 lb (70 kg)

Height 69 in. (175 cm)

▶ **Skin**

Dry appearing skin; (−) rashes or lesions

▶ **HEENT**

PERRLA, EOMI, head normocephalic, mucous membranes dry

▶ **Neck and Lymph Nodes**

(−) Nodules; (−) lymphadenopathy

▶ **Chest**

Clear to auscultation bilaterally

▶ **Cardiovascular**

RRR, normal S_1, S_2; no murmurs

▶ **Abdomen**

Not tender; not distended; (+) bowel sounds

▶ **Neurology**

Patient will open eyes to gentle stimulus; he is able to follow commands and move extremities

▶ **Genitourinary**

Normal external genitalia

▶ **Rectal**

No hemorrhoids

Laboratory Tests

	Conventional Units	SI Units
Na	142 mEq/L	142 mmol/L
K	4.7 mEq/L	4.7 mmol/L
Cl	108 mEq/L	108 mmol/L
CO_2	19 mEq/L	19 mmol/L
BUN	28 mg/dL	10 mmol/L
SCr	2.4 mg/dL	212 μmol/L
Glu	140 mg/dL	7.8 mmol/L
Ca	9.7 mg/dL	2.43 mmol/L
WBC	3.9×10^3/mm³	3.9×10^9/L
Neutrophils	78%	0.78
Bands	11%	0.11
Hgb	12.1 g/dL	121 g/L; 7.50 mmol/L
HCT	36.9%	0.369

Platelets	192×10^3/mm³	192×10^9/L
Urinalysis	Urine is yellow, cloudy	
pH	5.50	
Specific gravity	1.012	
WBC	>150 cells/mm³	$>150 \times 10^6$/L
RBC	48 cells/mm³	48×10^6/L
Protein	(+)	
Glucose	(−)	
Ketones	(−)	
Blood	Moderate	
Nitrate	(+)	
Casts	(−)	
Urine toxicology	(−)	

▶ **Blood Cultures**

(−) No growth

Urine cultures (obtained after placement of a foley catheter):

Klebsiella pneumoniae (>100,000 colonies/mL)—extended spectrum β-lactamase (ESBL) producing

Drug		MIC (mcg/mL or mg/L)
Amikacin	Susceptible	16
Ampicillin	Resistant	≥32
Cefepime	Susceptible	8
Ceftriaxone	Resistant	≥8
Cephazolin	Resistant	≥64
Ciprofloxacin	Resistant	≥4
Gentamicin	Resistant	≥4
Levofloxacin	Resistant	≥8
Imipenem	Susceptible	≤1
Meropenem	Susceptible	1
Nitrofurantoin	Susceptible	≤32
Piperacillin–tazobactam	Resistant	≥128/4
Trimethoprim–sulfamethoxazole	Resistant	≥16/304

Assessment

Seventy-four-year-old man with s/s, and laboratory tests consistent with a complicated UTI

Student Workup

Missing Information?

Evaluate:　Patient Database

Drug Therapy Problems

Care Plan (by Problem)

TARGETED QUESTIONS

1. What signs and symptoms does the patient have of a complicated UTI?

   Hint: See pp. 1307 and 1309 in PPP

2. What risk factors does the patient have for complicated UTI?

   Hint: See p. 1309 in PPP

3. On day 2, the patient serum creatinine has decreased to 1.8 mg/dL (159 μmol/L). On the basis of the patient's urine culture and clinical factors, what changes do you recommend to the patient's UTI therapy?

   Hint: See p. 1310 and Tables 79-2 and 79-3 in PPP

4. How should the patient be monitored for resolution of infection and ADEs?

   Hint: See p. 1313 and Table 79-4 in PPP

5. How long should the patient's UTI therapy be continued?

   Hint: See p. 1310 and Tables 79-2 and 79-3 in PPP

FOLLOW-UP

The patient's UTI symptoms improved and he was discharged from the hospital 4 days after admission. He received his UTI therapy as prescribed through a home health program at his assisted-living facility. Unfortunately, 2 months later he fell and fractured his left hip. An indwelling urinary catheter was inserted and 2 weeks later a urine culture is obtained when the catheter was being exchanged. The culture grew *Enterococcus* species (10,000–100,000 colonies/mL) and *Escherichia coli* (<10,000 colonies/mL). The urine sample has a pH 5.50, specific gravity 1.008, WBC 8 cells/mm³ (8×10^6/L), RBC 12 cells/mm³ (12×10^6/L), protein (+), glucose (−), ketones (−), and nitrate (−).

6. What would be the appropriate therapy for the patient?

   Hint: See p. 1313 in PPP

⊙ GLOBAL PERSPECTIVE

Worldwide the most common cause of nosocomial infection is associated with the use of urinary catheters that lead to UTIs.[1,2] Patients with an indwelling catheter have an estimated daily 5% incidence of UTIs. Therefore, the best way to avoid catheter-associated UTIs is to remove the catheter when no longer indicated as soon as possible based on the patient's clinical status. In addition, catheter-associated UTI have been estimated to cost more than four times the cost of a systematic UTIs in a patient without a catheter.[3]

REFERENCES

1. Hooton TM, Bradley SF, Cardenas DD, et al. Diagnosis, prevention, and treatment of catheter-associated urinary tract infection in adults: 2009 International Clinical Practice Guidelines from the Infectious Diseases Society of America. Clin Infect Dis 2010 50:625–663.

2. Gould CV, Umscheid CA, Agarwal RK, et al. Healthcare Infection Control Practices Advisory Committee: Guideline for prevention of catheter-associated urinary tract infections, 2009. http://www.cdc.gov/ncidod/dhqp/dpac_uti_pc.html. Accessed December 9, 2009.

3. Saint S. Clinical and economic consequences of nosocomial catheter-related bacteriuria. Am J Infect Control 2000 28:68–75.

CASE SUMMARY

- The patient's signs and symptoms are consistent with a complicated UTI.

- Although the majority of urinary tract infections are caused by *E. coli*, non-*E. coli* causes are more common in patients with complicated UTIs, patients with recurrent UTIs, and nosocomial UTIs.

- Recommended duration of therapy is usually longer for complicated UTIs and catheter-associated UTIs compared with uncomplicated UTIs.

For more information on the care plan and facilitator's guide please visit http://www.mhpharmacotherapy.com.

84 Syphilis

Patty Ghazvini   Angela Singh

CASE LEARNING OBJECTIVES

- Analyze the behavioral considerations and assess the importance of contraception with regard to the contributing factors
- Apply the "expedited partner treatment" method when recommending treatment
- Identify the patient populations that are epidemiologically affected
- Identify the clinical signs and symptoms associated with tertiary syphilis
- Select an appropriate therapy for the management of syphilitic meningitis
- Develop an appropriate treatment and monitoring plan for the management of syphilitic meningitis

PATIENT SUMMARY

Chief Complaint

"I have been feeling very dizzy and have had a severe headache since last night."

History of Present Illness

A 35-year-old Hispanic female presents to her physician with complaints of a severe headache accompanied by vomiting and dizziness that has been present for 2 days.

Past Medical History

Syphilis × 3 years

Depression × 5 years

GERD × 1 year

HIV × 1 month

HTN × 2 years

Recurrent yeast infections

Family History

Father had colon cancer and died at the age of 55. Mother is alive at age 65, with a history of alcoholism and depression. She has two sisters who are alive and healthy.

Social History

The patient came to the United States from Mexico at the age of 13. She is fluent in both English and Spanish. Currently, she is married and lives with her husband of 5 years; she has one child of age 3. She works at a retail clothing store.

Tobacco/Alcohol/Substance Abuse

Smokes 1 ppd × 15 years; (−) alcohol; (−) illicit drug use

Allergies/Intolerances/Adverse Drug Events

Penicillin (anaphylaxis)

Medications (Current)

Effexor XR 150 mg PO q 24 h

Yaz one tablet PO q 24 h

Lisinopril 40 mg PO q 24 h

Sustiva 600 mg PO q 24 h at bedtime

Truvada PO q 24 h

St. John's Wort one tablet PO daily

Tylenol 500 mg PO q 4 h PRN headache

Medications (Past)

Doxycycline 100 mg PO q 12 h × 14 days for the treatment of syphilis

Monistat 7

Vagistat-1

Diflucan 150 mg PO × two tablets

Review of Systems

Headache, not relieved with nonaspirin pain reliever; (−) tinnitus; (+) vertigo; (+) infection; (+) Kernig's sign; (+) Brudzinski's sign; (+) cervical rigidity; (+) photophobia; (−) history of seizures, syncope, or loss of consciousness; A&O × 3; (−) rash; (−) petechiae; (+) hyperpigmentation of palms.

Physical Examination

► **General**

Ill-appearing adult female in acute distress

► **Vital Signs**

BP 166/96, P 88, RR 16, T 40°C

Weight 180 lb (82 kg)

Height 60 in. (152 cm)

► **Skin**

(−) Rashes; (−) lesions

► **HEENT**

PERRLA; EOMI; (−) hemorrhages or papilledema

► **Neck**

(+) Cervical rigidity; (−) lymphadenopathy

► **Neurology**

(+) Kernig's sign; (+) Brudzinski's sign; A&O × 3

► **Chest**

Clear to auscultation

► **Breast**

Examination deferred

► **Abdomen**

Soft, nontender, nondistended

► **Genitourinary**

Examination deferred

► **Rectal**

Examination deferred

Laboratory Tests

	Conventional Units	SI Units
Na	141 mEq/L	141 mmol/L
K	4.5 mEq/L	4.5 mmol/L
Cl	103 mEq/L	103 mmol/L
BUN	9 mg/dL	3.2 mmol/L
SCr	0.9 mg/dL	80 mmol/L
Glucose	99 mg/dL	5.5 mmol/L
Hgb	13.5 g/dL	135 g/L; 8.38 mmol/L
Hct	41.2%	0.412
WBC	$3.5 \times 10^3/mm^3$	$3.5 \times 10^9/L$
Lymphocytes	46.1%	0.461
Monocytes	16.5%	0.165
Eosinophils	4.2%	0.042
Basophils	1%	0.01
Neutrophils	32.2%	0.322
ANC	$1.1 \times 10^3/mm^3$	$1.1 \times 10^9/L$
HIV RNA	Nondetectable	
CD4	360 cells/mm³	$360 \times 10^6/L$

► **Blood Cultures**

No growth

► **CSF Findings**

	Conventional Units	SI Units
WBC	100 cells/mm³	$100 \times 10^6/L$
Protein	68 mg/dL	680 mg/L
Glucose	35 mg/dL	1.9 mmol/L
Gram stain	Negative	
VDRL	1:32	

Assessment

A 35-year-old female with signs, symptoms, and laboratory tests consistent with syphilitic meningitis

---

Student Workup

Missing Information?

Evaluate: Patient Database

Drug Therapy Problems

Care Plan (by Problem)

TARGETED QUESTIONS

1. What is the causative agent associated with syphilis?

   Hint: See p. 1321 in PPP

2. What are the clinical signs and symptoms associated with neurosyphilis?

   Hint: Please refer to CDC Guidelines (2006), Sexually Transmitted Diseases Treatment Guidelines, at http://www.cdc.gov/mmwr/preview/mmwrhtml/rr5511a1.htm (see "Symptomatic Neurosyphilis" section)

3. Which form of penicillin is recommended for the management of neurosyphilis?

   Hint: See p. 1322 in PPP

4. Should the patient's husband be treated for syphilis?

   Hint: Please refer to CDC Guidelines (2006), Sexually Transmitted Diseases Treatment Guidelines, at http://www.cdc.gov/mmwr/preview/mmwrhtml/rr5511a1.htm (see "General Principles" and "Management of Sex Partners" sections)

5. What monitoring parameters should be implemented in the patient and what are our goals of therapy?

   Hint: See pp. 1324–1326 in PPP

FOLLOW-UP

After having a conversation with the physician, JR's spouse agrees to be tested for syphilis and his VDRL titer returns as 1:32.

6. Her husband requires treatment, what is the recommended therapy?

7. Penicillin is recommended for him, what formulation is used? Justify your answer.

8. An individual is allergic to penicillin, what would be the appropriate procedure for performing penicillin desensitization?

☉ GLOBAL PERSPECTIVE

STDs present a major public health concern in both industrialized and developing countries. However, since different countries have different types and levels of reporting systems of STD statistics, it is thought that many reports substantially underestimate the number of new STD cases because of social stigma and other factors prevent people from seeking health care. A WHO report published in 2001 provides estimates of the extent of the world's STD epidemics as they were in 1999, and as of early 2007, there were no more recent international estimates. Syphilis is a bacterial infection that is usually sexually transmitted, but may also be passed from an infected mother to an unborn child. It is a curable STD, which if left untreated, can eventually lead to irreversible damage to the heart and nervous system. An estimated 12.22 million cases of syphilis occurred worldwide in 1999, with an increase in incidence in Eastern Europe and Central Asia, Sub-Saharan Africa, Latin America, and the Caribbean. STDs are a major global cause of acute illness, infertility, long-term disability, and death, with severe medical and psychologic consequences for millions of men, women, and children. The WHO states that "in developing countries, STDs and their complications are amongst the top five disease categories for which adults seek health care. In women of childbearing age, STDs are second only to maternal factors as causes of disease and death." Many STDs can be treated and cured relatively easily and cheaply if diagnosed early enough. To combat these epidemics, patients must have access to testing and treatment facilities and become more educated about prevention of STDs.

CASE SUMMARY

- The patient with a history of syphilis is treated previously with doxycycline.

- Her current clinical presentation is consistent with syphilitic meningitis, and appropriate antibiotic therapy should be initiated.

- The patient may need to undergo desensitization due to her history of penicillin allergy.

For more information on the care plan and facilitator's guide please visit http://www.mhpharmacotherapy.com.

85 Gonorrhea, Chlamydia, and Herpes Simplex Type 2

Marlon S. Honeywell   Patty Ghazvini
Angela Singh

CASE LEARNING OBJECTIVES

- Recognize the signs and symptoms of gonorrhea, chlamydia, and herpes simplex type 2
- Identify the pertinent diagnostic techniques and goals of therapy
- Develop an appropriate treatment and monitoring plan for the infection(s)
- Select an appropriate pharmacologic agent to treat the infection(s)
- Educate the patient regarding the administration of medications and the importance of self-care

PATIENT PRESENTATION

Chief Complaint

"I have been having pain when I urinate. I tried an over-the-counter drug, but it didn't help. I just can't take it anymore. And please don't forget to refill all of my narcotics. Last time, the nurse only called in one of them."

History of Present Illness

CR is a 47-year-old Latin American female who regularly visits the local community health center for a myriad of health reasons, with the latest visit revolving around complaints of a purulent, vaginal discharge and pain on urination. After self-testing with Azo Test Strips and detecting a positive result, she subsequently began orally taking phenazopyridine for 4 days with minimal relief. She admits that her dysuric symptoms commenced approximately 10 days prior and have worsened over the past 2 days. Additionally, she admits to observing the resurgence of a cluster of small, painful, itchy bumps in her vaginal area. When asked by the clinician to describe her recent sexual history, she acknowledged that she does not have a steady boyfriend and that she currently engages in frequent sexual activity with two men, one of which she traveled to Hawaii with last week for vacation. Finally, as she requested a refill on her narcotics and her BP, cholesterol, and diabetic medications, she divulged that she felt "tingling" in her hands and feet and that she has been constipated for

3 days although she has been taking docusate sodium for 2 consecutive days.

Past Medical History

HTN diagnosed 7 years ago

Type 2 DM diagnosed 5 years ago

Hyperlipidemia diagnosed 1 year ago

Back pain from car accident that occured 3 months ago

Family History

The patient's father had a CAD and died of an MI at age 70. Her mother is alive at age 64 with HTN, diabetes, and osteoporosis. She has two sisters, one of which has been recently diagnosed with diabetes.

Social History

The patient migrated to the United States at age 16 from Mexico. She speaks fluent Spanish and English, and is a single mother, who lives alone with one son, age 20, from a previous marriage. As a result of the recession, her original job as a receptionist for a car dealership was terminated 4 months ago. She was recently hired (3 weeks prior to her visit) as a receptionist for a prominent law firm.

Tobacco/Alcohol/Substance Abuse

Social drinker; (−) tobacco or illicit drug use

Allergies/Intolerances/Adverse Drug Events

Tetracycline (rash as a child)

Propoxyphene (rash)

Medications

Glyburide 2.5 mg PO q AM

HCTZ 12.5 mg PO q AM

Amlodipine 2.5 mg PO q AM

Atorvastatin 40 mg PO q AM

Calcium carbonate one to two tablets PO q 8–12 h PRN

Docusate sodium 100 mg PO q AM

Hydrocodone 7.5 mg/acetaminophen 750 mg one to two tablets PO q 4–6 h PRN pain

Oxycodone 5 mg/acetaminophen 500 mg two tablets PO q 4–6 h PRN severe pain

Acetaminophen 325 mg one to two capsules PO q 4–6 h PRN pain

Review of Systems

Occasional headaches relieved by acetaminophen; (+) fever; (−) tinnitus and vertigo; increased urinary frequency with pain; (+) bowel distention on palpation; (−) history of seizures, syncope, or loss of consciousness; reports "tingling" in the extremities; (−) rhabdomyolysis; fruity breath; dry mucus membranes; deep and rapid breathing.

Physical Examination

▸ General

Overweight, middle-aged, Latin American woman in no acute distress

▸ Vital Signs

BP 150/97 mm Hg, P 74, RR 22, T 38.9°C (102.0°F)

Weight 190.3 lb (86.5 kg)

Height 66 in. (168 cm)

▸ Skin

Skin slightly dry; (−) rash or lesions

▸ HEENT

PERRLA; EOMI; TMs appear normal

▸ Neck and Lymph Nodes

Thyroid gland smooth and symmetrical; (−) thyroid nodules; (+) lymphadenopathy

▸ Chest

Clear to auscultation

▸ Breasts

Examination deferred

▸ Cardiovascular

RRR, normal S_1, S_2; (−) S_3 or S_4

▸ Abdomen

Non tender/distended; (−) organomegaly

▸ Neurology

Grossly intact; deep tendon reflexes normal

▸ Genitourinary

Cluster of vesicles

▸ Rectal

Examination deferred

Laboratory Tests

Fasting, obtained 3 months ago

	Conventional Units	SI Units
Na	139 mEq/L	139 mmol/L
K	4.4 mEq/L	4.4 mmol/L
Cl	103 mEq/L	103 mmol/L
CO_2	22 mEq/L	22 mmol/L
BUN	12 mg/dL	4.3 mmol/L
SCr	0.9 mg/dL	80 mmol/L
Glu	135 mg/dL	7.5 mmol/L
Ca	10.1 mg/dL	2.53 mmol/L
Mg	1.7 mEq/L	0.85 mmol/L
Phosphate	3.7 mg/dL	1.20 mmol/L
pH (arterial)	7.38	
Hgb	13 g/dL	130 g/L; 8.07 mmol/L
Hct	41%	0.41
WBC	$4.1 \times 10^3/mm^3$	$4.1 \times 10^9/L$
MCV	89 um³	89 fL
Albumin	3.9 g/dL	39 g/L
Total cholesterol	183 mg/dL	4.73 mmol/L
LDL cholesterol	91 mg/dL	2.35 mmol/L
HDL cholesterol	36 mg/dL	0.93 mmol/L
AST	45 IU/L	0.75 µkat/L
ALT	51 IU/L	0.85 µkat/L
HbA_{1C}	6.9%	0.069

Fasting, obtained yesterday

	Conventional Units	SI Units
Na	127 mEq/L	127 mmol/L
K	3.5 mEq/L	3.5 mmol/L
Cl	82 mEq/L	82 mmol/L
CO_2	18 mEq/L	18 mmol/L
BUN	40 mg/dL	14.3 mmol/L

SCr	1.6 mg/dL	141 mmol/L
Glu	180 mg/dL	10 mmol/L
Ca	10.1 mg/dL	2.53 mmol/L
Mg	1.8 mEq/L	0.90 mmol/L
Phosphate	3.8 mg/dL	1.23 mmol/L
pH (arterial)	7.21	
Urinalysis	(+) ketones	
Hgb	14 g/dL	140 g/L; 8.69 mmol/L
Hct	42%	0.42
WBC	$10.7 \times 10^3/mm^3$	$10.7 \times 10^9/L$
MCV	88 μm³	88 fL
Albumin	3.7 g/dL	37 g/L
Total cholesterol	185 mg/dL	4.78 mmol/L
LDL cholesterol	92 mg/dL	2.38 mmol/L
HDL cholesterol	34 mg/dL	0.88 mmol/L
AST	120 IU/L	2 μkat/L
ALT	130 IU/L	2.17 μkat/L
HbA$_{1C}$	10%	0.10

► **Urine Culture**

Ordered

Assessment

A 47-year-old woman with signs, symptoms, and laboratory tests consistent with a gonococcal infection.

Further, the patient has constipation and uncontrolled HTN and diabetes.

Student Workup

Missing Information?

Evaluate: Patient Database

Drug Therapy Problems

Care Plan (by Problem)

TARGETED QUESTIONS

1. What are the signs and symptoms of a gonococcal infection?

   Hint: See p. 1318 in PPP

2. Are there any other possible infections besides gonorrhea?

   Hint: See p. 1319 in PPP

3. When infected with gonorrhea, what is the probability of a coinfection?

   Hint: See p. 1320 in PPP

4. Does recent travel affect the selection of drug therapy?

   Hint: See p. 1319 in PPP

5. Should treatment be provided for her partner?

   Hint: See p. 1318 in PPP

6. What is the etiology of the elevated hepatic enzymes?

   Hint: Liver enzymes may be elevated for a variety of reasons. Since the patient's past medical history is inconsistent with hepatic damage, a medication-induced elevation of liver enzymes is a reasonable suspicion. See p. 394 in PPP

FOLLOW-UP

Twelve weeks later, the patient returns for a follow-up. Although reevaluation of her infection is not required, it is vital to express the importance of altering her sexual behaviors and reiterate the importance of practicing preventive measures (i.e., condoms, spermicides) and to determine whether her partners have received treatment. Essential to this process is an interaction between the patient and a knowledgeable, yet patient-friendly, clinician.

7. How can this be accomplished?

   Hint: See p. 1318 in PPP

Finally, the clinician and the patient must gain control of her HTN and diabetes by promoting a healthy diet, exercise, and continuous self-monitoring; effectively altering her medications to achieve optimal BP and glucose measurements; and scheduling the patient for education classes on diabetes.

⚙ GLOBAL PERSPECTIVE

Globally, new cases of STDs amenable to antimicrobial treatment amount to approximately 340 million per year. Evidence supports the need for better control of gonorrhea, especially with the emergence of fluoroquinolone-resistant strains of *Neisseria gonorrhoeae*. Such strains have been documented in several other countries, including Australia, China, India, Korea, and New Zealand. Another notable concern is the appearance of diminished gonococcal susceptibility to the third-generation cephalosporins, of which cefixime and ceftriaxone are commonly prescribed as effective options. Once 5% resistance or more to an antibiotic is recognized, the WHO recommends that the antibiotic be removed from the treatment recommendations for gonorrhea. Diminished susceptibility of *N. gonorhoeae* to drugs of choice has been attributed to the overuse and misuse of antibiotics in a nonregulated environment. Although instituting change may be complex, global integration of treatment measures may be more feasible than continuing to rely on antibiotics as the primary mechanism of control.

CASE SUMMARY

- Her clinical picture is consistent with a gonococcal infection and with herpes simplex type 2. Patient counseling and effective treatment measures are necessary. In addition to covering the primary organisms, treatment should also cover *Chlamydia trachomatis*.

- Ceftriaxone 125 mg IM and azithromycin 1 g PO as a one-time dose is reasonable for the coverage of gonorrhea and chlamydia. Administering a fluoroquinolone to this patient is inappropriate as the patient recently traveled to Hawaii, an area where resistant strains have been observed.

- Valacyclovir 1 g orally once daily for 7 days is appropriate for the treatment of herpes simplex.

- Expedited partner treatment should be instituted in this case.

For more information on the care plan and facilitator's guide please visit http://www.mhpharmacotherapy.com.

86 Acute Osteomyelitis

Melinda M. Neuhauser   Susan L. Pendland

CASE LEARNING OBJECTIVES

- Identify the goals of therapy for acute osteomyelitis
- Identify the clinical signs, symptoms, and laboratory/radiographic tests in the diagnosis and therapeutic monitoring of acute osteomyelitis
- Develop an appropriate treatment and monitoring plan for acute osteomyelitis
- Educate the patient regarding disease state and drug therapy

PATIENT PRESENTATION

Chief Complaint

"I have severe pain in my left arm, which was broken in a car accident last week. I've taken a few pain pills since then, but now it really hurts. Maybe I need a stronger pain pill."

History of Present Illness

Sam Cole is an 18-year-old Caucasian male who presented to the emergency department complaining of severe pain in his left upper arm. He met with a car accident 7 days ago and suffered an open fracture of the left proximal humerus. At that time, he was admitted to the surgical unit of the hospital and underwent irrigation and debridement. He received pre- and postoperative cefazolin, and was discharged after overnight observation on an oral antibiotic and PRN pain medications. At the time of discharge, the patient showed no sign of infection and required only occasional hydrocodone/acetaminophen for pain. He was scheduled for a follow-up office visit with the orthopedic surgeon in 1 week.

Past Medical History

Asthma, diagnosed in childhood
Allergic rhinitis, diagnosed in childhood

Family History

Father is 46 years old with type 2 DM and HTN, whereas mother is 43 years old with asthma. He has a younger sister in high school. Both sets of grandparents are alive.

Social History

The patient graduated from high school and currently attends community college. He lives with his parents and maintains a part-time job at a movie theater. His health insurance is covered under his father's insurance plan.

Tobacco/Alcohol/Substance Use

Occasionally drinks beer; denies tobacco and illicit drug use

Allergies/Intolerance/Adverse Drug Events

Benadryl causes him to be "jittery."

Medications (Current)

Cephalexin 500 mg one capsule PO q 6 h for 7 days

Ibuprofen 400 mg one tablet PO q 6 h PRN mild-to-moderate arm pain

Hydrocodone/acetaminophen 5/500 mg one tablet PO q 4 h PRN severe arm pain

Fluticasone/salmeterol 250/50 mg one puff twice daily

Albuterol one to two puffs q 4 h PRN wheezing (needs refill)

Loratadine 10 mg one tablet PO once daily

Fluticasone intranasal spray two puffs each nostril once daily PRN allergies

Acetaminophen 500 mg one to two tablets PO PRN headaches

Review of Systems

The patient experiences frequent headaches usually relieved with extra-strength acetaminophen, although he admits that he also uses some "sinus medication" that his grandparents bought at Walmart; he reports that his breathing is fine now, although he has had several hospital admissions for asthma in the past year, for which he received IV antibiotics, steroids, and nebulizer treatments. He has noticed that his breathing and allergies worsen when he spends a lot of time with his friends who smoke. He thought his arm had been getting better and attributed the recent severe pain to not keeping the arm immobile after going back to work.

Physical Examination

► General

Young adult male with arm in sling and experiencing acute pain in recently fractured arm

► Vital Signs

BP 117/76 mm Hg, P 85, RR 16, T 37.9°C

Weight 162.8 lb (74 kg)

Height 69 in. (175.3 cm)

Reports acute pain in fractured arm (pain 6/10)

► Skin

Swelling around the surgical wound

► HEENT

Swollen nasal mucosa; rhinorrhea

► Neck and Lymph Nodes

(−) Lymphadenopathy

► Chest

Mild expiratory wheezing on auscultation

► Cardiovascular

RRR, normal S_1, S_2; (−) S_3 or S_4

► Abdomen

Not tender/not distended

► Neurology

Grossly intact; deep tendon reflexes normal

► Genitourinary

Examination deferred

► Rectal

Examination deferred

Laboratory Tests

Obtained today in emergency department

	Conventional Units	SI Units
Na	141 mEq/L	141 mmol/L
K	3.9 mEq/L	3.9 mmol/L
Cl	101 mEq/L	101 mmol/L
CO_2	25 mEq/L	25 mmol/L
BUN	5 mg/dL	1.8 mmol/L
SCr	0.5 mg/dL	44 μmol/L
Glu	145 mg/dL	8 mmol/L
Hgb	15 g/dL	150 g/L; 9.31 mmol/L
Hct	43.7%	0.437
WBC	$10.1 \times 10^3/mm^3$	$10.1 \times 10^9/L$
ESR	119 mm/h	
CRP	68 mg/dL (680 mg/L)	

Microbiology

Blood culture (× 2): Pending

Bone biopsy: Gram stain shows Gram-positive cocci in clusters; culture pending

Imaging

Plain radiograph: Positive for soft-tissue swelling

Radionuclide bone scan: Positive for increased uptake in left proximal humerus

Assessment

An 18-year-old male with signs, symptoms, and laboratory and imaging tests consistent with acute osteomyelitis

Student Workup

Missing Information?

Evaluate: Patient Database

Drug Therapy Problems

Care Plan (by Problem)

TARGETED QUESTIONS

1. What antimicrobial agent(s), dosage regimen, and monitoring would you recommend for this patient?

   Hint: See p. 1341 in PPP

2. What duration of antimicrobial therapy do you anticipate for this patient?

   Hint: See pp. 1343–1344 in PPP

3. Is this patient an appropriate candidate for step-down oral therapy?

   Hint: See p. 1341 in PPP

4. What counseling topics would you discuss with this patient?

   Hint: See p. 1345 in PPP

FOLLOW-UP

The patient was started on an IV antimicrobial regimen through an outpatient infusion center. The bone aspirate grew *Staphylococcus aureus* (resistant to penicillin, oxacillin, cefazolin, clindamycin, erythromycin; sensitive to vancomycin, tetracycline, trimethoprim/sulfamethoxazole). Blood cultures were negative with no growth × 5 days. Following 1 week of therapy, he reports only minimal pain associated with extension of the arm that is necessary with certain daily functions (e.g., getting dressed). Laboratory tests were drawn yesterday.

Please answer the following questions with the assumption that the patient was started on IV vancomycin twice daily through an outpatient infusion center:

5. What, if any, modifications would you recommend regarding this patient's drug therapy if the vancomycin steady-state trough concentration was 10.5 mcg/mL (7.2 μmol/L)? Assume that renal function is stable, and a slight decline in ESR and CRP was observed following 1 week of IV therapy.

   Hint: See pp. 1344–1345 and Table 81-2 in PPP

6. What, if any, modifications would you recommend regarding this patient's drug therapy if the MIC of *S. aureus* against vancomycin was 2 mcg/mL (1.4 μmol/L)? Assuming that renal function is stable, a therapeutic vancomycin concentration was achieved, and a minimal decline in ESR, CRP, and WBC was observed following 1 week of IV therapy.

   Hint: See p. 1343 and Table 81-2 in PPP

7. The physician is considering completing the course of treatment with 2 weeks of oral therapy. What oral antimicrobial agents(s) would you recommend for this patient?

   Hint: See p. 1343 and Table 81-2 in PPP

☼ GLOBAL PERSPECTIVE

Acute osteomyelitis affects patients, particularly pediatric patients, throughout the world. In developing countries, the diagnosis of acute osteomyelitis may be more challenging with limited access to advanced imaging studies (e.g., nuclear medicine scans). Antimicrobial therapy may differ globally on the basis of local or regional susceptibility patterns, access to hospitals or infusion centers, and drug availability. For example, non–FDA-approved antistaphylococcal agents such as teicoplanin, fusidic acid, and fosfomycin are available in certain developed and developing countries outside the United States. Similarly, newer anti-MRSA agents such as linezolid or daptomycin may not be available in many developing countries.

CASE SUMMARY

- His clinical picture and diagnostic tests are consistent with acute osteomyelitis secondary to direct trauma.
- IV antimicrobial therapy should be initiated on the basis of microbiology culture and sensitivity results.
- An optimal dosage regimen should be utilized to obtain drug concentrations at the site of infection as well as effectiveness and safety parameters should be monitored to guide therapy.

For more information on the care plan and facilitator's guide please visit http://www.mhpharmacotherapy.com.

87 Sepsis Syndromes

Sara A. Stahle   Brian L. Erstad

CASE LEARNING OBJECTIVES

- Recognize the signs and symptoms of systemic inflammatory response syndrome (SIRS), sepsis, and severe sepsis
- Identify the initial goals of therapy for the treatment of patients with sepsis
- Devise an appropriate initial treatment plan, including fluid resuscitation and antibiotics, on the basis of patient characteristics and circumstances surrounding the patient's presentation
- Formulate a monitoring plan for the initial treatment while considering chosen therapies
- Determine the appropriateness of additional pharmacologic therapies for sepsis, including vasoactive agents, corticosteroids, and drotrecogin alfa, as well as adjunctive therapies

PATIENT PRESENTATION

Chief Complaint

"My father is confused and not responding to me. He looks pale and fatigued."

History of Present Illness

James Stallings is an 84-year-old male who was brought to the emergency department via emergency medical services (EMS) after his daughter found him sitting on the floor of his kitchen. She visits him at home twice a week to help him with his medications and other chores around the house, but he is normally very independent in his ADL despite having a stroke within the past year. She says that he has some small memory deficits post-stroke, but his current mental status is much more altered than his baseline. The last time she checked on him was 3 days ago when she took him to his primary care physician (PCP) for evaluation of difficult urination and an INR check. At that time, he was prescribed a short course of antibiotics. She believes that he is compliant with his medications since she puts them in a pill box for him and the medications are always gone when she returns. The EMS medic reports that the patient was hypotensive on arrival with SBPs in the 90s mm Hg and was subsequently given a 500-mL bolus of 0.9% sodium chloride en route to the emergency department. The medic also states that the patient would only intermittently answer questions, and was not aware of his current situation.

Past Medical History

BPH × 7 years
Type 2 DM × 9 months

HTN × 35 years
AF × 2 years
Cerebral vascular accident diagnosed 7 months ago
Depression × 4 years

Family History

Father died of a CVA at age 89. Mother died of bladder cancer at age 90. He has two brothers, one of which died at age 65 due to lung cancer and one alive at age 89 with a medical history that includes HTN, AF, and Parkinson's disease. He has two daughters, who are both alive and healthy.

Social History

Retired US Air Force and commercial airline pilot. Has lived alone since his wife passed away at age 80 due to colon cancer. Has two daughters, ages 57 and 54, five grandchildren, and two great-grandchildren.

Tobacco/Alcohol/Substance Use

Remote smoking history when he was in the US Air Force (approximately 50–60 years ago). Drinks an occasional beer socially. No history of illicit substance use

Allergies/Intolerances/Adverse Drug Events

Codeine (nausea)
Ramipril (cough)

Medications (Current)

Metformin 850 mg PO bid
Losartan 25 mg PO daily

Metoprolol succinate 50 mg PO daily

Sertraline 100 mg PO daily

Finasteride 5 mg PO daily

Terazosin 5 mg PO q hs

Warfarin 5 mg PO on Monday, Wednesday, and Friday; 7.5 mg PO on Tuesday, Thursday, Saturday, and Sunday

Nitrofurantoin 50 mg PO four times per day (prescribed 3 days ago by PCP)

Review of Systems

Unable to obtain secondary to the patient's current neurologic status. APACHE II score is 27. Glasgow Coma Score is 11.

Physical Examination

▶ **General**

Ill-appearing, elderly Caucasian male who is minimally responsive and communicative

▶ **Vital Signs**

BP 82/54 mm Hg, P 129, RR 26, T 39.5°C

Weight 172 lb (78 kg)

Height 70 in. (177.8 cm)

▶ **Skin**

Cold; (−) erythema; (−) rash

▶ **HEENT**

Scleral icterus; dry mucus membranes; pinpoint pupils

▶ **Neck and Lymph Nodes**

Minimal JVD; no nodules; minimal lymphadenopathy

▶ **Chest**

Decreased breath sounds; minimal wheezes bilaterally

▶ **Cardiovascular**

Sinus tachycardia; (−) M/R/G; (−) bruits; (+) femoral and pedal pulses

▶ **Abdomen**

Nontender, nondistended; (−) hepatosplenomegaly; (−) ascites

▶ **Neurology**

Unresponsive; obtunded

▶ **Genitourinary**

Mildly enlarged prostate

▶ **Rectal**

Decreased tone; (−) bright red blood per rectum (BRBPR)

Laboratory Tests

	Conventional Units	SI Units
Na	134 mEq/L	134 mmol/L
K	4.9 mEq/L	4.9 mmol/L
Cl	108 mEq/L	108 mmol/L
CO_2	18 mEq/L	18 mmol/L
BUN	45 mg/dL	16.1 mmol/L
sCr	2.6 mg/dL	230 μmol/L
Glucose	205 mg/dL	11.4 mmol/L
Ca	7.7 mg/dL	1.93 mmol/L
Mg	2.2 mEq/L	1.10 mmol/L
Phosphate	2.4 mg/dL	0.78 mmol/L
ABG		
pH	7.26	
pCO_2	25 mm Hg	3.3 kPa
pO_2	90 mm Hg	12.0 kPa
Hgb	11.2 g/dL	112 g/dL; 6.94 mmol/L
Hct	35.4%	0.354
WBC	$19.8 \times 10^3/\mu L$	$19.8 \times 10^9/L$
Platelets	$303 \times 10^3/\mu L$	$303 \times 10^9/L$
PT	37.5 s	
INR	3.6	

Assessment

An 84-year-old man with vital signs, physical examination, and laboratory tests consistent with sepsis

Student Workup

Missing Information?

Evaluate: Patient Database

Drug Therapy Problems

Care Plan (by Problem)

TARGETED QUESTIONS

1. What signs and symptoms of sepsis does this patient have?

   Hint: See p. 1349 in PPP

2. What potential pathogens should empiric antimicrobial therapy cover?

   Hint: See Table 82-2 and p. 1352 in PPP

3. What initial choice of IV fluids would be appropriate for this patient?

   Hint: See p. 1352 in PPP

4. What monitoring parameters should be utilized to determine if this patient is responding to initial therapy?

   Hint: See p. 1353 in PPP

5. Is this patient a candidate for drotrecogin alfa? Why or why not?

   Hint: See pp. 1356–1357 in PPP

FOLLOW-UP

After receiving several fluid boluses with IV crystalloid therapy, the patient remains hypotensive and tachycardic (BP 87/60 mm Hg; HR 130). The patient continues to be stable from a respiratory standpoint; however, his mental status has not improved. Cultures have been sent to the laboratory and are pending. The medical resident asks you if vasopressor and/or steroid therapy should be initiated in this patient.

6. If so, which medication, dose, and route would you recommend for this patient?

   Hint: See p. 1357 in PPP

⟳ GLOBAL PERSPECTIVE

Global treatment of sepsis and septic shock has been a topic of particular interest as of late with the prevalence of sepsis and the varying clinical approach to treatment. Initial results from the PROGRESS registry, which was designed to collect data that describe the management and outcomes of severe sepsis worldwide, detail the variability in mortality rate and use of treatment modalities.[1] Of participating countries and institutions, the highest overall hospital mortality rate was seen in Brazil (67.4%), whereas the lowest hospital mortality rate was seen in Australia (32.6%). Use of standard therapies such as antibiotics, mechanical ventilation, fluid resuscitation, and vasopressors was relatively consistent across participating institutions. There was relatively high usage of anticoagulants for venous thromboembolism prophylaxis, an increasing use of low-dose steroids, and a low usage of drotrecogin alfa overall.

Marked differences were seen in the choice of adjunctive therapies in specific countries, such as increased parenteral nutrition utilization in Germany and increased use of albumin for fluid resuscitation in Australia, India, and Malaysia. Initiation of programs such as PROGRESS will hopefully increase the global awareness of sepsis, provide data regarding the treatment and outcomes associated with sepsis, and contribute to improved outcomes in the treatment of patients with sepsis worldwide.

REFERENCE

1. Beale R, Reinhart K, Brunkhorst FM, Dobb G, Levy M, Martin G, et al. Promoting global research excellence in severe sepsis (PROGRESS): Lessons from an international sepsis registry. Infection 2009 37: 222–232.

CASE SUMMARY

- The patient's acute clinical picture is consistent with sepsis, likely due to an infectious process.
- Initial treatment of sepsis should include aggressive IV fluid resuscitation with crystalloids and/or colloids, as well as broad-spectrum antibiotic therapy targeted toward suspected sources of infection.
- Drotrecogin alfa therapy is recommended in patients with a high risk of death as evidenced by APACHE II score and organ failure; however, this therapy should not be used in patients with a low risk of death or a high risk of bleeding.
- Vasoactive agents should be initiated if initial fluid resuscitation is inadequate to reach a sufficient MAP.
- Adrenal insufficiency should be suspected in patients with an inadequate response to fluid resuscitation and vasopressor therapy, which should prompt initiation of hydrocortisone therapy.

For more information on the care plan and facilitator's guide please visit http://www.mhpharmacotherapy.com.

88 Dermatophytosis

Lauren S. Schlesselman

CASE LEARNING OBJECTIVES

- Recognize the signs and symptoms of tinea pedis and tinea cruris
- Identify the goals of therapy for tinea pedis and tinea cruris
- Develop an appropriate treatment and monitoring plan for tinea pedis and tinea cruris on the basis of individual patient characteristics
- Select an appropriate product for tinea pedis and tinea cruris therapy
- Properly educate a patient receiving tinea pedis and tinea cruris therapy

PATIENT PRESENTATION

Chief Complaint

"I have an itchy rash in my groin area. It looks like little red rings. By the way, I don't know if it is related but I have something similar on my feet … but I can't imagine why my feet and jock area would have the same rash. I have been rubbing petroleum jelly on the area, thinking that it might be chafing."

History of Present Illness

Edward Jacoby is a 26-year-old man who presents to the physician's clinic complaining of severe inguinal itching and soreness, accompanied by a red ring-shaped rash. Thinking that the rash may be due to chafing, he has been applying petroleum jelly to the area. He is an otherwise healthy male who has never been to the clinic before today. Other than petroleum jelly for prevention of chafing, he has not tried any over-the-counter products for the rash. He also expresses concern about the presence of a similar red, itchy rash on his feet.

Past Medical History

No significant medical history

FAMILY HISTORY

Father is alive at age 50 with no significant medical history. Mother is alive at age 48 and has HTN. He has one sister who is 24 years old with no significant medical history.

Social History

Single and lives with a roommate; has no children. Employed as a physical trainer at Fitness World and Pool.

Tobacco/Alcohol/Substance Use

Denies alcohol, tobacco, or illicit drug use

Allergies/Intolerances/Adverse Drug Events

No known drug allergies

Medications

No current oral medications

Petroleum jelly to groin area PRN

Review of Systems

▶ *General*

Healthy and fit-appearing, Caucasian man in no acute distress

▶ *Vital Signs*

BP 115/65 mm Hg, P 60, RR 12, T 36.2°C

Weight 180 lb (81.8kg)

Height 72 in. (183 cm)

Denies pain

▶ *Skin*

Follicular papules and pustules on medial thigh and inguinal folds; fissures and maceration present between toes

▶ *HEENT*

PERRLA, EOMI; (−) sinus tenderness; TMs appear normal

▶ *Neck and Lymph Nodes*

Thyroid gland symmetrical; (−) nodules; (−) lymphadenopathy; (−) carotid bruits

▸ **Chest**

Clear to auscultation

▸ **Cardiovascular**

RRR, normal S_1, S_2; (−)S_3 or S_4

▸ **Abdomen**

Not tender; not distended; (−) organomegaly

▸ **Neurology**

Grossly intact; deep tendon reflexes normal

▸ **Genitourinary**

Follicular papules and pustules on medial thigh and inguinal folds

▸ **Rectal**

Examination deferred

Laboratory Tests

	Conventional Units	SI Units
Na	140 mEq/L	140 mmol/L
K	3.7 mEq/L	3.7 mmol/L
Cl	98 mEq/L	98 mmol/L
CO_2	24 mEq/L	24 mmol/L
BUN	12 mg/dL	4.3 mmol/L
SCr	0.7 mg/dL	62 mmol/L
Glu	105 mg/dL	5.8 mmol/L

Assessment

A 26-year-old man with signs and symptoms consistent with tinea pedis and tinea cruris

Student Workup

Missing Information?

Evaluate: Patient Database

Drug Therapy Problems

Care Plan (by Problem)

TARGETED QUESTIONS

1. What signs and symptoms of tinea pedia and tinea cruris does the patient have?

   Hint: See p. 1369 in PPP

2. What treatment options are available for treating tinea pedis and tinea cruris?

   Hint: See p. 1371 in PPP

3. What risk factors does the patient have for tinea pedia and tinea cruris?

   Hint: See p. 1369 and Table 83-5 in PPP

4. What risks and adverse effects of therapy would you discuss with the patient?

   Hint: See p. 1372 in PPP

FOLLOW-UP

5. What nonpharmacologic treatment options should be recommended to the patient?

   Hint: See p. 1370 in PPP

6. Would the treatment plan change if the infection site was significantly inflamed and macerated?

   Hint: See p. 1371 and Table 83-5 in PPP

7. How would hyperkeratosis of the site alter the treatment plan?

   Hint: See p. 1371 and Table 83-5 in PPP

⊙ GLOBAL PERSPECTIVE

Mycotic infections of the skin, hair, and nails are superficial fungal infections in which the pathogen remains within the keratinous layers. These infections, typically named for the affected body part, are commonly referred to as ringworm due to the characteristic circular lesions, although they can vary from rings to scales to lesions. Tinea infections are second only to acne in frequency of reported skin disease. They are primarily caused by dermatophytes such as *Trichophyton*, *Microsporum*, and *Epidermophyton* species.

CASE SUMMARY

- His current clinical picture is consistent with tinea pedis and tinea cruris. Antifungal therapy should be initiated.

- For the treatment of tinea pedis, clotrimazole, tolnaftate, or terbinafine cream applied one to two times daily for 4 weeks is recommended.

- For the treatment of tinea cruris, clotrimazole or terbinafine cream or solution applied one to two times daily for 2 weeks is recommended.

- Treatment should be continued at least 1 week after resolution of symptoms.

- Systemic therapy should be reserved for refractory cases or widespread lesions.

For more information on the care plan and facilitator's guide please visit http://www.mhpharmacotherapy.com.

89 Vaginal Candidiasis

Lauren S. Schlesselman

CASE LEARNING OBJECTIVES

- Recognize the signs and symptoms of vaginal candidiasis
- Identify the goals of therapy for vaginal candidiasis
- Develop an appropriate treatment and monitoring plan for vaginal candidiasis on the basis of individual patient characteristics
- Select an appropriate product for vaginal candidiasis therapy
- Properly educate a patient receiving vaginal candidiasis therapy

PATIENT PRESENTATION

Chief Complaint

"My private area is really itchy and sore. I think I have another one of those infections."

History of Present Illness

Lilly Hayes is a 39-year-old woman who presents to the physician's clinic complaining of severe vaginal itching and soreness, accompanied by a thick vaginal discharge. Her first visit to the clinic was 4 days earlier for an *Escherichia coli* UTI. For the UTI, she was prescribed ciprofloxacin 250 mg twice daily for 3 days. After initiating the antibiotic therapy, the patient noted the development of the vaginal discharge, followed by vaginal itching and soreness. Although records are not currently available from her previous physician, the patient reports a history of recurrent vaginal candidiasis, including five episodes in the last year (excluding this episode). She expresses frustration with the repeated infections, especially since she cannot afford over-the-counter medications and therefore must make time to go to the physician's office to get a prescription medication that is covered on her assistance plan.

Past Medical History

Type 2 DM, diagnosed 5 years ago
Obesity
Dysmenorrhea, diagnosed 10 years ago
h/o UTI, diagnosed 4 days ago

Family History

Father is alive at age 65 with no significant medical history. Mother had DM, dyslipidemia, CAD, and died of complications due to DM at age 60. She has one sister who is 44 and has type 2 DM.

Social History

Single and lives with her sister; has no children. Has been unemployed for 5 years

Tobacco/Alcohol/Substance Use

Drinks one to two beers on the weekend; (−) tobacco or illicit drug use

Allergies/Intolerances/Adverse Drug Events

No known drug allergies

Medications (Current)

Glipizide 5 mg PO q 24 h
Metformin 850 mg PO q 24 h
Ortho Tri-Cyclen LO PO q 24 h

Review of Systems

► *General*

Well-appearing, obese Caucasian woman in no acute distress

► *Vital Signs*

BP 124/69 mm Hg, P 68, RR 14, T 36.2°C (97.2°F)
Weight 175 lb (80 kg)
Height 66 in. (168 cm)
Denies pain

► *Skin*

Dry-appearing skin; (−) rashes or lesions

▶ **HEENT**

PERRLA, EOMI; (−) sinus tenderness; TMs appear normal

▶ **Neck and Lymph Nodes**

Thyroid gland symmetrical; (−) nodules; (−) lymphadenopathy; (−) carotid bruits

▶ **Chest**

Clear to auscultation

▶ **Breast**

Examination deferred

▶ **Cardiovascular**

RRR, normal S_1, S_2; (−) S_3 or S_4

▶ **Abdomen**

Not tender; not distended; (−) organomegaly

▶ **Neurology**

Grossly intact; deep tendon reflexes normal

▶ **Genitourinary**

White exudate; (+) thick, curd-like discharge

▶ **Rectal**

Examination deferred

Laboratory Tests

	Conventional Units	SI Units
Na	140 mEq/L	140 mmol/L
K	3.7 mEq/L	3.7 mmol/L
Cl	98 mEq/L	98 mmol/L
CO_2	24 mEq/L	24 mmol/L
BUN	12 mg/dL	4.3 mmol/L
SCr	1.2 mg/dL	106 μmol/L
Glu	175 mg/dL	9.7 mmol/L
Vaginal smear	(+) *Candida albicans*	

Assessment

A 39-year-old woman with signs, symptoms, and laboratory tests consistent with vulvovaginal candidiasis

Student Workup

Missing Information?

Evaluate: Patient Database

Drug Therapy Problems

Care Plan (by Problem)

TARGETED QUESTIONS

1. What signs and symptoms of vaginal candidiasis does the patient have?

   Hint: See p. 1362 in PPP

2. What treatment options are available for treating vaginal candidiasis?

   Hint: See pp. 1362 and 1363 in PPP

3. What risk factors does the patient have for vaginal candidiasis?

   Hint: See p. 1362 and Table 83-1 in PPP

4. What risks and adverse effects of therapy would you discuss with the patient?

   Hint: See pp. 1364 and 1365 in PPP

5. Is the patient a candidate for suppressive therapy and why?

   Hint: See p. 1364 in PPP

FOLLOW-UP

Six months later, the patient tells her primary care physician that she is trying to conceive a child. However, she is concerned about the treatment of vaginal candidiasis if she becomes pregnant.

6. What treatment options would be recommended if the patient was pregnant?

   Hint: See p. 1365 in PPP

7. Would the treatment plan for the acute infection be changed if the patient was taking theophylline?

   Hint: See p. 1364 in PPP

8. What treatment plan for suppressive therapy should be changed if the patient was taking warfarin?

   Hint: See p. 1364 in PPP

⟳ GLOBAL PERSPECTIVE

Vulvovaginal candidiasis is a common form of vaginitis with *C. albicans* accounting for more than 90% of cases across the world. Nearly 50% of women will experience one or more episodes by the age of 25 years. Uncontrolled diabetes, antibiotic use, hormonal contraceptives, obesity, pregnancy, and debilitation are all risk factors for developing candidiasis, which do vary across the world. Recurrent candidiasis, defined as four or more infections per year, occurring in less than 5% of women, is distinguishable from a persistent infection by the presence of a symptom-free interval between infections.

CASE SUMMARY

- Her current clinical picture is consistent with vaginal candidiasis, and antifungal therapy should be initiated.
- A single dose of fluconazole 150 mg orally is recommended. The dose can be repeated in 3 days.

- The patient is unable to afford over-the-counter antifungal agents, but fluconazole would be covered by her insurance.
- Suppressive therapy of weekly fluconazole should be considered due to her history of recurrent candidiasis.

For more information on the care plan and facilitator's guide please visit http://www.mhpharmacotherapy.com.

90 Invasive Fungal Infection

Russell E. Lewis

CASE LEARNING OBJECTIVES

- Recognize the host risk factors that predispose patients to invasive fungal infections
- Identify the common patterns of antifungal resistance that affect the selection and dosing of antifungal therapy
- Develop an appropriate treatment and monitoring plan for the management of invasive candidiasis
- Compare and contrast the relative strengths and weaknesses of current systemic antifungal agents for the empiric treatment of an invasive fungal pathogen
- Properly educate patients on potential drug interactions and adverse effects of triazole antifungal agents

PATIENT PRESENTATION

Chief Complaint

"Patient in the intensive care unit has persistent fever despite broad-spectrum antibiotic therapy."

History of Present Illness

Steven Johnson is a 49-year-old male who presented to the emergency department 5 days ago with a history of worsening diffuse abdominal pain and vomiting. During the workup in the emergency department, a contrast-enhanced CT scan of the abdomen was ordered that showed inflammation and necrosis involving less than 15% of the pancreas. The patient was started on IV fluids, meropenem 1 g q 8 h plus vancomycin 1 g q 12 h. The patient underwent an exploratory abdominal laparotomy, which revealed inflammation of the common bile and stones in the gallbladder requiring cholecystectomy. The patient was subsequently transferred to the surgical ICU for postsurgical care where he remained in a guarded condition and extubated, but has developed a new fever in the last 24 hours on broad-spectrum antibiotic therapy.

Past Medical History

HTN

Hyperlipidemia

Family History

Father had CAD and died of an MI at age 56. Mother is alive at age 70 with type 2 DM and osteoporosis.

Social History

Construction worker in Chicago. No recent travel or unusual exposures. Married and lives with wife of 18 years, has two kids, ages 12 and 15, and two pet dogs.

Tobacco/Alcohol Substance Abuse

Social drinker; occasional cigars; (−) illicit drug use

Allergies/Intolerances/Adverse Drug Events

None

Medications (Current)

Meropenem 1 g IV q 8 h

Vancomycin 1 g IV q 12 h

Normal saline, IV, 50 mL/h

Fentanyl 75 mcg/h IV

Lorazepam 0.05 mg/kg/h IV

Tube feeds q 6 h via Dobhoff catheter as tolerated

Pantoprazole 40 mg IV daily

HCTZ 25 mg PO daily (on hold)

Atorvastatin 40 mg PO daily (on hold)

Acetaminophen 500 mg PO q 6 h PRN

Diphenhydramine 50 mg PO q 4–6 h PRN

Docusate sodium liquid 100 mg PO twice daily

Review of Systems

The patient is somewhat difficult to arouse and appears to be developing a nonconfluent rash across the chest and upper back.

Physical Examination

► General

Somewhat ill-appearing, difficult-to-arouse male in late forties with extremities that are cool to touch. The patient is not intubated.

► Vital Signs

BP 108/76 mm Hg, P 88, RR 17, T 38.4°C

Weight 218 lb (99 kg)

Height 69 in. (175 cm)

► Skin

Decreased skin turgor. Peripherally inserted central catheter (PICC) site is not indurated or inflamed. A light diffuse morbilliform rash evident on the upper chest that is spreading on the arms, neck, and back. Rash has slowly developed over the last 72 hours to involve the back. Surgical sites are clean and dressed without signs of erythema or pus.

► HEENT

PEERLA, EOMI; (−) sinus tenderness; TMs appear normal; mucus membranes dry

► Neck and Lymph Nodes

(−) Evidence of lymphadenopathy; thyroid nodules; (−) carotid bruits

► Chest

Dullness to percussion in lower right and left bases; (−) wheezes; (+) crackles during inspiration

► Cardiovascular

RRR, normal S_1, S_2; (−) S_3 or S_4

► Abdomen

Tender, not distended

► Neurology

The patient moderately sedated and not well oriented to person, place, or time

► Genitourinary

Foley catheter present

► Rectal

Examination deferred

Laboratory Tests

	Conventional Units	SI Units
Na	138 mEq/L	138 mmol/L
K	3.6 mEq/L	3.6 mmol/L
Cl	101 mEq/L	101 mmol/L
CO_2	23 mEq/L	23 mmol/L
BUN	23 mg/dL	8.2 mmol/L
SCr	1.5 mg/dL	133 μmol/L
Glu	122 mg/dL	6.8 mmol/L
Ca	9.4 mg/dL	2.35 mmol/L
Mg	1.2 mEq/L	0.60 mmol/L
Phos	3.3 mg/dL	1.07 mmol/L
Albumin	3.8 g/dL	38 g/L
AST	77 IU/L	1.28 μkat/L
ALT	92 IU/L	1.53 μkat/L
ALP	250 IU/L	4.17 μkat/L
Total bilirubin	2.6 mg/dL	44.5 μmol/L
Hgb	11 g/dL	110 g/L; 6.83 mmol/L
Hct	58%	0.58
WBC	$13.5 \times 10^3/mm^3$	13.5×10^9
Segs	50%	0.50
Bands	8%	0.08
Lymphocytes	28%	0.28
Monocytes	6%	0.06
Eosinophils	8%	0.08
Platelets	$290 \times 10^3/mm^3$	$290 \times 10^9/L$

► Culture Results

Blood: (−) no growth

Urine: (+) yeast

Wound swab: (+) coagulase-negative Gram-positive cocci

Urinalysis: Na 15 mEq/L (15 mmol/L); osmolality 500 mOsmol/kg (500 mmol/kg); hyaline casts; WBC (−); RBC (−); protein (−)

Assessment

A 49-year-old male s/p abdominal laparotomy with fever on broad-spectrum antibiotic therapy (suspected fungal infection), hypotension, and renal insufficiency

Student Workup

Missing Information?

Evaluate: Patient Database

Drug Therapy Problems

Care Plan (by Problem)

TARGETED QUESTIONS

1. What are the patient's risk factors for developing an opportunistic mycosis? Which fungal pathogen is most likely?

   Hint: See p. 1382 in PPP

2. In the absence of definitive microbiologic data, what antifungal therapy should be started in this patient?

   Hint: See p. 1383 and Table 84-3 in PPP

3. If blood cultures acquired the following day come back positive for a germ-tube-negative yeast, how would this influence the selection of the antifungal agent?

   Hint: See p. 1384 in PPP

4. Is the (+) yeast culture from the urine indicative of true infection or colonization in this patient?

   Hint: Review results of the urinalysis and see p. 1385 in PPP

5. What is the most likely explanation of this patient's rash?

   Hint: Review the CBC with differential

FOLLOW-UP

Three days after starting the antifungal therapy, the patient has defervesced, and renal function is improving. Fluconazole susceptibility test results for the yeast isolated from the blood (*Candida glabrata*) show an MIC of 64 mcg/mL (64 mg/L), which is considered resistant to fluconazole. The attending physician asks you if the patient can be transitioned from IV antifungal therapy to voriconazole oral solution to complete the treatment course for candidemia.

6. What is your recommendation?

   Hint: See p. 1385 in PPP

⟳ GLOBAL PERSPECTIVE

Candida species are the third to fourth most commonly isolated bloodstream pathogens in hospitalized patients associated with crude mortality rates approaching 30% to 40%. Like many opportunistic invasive fungal pathogens,

invasive candidiasis can be difficult to diagnose early. Therefore, early suspicion of infection in patients with multiple risk factors for infection (e.g., central venous catheters, broad-spectrum antibiotic therapy, recent intra-abdominal surgery, colonization with *Candida* at multiple sites) should prompt empiric treatment during the diagnostic workup, as delays in the initiation of appropriate antifungal therapy have been associated with increased patient mortality. Antifungal therapy selection is determined by local epidemiology (i.e., prevalence of *C. glabrata* and *C. krusei* in the institution), previous antifungal exposures, and underlying comorbidities of the host. For most patients, initial therapy with either appropriately dosed IV fluconazole (lower risk) or an echinocandin antifungal (higher risk) is recommended until pathogen identification and clinical response can be assessed.

CASE SUMMARY

- The patient's clinical picture is consistent with invasive candidiasis with developing sepsis, requiring immediate empiric antifungal therapy.

- Because the patient is at relatively higher risk, initial therapy with an echinocandin would be appropriate (i.e., IV caspofungin 70 mg on day 1 and then 50 mg/d thereafter). The patient should receive at least 2 weeks of therapy and have the PICC line replaced.

- Because the patient has a fluconazole-resistant *C. glabrata*, he should not be considered as a candidate for step-down (oral) fluconazole therapy.

For more information on the care plan and facilitator's guide please visit http://www.mhpharmacotherapy.com.

91 Pediatric Immunizations

Hanna Phan   Lynn C. Nelson

CASE LEARNING OBJECTIVES

- Evaluate pediatric immunization records and identify missing immunizations
- Recognize appropriate contraindications for holding immunizations until a subsequent visit
- Develop an appropriate plan for vaccine catch-up including selection of appropriate vaccine products for pediatric immunizations
- Properly educate caregivers regarding premedication, adverse effects of vaccines, and vaccine controversies, such as autism

PATIENT PRESENTATION

Date of Clinic Visit: August 1, 2009, at 10:00

Chief Complaint

"Lately my son has been fussy and doesn't sleep very well. His forehead was warm to the touch last night and I am concerned that he may be coming down with something."

History of Present Illness

Kyle Smith is an 18-month-old male toddler who was brought into his pediatrician's office by his mother. The mother notes that her son has been irritable and demonstrates difficulty sleeping over the past few days. Additionally, she reports that he has been eating less with meals over the past week and has been tugging on his right ear on occasion. His mother has no other complaints at this time.

Past Medical History

Normal spontaneous vaginal delivery (NSVD) at 37 weeks' gestation. No hospitalizations or complications since birth.

Social History

The patient lives at home with mother and father. He attends day care during the weekdays as both parents work full time. Siblings include a 4-year-old sister who also attends day care as well as preschool.

Allergies/Intolerances/Adverse Drug Events

Green jello ("itching" per mother)

Medications (Current)

Acetaminophen infant drops 130 mg PO q 6 h PRN fever, last dose given at 21:00 last night

Immunizations

Please see attached immunization record for this patient.

Per mother, the patient has not experienced any adverse reactions with immunizations except for some mild erythema with the Pediarix vaccine.

Review of Systems

Positive for fever and decreased appetite; negative for rashes, bruises, recent trauma, or accidental falls; negative for discharge from the eyes or ear pulling; negative for nausea, vomiting, or changes in bowel or urinary patterns; positive for decreased oral intake; negative for lethargy

Physical Examination

▶ *General*

Irritable and fussy 18-month-old male in no acute distress

▶ *Vital Signs*

BP 100/55 mm Hg, P 95, RR 24, T 37°C

Weight 28 lb (12.7 kg)

Height 33 in. (84 cm)

▶ *Skin*

No abnormalities noted; normal skin turgor

► HEENT

PERRLA, EOMI; moist mucous membranes (MMM); discolored, bulging eardrum on right; pneumatic otoscopy demonstrates eardrum immobility on right side.

► Neck and Lymph Nodes

(−) Lymphadenopathy

► Chest

Clear to auscultation

► Cardiovascular

RRR, normal S_1, S_2; (−) S_3 or S_4

► Abdomen

Not tender/not distended; (−) organomegaly

► Neurology

Grossly intact; deep tendon reflexes normal

► Genitourinary

Examination deferred

► Rectal

Examination deferred

Laboratory Tests

Obtained during routine clinic visit on 1/5/2009

	Conventional Units	SI Units
Na	140 mEq/L	140 mmol/L
K	4.1 mEq/L	4.1 mmol/L
Cl	105 mEq/L	105 mmol/L
CO_2	23 mEq/L	23 mmol/L
BUN	5 mg/dL	1.8 mmol/L
SCr	0.3 mg/dL	27 μmol/L
Glu	70 mg/dL	3.9 mmol/L
Ca	9.7 mg/dL	2.43 mmol/L
Mg	1.8 mEq/L	0.90 mmol/L
Phosphate	6 mg/dL	1.94 mmol/L
Hgb	12.2 g/dL	122 g/L; 7.57 mmol/L
Hct	36.7%	0.367
WBC	$15.2 \times 10^3/mm^3$	$15.2 \times 10^9/L$
MCV	74 μm³	74 fL
Albumin	4.2 g/dL	42 g/L

Assessment

An 18-month-old male with signs and symptoms consistent with AOM of the right ear. Pharmacist to review immunization record.

Student Workup

Missing Information?

Evaluate: Patient Database
         Drug Therapy Problems
         Care Plan (by Problem)

TARGETED QUESTIONS

1. What signs and symptoms would the physician evaluate to determine if Kyle should receive immunizations today?

   Hint: See Guide to Vaccine Contraindications and Precautions (by the CDC), http://www.cdc.gov/vaccines/recs/vac-admin/contraindications.htm -or- http://www.cdc.gov/vaccines/recs/vac-admin/downloads/contraindications-guide-508.pdf

2. What adverse effects should the mother be educated about regarding Kyle's immunizations?

   Hint: See pp. 1414 and 1415 in PPP

3. What combination vaccines were used for Kyle's immunizations based on review of his record and what vaccines are contained in these combination products?

   Hint: See pp. 1413 and 1414 in PPP

4. What would you educate the mother about in regard to thimerosal and vaccines?

   Hint: See p. 1415 in PPP

5. Which of Kyle's missing vaccines is/are likely to cause body temperature elevation?

   Hint: See p. 1415 in PPP

FOLLOW-UP

Kyle and his mother return to the clinic for a routine checkup a couple months later that year in October. Kyle is well developed, not in distress, no present illnesses. The pediatrician asks you what vaccine(s) he should receive.

6. Which vaccine(s) should be given and why?

   Hint: See p. 1414 and Table 86-2 in PPP

☼ GLOBAL PERSPECTIVE

Immunization of children remains a significant public health concern internationally. According to the WHO, immunizations do not reach every child worldwide, resulting in an estimated 1.3 million deaths from pneumococcal disease and rotavirus as well as a considerable number of deaths from other vaccine preventable diseases. An estimated 2.5 million deaths of children due to diphtheria, tetanus, pertussis, and measles are prevented by immunizations each year. Measles mortality across the globe has decreased by 74% between 2000 and 2007 as a result of intensified vaccination campaigns.[1] Due to growing immunization programs, improved access to clean water, improved

IMMUNIZATION RECORD

Name: Kyle R. Smith

Birthdate: 1/1/2008

Vaccine	Product Name	Date Given	Route and Site	Vaccinator Signature/Initials
Hepatitis B	Recombivax HB	1/1/2008	IM RT	*A.R.*
	Pediarix	3/5/2008	IM RT	*B.C.*
	Pediarix	5/16/2008	IM LT	*A.B.*
	Pediarix	7/23/2008	IM LT	*A.B.*
Diptheria, tetanus, pertussis	Pediarix	3/5/2008	IM RT	*B.C.*
	Pediarix	5/16/2008	IM LT	*A.B.*
	Pediarix	7/23/2008	IM LT	*A.B.*
Haemophilus influenzae type b	PedvaxHIB	3/5/2008	IM LT	*B.C.*
	PedvaxHIB	5/16/2008	IM RT	*A.B.*
	PedvaxHIB	1/5/2009	IM LT	*P.T.*
Polio	Pediarix	3/5/2008	IM RT	*B.C.*
	Pediarix	5/16/2008	IM LT	*A.B.*
	Pediarix	7/23/2008	IM LT	*A.B.*
Pneumococcal	Prevnar	3/5/2008	IM LT	*B.C.*
	Prevnar	5/16/2008	IM LT	*A.B.*
	Prevnar	7/23/2008	IM RT	*A.B.*
	Prevnar	1/5/2009	IM RT	*P.T.*
Rotavirus	Rotarix	3/5/2008	PO	*B.C.*
	Rotarix	5/16/2008	PO	*A.B.*
Measles, mumps, rubella	ProQuad	1/5/2009	SC LT	*P.T.*
Varicella	ProQuad	1/5/2009	SC LT	*P.T.*
Hepatitis A				
Meningococcal				
Influenza				

IM, intramuscular; SC, subcutaneous; PO, oral; LT, left thigh; RT, right thigh.

Adapted from the Immunization Action Coalition Vaccine Administration Record for Children and Teens.

nutrition, and sanitary living conditions by public health organizations, such as the WHO, the number of children dying every year has fallen below 10 million.[2] Optimal outreach of immunizations to the world's children is faced with challenges in financial support, logistics of organizing national and local public health groups, and support of caregivers regarding the importance of immunization for individual and community health.

REFERENCES

1. http://www.who.int/features/factfiles/immunization/en/index.html. Accessed March 7, 2010.

2. WHO, UNICEF, World Bank. State of the World's Vaccines and Immunization, 3rd ed. Geneva, World Health Organization, 2009. http://whqlibdoc.who.int/publications/2009/9789241563864_eng.pdf. Accessed March 7, 2010.

CASE SUMMARY

- Kyle presents to the clinic with AOM of his right ear and will likely receive antibiotic therapy.

- Kyle is in no acute distress and has a history of possible low-grade fever based on tactile observation by his mother, treated with acetaminophen.

- Patients should be reviewed for missing scheduled or recommended immunizations on each visit to the primary care provider as each visit is an opportunity to maintain adherence to the recommended immunization schedule by the Advisory Committee on Immunization Practices (ACIP) within the CDC.

- The decision to vaccinate Kyle should be based on which vaccine(s) is(are) missing and clinical judgment of the patient's current clinical status and ability to receive immunizations today.

For more information on the care plan and facilitator's guide please visit http://www.mhpharmacotherapy.com.

92 Adult Immunizations

Kathryn R. Matthias

CASE LEARNING OBJECTIVES

- Evaluate adult immunization records and identify missing recommended vaccinations based on patient's age, comorbid conditions, risk factors, and time since previous vaccinations
- Recognize appropriate contraindications and precautions for administration of immunizations in adult patients
- Develop an appropriate plan for vaccine catch-up including an evaluation of which vaccines can be administered at the same time
- Describe appropriate patient education for potential benefits and adverse reactions of vaccines

PATIENT PRESENTATION

Chief Complaint

"I was told to see my physician after being discharged from XYZ Hospital. I was admitted to the hospital for 4 days because I broke my arm after a bad car accident."

History of Present Illness

Eric Jones is a 22-year-old college student who was a restrained driver in a MVA 7 days ago on December 2nd, 2009. He was not ejected from the car and had no loss of consciousness. In the ED, he was found to have a left mid-shaft humerus fracture and spleen laceration. He was taken emergently to the operating room and a splenectomy was performed due to uncontrollable bleeding. The rest of his hospital stay was uneventful but he was told to see his primary care physician (PCP) after discharge for follow-up and to make an appointment with an orthopedic specialist for his humerus fracture. During his initial visit to his PCP, his physician asks the clinic's pharmacist to review his immunization history.

Past Medical History

Migraines diagnosed 5 years ago
Left humerus fracture 7 days ago

Past Surgical History

Splenectomy 7 days ago

Family History

Mother and father are both alive. Father is 52 and has a history of T2DM. Mother is 48 and has no significant past medical history. He has no siblings.

Social History

Patient is currently a third year college student (psychology major) and lives off-campus in an apartment with his girlfriend and two other roommates. He has two healthy indoor-only cats. He denies smoking and IV drug use. He drinks alcohol socially (3–4 beers per week).

Allergies/Intolerances/Adverse Drug Events

NKDA

Medications (Current—No Medications Prior to Car Accident)

Acetaminophen 650 mg PO q 4 h PRN musculoskeletal pain

Docusate 100 mg PO q 12 h

Famotidine 20 mg PO q 12 h

Oxycodone (oral solution) 5–10 mg PO q 4 h PRN pain

Immunizations

Most recent photocopy from 06/20/2008 of immunization record in patient's medical chart at clinic:

IMMUNIZATION RECORD

Name: Eric P. Jones
Birthdate: 2/8/1987

Vaccine	Date Given	Vaccinator Signature/ Initials
Hepatitis B	8/15/1996	F.G.
	9/21/1996	F.G.
	2/17/1997	F.G.
Diphtheria, tetanus, pertussis	3/9/1987	S.M.
	4/20/1987	S.M.
	8/10/1987	S.M.
	8/15/1988	S.M.
	4/8/1991	F.G.
Diphtheria and tetanus	7/29/1998	F.G.
	9/15/2007	H.J.
Polio	3/9/1987	S.M.
	4/20/1987	S.M.
	8/10/1987	S.M.
	8/15/1988	S.M.
	4/8/1991	F.G.
Pneumococcal	3/9/1987	S.M.
	4/20/1987	S.M.
	8/15/1988	S.M.
Measles, mumps, rubella	6/20/1988	S.M.
	1/30/1998	F.G.
Varicella	1/5/1996	F.G.
	4/10/1996	F.G.
Influenza [LAIV (live attenuated influenza vaccine)]	9/15/2006	P.M.
	10/24/2007	S.C.

As per the patient's discharge paperwork from XYZ Hospital, he received a diphtheria, tetanus, pertussis (DTaP) vaccination on 12/2/2009. No other administered vaccinations were listed. The patient states that he got his annual influenza vaccine that was administered into his "nose rather than a shot" last month at a Flu Clinic on his college campus. He does not remember the exact date and did not bring an immunization record with him to clinic today but thinks it was mid-November.

Review of Systems

Mild left arm pain; arm is in a sling. Minor abrasions over flank, arms, and face.

Physical Examination

▶ General

Twenty-two-year-old Caucasian man in no acute distress

▶ Vital Signs

BP 126/74 mm Hg, P 88, RR 18, T 37.1°C

Weight 162 lb (73.6 kg)

Height 71 in. (180 cm)

Pain 2/10 (left arm)

▶ Skin

Multiple healing abrasions over flank, arms, and face. Three healing 2-inch (5 cm) surgical wounds on abdomen from splenectomy with no signs of infection.

▶ Neck and Lymph Nodes

(−) Lymphadenopathy

▶ Chest

Clear to auscultation

▶ Cardiovascular

RRR, normal S_1, S_2; (−) S_3 or S_4

▶ Abdomen

Slight tenderness around surgical wound site

▶ Neurology

Grossly intact; DTRs normal

▶ Genitourinary

Examination deferred

▶ Rectal

Examination deferred

Laboratory Tests

Obtained 4 days ago

	Conventional Units	SI Units
Na	135 mEq/L	135 mmol/L
K	4.3 mEq/L	4.3 mmol/L
Cl	102 mEq/L	102 mmol/L
CO_2	25 mEq/L	25 mmol/L
BUN	5 mg/dL	1.8 mmol/L
SCr	0.6 mg/dL	54 μmol/L
Glu	105 mg/dL	5.9 mmol/L
Ca	9.7 mg/dL	2.43 mmol/L
Hgb	13.9 g/dL	139 g/L; 8.63 mmol/L
HCT	39.7%	0.397
MCV	95 μm³	95 fL
Platelets	$253 \times 10^3/mm^3$	$253 \times 10^9/L$
WBC	$6.8 \times 10^3/mm^3$	$6.8 \times 10^9/L$

Assessment

Twenty-two-year-old man in no acute distress with left humerus fracture and splenectomy 7 days ago after a MVA. Pharmacist to review immunization record.

Student Workup

Missing Information?

Evaluate:	Patient Database
	Drug Therapy Problems
	Care Plan (by Problem)

TARGETED QUESTIONS

1. Which comorbid conditions and lifestyle risk factors put the patient at higher risk of infection that can be prevented by vaccination?

   Hint: See p. 1411 in PPP

   Hint: See guide to Vaccine-Preventable Adult Diseases (by the CDC), http://www.cdc.gov/vaccines/vpd-vac/adult-vpd.htm

2. Why and when should adult asplenia patients receive additional vaccines beyond the recommended adult immunization schedule?

   Hint: See p. 1411 in PPP

   Hint: See Adult Immunization Schedule (by the CDC), http://www.cdc.gov/vaccines/recs/schedules/adult-schedule.htm

3. Does the patient have any comorbid conditions that would contraindicate him from receiving live or inactivated vaccinations today?

   Hint: See pp. 1414 and 1415 in PPP

   Hint: See Guide to Vaccine Contraindications and Precautions (by the CDC), http://www.cdc.gov/vaccines/recs/vac-admin/contraindications.htm or http://www.cdc.gov/vaccines/recs/vac-admin/downloads/contraindications-guide-508.pdf

4. Which recommended vaccinations are missing from the patient's immunization record and when should they be administered?

   Hint: See p. 1414 in PPP

   Hint: See Adult Immunization Schedule (by the CDC), http://www.cdc.gov/vaccines/recs/schedules/adult-schedule.htm

5. What are the common and serious potential adverse effects of recommended vaccines determined in question 4?

   Hint: See pp. 1414 and 1415 and Table 86-2 in PPP

FOLLOW-UP

Eric receives all immunizations as per the pharmacist and physician recommendations. He returns to his PCP 9 months later for his annual checkup. He had no further complications related to the motor vehicle accident and his left arm healed well. His physician asks the clinic pharmacist to evaluate his immunization record for any missing vaccinations.

6. Which vaccine(s) should be recommended and why?

   Hint: See p. 1414 in PPP

   Hint: See Adult Immunization Schedule (by the CDC), http://www.cdc.gov/vaccines/recs/schedules/adult-schedule.htm

🌎 GLOBAL PERSPECTIVE

An annual review of immunizations reports from countries and territories from across the world is conducted by the World Health Organization (WHO) and United Nations Children's Fund (UNICEF).[1] Although global rates of certain immunizations have increased dramatically over the past 30 years, many vaccines on the United States' Immunization Schedule are not yet recommended in other countries' national immunization schedules. Although the United States and other industrialized countries have estimated vaccinated target populations (by antigen) above 90% based on childhood recommended immunization schedule, missed opportunities to vaccinate adult patients often occur. In a case-cohort study of two large tertiary medical centers in Australia only 2.3% of patients had their vaccination status for influenza or pneumococcal determined during a hospital visit.[2] In another study of adult patients who developed invasive pneumococcal disease, it was determined that 92% of these patients had at least one missed opportunity for vaccination such as a hospital, emergency department, or primary care visit in the 2 years prior to infection.[3] Due to high rates of missed opportunities to vaccinate, the Advisory Committee on Immunization Practices (ACIP) through the Centers for Disease Control (CDC) has recommended the use of institution protocols for standing order immunization programs for administration of vaccines by nurses or pharmacists to decrease rates of eligible, unvaccinated patients.[4]

REFERENCES

1. World Health Organization: Immunization surveillance, assessment and monitoring. http://www.who.int/immunization_monitoring/data/en/. Accessed February 10, 2010.
2. Skull SA, Andrews RM, Byrnes GB, et al. Missed opportunities to vaccinate a cohort of hospitalized elderly with pneumococcal and influenza vaccines. Vaccine 2007 25:5146–5154.
3. Kyaw MH, Greene CM, Schaffner W, et al. Adults with invasive pneumococcal disease: Missed opportunities for vaccination. Am J Prev Med 2006 31(4):286–292.

4. Centers for Disease Control and Prevention. Use of standing orders programs to increase adult vaccination rates. MMWR 2000 49(No. RR-1):15–26.

CASE SUMMARY

- Eric presents to his PCP 7 days after a motor vehicle accident and splenectomy. Despite receiving diphtheria/tetanus/pertussis vaccination while admitted to XYZ Hospital, additional immunizations were missed during the hospital admission.

- Eric is in no acute distress but certain medical conditions and lifestyle put him at higher risk of certain infections that could be prevented by vaccination.
- Eric should receive his missing immunizations as per the recommended adult immunization schedule by the ACIP within the CDC.
- Eric should be counseled on potential adverse effects of recommended vaccines.

For more information on the care plan and facilitator's guide please visit http://www.mhpharmacotherapy.com.

93 Human Immunodeficiency Virus

Amanda H. Corbett   Colin I. Sheffield

CASE LEARNING OBJECTIVES

- Identify the typical and atypical signs and symptoms of acute and chronic human immunodeficiency virus (HIV) infection
- Identify the desired therapeutic outcomes for patients with HIV infection
- Recommend appropriate first-line pharmacotherapy interventions for patients with HIV infection
- Describe the components of a monitoring plan to assess the effectiveness and adverse effects of pharmacotherapy for HIV infection
- Educate patients about the disease state, appropriate lifestyle modifications, and drug therapy required for effective treatment

PATIENT PRESENTATION

Chief Complaint

"I am ready to start medications."

History of Present Illness

Kim Jones is a 35-year-old African American female recently diagnosed with HIV after presenting with *Pneumocystis jiroveci* pneumonia. *P. jiroveci* pneumonia was diagnosed 1 month ago when she presented to the hospital with increased weight loss, SOB, insomnia, nonproductive cough, and unremarkable chest x-ray. During her hospitalization, antiretroviral therapy was discussed but the patient was not ready to start taking it yet. She also had no insurance or way to pay for her medications at the time.

Past Medical History

P. jiroveci pneumonia (PJP) diagnosed 1 month ago

Depression × 5 years

HTN × 5 years

Family History

She has not seen her father in more than 15 years and her mother is alive with a history of stroke and HTN.

Social/Work History

She is currently unemployed and lives with her mother.

Tobacco/Alcohol/Substance Use

Smokes 2 ppd; drinks about 10 to 12 drinks a week; former crack/cocaine use, but clean for 6 months

Allergy/Intolerance/Adverse Drug Events

Sulfur drugs

Medication (Current)

Dapsone 100 mg PO q 24 h

Azithromycin 1,200 mg PO weekly

Enalapril 10 mg PO q 24 h

Bupropion XL 150 mg PO q 24 h

Review of Systems

(+) Weight loss; decreased appetite; (+) insomnia; (−) SOB; chest pain

Physical Examination

▶ *General*

Well-appearing African American woman in no acute distress

► **Vital Signs**

BP 130/86 mm Hg, P 72, RR 13, T 36.4°C

Weight 130 lb (59 kg)

Height 65 in. (165.1 cm)

No pain

► **Skin**

Supple; (−) rashes

► **HEENT**

PERRL; no evidence of retinopathy. Oropharynx, no evidence of thrush

► **Neck and Lymph Nodes**

Neck supple; no lymphadenopathy

► **Chest**

Clear to auscultation bilaterally

► **Breasts**

Breast nontender and (−) nodules

► **Cardiovascular**

RRR, normal S_1, S_2; (−) murmurs, rubs, or gallops

► **Abdomen**

Not tender/not distended; (−) organomegaly

► **Neurology**

Grossly intact; deep tendon reflexes normal

► **Extremities**

Thin, dry upper and lower extremities with no edema

► **Genitourinary**

Examination deferred

► **Rectal**

Examination deferred

Laboratory Tests

Fasting, obtained 2 weeks ago in hospital

	Conventional Units	SI Units
Na	137 mEq/L	137 mmol/L
K	4 mEq/L	4 mmol/L
Cl	101 mEq/L	101 mmol/L
CO_2	25 mEq/L	25 mmol/L
BUN	12 mg/dL	4.3 mmol/L
SCr	0.9 mg/dL	80 μmol/L
Glucose	85 mg/dL	4.7 mmol/L
Hg	14 g/dL	140 g/L; 8.69 mmol/L
Hct	38%	0.38
WBC	$4.4 \times 10^3/mm^3$	$4.4 \times 10^9/L$
Absolute lymphocyte count (ALC)	$0.9 \times 10^3/mm^3$	$0.9 \times 10^9/L$
ANC	$2.9 \times 10^3/mm^3$	$2.9 \times 10^9/L$
Platelets	$425 \times 10^3/mm^3$	$425 \times 10^9/L$
HIV RNA	23,000 copies/mL	
$CD4^+$ T-cell count	35 cells/mm^3	$0.035 \times 10^9/L$
HIV genotype	Wild-type virus	

Assessment

A 35-five-year-old woman with diagnosis of HIV in clinic ready to start her new antiretroviral regimen. She was initially prescribed as her first regimen Truvada (tenofovir 300 mg/zemtricitabine 200 mg) one tablet by mouth once a day and Kaletra (lopinavir 200 mg/ritonavir 50 mg) four tablets by mouth once a day.

Student Workup

Missing Information?

Evaluate:	Patient Database
	Drug Therapy Problems
	Care Plan (by Problem)

TARGETED QUESTIONS

1. What signs and symptoms (typical or atypical) of HIV infection does this patient have?

   Hint: See pp. 1422 and 1423 in PPP

2. What monitoring goals (treatment and adverse effects of medications) should be discussed with this patient?

   Hint: See p. 1436 and Tables 87-2 and 87-5 in PPP

3. What medication(s) could be causing side effects that would preclude her from taking her regimen properly?

   Hint: See Table 87-5 in PPP

4. What risks and adverse effects of using efavirenz on this patient would you discuss with the patient and/or provider?

   Hint: Teratogenicity with women of childbearing age and this patient's history of depression. See Table 87-5 in PPP

5. In choosing a protease inhibitor (PI) for this patient, would using Lexiva (fosamprenavir) or Prezista (darunavir) be a prudent choice? Why or why not?

> Hint: Both are drugs that have a sulfa base, and with this patient's history of a sulfa allergy, there would be risk of allergic reaction to these medications. See Table 87-5 in PPP

FOLLOW-UP

She went to her local pharmacy 2 months after starting new antiretrovirals requesting refills for all her medications. The pharmacist noted that she was also purchasing a pregnancy test, St. John's Wort, and Prilosec (omeprazole). The pharmacist contacted the clinic provider and pharmacist, informed them of the patient's purchases, and stated that the patient was late on her refills last month. Her HIV RNA 2 weeks after starting medications decreased by 1 log copy/mL (23,000–2,000 copies/mL). She reported side effects of stomach upset and some nausea.

6. What discussions of sexual behavior should be addressed in this patient, and if this patient becomes pregnant, what considerations must occur so that the baby can be taken to full term?

> Hint: There should be discussions of contraceptive use and the effect of antiretrovirals on oral contraceptives and barrier protection. Discussions of risk of transmission of HIV between partners with unprotected sex and making sure that the mother is virologically suppressed and taking her regimen during pregnancy is also important. See p. 1434 in PPP

7. What drug–drug interactions must be evaluated with the patient and how could the pharmacist intervene by counseling the patient and discussing with the provider?

> Hint: St. John's Wort can significantly decrease concentrations of protease inhibitors (including lopinavir/ritonavir). The patient should be advised not to use St. John's Wort. Also, if she is still having uncontrolled depression, as suggested by purchasing St. John's Wort, her antidepressant therapy should be evaluated. In addition, omeprazole can interact with certain antiretrovirals, so this should be evaluated if she changes antiretroviral therapy in the future (i.e., atazanavir). See Table 87-5 in PPP

8. What discussions should the pharmacist have concerning adherence with her current regimen and goals of treatment?

> Hint: A discussion should take place concerning the importance of not missing doses and intervening with the patient to find out why she is missing doses (late refills). An initial VL of 23,000 copies/mL and 2 months of therapy should result in an undetectable (<50 copies/mL) HIV RNA. See pp. 1433 and 1434 in PPP

☉ GLOBAL PERSPECTIVE

HIV is a global pandemic that affects the entire population. Access to care in resource-poor countries is much limited compared to those treated in the United States and other industrialized countries. Most resource-poor countries follow WHO guidelines with country-specific antiretroviral therapy recommendations. Many countries rely on generic antiretrovirals that are still under the US FDA patent or funding from countries, including the United States, through programs such as PEPFAR (US President's Emergency Plan for AIDS Relief). Pharmaceutical industry also provides resources for countries. Not only are therapies limited, but often only first-line therapy is available with second-line therapy less readily available. Criterion for when to treat is also variable and typically delayed until CD4+ T-cell counts are lower than what is recommended in the United States Department of Health and Human Services (DHHS) guidelines.

CASE SUMMARY

- This is an HIV-infected patient that meets criteria for starting antiretrovirals, and combination HAART should be started.
- Multiple first-line therapies are available; however, the combination of tenofovir/emtricitabine 300/200 mg once daily + lopinavir/ritonavir (200/50 mg tablets) four tablets once daily is an acceptable choice for this patient.
- Continued adherence consultations with this patient are needed and should be reinforced by the pharmacist at each visit to the clinic and her local pharmacy.

For more information on the care plan and facilitator's guide please visit http://www.mhpharmacotherapy.com.

94 Breast Cancer

Christopher J. Campen   Leona Downey

CASE LEARNING OBJECTIVES

- List the known risk factors in the development of breast cancer
- Assess the manifestations of locally advanced and metastatic breast cancer
- Identify the goals of therapy for a patient with locally advanced and metastatic disease
- Choose an appropriate personalized monitoring plan for patients on multimodal therapies for breast cancer
- Devise educational information for patients on systemic therapies for breast cancer

PATIENT PRESENTATION

Chief Complaint

"I noticed a lump on my breast. It doesn't hurt, but I am worried it might be cancer."

History of Present Illness

Cindy Thomas is a 56-year-old premenopausal woman who presents to her primary care physician (PCP) complaining of a new breast lump. She noticed this while trying on new clothes a week ago. There does not appear to be any pain associated with the lump. She last had a mammography 3 years ago, which showed no evidence of breast cancer.

Past Medical History

Depression diagnosed 14 years ago
HTN diagnosed 12 years ago

Family History

Her mother was diagnosed with early breast cancer at age 64. She underwent a total mastectomy followed by adjuvant chemotherapy and is currently free of cancer at age 78. Her father is currently in excellent health. She currently has no children.

Social History

She is married to her husband of 34 years. She has lived outside of San Francisco for nearly all of her life. She is the head of a small IT company and works 60 to 80 h/wk.

Tobacco/Alcohol/Substance Use

Past history of smoking for 6 years. Uses alcohol; four to six hard alcoholic drinks/wk. No illicit drug use

Allergies/Intolerances/Adverse Drug Events

No known drug allergies

Medications (Current)

Fluoxetine 40 mg PO q 24 h
HCTZ 12.5 mg PO q 24 h
Lisinopril 10 mg PO q 24 h
MVI one tablet PO daily

Review of Systems

Slightly distressed female with new-onset painless breast lump. No complaints of pain, soreness, or fatigue at this time

Physical Examination

▶ **General**

Slightly overweight woman in no acute distress

▶ **Vital Signs**

BP 152/96 mm Hg, P 78, RR 12, T 36.3°C
Weight 182 lb (82.7 kg)
Height 66 in. (167.6 cm)
Denies pain (pain 0/10)

▶ **Skin**

No suspicious lesions

▶ **HEENT**

PERRLA, EOMI

▶ **Lymph Nodes**

No palpable cervical, axillary, or clavicular adenopathy

▶ **Breasts**

Right: No masses or tenderness noted. Nipple everted. No abnormalities

Left: Breast lump approximately 5 cm palpable at the one o'clock position about 3 cm from the nipple. No nipple abnormalities or skin changes

▶ **Lungs**

Clear to auscultation and percussion. Good diaphragmatic movement

▶ **Cardiovascular**

RRR with normal S_1, S_2. Carotids without bruits

▶ **Abdomen**

Soft and nontender without hepatosplenomegaly or masses. Normal bowel sounds

▶ **Extremities**

No pedal edema

▶ **Neurology**

Grossly intact; reflexes normal

▶ **Psychiatric**

Mental status oriented × 3. Mood affect: slightly absent affect

Laboratory Tests

	Conventional Units	SI Units
Na	138 mEq/L	138 mmol/L
K	3.9 mEq/L	3.9 mmol/L
Cl	101 mEq/L	101 mmol/L
CO_2	23 mEq/L	23 mmol/L
BUN	12 mg/dL	4.3 mmol/L
SCr	0.8 mg/dL	71 μmol/L
Glu	110 mg/dL	6.1 mmol/L
Ca	9.2 mg/dL	2.30 mmol/L
Mg	2 mEq/L	1 mmol/L
Phosphate	4 mg/dL	1.29 mmol/L
Hgb	13.3 g/dL	133 g/L; 8.26 mmol/L
Hct	39.3%	0.393
WBC	$7.6 \times 10^3/mm^3$	$7.6 \times 10^9/L$
Platelet	$340 \times 10^3/mm^3$	$340 \times 10^9/L$
Albumin	4.1 g/dL	41 g/L

Pathology results

Invasive ductal carcinoma

Tumor size 5.3 cm at maximum dimension

Estrogen receptor (ER)/progresterone receptor (PR)+; HER2/neu+; no distant metastases seen

Diagnosed with T3N1M0 disease

ER	+ (95%)
PR	slightly + (45%)
HER2	+ (3+ out of 3+) via immunohistochemistry (IHC)

MRI results

Tumor size	$5.3 \times 2.8 \times 3.7$ cm
	Two lymph nodes appear positive in the ipsilateral axillary region

Assessment

A 56-year-old premenopausal woman presents with new-onset breast cancer. She first undergoes a left total mastectomy with axillary lymph node dissection and is diagnosed with T3N1M0 breast cancer. The physician decides to initiate adjuvant chemotherapy with doxorubicin/cyclophosphamide (AC) for four cycles followed by paclitaxel (T) and trastuzumab (Herceptin) weekly for 12 weeks. This will be followed by trastuzumab for a total of 1 year and tamoxifen for a total of 5 years. For the prevention of nausea/vomiting, she will be given ondansetron and dexamethasone, prior to AC, and prochlorperazine for breakthrough nausea/vomiting.

Student Workup

Missing Information?

Evaluate: Patient Database

Drug Therapy Problems

Care Plan (by Problem)

TARGETED QUESTIONS

1. What are the common early signs and symptoms of breast cancer?

    Hint: See p. 1478 in PPP

2. What stage is this patient diagnosed as?

    Hint: See pp. 1479–1480 and Table 89-3 in PPP

3. Discuss the positive and negative prognostic factors for this patient.

    Hint: See p. 1480 in PPP

4. Compare and contrast the use of adjuvant or neoadjuvant chemotherapy for this patient.

   Hint: See p. 1482 in PPP

5. What are some of the common toxicities and counseling points for anthracyclines, alkylating agents, and taxanes?

   Hint: See Table 89-7 in PPP

6. What are the counseling points for patients taking tamoxifen?

   Hint: See Table 89-9 in PPP

FOLLOW-UP

Three weeks later, the patient returns for the second course of doxorubicin and cyclophosphamide. She complains of significant nausea/vomiting lasting approximately 4 days following the first course, and is very fearful of this occurring again.

7. What are the patient-specific risk factors for nausea/ vomiting, and what are the risks of uncontrolled nausea? What antiemetic options are available for the prevention of anticipatory, acute, and delayed nausea/vomiting in this patient?

   Hint: See p. 1485 in PPP

☉ GLOBAL PERSPECTIVE

Breast cancer is the number one cause of cancer-related deaths in women globally. In many underdeveloped countries, infectious diseases are the primary threat, making cancer a low priority for resources. Unfortunately, a lack of screening and prevention results in significant resources required to manage patients that more often present with late-stage or advanced disease. The most effective strategy is to develop programs that will result in early diagnosis and intervention. The use of local–regional treatment and systemic therapy depends on the level of resources available, and is often region and country specific.

CASE SUMMARY

- The patient was diagnosed with locally advanced breast cancer, and multimodal therapy consisting of surgery, radiotherapy, and systemic therapy is indicated.

- The initial systemic chemotherapy regimen is appropriate given her diagnosis. Consider her pathology results when choosing additional endocrine and biologic therapy.

For more information on the care plan and facilitator's guide please visit http://www.mhpharmacotherapy.com.

95 Colon Cancer

Patrick J. Medina   Emily B. Borders

CASE LEARNING OBJECTIVES

- Identify the risk factors for colon cancer
- Recognize the signs and symptoms of colon cancer
- Describe the treatment options for colon cancer on the basis of patient-specific factors, such as stage of disease, age of the patient, and previous treatment received
- Develop a monitoring plan to assess the efficacy and toxicity of agents used in colon cancer
- Educate patients about the adverse effects of chemotherapy that require patient-specific counseling

PATIENT PRESENTATION

Chief Complaint

"I've been tired for the past 3 months and have this pain in my stomach that is getting worse. Today I noticed some blood in my stool and got scared. I'm not sure what is going on."

History of Present Illness

John Braxton is a 59-year-old Caucasian male who presented to his primary care physician with generalized fatigue for 3 months, abdominal pain, and new blood in his stool. Over-the-counter famotidine had been recommended for the abdominal pain, and provided no relief. He also reports that he has not been able to eat like he normally does due to "feeling full all the time" and constipation. A CBC revealed microcytic anemia and iron profile was consistent with iron deficiency. Fecal occult blood test was positive. Colonoscopy demonstrated a 5-cm (2-inch) frond-like, nonobstructing, villous lesion arising from the descending colon. Biopsies were positive for low-grade, moderately differentiated adenocarcinoma. Tumor marker carcinoembryonic antigen (CEA) was 80 ng/mL (80 mcg/L) [normal 0–5 ng/mL (0–5 mcg/L)]. There was no evidence of metastatic disease on staging CT scans. Pathology revealed 4.5-cm (1.8-inch), low-grade, moderately differentiated adenocarcinoma invading into the muscularis propria. Twenty-four lymph nodes were removed and four were positive for malignancy. The final diagnosis was stage III colon cancer. Postoperatively, CEA decreased to <0.1 ng/mL (<0.1 mcg/L). He underwent surgical resection with clear margins and is being evaluated 4 weeks later in your clinic for adjuvant treatment regimens.

Past Medical History

HTN

Hypercholesterolemia

Past Surgical History

Left-sided hemicolectomy for the colon mass

Family History

Mother deceased at age 75 with MI. Father deceased at age 60 with colon cancer diagnosed at the age of 58. Sister diagnosed with breast cancer at the age of 52; no additional family history of cancer in family per the patient's report.

Social History

The patient is a lifelong resident of the state of Florida. He currently works as a piano teacher. He is married and has two children.

Tobacco/Alcohol/Substance Use

The patient has been a lifetime nonsmoker, drinks alcohol socially, and denies any drug use.

Allergies/Intolerances/Adverse Drug Events

Not known

Medications (Current)

Atenolol 50 mg PO q 24 h

Atorvastatin 10 mg PO q 24 h

Famotidine 20 mg PO PRN abdominal pain

Hydrocodone/acetaminophen 5/325 mg PO PRN pain

Review of Systems

Abdominal pain/constipation with minor relief with famotidine; the patient has moderate postsurgical pain relieved with as-needed hydrocodone/acetaminophen. He denies any other symptoms, and additional review of symptoms is negative.

Physical Examination

▶ *General*

Thinly built, well-dressed, white male in no acute distress

▶ *Vital Signs*

BP 104/74 mm Hg, P 64, RR 13, T 36.4°C

Weight 165.3 lb (75.1 kg)

Height 69 in. (175.3 cm)

Mild abdominal and postsurgical pain

▶ *Skin*

Normal color with good turgor; (−) lesions or pigments noted

▶ *HEENT*

PERRLA; (−) pallor, icterus; oropharynx clear

▶ *Neck*

Supple; no jugular venous distention; no significant lymphadenopathy

▶ *Respiratory*

Clear to auscultation

▶ *Cardiovascular*

RRR; no murmurs

▶ *Abdomen*

Soft; tender on palpation; ostomy site clean; normal BS; (−) organomegaly

▶ *Extremities*

(−) Edema, cyanosis, clubbing

▶ *Neurology*

AAO × 3; CNs grossly intact; no focal deficits noted

▶ *Rectal*

Stool is guaiac (+).

Laboratory Tests

Fasting, obtained 5 days ago. S/p surgery 4 weeks ago

	Conventional Units	SI Units
Na	146 mEq/L	146 mmol/L
K	3.9 mEq/L	3.9 mmol/L
Cl	106 mEq/L	106 mmol/L
CO_2	24 mEq/L	24 mmol/L
BUN	18 mg/dL	6.4 mmol/L
SCr	0.9 mg/dL	80 μmol/L
Glu	117 mg/dL	6.5 mmol/L
Ca	8.8 mg/dL	2.20 mmol/L
Mg	1.9 mEq/L	0.95 mmol/L
WBC	$6 \times 10^3/mm^3$	$6 \times 10^9/L$
Hgb	13.4 g/dL	134 g/L; 8.31 mmol/L
Hct	38.2%	0.382
Platelets	$295 \times 10^3/mm^3$	$295 \times 10^9/L$
Albumin	3.1 g/dL	31 g/L
Total cholesterol	192 mg/dL	4.97 mmol/L
LDL cholesterol	140 mg/dL	3.62 mmol/L
HDL cholesterol	32 mg/dL	0.84 mmol/L
Total bilirubin	1.1 mg/dL	18.8 μmol/L
CEA	0.4 ng/mL	0.4 mcg/L

Assessment

A 59-year-old male with signs, symptoms, and pathology results diagnostic of stage III colon cancer

Student Workup

Missing Information?

Evaluate:	Patient Database
	Drug Therapy Problems
	Care Plan (by Problem)

TARGETED QUESTIONS

1. What are the signs and symptoms this patient has for colon cancer?

   Hint: See pp. 1521 and 1522 in PPP

2. What risk factors did this patient have for the development of colon cancer?

   Hint See pp. 1518 and 1519 in PPP

3. Why does this patient require adjuvant therapy?

   Hint: See pp. 1522 and 1524 in PPP

4. Why is FOLFOX the recommended regimen in this patient?

   Hint: See p. 1530 in PPP

5. What risk factors and adverse effects of therapy would you discuss with this patient?

   Hint: See pp. 1531 and 1532 in PPP; may also refer to individual chemotherapy summaries in Chapter 91 of PPP

FOLLOW-UP

The patient has been receiving the FOLFOX regimen for 4 months (eight cycles) with minimal adverse effects. During routine follow-up prior to his ninth cycle, he discusses a slight tingling in his fingers and toes.

6. What is most likely causing this problem? What actions, if any, would you take?

   Hint: See p. 1525 in PPP

⟲ GLOBAL PERSPECTIVE

Colon cancer is one of the most common cancers in the United States. The rate of colon cancer also is high in other industrialized countries in North America and Europe. Industrialized countries tend to have diets high in fat that partially explains the increased incidence, though other dietary and genetic factors play a role in its development. Early stage colon cancer (stages I–III) is curable with either surgery alone or surgery in combination with chemotherapy. Most patients receive 6 months of adjuvant chemotherapy following surgical resection of the tumor. Metastatic disease (stage IV) is currently incurable. The initial treatment for most patients is the same, though some of the chemotherapy agents (e.g., 5-fluorouracil, irinotecan) have pharmacogenomic factors that partially determine their efficacy and toxicity.

CASE SUMMARY

- The patient is diagnosed with stage III colon cancer requiring adjuvant chemotherapy.
- The initial regimen of FOLFOX is a reasonable choice, with 6 months of therapy recommended.
- Cumulative toxicities of the chemotherapy regimen should be evaluated at each clinic visit.

For more information on the care plan and facilitator's guide please visit http://www.mhpharmacotherapy.com.

96 Acute Lymphocytic Leukemia

Nancy H. Heideman   Richard L. Heideman

CASE LEARNING OBJECTIVES

- Recognize the major prognostic factors in childhood pre–B-cell acute lymphocytic leukemia
- Identify the treatment-related complications associated with the therapy for acute lymphocytic leukemia
- Identify the role of thiopurine methyltransferase metabolism with respect to 6-mercaptopurine toxicity
- Develop a plan to evaluate the patient's current problems and determine if they are related to his ability to metabolize 6-mercaptopurine and select an appropriate new dose for this patient
- Describe the late effects of chemotherapy related to the treatment of acute lymphocytic leukemia

PATIENT PRESENTATION

Chief Complaint (Mother's)

"My son keeps having repeated episodes of infection and low blood counts. He needs to be transfused more often than the other patients I know who are on the same protocol."

History of Present Illness

MC is a 12-year-old Hispanic male who was diagnosed with pre–B-cell acute lymphoblastic leukemia (ALL) diagnosed at age 11 years. His presenting WBC count was $7.5 \times 10^3/\text{mm}^3$ ($7.5 \times 10^9/\text{L}$) with 80% leukemic cells. He had no testicular disease and his cerebrospinal fluid showed no leukemic cells. Cytogenetic evaluation of his leukemic cells showed random chromosomal loss and gain. Tumor-cell ploidy showed a DNA content of 1.15. He had a prompt response to induction therapy with a morphologic remission at day 8. His end-of-induction minimal residual disease (MRD) was low. He recently completed his final "delayed intensification" treatment module and began "maintenance" treatment 5 months ago. Since the start of maintenance, he has had two admissions for fever of 101.3°F (38.5°C) and ANC of 250 to 300/mm³ ($0.25–0.30 \times 10^9/\text{L}$), each lasting 7 days. Both episodes were associated with negative blood cultures. On each occasion, his maintenance chemotherapy [daily oral 6-mercaptopurine (6MP) and weekly oral methotrexate] was stopped until his ANC was above 500/mm³ ($0.50 \times 10^9/\text{L}$), and he was afebrile for 48 hours.

Past Medical History

Full-term infant, uncomplicated birth, and neonatal history

ALL s/p chemotherapy; history of one previous admission for fever and neutropenia during the delayed intensification phase of treatment. He has received two prior platelet transfusions, one each during induction and delayed intensification phases of treatment. He has received three prior RBC transfusions, the last of which was greater than 3 months ago

Completely up-to-date on childhood immunizations for his age up to the time of his diagnosis for ALL

Family History

Noncontributory

Social/Work History

The patient is currently in seventh grade at an elementary school in a disadvantaged neighborhood where the first language of many residents is Spanish. He is a good student, and his parents were involved in his school and community in a positive way. There are two additional siblings in the home: a 6-year-old sister in kindergarten and a 9-year-old brother in fifth grade. All the children and parents are bilingual; even so, the parents are more comfortable in and prefer Spanish for oral and written communication.

Tobacco/Alcohol/Substance Use

Noncontributory

Allergies/Intolerances/Adverse Drug Events

None known

Medications (Current)

6MP 100 mg/m² PO daily

Methotrexate 33.75 mg/m² PO once weekly

Vincristine 2 mg/m² IV once monthly

Dexamethasone 4 mg PO bid 5 days each month

Docusate 50 mg at bedtime PRN constipation

Review of Systems

The patient has chronic and troublesome constipation, assumed to be related to vincristine. This is moderated by the administration of docusate at bedtime, but never completely resolves. He was discharged from the inpatient service 2 weeks ago for a culture-negative episode of fever and neutropenia, for which he received 3 days of IV cefepime. He has had no recent fevers and has resumed his oral 6MP and methotrexate after being off these agents for almost 2 weeks. He does complain that his hips are increasingly "sore" over the last 4 to 6 weeks and he takes acetaminophen as often as six times a day for these symptoms. There are no other systemic symptoms.

Physical Examination

▶ General

Well appearing in no acute distress

▶ Vital Signs

BP 98/56 mm Hg, P 75, RR 18, T 99.7°F (37.6°C)

Weight 94.6 lb (43 kg)

Height 59 in. (150 cm)

Pain 6/10

▶ Skin

Warm, soft, supple, without rash

▶ HEENT

Partial alopecia; other within normal limits

▶ Neck and Lymph Nodes

No palpable adenopathy; no palpable thyroid gland

▶ Chest

Clear to auscultation; port site in right upper chest clean, dry, and intact

▶ Cardiovascular

Normal sinus rate and rhythm; good capillary refill; no murmurs appreciated

▶ Abdomen

Nontender, nondistended, palpable stool in left lower quadrant. Liver and spleen are not palpable.

▶ Extremities

Range of motion normal. No deformities noted. Some tenderness associated with extremes of motion and weight bearing, particularly on the right side. Some nonquantifiable discomfort associated with deep palpation at hip joint.

▶ Neurology

Unremarkable, except for loss of deep tendon reflexes at knees and somewhat flat-footed gait. Other within normal limits.

▶ Genitourinary

Unremarkable; testes normal size and texture for age

▶ Rectal

Small, healing perirectal tear with mild and perilesional erythema. No discharge or flatulence.

Laboratory Tests

	Conventional Units	SI Units
Na	137 mEq/L	137 mmol/L
K	4.2 mEq/L	4.2 mmol/L
BUN	9 mg/dL	3.2 mmol/L
SCr	0.35 mg/dL	31 μmol/L
Mg	1.9 mEq/L	0.95 mmol/L
Phosphate	3.8 mg/dL	1.23 mmol/L
AST	51 IU/L	0.85 μkat/L
ALT	44 IU/L	0.73 μkat/L
Total bilirubin	0.9 mg/dL	15.4 μmol/L
Direct bilirubin	0.45 mg/dL	7.7 μmol/L
Hgb	11.8 g/dL	118 g/L; 7.32 mmol/L
Hct	34%	0.34
WBC	1.2×10^3/mm³	1.2×10^9/L
ANC	675/mm³	0.675×10^9/L
MCV	85 μm³	85 fL
Platelet count	98,000/mm³	98×10^9/L

▶ Urinalysis

Pale color

Specific gravity 1.010

No RBCs or WBCs seen

Nitrate negative

▶ Radiology

X-ray of hips shows some sclerosis of both femoral heads and partial collapse on the right.

Assessment

A 12-year-old boy with acute pre–B-cell ALL in the maintenance phase of treatment with two recent episodes of fever and neutropenia and a current somewhat low ANC. The history and current laboratory tests suggest repeated episodes of excessive hematologic toxicity. He additionally has chronic constipation that causes periodic rectal pain despite laxative use. Further, he complains of pain in both hips, which has been increasing in severity over the last 4 to 6 weeks.

Student Workup

Missing Information?

Evaluate:	Patient Database
	Drug Therapy Problems
	Care Plan (by Problem)

TARGETED QUESTIONS

1. Evaluate the prognostic factors for ALL and evaluate the patient's potential risk for relapse.

   Hint: See pp. 1583 and 1584 in PPP

2. What do the patient's current CBC and prior problems with fever and neutropenia suggest with respect to potential drug toxicity?

   Hint: See p. 1589 in PPP

3. What additional testing should be considered to determine if there is an underlying problem in drug metabolism?

   Hint: See p. 1589 in PPP

4. Is there a potential role for interviewing the patient's mother/father through a Spanish interpreter?

   Hint: See patient/family's preferred language in "Social/ Work History" for this case

5. Are there any medications missing from the patient's treatment profile?

   Hint: See p. 1594 in PPP

6. What is the likely cause of the patient's bilateral hip pain?

   Hint: See p. 1595 in PPP

FOLLOW-UP

The patient returns at 2 and 4 weeks after a 90% dose reduction in 6MP dose was started. His WBC counts at these points were 2.3 and 3.0×10^3/mm^3 (2.3 and 3.0×10^9/L), respectively, with corresponding ANCs of 1,600 and 2,000/mm^3 (1.6 and 2.0×10^9/L). At 3 months after the initial dose reduction, the WBC count is 4.8×10^3/mm^3 (4.8×10^9/L), the ANC is 3,000/mm^3 (3.0×10^9/L), and the patient has a normal hemoglobin, hematocrit, and platelet count.

7. What does this potentially say about you are the degree of your dose reduction?

   Hint: The WBC and ANC recovery are consistent with a thiopurine methyltransferase (TPMT) genotype associated with diminished drug inactivation. The initial 90% dose reductions may have been too much and the latest laboratory values suggest insufficient drug activity. Another possibility is that the family/patient have been giving even less 6MP because they were worried about toxicity. Check for compliance and consider adjusting the 6MP dose to 50% of the original dose. A 90% reduction is done only for patients with TPMT alleles with very diminished activity; 50% reductions are done in those with intermediate enzyme activity. After starting an additional drug for Pneumocystis jiroveci pneumonia (PJP) prophylaxis, the patient developed a pruritic, maculopapular rash over his chest and extremities.

8. What drug is the most likely cause for this problem and what recommendations would you make regarding a change in therapy?

   Hint: The most common agent used for PJP prophylaxis and the medication missing from the patient's profile is trimethoprim/sulfamethoxazole (TMP/SMX). Most patients tolerate this drug well; however, some develop an allergy to the drug, which is most typically a maculopapular rash. The drug should be discontinued. The patient's chart and records should also be labeled as "TMP/SMX and sulfa allergic." Because of the patient's age, he is a good candidate for monthly inhaled pentamidine as a substitute.

⟳ GLOBAL PERSPECTIVE

Risk assessment (for relapse) is important in the treatment of ALL, and virtually all other malignancies. Knowing this allows for appropriate risk (toxicity of treatment) and reward (diminished risk of relapse) to be determined and thus the selection of a protocol with appropriate treatment intensity. Hematologic toxicity is common in patients receiving chemotherapy. Excessive toxicity may suggest an underlying problem with drug metabolism, clearance, or an incorrect dose. Likewise, the lack of expected myelosuppression may be an indicator of insufficient or absent doses. The etiologic distinction between drug interactions, incorrect dosing by the patient or family, or individual drug metabolic capacity can be difficult to determine, especially with oral medications. 6MP bioavailability is affected by the time of day the drug is given as well as the proximity to food and dairy products. Further, older children and adolescents may "game" their caretakers by not taking their medications ("cupping" their pills in their hand or holding them in their mouth without swallowing them and only later to dispose of them) or by only occasionally taking their medications. Also, there is also great potential for misunderstanding the dose and schedule of administration among patients and families whose primary language is different than the prescriber's; frequent questioning confirming the dose and timing is needed to assure compliance. It should also be kept in mind that, at times, the caretaker may change from the parent to a grandparent or other person during times when medications are due. The understanding and willingness of these persons to give the dose can be another source of problems. Related to this are cultural beliefs; other caretakers may possess beliefs contrary to the parents' and conventional medical advice. This can make them reluctant to give what they consider "toxic" medications and/or add the use of traditional remedies that have the potential to affect drug absorption, metabolism, and toxicity. Drug metabolism problems are the least frequent cause of toxicity than the other reasons noted above, and for the same reason, often the last to be considered as a cause for toxicity. For 6MP in particular, and other maintenance drugs for ALL, monitoring the WBC and ANC is an effective way to spot problems. Virtually all patients began treatment at a dose that assumes that they are among the 90% or more of patients who have normal drug-metabolizing activity. In these patients, excessive toxicity is rare, and monitoring WBC and ANC to make empiric and protocol-specific changes to the dose is effective and easy. In patients who show early and excessive toxicity, the likelihood of drug metabolism issues is heightened. In the absence of pretreatment genotyping for alleles associated with altered metabolism (a reasonable, but controversial, issue), these patients are best investigated with the use of 6MP metabolites and a determination of TPMT genotype. Both of these can be easily obtained from a patient's RBCs. However, the RBCs should not represent transfused cells; a minimum of 2 to 3 months since the last RBC transfusion is necessary to obtain reliable results.

CASE SUMMARY

- The patient's clinical findings at diagnosis put him into a particular "risk" category for relapse.

- He has generally done well with aggressive therapy until the time he began daily 6MP and weekly methotrexate during his "maintenance" phase of treatment. His recent course and laboratory results are consistent with 6MP toxicity. This could be from potential overdosing as a result of poor provider/patient communication or inheritance of a polymorphism that limits drug metabolism and results in excessive levels of active metabolites. Given his "risk" category, his recent clinical course and laboratory results may warrant modification of the current treatment.

- A significant alteration in his 6MP dose was made that appears to have markedly diminished the patient's toxic episodes. However, his WBC and ANC seem to suggest that the dose reduction may have been too much or that some other problem has developed. A search for these problems and potential adjustments to the patient's dose may be needed to improve his antileukemic therapy and prevent relapse. Some critical tests and patient/family interviews are needed to determine what should be done next.

For more information on the care plan and facilitator's guide please visit http://www.mhpharmacotherapy.com.

97 Parenteral Nutrition

Michael D. Kraft   Imad F. Btaiche

CASE LEARNING OBJECTIVES

- List the appropriate indication(s) for the use of parenteral nutrition (PN)
- List the elements of a nutrition assessment and factors considered in assessing a patient's nutritional status and nutritional requirements
- Develop a plan to design, initiate, and adjust a PN formulation using patient-specific factors
- Describe the etiology and risk factors for the refeeding syndrome
- Design a plan to monitor and correct fluid, electrolyte, vitamin, and trace-element abnormalities in patients receiving PN
- Design a plan to monitor and assess the efficacy and safety of PN therapy

PATIENT PRESENTATION

Chief Complaint

"I've had an upset stomach and pain which has been getting worse for about 10 days, and I started vomiting about 3 days ago. I can't keep any food or liquids down."

History of Present Illness

Alex Rocker is a 46-year-old man with a history of morbid obesity s/p Roux-en-Y gastric bypass surgery in February 2007 for morbid obesity, who was admitted to the hospital 5 days ago on November 2, 2009, with abdominal pain, nausea, vomiting, and inability to tolerate oral intake. His postoperative course was complicated by anastomotic leak, peritonitis, sepsis, and high-output enterocutaneous (EC) fistula. He was initially placed nothing per os (NPO) with home PN and wound care for 6 months, and afterward underwent surgery for EC fistula takedown and small bowel resection with primary anastamosis. The patient has also had recurrent partial and total small bowel obstructions due to adhesions and had two other surgeries (exploratory laparotomies) for lysis of adhesions (in May 2008 and September 2009). Since his initial gastric bypass surgery, the patient lost approximately 100 lb (~46 kg) of his original pregastric bypass weight of 295 lb (134 kg). For the past 10 days before presentation to the emergency department, he has had worsening nausea and abdominal pain that initially developed after eating a meal and appeared to get worse after eating. The abdominal pain gradually worsened, was associated with vomiting for the past 3 days, and he could not keep any food or liquids down. He described his symptoms as similar to the last time he had a bowel obstruction, but they now seem worse.

The patient was subsequently admitted to the GI surgery service for further management. Initially, he was managed conservatively by placing a NG tube for gastric fluid suctioning and bowel decompression, was placed NPO, and started on IV fluids for hydration. After 2 days of conservative management, the patient did not show any signs of improvement of his GI symptoms. A CT scan with oral contrast was done and demonstrated a complete small bowel obstruction. The surgical team decided on observing the patient and continuing conservative management for about a week until the patient's symptoms would resolve or otherwise would necessitate surgical intervention. Because the patient has had poor nutritional intake for about 12 days since the beginning of his symptoms, is currently NPO, has a complete bowel obstruction, and has had significant chronic weight loss since his gastric bypass surgery, he had a peripherally inserted central catheter (PICC) placed for PN therapy to be initiated.

PN therapy was initiated and then advanced to full nutritional goal on the second day. On the third day of PN therapy, he developed some confusion, and his biochemical workup showed multiple serum electrolyte abnormalities.

Past Medical History

Type 2 DM × 5 years

Morbid obesity for "most of his life" per patient

Past Surgical History

Gastric bypass surgery (Roux-en-Y procedure) in February 2007

Exploratory laparotomies and lysis of adhesions in May 2008 and September 2009

Family History

Remarkable for obesity and type 2 DM (mother and father), HTN (mother and father), and hyperlipidemia (father)

Social History

Married, lives with his wife

Tobacco/Alcohol/Substance Abuse

Drinks alcohol occasionally/socially; no history of smoking

Allergies/Intolerances/Adverse Drug Events

No known drug allergies

Medications (Current)

Heparin 5,000 units SC tid

Pantoprazole 40 mg IV daily

Bisacodyl 10 mg suppository per rectum daily PRN constipation

Morphine sulfate 5 to 10 mg IV q 4 h PRN pain

Prochlorperazine 10 mg IV q 6 h PRN nausea

Regular insulin q 6 h, dosage per capillary blood glucose measurements (chemsticks)

Medications Prior to Admission

Glipizide XL 10 mg PO daily

Metformin XR 1,000 mg PO daily

Review of Systems

Subjectively reporting ongoing abdominal pain, nausea, vomiting, no appetite. Also complains of dry mouth, feels thirsty, and abdomen feels bloated. (+) Dry mucus membranes. Denies fever, chills, or other pain.

Physical Examination

► General

Middle-aged, slightly overweight African American man, uncomfortable because of abdominal pain, nausea, and vomiting

► Vital Signs

BP 134/84 mm Hg, P 92, RR 17, T 37.6°C

Weight 194 lb (88 kg)

Height 69 in. (175 cm)

Per patient, weight in 2006 prior to gastric bypass surgery 295 lb (~134 kg); weight in January 2009 reported to be 220 lb (100 kg)

Patient reports abdominal pain rated as 4–6/10, some relief with morphine and prochlorperazine

► Skin

Dry

► HEENT

PERRLA, EOMI, anicteric sclerae, mucus membranes dry

► Chest

Clear to auscultation bilaterally

► Cardiovascular

RRR; no murmurs, rubs, or gallops

► Abdomen

(+) Distention, hypoactive/absent bowel sounds, diffuse tenderness throughout all quadrants

► Neurology

A&O × 3; CNs II to XII intact

► Extremities

(−) Cyanosis, good pulse

► Genitourinary

Examination deferred

► Rectum

Examination deferred

Laboratory Tests

On admission

	Conventional Units	SI Units
Na	138 mEq/L	138 mmol/L
K	3.6 mEq/L	3.6 mmol/L
Cl	94 mEq/L	94 mmol/L
CO_2	28 mEq/L	28 mmol/L
BUN	12 mg/dL	4.3 mmol/L
SCr	0.5 mg/dL	44 μmol/L
Ca	7.6 mg/dL	1.90 mmol/L
Mg	1.7 mEq/L	0.85 mmol/L
Phos	3.1 mg/dL	1 mmol/L
Glu	152 mg/dL	8.4 mmol/L
Hgb	14.1 g/dL	141 g/L; 8.74 mmol/L
Hct	41.7%	0.417
Platelet	$348 \times 10^3/mm^3$	$348 \times 10^9/L$
WBC	$7.4 \times 10^3/mm^3$	$7.4 \times 10^9/L$

AST	17 IU/L	0.28 μkat/L
ALT	21 IU/L	0.35 μkat/L
Alk phos	31 IU/L	0.52 μkat/L
Total bilirubin	0.6 mg/dL	10.3 μmol/L
Alb	2.4 g/dL	24 g/L
Total protein	5.6 g/dL	56 g/L

Laboratory Tests

On hospital day 5 (day 3 of PN)

	Conventional Units	SI Units
Na	135 mEq/L	135 mmol/L
K	2.9 mEq/L	2.9 mmol/L
Cl	92 mEq/L	92 mmol/L
CO_2	38 mEq/L	38 mmol/L
BUN	19 mg/dL	6.8 mmol/L
SCr	0.6 mg/dL	53 μmol/L
Glu	207 mg/dL	11.5 mmol/L
Ca	7.1 mg/dL	1.78 mmol/L
Mg	1.2 mEq/L	0.60 mmol/L
Phos	1.1 mg/dL	0.36 mmol/L
Hgb	13.2 g/dL	132 g/L; 8.18 mmol/L
Hct	38.4%	0.384
Platelet	$297 \times 10^3/mm^3$	$297 \times 10^9/L$
WBC	$8.9 \times 10^3/mm^3$	$8.9 \times 10^9/L$
AST	18 IU/L	0.30 μkat/L
ALT	19 IU/L	0.32 μkat/L
Alk phos	34 IU/L	0.57 μkat/L
Total bilirubin	0.9 mg/dL	15.4 μmol/L
Alb	2.1 g/dL	21 g/L
Total protein	5.2 g/dL	52 g/L

► Radiology

CT scan with oral contrast demonstrates a complete small bowel obstruction

Assessment

This is a 46-year-old man with a history of morbid obesity and type 2 DM, who is s/p Roux-en-Y gastric bypass surgery, gradual weight loss of approximately 100 lb (~46 kg) over the past 32 months, and weight loss of approximately 26 lb (~12 kg) since January; he was admitted to the hospital with abdominal pain and nausea for 10 days and vomiting for 3 days. The results of his abdominal CT scan and his symptoms are consistent with recurrent complete small bowel obstruction. Given the patient's medical and surgical history, the attending surgeon did not believe the patient was an optimal candidate for immediate surgery and decided to continue conservative management by keeping the patient NPO, continue with an NG tube to suction, supportive care, symptomatic treatment, and PN for nutrition support. After 3 days of PN, he developed signs and symptoms consistent with refeeding syndrome.

Student Workup

Missing Information?

Evaluate:	Patient Database
	Drug Therapy Problems
	Care Plan (by Problem)

TARGETED QUESTIONS

1. Why is this patient at risk for refeeding syndrome?

   Hint: See pp. 1697–1698 and reference 45 in Chapter 100 in PPP

2. Does this patient have an appropriate indication for PN therapy?

   Hint: See p. 1682, Table 100-1, and references 1, 2, and 6 in Chapter 100 in PPP

3. What signs, symptoms, and laboratory abnormalities does this patient have that are consistent with refeeding syndrome?

   Hint: See pp. 1697–1698 and reference 45 in Chapter 100 in PPP

4. What steps would you take to treat refeeding syndrome in this patient?

   Hint: See pp. 1697–1698 and references 45 and 49 in Chapter 100 in PPP

5. Given that this patient has a complete small bowel obstruction and is NPO, what treatment would you recommend for his hyperglycemia? What target range for serum glucose concentrations would you recommend?

   Hint: See pp. 1694–1695 and references 32–35 in Chapter 100 in PPP

6. Is this patient receiving any medications that do not have an appropriate indication?

FOLLOW-UP

The surgical team takes your recommendations, and the patient's symptoms and electrolyte abnormalities have resolved. His bowel obstruction has still not resolved, and the team wants to continue PN therapy. You found that the patient was receiving the following IV fluids: 5% dextrose and 0.45% sodium chloride in water (D_5W ½ NS) at 80 mL/h prior to PN and then decreased to 20 mL/h when PN was started. He was also receiving the following PN prescription at goal (day 2 of PN):

Two-in-one PN formulation (IV lipid emulsion infused separately from dextrose/amino acid/micronutrient admixture at Y-site)

20% lipid emulsion = 384 mL/d (16 mL/h)

PN volume (dextrose/amino acid/micronutrient admixture) = 2,160 mL (90 mL/h)

Dextrose = 450 g/d

Amino acids = 130 g/d

Potassium chloride = 80 mEq/d (80 mmol/d)

Sodium chloride = 20 mEq/d (20 mmol/d)

Sodium acetate = 60 mEq/d (60 mmol/d)

Sodium phosphate = 20 mmol/d

Calcium gluconate = 10 mEq/d (5 mmol/d)

Magnesium sulfate = 10 mEq/d (5 mmol/d)

Parenteral adult multivitamin = 10 mL/d

Multitrace element (concentrate) = 1 mL/d

7. What recommendations would you have about resuming PN in this patient? Develop a goal PN regimen, as well as a plan to initiate PN, advance PN to goal, and monitor PN therapy while in the hospital.

> *Hint: Calculate total calories and protein in the above PN prescription; note amounts of electrolytes (especially phosphate, potassium, magnesium, and sodium), total fluid, and any supplemental vitamins and trace elements; evaluate the patient's fluid needs and assess any abnormal fluid and electrolyte losses (e.g., GI losses); see pp. 1684–1687, 1697–1698, and references 45 and 49 in Chapter 100 in PPP*

⊙ GLOBAL PERSPECTIVE

The refeeding syndrome is a constellation of metabolic derangements that can occur in patients who are malnourished or who have had a prolonged period of inadequate nutrition with significant weight loss. Refeeding syndrome can lead to serious complications, including death, and it is one of the few true emergencies associated with nutrition support. In developing countries or areas where malnutrition is prevalent and nutrient and vitamin deficiencies are common, refeeding syndrome could be a significant concern if the person were to receive a more abundant source of nutrition (orally or parenterally). These individuals with severe protein and calorie malnutrition may be more likely to have underlying vitamin and trace element deficiencies that could complicate or worsen symptoms of refeeding syndrome (e.g., thiamine, folic acid, vitamin B_{12}, vitamin D, iron, selenium, zinc, copper).

This could be especially concerning in growing children with poor body protein and energy reserves and pregnant women who have added energy and nutrient demands. A good rule of thumb in individuals with moderate-to-severe malnutrition is to "start low and go slow" when initiating any type of nutrition whether PN, enteral nutrition, or oral diet. This slow-and-gradual approach is essential to avoid the complications of refeeding syndrome that may severely affect the cardiac, respiratory, neurologic, and neuromuscular systems. It is also important to provide aggressive supplementation of electrolytes, vitamins, and trace elements *before* initiating nutrition, and regularly as needed during nutrition advancement guided by serum electrolyte concentrations and clinical status.

CASE SUMMARY

- The patient is exhibiting signs and symptoms consistent with refeeding syndrome. Even though he may not have the traditional marasmic appearance (i.e., "skin and bone"), he has experienced dramatic weight loss and has had little or no nutrition intake for approximately 10 days. Individuals at risk for refeeding syndrome should be first identified, and electrolyte supplementation provided immediately with supportive treatment provided when necessary to avoid comorbidities and possibly death. A specific prevention and treatment plan should be outlined.

- PN should be restarted very cautiously, and a treatment plan should be developed to avoid signs and symptoms of refeeding syndrome from recurring.

- The patient also has type 2 DM, and is NPO with a complete small bowel obstruction. Therefore, a plan must be developed to adequately treat hyperglycemia while he is NPO and receiving PN in the hospital.

> **For more information on the care plan and facilitator's guide please visit http://www.mhpharmacotherapy.com.**

98 Obesity

Maqual R. Graham

CASE LEARNING OBJECTIVES

- Identify parameters utilized to diagnose obesity and other objective information that indicates the severity of disease
- Identify desired therapeutic goals for patients who are obese
- Recommend appropriate nonpharmacologic and pharmacologic therapeutic interventions for obese patients
- Implement a monitoring plan that will assess both the efficacy and safety of therapy initiated
- Educate the patient about the disease state and associated risks, appropriate lifestyle modifications, and drug therapy options necessary for effective treatment

PATIENT PRESENTATION

Chief Complaint

"I will be 60 years old very soon. I am tired of being tired. I want more energy; I want to feel young again."

History of Present Illness

Joseph Michelson is a 59-year-old male patient presenting to the Cardiovascular Disease Risk Reduction Clinic for an initial evaluation. He was referred by his primary care provider for aggressive weight management. The patient states that he rarely eats healthy, even though his wife continually suggests healthier food choices. He prefers to eat meals high in fat and carbohydrates. He defines himself as a meat and potato type of guy. He snacks on corn and potato chips several times per day. He usually follows his salty snack with sweet-tasting foods, such as cookies or candy. He rarely consumes fruit. He drinks a glass of orange juice every morning. Throughout the day, he generally craves soda that is usually dark in color and caffeinated. Because of his work schedule, he finds it difficult to exercise. If he does have time to exercise in the evening, he lacks motivation. He has lost weight many times in the past. Each drop in weight resulted in him feeling more energetic and thus he appears ready to lose weight.

Past Medical History

HTN diagnosed 5 years ago
GERD diagnosed 10 years ago

Family History

Father had CHD and died following a second MI at age 63. Mother is alive at age 89 with type 2 DM and hypothyroidism.

He has three sisters and one brother who are all alive. His brother was recently hospitalized with cardiac chest pain (age 61).

Social History

The patient is married and lives with his wife of 41 years. He has two children (ages 35 and 39). He owns a small business that specializes in floor covering.

Tobacco/Alcohol/Substance Use

The patient denies tobacco use. He occasionally drinks alcohol, one to two beers on the weekend. No current or past illicit drug use.

Allergies/Intolerances/Adverse Drug Events

None

Medications (Current)

Metoprolol 25 mg PO twice daily
Diltiazem 360 mg PO once daily
Aspirin 325 mg PO once daily
Ranitidine 75 mg PO twice daily

Review of Systems

▶ *General*

The patient has gained 10 lb (4.5 kg) in the last year.

▶ *Skin*

No rashes or other skin changes

▶ **HEENT**

Hearing good; (−) tinnitus; (−) infections. The patient reports two mild colds in the last year.

▶ **Neck**

(−) Lumps, goiter

▶ **Respiratory**

(−) Cough, wheezing, SOB

▶ **Cardiovascular**

(−) Dyspnea, chest pain, palpitations

▶ **Gastrointestinal**

Appetite good; (−) nausea, vomiting; (+) daily bowel movements. Occasional reflux symptoms following very high fat meals

▶ **Urinary**

(−) Change in urinary frequency, hematuria

▶ **Neurologic**

(−) Syncope; (−) loss of consciousness

Physical Examination

▶ **General**

Well-developed, middle-aged male in no acute distress

▶ **Vital Signs**

BP 132/74 mm Hg, P 58 bpm, RR 12 rpm, T 96.8°F (36.0°C)

Weight 225 lb (102.3 kg)

Height 65 in. (165.1 cm)

Waist circumference 46.5 inch (118 cm)

Pain 0/10

▶ **Skin**

(−) Lesions; nails without clubbing or cyanosis

▶ **HEENT**

PERRLA, EOMI; (−) sinus tenderness; TM appears normal bilaterally; oral mucosa pink

▶ **Neck and Lymph Nodes**

Neck supple; (−) lymphadenopathy; trachea midline; (−) enlarged thyroid, (−) thyroid nodules; (−) carotid bruits

▶ **Chest**

Clear to auscultation bilaterally

▶ **Cardiovascular**

Regular rhythm, bradycardic, (−) S_3 or S_4

▶ **Abdomen**

Nontender, nondistended, bowel sounds active in all four quadrants, no masses detected

▶ **Neurology**

CNs II to XII intact; strength 5/5; normal gait; (−) Romberg, normal reflexes

▶ **Extremities**

Warm and without edema bilaterally

▶ **Genitourinary**

Examination deferred

▶ **Rectal**

Examination deferred

Laboratory Tests

Fasting

	Conventional Units	SI Units
Na	140 mEq/L	140 mmol/L
K	4.6 mEq/L	4.6 mmol/L
Cl	106 mEq/L	106 mmol/L
CO_2	24 mEq/L	24 mmol/L
BUN	12 mg/dL	4.3 mmol/L
SCr	0.9 mg/dL	80 μmol/L
Glu	96 mg/dL	5.3 mmol/L
Ca	9.7 mg/dL	2.43 mmol/L
Lipase	26 U/L	0.43 μkat/L
Amylase	36 U/L	0.60 μkat/L
Hgb	14.9 g/dL	149 g/L; 9.24 mmol/L
Hct	44%	0.44
WBC	$5.4 \times 10^3/mm^3$	$5.4 \times 10^9/L$
Platelets	$156 \times 10^3/\mu L$	$156 \times 10^9/L$
AST	29 U/L	0.48 μkat/L
ALT	38 U/L	0.63 μkat/L
TSH	1.498 μIU/mL	1.498 mIU/L
Total cholesterol	274 mg/dL	7.09 mmol/L
LDL cholesterol	201 mg/dL	5.20 mmol/L
HDL cholesterol	31 mg/dL	0.80 mmol/L
Triglycerides	272 mg/dL	3.07 mmol/L

Assessment

A 59-year-old obese male in need of reduced cardiovascular disease (CVD) risk

Student Workup

Missing Information?

Evaluate: Patient Database

Drug Therapy Problems

Care Plan (by Problem)

TARGETED QUESTIONS

1. How would you classify this patient s BMI?

    Hint: See p. 1721 in PPP

2. Does this patient have a high-risk waist circumference?

    Hint: See p. 1721 in PPP

3. Does this patient have CV risk factors, and if so, which one(s)?

    Hint: See Table 102-3 in PPP

4. Is this patient a candidate for weight loss, and if so, what is the initial weight loss goal?

    Hint: See p. 1721 in PPP

5. Is nonpharmacologic therapy, pharmacologic therapy, or both recommended for this patient?

    Hint: See pp. 1722–1728 in PPP

6. What patient parameters need to be assessed when this patient returns for follow-up?

    Hint: See pp. 1728–1729 in PPP

FOLLOW-UP

The patient has returned for all scheduled follow-up assessment visits in the CVD Risk Reduction Clinic. By the 6-month follow-up visit, the patient's weight was reduced by 10 lb (4.5 kg). His waist circumference is now 45.5 inch (116 cm). He appears compliant with the therapy previously recommended. He feels a little more energetic; however, he wishes that he was closer to his weight loss goal.

7. Should the initial therapeutic recommendations be altered, and if so, how?

    Hint: See pp. 1728–1729 in PPP

GLOBAL PERSPECTIVE

Energy imbalance, or energy intake greater than energy expenditure, is a key factor in the development of obesity. The longer the imbalance occurs, the greater the extent of obesity. Height and weight can easily be assessed anytime a patient–provider interaction occurs. From these two parameters, BMI can be determined. Waist circumference should also be evaluated as well as presence of other comorbidities and CV risk factors. Weight reduction, maintaining weight loss, and preventing weight gain are the general therapeutic goals for obese patients. Controlling related risks is an additional goal in the management of obesity. Lifestyle changes (dietary modification, increased physical activity, and behavioral therapy), drug treatment, surgery, or a combination of strategies are necessary for meeting desired outcomes. Frequent monitoring is necessary to determine the success or failure of the treatment plan.

CASE SUMMARY

- JM is a class 2 obese patient with a high-risk waist circumference and CV risk factors that include male gender and age 45 years or older, HTN, high LDL cholesterol, and low HDL cholesterol.

- Lifestyle changes are recommended to reduce his weight by 22 lb (10 kg) in 6 months at a rate of 1 to 2 lb (0.45–0.9 kg)/wk.

- Aggressive management of related risks (BP, LDL cholesterol, and HDL cholesterol) is necessary for overall effective treatment of the obese patient.

For more information on the care plan and facilitator's guide please visit http://www.mhpharmacotherapy.com.

Appendix A: Conversion Factors and Anthropometrics*

CONVERSION FACTORS

SI Units

SI (*le Systéme International d'Unités*) units are used in *many* countries to express clinical laboratory and serum drug concentration data. Instead of employing units of mass (such as micrograms), the SI system uses moles (mol) to represent the amount of a substance. A molar solution contains 1 mole (the molecular weight of the substance in grams) of the solute in 1 L of solution. The following formula is used to convert units of mass to moles (mcg/mL to µmol/L or, by substitution of terms, mg/mL to mmol/L or ng/mL to nmol/L).

▶ *Micromoles per Liter*

Micromoles per liter (µmol/L)

$$= \frac{\text{drug concentration (mcg/mL)} \times 1{,}000}{\text{molecular weight of drug (g/mol)}}$$

▶ *Milliequivalents*

An equivalent weight of a substance is that weight which will combine with or replace 1 g of hydrogen; a milliequivalent is 1/1,000 of an equivalent weight.

Milliequivalents per Liter

Milliequivalents per liter (mEq/L)

$$= \frac{\text{weight of salt (g)} \times \text{valence of ion} \times 1{,}000}{\text{molecular weight of salt}}$$

Weight of salt (g)

$$= \frac{\text{mEq/L} \times \text{molecular weight of salt}}{\text{valence of ion} \times 1{,}000}$$

Approximate Milliequivalents: Weight Conversions for Selected Ions		
Salt	mEq/g Salt	mg Salt/ mEq
Calcium carbonate ($CaCO_3$)	20.0	50.0
Calcium chloride ($CaCl_2 \cdot 2H_2O$)	13.6	73.5
Calcium gluceptate ($Ca[C_7H_{13}O_8]_2$)	4.1	245.2
Calcium gluconate ($Ca[C_6H_{11}O_7]_2 \cdot H_2O$)	4.5	224.1
Calcium lactate ($Ca[C_3H_5O_3]_2 \cdot 5H_2O$)	6.5	154.1
Magnesium gluconate ($Mg[C_6H_{11}O_7]_2 \cdot H_2O$)	4.6	216.3
Magnesium oxide (MgO)	49.6	20.2
Magnesium sulfate ($MgSO_4$)	16.6	60.2
Magnesium sulfate ($MgSO_4 \cdot 7H_2O$)	8.1	123.2
Potassium acetate ($K[C_2H_3O_2]$)	10.2	98.1
Potassium chloride (KCl)	13.4	74.6
Potassium citrate ($K_3[C_6H_5O_7] \cdot H_2O$)	9.2	108.1
Potassium iodide (KI)	6.0	166.0
Sodium acetate ($Na[C_2H_3O_2]$)	12.2	82.0
Sodium acetate ($Na[C_2H_3O_2] \cdot 3H_2O$)	7.3	136.1
Sodium bicarbonate ($NaHCO_3$)	11.9	84.0
Sodium chloride (NaCl)	17.1	58.4
Sodium citrate ($Na_3[C_6H_5O_7] \cdot 2H_2O$)	10.2	98.0
Sodium iodide (NaI)	6.7	149.9
Sodium lactate ($Na[C_3H_5O_3]$)	8.9	112.1
Zinc sulfate ($ZnSO_4 \cdot 7H_2O$)	7.0	143.8

*This appendix contains information from Appendices 1 and 2 of Anderson PO, Knoben JE, Troutman WG, et al (eds). *Handbook of Clinical Drug Data*, 10th ed. New York: McGraw-Hill, 2002:1053–1058, with permission.

Valences and Atomic Weights of Selected Ions

Substance	Electrolyte	Valence	Molecular Weight
Calcium	Ca^{2+}	2	40.1
Chloride	Cl^-	1	35.5
Magnesium	Mg^{2+}	2	24.3
Phosphate (pH = 7.4)	HPO_4^- (80%) $H_2PO_4^-$ (20%)	1.8	96.0^a
Potassium	K^+	1	39.1
Sodium	Na^+	1	23.0
Sulfate	SO_4^-	2	96.0^a

^{a}The molecular weight of phosphorus only is 31; that of sulfur only is 32.1.

Anion Gap

The anion gap is the concentration of plasma anions not routinely measured by laboratory screening. It is useful in the evaluation of acid–base disorders. The anion gap is greater with increased plasma concentrations of endogenous species (e.g., phosphate, sulfate, lactate, and ketoacids) or exogenous species (e.g., salicylate, penicillin, ethylene glycol, ethanol, and methanol). The formulas for calculating the anion gap are as follows:

$$\text{Anion gap} = (Na^+ + K^+) - (Cl^- + HCO_3^-)$$

or

$$\text{Anion gap} = Na^+ - (Cl^- + HCO_3^-)$$

where the expected normal value for the first equation is 11 to 20 mmol/L and that for the second equation is 7 to 16 mmol/L. Note that there is a variation in the upper and lower limits of the normal range.

Temperature

Fahrenheit to Centigrade: $(°F - 32) \times 5/9 = °C$
Centigrade to Fahrenheit: $(°C \times 9/5) + 32 = °F$
Centigrade to Kelvin: $°C + 273 = °K$

Calories

1 calorie = 1 kilocalorie = 1,000 calories = 4.184 kilojoules (kJ)
1 kilojoule = 0.239 calories = 0.239 kilocalories = 239 calories

Weights and Measures

▶ Metric Weight Equivalents

1 kilogram (kg) = 1,000 grams
1 gram (g) = 1,000 milligrams
1 milligram (mg) = 0.001 gram
1 microgram (mcg, μg) = 0.001 milligram
1 nanogram (ng) = 0.001 microgram
1 picogram (pg) = 0.001 nanogram
1 femtogram (fg) = 0.001 picogram

▶ Metric Volume Equivalents

1 liter (L) = 1,000 milliliters
1 deciliter (dL) = 100 milliliters
1 milliliter (mL) = 0.001 liter
1 microliter (μL) = 0.001 milliliter
1 nanoliter (nL) = 0.001 microliter
1 picoliter (pL) = 0.001 nanoliter
1 femtoliter (fL) = 0.001 picoliter

▶ Apothecary Weight Equivalents

1 scruple (ว) = 20 grains (gr)
60 grains (gr) = 1 dram (ʒ)
8 drams (ʒ) = 1 ounce (fl ʒ)
1 ounce (ʒ) = 480 grains (gr)
12 ounces (ʒ) = 1 pound (lb)

▶ Apothecary Volume Equivalents

60 minims (m) = 1 fluidram (fl ʒ)
8 fluidrams (fl ʒ) = 1 fluid ounce (fl ʒ)
1 fluid ounce (fl ʒ) = 480 minims (m)
16 fluid ounces (fl ʒ) = 1 pint (pt)

▶ Avoirdupois Equivalents

1 ounce (oz) = 437.5 grains
16 ounces (oz) = 1 pound (lb)

▶ Weight/Volume Equivalents

1 mg/dL = 10 mcg/mL
1 mg/dL = 1 mg%
1 ppm = 1 mg/L

▶ Conversion Equivalents

1 gram (g) = 15.43 grains (gr)
1 grain (gr) = 64.8 milligrams (mg)
1 ounce (ʒ) = 31.1 grams (g)
1 ounce (oz) = 28.35 grams (g)
1 pound (lb) = 453.6 grams (g)
1 kilogram (kg) = 2.2 pounds (lb)
1 milliliter (mL) = 16.23 minims (m)
1 minim (m) = 0.06 milliliter (mL)
1 fluid ounce (fl oz) = 29.57 milliliters (mL)
1 pint (pt) = 473.2 milliliters (mL)
1 US gallon = 3.78 liters (L)
1 Canadian gallon = 4.55 liters (L)
0.1 milligram = 1/600 grain
0.12 milligram = 1/500 grain
0.15 milligram = 1/400 grain
0.2 milligram = 1/300 grain
0.3 milligram = 1/200 grain
0.4 milligram = 1/150 grain
0.5 milligram = 1/120 grain
0.6 milligram = 1/100 grain
0.8 milligram = 1/80 grain
1 milligram = 1/65 grain

▶ Metric Length Conversion Equivalents

2.54 cm = 1 inch
30.48 cm = 1 foot
1 m = 3.28 feet
1.6 km = 1 mile

ANTHROPOMETRICS

Creatinine Clearance Formulas

▶ Formulas for Estimating Creatinine Clearance in Patients with Stable Renal Function

Cockcroft-Gault Formula

Adults (age 18 years and older)[1]:

$$\text{CrCl (males)} = \frac{(140 - \text{age}) \times \text{weight}}{\text{SCr} \times 72}$$

CrCl (females) = 0.85 × above value*

*Some studies suggest that the predictive accuracy of this formula for women is better *without* the correction factor of 0.85.

where CrCl is creatinine clearance (in mL/minute), SCr is serum creatinine (in mg/dL [or μmol/L divided by 88.4]), age is in years, and weight is in kilograms.

Traub-Johnson Formula

Children (age 1–18 years)[2]:

$$\text{CrCl} = \frac{0.48 \times \text{height} \times \text{BSA}}{\text{SCr} \times 1.73}$$

where BSA is body surface area (in m[2]), CrCl is creatinine clearance (in mL/minute), SCr is serum creatinine (in mg/dL [or μmol/L divided by 88.4]), and height is in centimeters.

▶ Formula for Estimating Creatinine Clearance From a Measured Urine Collection

$$\text{CrCl (mL/minute)} = \frac{U \times V^*}{P \times T}$$

where U is the concentration of creatinine in a urine specimen (in same units as P such as mg/dL), V is the volume of urine (in mL), P is the concentration of creatinine in serum at the midpoint of the urine collection period (in same units as U), and T is the time of the urine collection period in minutes (e.g., 6 hours = 360 minutes; 24 hours = 1,440 minutes).

*The product of $U \times V$ equals the production of creatinine during the collection period and, at steady state, should equal 20 to 25 mg/kg/day for ideal body weight (IBW) in males and 15 to 20 mg/kg/day for IBW in females. If it is less than this, in adequate urine collection may have occurred, and CrCl will be underestimated.

▶ MDRD Formula for Estimating Glomerular Filtration Rate (From the Modification of Diet in Renal Disease Study)[3]

Conventional calibration MDRD equation [used only with those creatinine methods that have not been recalibrated to be traceable to isotope dilution mass spectrometry (IDMS)]

For creatinine in mg/dL:

$$X = 186 \text{ creatinine}^{-1.154} \times \text{age}^{-0.203} \times \text{constant}$$

For creatinine in μmol/L:

$$X = 32,788 \times \text{creatinine}^{-1.154} \times \text{age}^{-0.203} \times \text{constant}$$

where X is the glomerular filtration rate (GFR), constant for white males is 1 and for females is 0.742, and constant for African Americans is 1.21. Creatinine levels in μmol/L can be converted to mg/dL by dividing by 88.4.

▶ IDMS-Traceable MDRD Equation (Used Only With Creatinine Methods That Have Been Recalibrated to Be Traceable to IDMS)

For creatinine in mg/dL:

$$X = 175 \times \text{creatinine}^{-1.154} \times \text{age}^{-0.203} \times \text{constant}$$

For creatinine in μmol/L:

$$X = 175 \times (\text{creatinine}/88.4)^{-1.154} \times \text{age}^{-0.203} \times \text{constant}$$

where X is the GFR, constant for white males is 1 and for females is 0.742, and constant for African Americans is 1.21.

Ideal Body Weight

IBW is the weight expected for a nonobese person of a given height. The IBW formulas below and various life insurance tables can be used to estimate IBW. Dosing methods described in the literature may use IBW as a method in dosing obese patients.

Adults (age 18 years and older)[4]:

IBW (males) = 50 + (2.3 × height in inches over 5 ft)

IBW (females) = 45.5 + (2.3 × height in inches over 5 ft)

where IBW is in kilograms.

Children (age 1–18 years)[2]:
Under 5 ft tall:

$$\text{IBW} = \frac{\text{height}^2 \times 1.65}{1,000}$$

where IBW is in kilograms and height is in centimeters.

Five feet or taller:

IBW (males) = 39 + (2.27 × height in inches over 5 ft)

IBW (females) = 42.2 + (2.27 × height in inches over 5 ft)

where IBW is in kilograms.

REFERENCES

1. Cockcroft DW, Gault MH. Prediction of creatinine clearance from serum creatinine. Nephron 1976;16:31-41.
2. Traub SI, Johnson CE. Comparison of methods of estimating creatinine clearance in children. Am J Hosp Pharm 1980;37:195-201.
3. Levey AS, Bosch JP, Lewis JB, et al. A more accurate method to estimate glomerular filtration rate from serum creatinine: A new prediction equation. Modification of Diet in Renal Disease Study Group. Ann Intern Med 1999;130:461-470.
4. Devine BJ. Gentamicin therapy. Drug Intell Clin Pharm 1974;8:650-655.

Appendix B: Common Laboratory Tests

The following table is an alphabetical listing of some common laboratory tests and their reference ranges for adults as measured in plasma or serum (unless otherwise indicated). Reference values differ among laboratories, so readers should refer to the published reference ranges used in each institution. For some tests, both the Système International Units and Conventional Units are reported.

Lab	Conventional Units	Conversion Factor	Système International Units
Acid phosphatase			
Male	2–12 units/L	16.7	33–200 nkat/L
Female	0.3–9.2 units/L	16.7	5–154 nkat/L
Activated partial thromboplatin time (aPTT)	25–40 seconds		
Adrenocorticotropic hormone (ACTH)	15–80 pg/mL or ng/L	0.2202	3.3–176 pmol/L
Alanine aminotransferase (ALT, SGPT)	7–53 IU/L	0.01667	0.12–0.88 μkat/L
Albumin	3.5–5.0 g/dL	10	35–50 g/L
Albumin:creatinine ratio (urine)			
Normal	Less than 30 mg/g creatinine		
Microalbuminuria	30–300 mg/g creatinine		
Proteinuria	Greater than 300 mg/g creatinine		
or	or		
Normal			
Male	Less than 2.0 mg/mmol creatinine		
Female	Less than 2.8 mg/mmol creatinine		
Microalbuminuria			
Male	2.0–20 mg/mmol creatinine		
Female	2.8–28 mg/mmol creatinine		
Proteinuria			
Male	Greater than 20 mg/mmol creatinine		
Female	Greater than 28 mg/mmol creatinine		
Alcohol			
See under Ethanol			
Aldosterone			
Supine	Less than 16 ng/dL	27.7	Less than 444 pmol/L
Upright	Less than 31 ng/dL	27.7	Less than 860 pmol/L

(Continued)

Lab	Conventional Units	Conversion Factor	Système International Units
Alkaline phosphatase			
10–15 years	130–550 IU/L	0.01667	2.17–9.17 µkat/L
16–20 years	70–260 IU/L	0.01667	1.17–4.33 µkat/L
Greater than 20 years	38–126 IU/L	0.01667	0.13–2.10 µkat/L
a-fetoprotein (AFP)	Less than 15 ng/mL	1	Less than 15 mcg/L
a-1-antitrypsin	80–200 mg/dL	0.01	0.8–2.0 g/L
Amikacin, therapeutic (traditional dosing)			
Peak	15–30 mg/L	1.71	25.6–51.3 µmol/L
Trough	Less than or equal to 8 mg/L	1.71	Less than or equal to 13.7 µmol/L
Amitriptyline	80–200 ng/mL or mcg/L	3.4	272–680 nmol/L
Ammonia (plasma)	15.33–56.20 mcg NH_3/dL	0.5872	9–33 µmol NH_3/L
Amylase	25–115 IU/L	0.01667	0.42–1.92 µkat/L
Androstenedione	50–250 ng/dL	0.0349	1.7–8.7 nmol/L
Angiotensin converting enzyme	15–70 units/L	16.67	250–1167 nkat/L
Anion gap	7–16 mEq/L	1	7–16 mmol/L
Anti-double stranded DNA (anti-ds DNA)	Negative		
Anti-HAV	Negative		
Anti-HBc	Negative		
Anti-HBs	Negative		
Anti-HCV	Negative		
Anti-Sm antibody	Negative		
Antinuclear antibody (ANA)	Negative		
Apolipoprotein A-1			
Male	95–175 mg/dL	0.01	0.95–1.75 g/L
Female	100–200 mg/dL	0.01	1.0–2.0 g/L
Apolipoprotein B			
Male	50–110 mg/dL	0.01	0.5–1.10 g/L
Female	50–105 mg/dL	0.01	0.5–1.05 g/L
Aspartate aminotransferase (AST, SGOT)	11–47 IU/L	0.01667	0.18–0.78 µkat/L
β_2-microglobulin	Less than 0.2 mg/dL	10	2 mg/L
Bicarbonate	22–26 mEq/L	1	22–26 mmol/L
Bilirubin			
Total	0.3–1.1 mg/dL	17.1	5.13–18.80 µmol/L
Direct	0–0.3 mg/dL	17.1	0–5.1 µmol/L
Indirect	0.1–1.0 mg/dL	17.1	1.71–17.1 µmol/L
Bleeding time	3–7 minutes		
Blood gases (arterial)			
pH	7.35–7.45	1	7.35–7.45
PO_2	80–105 mmHg	0.133	10.6–14.0 kPa
PCO_2	35–45 mmHg	0.133	4.7–6.0 kPa
HCO_3	22–26 mEq/L	1	22–26 mmol/L
O_2 saturation	Greater than or equal to 0.95	0.01	0.95
Blood urea nitrogen (BUN)	8–25 mg/dL	0.357	2.9–8.9 mmol/L
B-type natriuretic peptide (BNP)	0–99 pg/mL	1	0–99 ng/L
		0.289	0–29 pmol/L
BUN-to-creatinine ratio	10:1 to 20:1		

(Continued)

Lab	Conventional Units	Conversion Factor	Système International Units
C-peptide	0.51–2.70 ng/mL	331	170–894 pmol/L
		0.331	0.17–0.89 nmol/L
C-reactive protein	Less than 0.8 mg/dL	10	Less than 8 mg/L
CA-125	Less than 35 units/mL	1	Less than 35 kU/L
CA 15–3	Less than 30 units/mL	1	Less than 30 kU/L
CA 19–9	Less than 37 units/mL	1	Less than 37 kU/L
CA 27.29	Less than 38 units/mL	1	Less than 38 kU/L
Calcium			
Total	8.6–10.3 mg/dL	0.25	2.15–2.58 mmol/L
	4.3–5.16 mEq/L	0.50	2.15–2.58 mmol/L
Ionized	4.5–5.1 mg/dL	0.25	1.13–1.28 mmol/L
	2.26–2.56 mEq/L	0.50	1.13–1.28 mmol/L
Carbamazepine, therapeutic	4–12 mg/L	4.23	17–51 µmol/L
Carboxyhemoglobin (nonsmoker)	Less than 2%	0.01	Less than 0.02
Carcinoembryonic antigen (CEA)			
Nonsmokers	Less than 2.5 ng/mL	1	Less than 2.5 mcg/L
Smokers	Less than 5 ng/mL	1	Less than 5 mcg/L
CD4 lymphocyte count	31–61% of total lymphocytes		
CD8 lymphocyte count	18–39% of total lymphocytes		
Cerebrospinal fluid (CSF)			
Pressure	75–175 mm H_2O		
Glucose	40–70 mg/dL	0.0555	2.2–3.9 mmol/L
Protein	15–45 mg/dL	0.01	0.15–045 g/L
WBC	Less than 10/mm^3		
Ceruloplasmin	18–45 mg/dL	10	180–450 mg/L
		0.063	1.1–2.8 µmol/L
Chloride	97–110 mEq/L	1	97–110 mmol/L
Cholesterol			
Desirable	Less than 200 mg/dL	0.0259	Less than 5.18 mmol/L
Borderline high	200–239 mg/dL	0.0259	5.18–6.19 mmol/L
High	Greater than or equal to 240 mg/dL	0.0259	Greater than or equal to 6.2 mmol/L
Chorionic gonadotropin (ß-hCG)	Less than 5 mIU/mL	1	Less than 5 units/L
Clozapine, minimum trough	300–350 ng/mL or mcg/L	3.06	918–1,071 nmol/L
		0.003	0.92–1.07 µmol/L
CO_2 content	22–30 mEq/L	1	22–30 mmol/L
Complement component 3 (C3)	70–160 mg/dL	0.01	0.7–1.6 g/L
Complement component 4 (C4)	20–40 mg/dL	0.01	0.2–0.4 g/L
Copper	70–150 mcg/dL	0.157	11–24 µmol/L
Cortisol (fasting, morning)	5–25 mcg/dL	27.6	138–690 nmol/L
Cortisol (free, urinary)	10–100 mcg/d	2.76	28–276 nmol/d
Creatine kinase			
Male	30–200 IU/L	0.01667	0.50–3.33 µkat/L
Female	20–170 IU/L	0.01667	0.33–2.83 µkat/L
MB fraction	0–7 IU/L	0.01667	0.0–0.12 µkat/L
Creatinine clearance (CrCl) (urine)	85–135 mL/minute/1.73 m^2	0.00963	0.82–1.3 mL/s/m^2

(Continued)

Lab	Conventional Units	Conversion Factor	Système International Units
Creatinine			
Male 4–20 years	0.2–1.0 mg/dL	88.4	18–88 µmol/L
Female 4–20 years	0.2–1.0 mg/dL	88.4	18–88 µmol/L
Male (adults)	0.7–1.3 mg/dL	88.4	62–115 µmol/L
Female (adults)	0.6–1.1 mg/dL	88.4	53–97 µmol/L
Cyclosporine			
Renal, cardiac, liver, or pancreatic transplant	100–400 ng/mL or mcg/L	0.832	83–333 nmol/L
Cryptococcal antigen	Negative		
D-dimers	Less than 250 ng/mL	1	Less than 250 mcg/L
Desipramine	75–300 ng/mL or mcg/L	3.75	281–1125 nmol/L
Dexamethasone suppression test (DST) (overnight), 8:00 AM cortisol	Less than 5 mcg/dL	0.0276	Less than 0.14 µmol/L
DHEAS (dehydroepiandrosterone sulfate)			
Male	170–670 mcg/dL	0.0271	4.6–18.2 µmol/L
Female			
Premenopausal	50–540 mcg/dL	0.0271	1.4–14.7 µmol/L
Postmenopausal	30–260 mcg/dL	0.0271	0.8–7.1 µmol/L
Digoxin, Therapeutic (heart failure)	0.5–0.8 ng/mL or mcg/L	1.28	0.6–1.3 nmol/L
Therapeutic (Atrial Fibrillation)	0.8–2.0 ng/mL or mcg/L	1.28	0.8–2.6 nmol/L
Erythrocyte count (blood)			
See under Red Blood Cell count			
Erythrocyte sedimentation rate (ESR)			
Westergren			
Male	0–20 mm/h		
Female	0–30 mm/h		
Wintrobe			
Male	0–9 mm/h		
Female	0–15 mm/h		
Erythropoietin	2–25 mlU/mL	1	2–25 IU/L
Estradiol			
Male	10–36 pg/mL	3.67	37–132 pmol/L
Female	34–170 pg/mL	3.67	125–624 pmol/L
Ethanol, legal intoxication (depends on location)	Greater than or equal to 50–100 mg/dL	0.217	10.9–21.7 mmol/L
	Greater than or equal to 0.05–0.1%	217	10.9–21.7 mmol/L
Ethosuccimide, therapeutic	40–100 mg/L or mcg/mL	7.08	283–708 µmol/L
Factor VIII or Factor IX			
Severe hemophilia	Less than 1 IU/dL	0.01	Less than 0.01 units/mL
Moderate hemophilia	1–5 IU/dL	0.01	0.01–0.05 units/mL
Mild hemophilia	Greater than 5 IU/dL	0.01	Greater than 0.05 units/mL
Usual adult levels	60 to 140 IU/dL	0.01	0.60 to 1.40 units/mL
Ferritin			
Male	20–250 ng/mL	1	20–250 mcg/L
Female	10–150 ng/mL	1	10–150 mcg/L
Fibrin degradation products (FDP)	2–10 mg/L		
Fibrinogen	200–400 mg/dL	0.01	2.0–4.0 g/L
Folate (plasma)	3.1–12.4 ng/mL	2.266	7.0–28.1 nmol/L

(Continued)

Lab	Conventional Units	Conversion Factor	Système International Units
Folate (RBC)	125–600 ng/mL	2.266	283–1,360 nmol/L
Follicle-stimulating hormone (FSH)			
Male	l–7 mlU/mL	1	1–7 IU/L
Female			
Follicular phase	1–9 mlU/mL	1	1–9 IU/L
Midcycle	6–26 mlU/mL	1	6–26 IU/L
Luteal phase	1–9 mlU/mL	1	1–9 IU/L
Postmenopausal	30–118 mlU/mL	1	30–118 IU/L
Free thyroxine index (FT_4I)	6.5–12.5		
Gamma glutamyl transferase (GGT)	0–30 IU/L	0.01667	0–0.5 μkat/L
Gastrin (fasting)	0–130 pg/mL	1	0–130 ng/L
Gentamicin, therapeutic (traditional dosing)			
Peak	4–10 mg/L	2.09	8.4–21 μmol/L
Trough	Less than or equal to 2 mg/L	2.09	Less than or equal to 4.2 μmol/L
Globulin	2.3–3.5 q/dL	10	23–35 g/L
Glucose (fasting, plasma)	65–109 mg/dL	0.0555	3.6–6.00 mmol/L
Glucose, two hour postprandial blood (PPBG)	Less than 140 mg/dL	0.0555	Less than 7.8 mmol/L
Granulocyte count	$1.8–6.6 \times 10^3/mm^3$	10^6	$1.8–6.6 \times 10^9/L$
Growth hormone (fasting)			
Male	Less than 5 ng/mL	1	Less than 5 mcg/L
Female	Less than 10 ng/mL	1	Less than 10 mcg/L
Haptoglobin	60–270 mg/dL	0.01	0.6–2.7 g/L
HBeAg	Negative		
HbsAg	Negative		
HBV DNA	Negative		
Hematocrit			
Male	40.7–50.3 %	0.01	0.407–0.503
Female	36.1–44.3 %	0.01	0.361–0.443
Hemoglobin (Blood)			
Male	13.8–172 g/dL	10	138–172 g/L
		0.62	8.56–10.67 mmol/L
Female	12.1–15.1 g/dL	10	121–151 g/L
		0.62	75–9.36 mmol/L
Hemoglobin A1$_c$	4.0–6.0 %	0.01	0.04–0.06
Heparin			
Via protamine titration method	0.2–0.4 units/mL		
Via antifactor Xa assay	0.3–0.7 units/mL		
High-density lipoprotein (HDL) cholesterol	Greater than 35 mg/dL	0.0259	Greater than 0.91 mmol/L
Homocysteine	3.3–104 μmol/L		
Ibuprofen			
Therapeutic	10–50 mcg/mL	4.85	49–243 μmol/L
Toxic	100–700 mcg/mL or more	4.85	485–3,395 μmol/L or more
Imipramine, therapeutic	100–300 ng/mL or mcg/L	3.57	357–1,071 nmol/L

(Continued)

Lab	Conventional Units	Conversion Factor	Système International Units
Immunoglobulin A (IgA)	85–385 mg/dL	0.01	0.85–3.85 g/L
Immunoglobulin G (IgG)	565–1,765 mg/dL	0.01	5.65–17.65 g/L
Immunoglobulin M (IgM)	53–375 mg/dL	0.01	0.53–3.75 g/L
Insulin (fasting)	2–20 μU/mL or mU/L	7.175	14.35–143.5 pmol/L
International normalized ratio (INR), therapeutic	2.0–3.0 (2.5–3.5 for some indications)		
Iron			
Male	45–160 mcg/dL	0.179	8.1–28.6 μmol/L
Female	30–160 mcg/dL	0.179	5.4–28.6 μmol/L
Iron binding capacity (Total)	220–420 mcg/dL	0.179	39.4–75.2 μmol/L
Iron saturation	15–50 %	0.01	0.15–0.50
Itraconazole, therapeutic			
Trough	0.5–1 mcg/mL	1	0.5–1 mg/L
Lactate (plasma)	0.7–2.1 mEq/L	1	0.7–2.1 mmol/L
	6.3–18.9 mg/dL	0.111	0.7–2.1 mmol/L
Lactate dehydrogenase (LDH)	100–250 IU/L	0.01667	1.67–4.17 μkat/L
Lead	Less than 25 mcg/dL	0.0483	Less than 1.21 μmol/L
Leukocyte count	3.8–9.8 × 10³/mm³	10⁶	3.8–9.8 × 10⁹/L
Lidocaine, therapeutic	1.5–6.0 mcg/mL or mg/L	4.27	6.4–25.6 μmol/L
Lipase	Less than 100 IU/L	0.01667	1.7 μkat/L
Lithium, therapeutic	0.5–1.25 mEq/L	1	0.5–1.25 mmol/L
Low-density lipoprotein (LDL) cholesterol			
Target for very high-risk patients	Less than 70 mg/dL	0.0259	Less than 1.81 mmol/L
Target for high-risk patients (optimal)	Less than 100 mg/dL	0.0259	Less than 2.59 mmol/L
Desirable	Less than 130 mg/dL	0.0259	Less than 3.36 mmol/L
Borderline high risk	130–159 mg/dL	0.0259	3.36–4.11 mmol/L
High risk	Greater than or equal to 160 mg/dL	0.0259	Greater than or equal to 4.13 mmol/L
Luteinizing hormone (LH)			
Male	1–8 mU/mL	1	1–8 units/L
Female			
Follicular phase	1–12 mU/mL	1	1–12 units/L
Midcycle	16–104 mU/mL	1	16–104 units/L
Luteal phase	1–12 mU/mL	1	1–12 units/L
Postmenopausal	16–66 mU/mL	1	16–66 units/L
Lymphocyte count	1.2–3.3 × 10³/mm³	10⁶	1.2–3.3 × 10⁹/L
Magnesium	1.3–2.2 mEq/L	0.5	0.65–1.10 mmol/L
	1.58–2.68 mg/dL	0.411	0.65–1.10 mmol/L
Mean corpuscular volume	80.0–97.6 μm³	1	80.0–976 fl
Mononuclear cell count	0.2–0.7 × 10³/mm³	10⁶	0.2–0.7 × 10⁹/L
Nortriptyline, therapeutic	50–150 ng/mL or mcg/L	3.8	190–570 nmol/L
Osmolality (serum)	275–300 mOsm/kg	1	275–300 mmol/kg
Osmolality (urine)	250–900 mOsm/kg	1	250–900 mmol/kg
Parathyroid hormone (PTH), Intact	10–60 pg/mLor ng/L	0.107	1.1–6.4 pmol/L
PTH, N-terminal	8–24 pg/mL or ng/L		
PTH, C-terminal	50–330 pg/mL or ng/L		
Phenobarbital, therapeutic	15–40 mcg/mL or mg/L	4.31	65–172 μmol/L

(Continued)

Lab	Conventional Units	Conversion Factor	Système International Units
Phenytoin, therapeutic	10–20 mcg/mL or mg/L	3.96	40–79 µmol/L
Phosphate	2.5–4.5 mg/dL	0.323	0.81–1.45 mmol/L
Platelet count	140–440 × 10^3/mm^3	10^6	140–440 × 10^9/L
Potassium (plasma)	3.3–4.9 mEq/L	1	3.3–4.9 mmol/L
Prealbumin (adult)	19.5–35.8 mg/dL	10	195–358 mg/L
Primidone, therapeutic	5–12 mcg/mL or mg/L	4.58	23–55 µmol/L
Procainamide, therapeutic	4–10 mcg/mL or mg/L	4.23	17–42 µmol/L
Progesterone			
Male	13–97 ng/dL	0.0318	0.4–3.1 nmol/L
Female			
Follicular phase	15–70 ng/dL	0.0318	0.5–2.2 nmol/L
Luteal phase	200–2,500 ng/dL	0.0318	6.4–79.5 nmol/L
Prolactin	Less than 20 ng/mL	1	Less than 20 mcg/L
Prostate-specific antigen (PSA)	Less than 4 ng/mL	1	Less than 4 mcg/L
Protein, total	6.0–8.0 g/dL	10	60–80 g/L
Prothrombin time (PT)	10–12 seconds		
Quinidine, therapeutic	2–5 mcg/mL or mg/L	3.08	6.2–15.4 µmol/L
Radioactive iodine uptake (RAIU)	Less than 6% in 2 hours		
Red blood cell (RBC) count (blood)			
Male	4–6.2 × 10^6/mm^3	10^6	4–6.2 × 10^{12}/L
Female	4–6.2 × 10^6/mm^3	10^6	4–6.2 × 10^{12}/L
Pregnant			
Trimester 1	4–5 × 10^6/mm^3	10^6	4–5 × 10^{12}/L
Trimester 2	3.2–4.5 × 10^6/mm^3	10^6	3.2–4.5 × 10^{12}/L
Trimester 3	3–4.9 × 10^6/mm^3	10^6	3–4.9 × 10^{12}/L
Postpartum	3.2–5 × 10^6/mm^3	10^6	3.2–5 × 10^{12}/L
Red blood cell distribution width (RDW)	11.5–14.5%	0.01	0.115–0.145
Reticulocyte count			
Male	0.5–1.5% of total RBC count	0.01	0.005–0.015
Female	0.5–2.5% of total RBC count	0.01	0.005–0.025
Retinol-binding protein (RBP)	2.7–7.6 mg/dL	10	27–76 mg/L
Rheumatoid factor (RF) titer	Negative		
Salicylate, therapeutic	150–300 mcg/mL or mg/L	0.00724	1.09–2.17 mmol/L
	15–30 mg/dL	0.0724	1.09–2.17 mmol/L
Sirolimus (renal transplant)	4–20 ng/mL	1	4–20 mcg/L
Sodium	135–145 mEq/L	1	135–145 mmol/L
Tacrolimus			
Renal, cardiac, liver, or pancreatic transplant	5–20 ng/mL	1	5–20 mcg/L
Testosterone (total)			
Men	300–950 ng/dL	0.0347	10.4–33.0 nmol/L
Women	20–80 ng/dL	0.0347	0.7–2.8 nmol/L
Testosterone (free)			
Men	9–30 ng/dL	0.0347	0.31–1.04 nmol/L
Women	0.3–1.9 ng/dL	0.0347	0.01–0.07 nmol/L
Theophylline			
Therapeutic	5–15 mcg/mL or mg/L	5.55	28–83 µmol/L
Toxic	20 mcg/mL or mg/L or more	5.55	111 µmol/L or more

(Continued)

Lab	Conventional Units	Conversion Factor	Système International Units
Thiocyanate	Toxic level unclear. Units are mcg/mL or mg/L	17.2	μmol/L
Thrombin time	20–24 seconds		
Thyroglobulin	Less than 42 ng/mL	1	Less than 42 mcg/L
Thyroglobulin antibodies	Negative		
Thyroxine-binding globulin (TBG)	1.2–2.5 mg/dL	10	12–25 mcg/L
Thyroid-stimulating hormone (TSH)	0.35–6.20 μU/mL	1	0.35–6.20 mU/L
TSH receptor antibodies (TSH Rab)	0–1 units/mL		
Thyroxine (T_4)			
Total	4.5–12.0 mcg/dL	12.87	58–154 nmol/L
Free	0.7–1.9 ng/dL	12.87	9.0–24.5 pmol/L
Thyroxine index, free (FT_4I)	6.5–12.5		
TIBC—see Iron Binding Capacity (total)			
Tobramycin, therapeutic (traditional dosing)			
Peak	4–10 mcg/mL or mg/L	2.14	8.6–21.4 μmol/L
Trough	Less than or equal to 2 mcg/mL or mg/L	2.14	Less than or equal to 4.28 μmol/L
Transferrin	200–430 mg/dL	0.01	2.0–4.3 g/L
Transferrin saturation	30–50%	0.01	0.30–0.50
Triglycerides (fasting)	Less than 160 mg/dL	0.0113	Less than 1.8 mmol/L
Triiodothyronine (T_3)	45–132 ng/dL	0.0154	0.91–2.70 nmol/L
Triiodothyronine (T_3) resin uptake	25–35%		
Uric acid	3–8 mg/dL	59.48	179–476 nmol/L
Urinalysis (urine)			
pH	4.8–8.0		
Specific gravity	1.005–1.030		
Protein	Negative		
Glucose	Negative		
Ketones	Negative		
RBC	1–2 per low-power field		
WBC	Less than 5 per low-power field		
Valproic acid, therapeutic	50–100 mcg/mL or mg/L	6.93	346–693 nmol/L
Vancomycin, therapeutic			
Peak	20–40 mcg/mL or mg/L	0.690	14–28 μmol/L
Trough	5–20 mcg/mL or mg/L	0.690	3–14 μmol/L
Trough for CNS infections	15–20 mcg/mL or mg/L	0.690	10–14 μmol/L
Vitamin A (retinol)	30–95 mcg/dL	0.0349	1.05–3.32 μmol/L
Vitamin B_{12}	180–1,000 pg/mL	0.738	133–738 pmol/L
Vitamin D_3, 1, 25-dihydroxy	20–76 pg/mL	2.4	48–182 pmol/L
Vitamin D_3, 25-hydroxy	10–50 ng/mL	2.496	25–125 nmol/L
Vitamin E (*a*-tocopherol)	0.5–2.0 mg/dL	23.22	12–46 μmol/L
WBC count	$4–10 \times 10^3/mm^3$	10^6	$4–10 \times 10^9/L$
WBC differential (peripheral blood)			
Polymorphonuclear neutrophils	50–65%		
Band neutrophils	0–5%		
Eosinophils	0–3%		
Basophils	1–3%		
Lymphocytes	25–35%		
Monocytes	2–6%		

(Continued)

Lab	Conventional Units	Conversion Factor	Système International Units
WBC differential (bone marrow)			
Polymorphonuclear neutrophils	3–11%		
Band neutrophils	9–15%		
Metamyelocytes	9–25%		
Myelocytes	8–16%		
Promyelocytes	1–8%		
Myeloblasts	0–5%		
Eosinophils	1–5%		
Basophils	0–1%		
Lymphocytes	11–23%		
Monocytes	0–1%		
Zinc	60–150 mcg/dL	0.153	9.2–23.0 µmol/L

This table is a modification of the Medical Algorithms Project (Chapter 40), unit conversions of the following Excel worksheets: Conversion of Conventional to SI units: Blood Chemistries; Conversion of Conventional to SI units: Urine Chemistries; Conversion of Conventional to SI units: Hematology and Coagulation; and Conversion of Conventional to SI units: Therapeutic Drug Monitoring. Available at http://www.medal.org/visitor/www/active/ch40/ch40.aspx; accessed November 17, 2010.

Other references (conventional and SI units from the preceding table were double-checked against the following references and modified as needed):

Système International (SI) Conversion Table. JAMA 2005;294(1):119. Available at http://jama.ama-assn.org/content/vol294/issue1/images/data/119/DC6/JAMA_auinst_sitable.dtl; accessed November 17, 2010.

Laboratory Test Handbook (DS Jacobs, DK Oxley, WR DeMott, eds.) Lexi-Comp, Inc., Hudson OH, 2001.

Reviewed and updated by: Edward W. Randell and Rebecca M.T. Law.

Appendix C: Common Medical Abbreviations

These are the abbreviations used commonly in medical practice both in verbal communication and in the medical record.

A&O	Alert and oriented
A&O×3	Awake (or alert) and oriented to person, place, and time
A&O×4	Awake (or alert) and oriented to person, place, time, and situation
A&P	Auscultation and percussion; anterior and posterior; assessment and plans; active and plans
A&W	Alive and well
A1C	Hemoglobin A1C
AA	Aplastic anemia; Alcoholics Anonymous
AAA	Abdominal aortic aneurysm
AAO	Awake, alert, and oriented
AAO×3	Awake and orientated to time, place, and person
ABC	Absolute band counts; absolute basophil count; apnea, bradycardia, and cytology; aspiration, biopsy, and cytology; artificial beta cells
Abd	Abdomen
ABG	Arterial blood gases
ABO	Blood group system (A, AB, B, and O)
ABP	Arterial blood pressure
ABW	Actual body weight
ABx	Antibiotics
AC	Before meals (*ante cibos*)
ACE	Angiotensin-converting enzyme
ACE-I	Angiotensin-converting enzyme inhibitor
ACLS	Advanced cardiac life support
ACS	Acute coronary syndromes
ACTH	Adrenocorticotropic hormone
AD	Alzheimer's disease; right ear (*auris dextra*)
ADA	American Diabetes Association; adenosine deaminase
ADE	Adverse drug effect (or event)
ADH	Antidiuretic hormone
ADHD	Attention-deficit hyperactivity disorder
ADL	Activities of daily living
ADR	Adverse drug reaction
AF	Atrial fibrillation
AFB	Acid-fast bacillus; aortofemoral bypass; aspirated foreign body
AFEB	Afebrile
AI	Aortic insufficiency
AIDS	Acquired immune-deficiency syndrome
AKA	Above-knee amputation; alcoholic ketoacidosis; all known allergies; also known as
AKI	Acute kidney injury
ALFT	Abnormal liver function test
ALL	Acute lymphoblastic leukemia; acute lymphocytic leukemia
ALP	Alkaline phosphatase
ALS	Amyotrophic lateral sclerosis
ALT	Alanine transaminase (SGPT); alanine aminotransferase
AMA	Against medical advice; American Medical Association; antimitochondrial antibody
AMI	Acute myocardial infarction
AML	Acute myelogenous leukemia
Amp	Ampule
ANA	Antinuclear antibody
ANC	Absolute neutrophil count
ANLL	Acute nonlymphocytic leukemia
AODM	Adult-onset diabetes mellitus
AOM	Acute otitis media
AP	Anteroposterior
APAP	Acetaminophen (acetyl-*p*-aminophenol)
aPTT	Activated partial thromboplastin time
ARB	Angiotensin receptor blocker
ARC	AIDS-related complex
ARD	Acute respiratory disease; adult respiratory disease; antibiotic removal device; aphakic retinal detachment
ARDS	Adult respiratory distress syndrome
ARF	Acute renal failure; acute respiratory failure; acute rheumatic fever
AROM	Active range of motion
AS	Left ear (*auris sinistra*)
ASA	Aspirin (acetylsalicylic acid)
ASCVD	Arteriosclerotic cardiovascular disease
ASD	Atrial septal defect
ASH	Asymmetric septal hypertrophy

ASHD	Arteriosclerotic heart disease
AST	Aspartate transaminase (SCOT); aspartate aminotransferase
ATG	Antithymocyte globulin
ATN	Acute tubular necrosis
AU	Each ear (*auris uterque*)
AV	Arteriovenous; atrioventricular; auditory visual
AVR	Aortic valve replacement
BBB	Bundle-branch block; blood-brain barrier
BC	Blood culture
BCOP	Board Certified Oncology Pharmacist
BCP	Birth control pill
BCPP	Board Certified Psychiatric Pharmacist
BCPS	Board Certified Pharmacotherapy Specialist
BE	Barium enema
BG	Blood glucose
BID	Twice daily (*bis in die*)
BKA	Below-knee amputation
BM	Bone marrow; bowel movement; an isoenzyme of creatine phospokinase
BMC	Bone marrow cells
BMD	Bone mineral density
BMI	Body mass index
BMP	Basic metabolic panel
BMR	Basal metabolic rate
BMT	Bone marrow transplantation
BP	Blood pressure
BPD	Bronchopulmonary dysplasia
BPH	Benign prostatic hyperplasia
bpm	Beats per minute
BR	Bed rest
BS	Bowel sounds; breath sounds; blood sugar
BSA	Body surface area
BUN	Blood urea nitrogen
Bx	Biopsy
C&S	Culture and sensitivity
CA	Cancer; calcium
CABG	Coronary artery bypass grafting
CAD	Coronary artery disease
CAH	Chronic active hepatitis
CAM	Complementary and alternative medicine
CAPD	Continuous ambulatory peritoneal dialysis
CBC	Complete blood count
CBD	Common bile duct
CBG	Capillary blood gas; corticosteroid-binding globulin
CC	Chief complaint
CCA	Calcium channel antagonist
CCB	Calcium channel blocker
CCE	Clubbing, cyanosis, edema
CCK	Cholecystokinin
CCU	Coronary care unit
CF	Cystic fibrosis
CFS	Chronic fatigue syndrome
CFU	Colony-forming unit
CHD	Coronary heart disease

CHF	Congestive heart failure; chronic heart failure
CHO	Carbohydrate
CI	Cardiac index
CIWA	Clinical Institute Withdrawal Assessment
CK	Creatine kinase
CKD	Chronic kidney disease
ClCr	Creatinine clearance
CLL	Chronic lymphocytic leukemia
CM	Costal margin
CMG	Cystometrogram
CML	Chronic myelogenous leukemia
CMV	Cytomegalovirus
CN	Cranial nerve
CNS	Central nervous system
C/O, c/o	Complains of
CO	Cardiac output; carbon monoxide
COLD	Chronic obstructive lung disease
COPD	Chronic obstructive pulmonary disease
CP	Chest pain; cerebral palsy
CPAP	Continuous positive airway pressure
CPK	Creatine phosphokinase (BB, MB, and MM are isoenzymes)
CPP	Cerebral perfusion pressure
CPR	Cardiopulmonary resuscitation
Cr	Creatinine
CrCl	Creatinine clearance
CRF	Chronic renal failure; corticotropin-releasing factor
CRH	Corticotropin-releasing hormone
CRI	Chronic renal insufficiency; catheter-related infection
CRNA	Certified Registered Nurse Anesthetist
CRNP	Certified Registered Nurse Practitioner
CRP	C-reactive protein
CRTT	Certified Respiratory Therapy Technician
CSF	Cerebrospinal fluid; colony-stimulating factor
CT	Computed tomography; chest tube
cTnI	Cardiac troponin I
CTZ	Chemoreceptor trigger zone
CV	Cardiovascular
CVA	Cerebrovascular accident
CVC	Central venous catheter
CVP	Central venous pressure
Cx	Culture; cervix
CXR	Chest x-ray
D&C	Dilatation and curettage
D_5W	5% Dextrose in water
DBP	Diastolic blood pressure
D/C	Discontinue; discharge
DCC	Direct-current cardioversion
DI	Diabetes insipidus
DIC	Disseminated intravascular coagulation
Diff	Differential
DJD	Degenerative joint disease
DKA	Diabetic ketoacidosis
dL	Deciliter

DM	Diabetes mellitus
DNA	Deoxyribonucleic acid
DNR	Do not resuscitate
DO	Doctor of Osteopathy
DOA	Dead on arrival; date of admission; duration of action
DOB	Date of birth
DOE	Dyspnea on exertion
DOT	Directly observed therapy
DPGN	Diffuse proliferative glomerulonephritis
DPI	Dry powder inhaler
DRE	Digital rectal examination
DRG	Diagnosis-related group
DS	Double strength
d/t	Due to
DTP	Diphtheria-tetanus-pertussis
DTR	Deep-tendon reflex
DVT	Deep-vein thrombosis
Dx	Diagnosis
EBV	Epstein-Barr virus
EC	Enteric-coated
ECF	Extracellular fluid
ECG	Electrocardiogram
ECHO	Echocardiogram
ECT	Electroconvulsive therapy
ED	Emergency department
EEG	Electroencephalogram
EENT	Eyes, ears, nose, throat
EF	Ejection fraction
EGD	Esophagogastroduodenoscopy
EIA	Enzyme immunoassay
EKG	Electrocardiogram
EMG	Electromyogram
EMT	Emergency Medical Technician
Endo	Endotracheal, endoscopy
EOMI	Extraocular movements (or muscles) intact
EPO	Erythropoietin
EPS	Extrapyramidal symptoms
ER	Emergency room
ERCP	Endoscopic retrograde cholangiopancreatography
ERT	Estrogen-replacement therapy
ESKD	End-stage kidney disease
ESLD	End-stage liver disease
ESR	Erythrocyte sedimentation rate
ESRD	End-stage renal disease
ET	Endotracheal
EtOH	Ethanol
FB	Finger-breadth; foreign body
FBS	Fasting blood sugar
FDA	Food and Drug Administration
FEF	Forced expiratory flow rate
FEV_1	Forced expiratory volume in 1 second
FFP	Fresh-frozen plasma
FH	Family history
FiO_2	Fraction of inspired oxygen
FOBT	Fecal occult blood test
FPG	Fasting plasma glucose
FPIA	Fluorescence polarization immunoassay
FSH	Follicle-stimulating hormone
FTA	Fluorescent treponemal antibody
F/U	Follow-up
FUO	Fever of unknown origin
Fx	Fracture
FT_4	Free T_4
g	grams
G-CSF	Granulocyte colony-stimulating factor
G6PD	Glucose-6-phosphate dehydrogenase
GB	Gall bladder
GBS	Group B *Streptococcus*; Guillain-Barré syndrome
GC	Gonococcus
GDM	Gestational diabetes mellitus
GE	Gastroesophageal; gastroenterology
GERD	Gastroesophageal reflux disease
GFR	Glomerular filtration rate
GGT	γ-Glutamyl transferase
GGTP	γ-Glutamyl transpeptidase
GI	Gastrointestinal
GM-CSF	Granulocyte-macrophage colony-stimulating factor
GN	Glomerulonephritis; graduate nurse
gr	Grain
GT	Gastrostomy tube
gtt	Drops (*guttae*)
GTT	Glucose tolerance test
GU	Genitourinary
GVHD	Graft-versus-host disease
GVL	Graft-versus-leukemia
Gyn	Gynecology
H&H	Hemoglobin and hematocrit
H&P	History and physical examination
HA	Headache
H_2RA	H_2 receptor antagonist
HAART	Highly-active antiretroviral therapy
HAMD	Hamilton Rating Scale for Depression
HAV	Hepatitis A virus
Hb, hgb	Hemoglobin
HbA_{1c}	Glycosylated hemoglobin (hemoglobin A_{1c})
HBIG	Hepatitis B immune globulin
HBP	High blood pressure
HBsAg	Hepatitis B surface antigen
HBV	Hepatitis B virus
HC	Hydrocortisone, home care
HCG	Human chorionic gonadotropin
HCO_3	Bicarbonate
Hct	Hematocrit
HCTZ	Hydrochlorothiazide
HCV	Hepatitis C virus
HD	Hodgkin's disease; hemodialysis
HDL	High-density lipoprotein
HEENT	Head, eyes, ears, nose, and throat
HF	Heart failure
HFA	Hydrofluouroalkane

H flu	*Haemophilus influenzae*	IVC	Inferior vena cava; intravenous cholangiogram
HGH	Human growth hormone	IVDA	Intravenous drug abuse
HH	Hiatal hernia	IVDU	Injection drug use; intravenous drug use
H/H	Hemoglobin and hematocrit	IVF	Intravenous fluids
Hib	*Haemophilus influenzae* type b	IVIG	Intravenous immunoglobulin
HIT	Heparin-induced thrombocytopenia	IVP	Intravenous pyelogram; intravenous push
HIV	Human immunodeficiency virus	JODM	Juvenile-onset diabetes mellitus
HJR	Hepatojugular reflux	JRA	Juvenile rheumatoid arthritis
HLA	Human leukocyte antigen; human lymphocyte antigen	JVD	Jugular venous distension
HMG-CoA	Hydroxy-methylglutaryl coenzyme A	JVP	Jugular venous pressure
H/O, h/o	History of	K	Potassium
HOB	Head of bed	kcal	Kilocalorie
HPA	Hypothalamic-pituitary axis	KCl	Potassium chloride
hpf	High power field	KOH	Potassium hydroxide
HPI	History of present illness	KUB	Kidney, ureter, and bladder
HR	Heart rate	KVO	Keep vein open
HRSD	Hamilton Rating Scale for Depression	L	Liter
HRT	Hormone-replacement therapy	LABA	Long-acting beta agonist
HS	At bedtime (*hora somni*)	LAD	Left anterior descending; left axis deviation
HSV	Herpes simplex virus	LAO	Left anterior oblique
HTN	Hypertension	LBBB	Left bundle branch block
Hx	History	LBP	Low-back pain
I&D	Incision and drainage	LDH	Lactate dehydrogenase
I&O	Intake and output	LDL	Low-density lipoprotein
IBD	Inflammatory bowel disease	LE	Lower extremity
IBW	Ideal body weight	LES	Lower esophageal sphincter
ICD	Implantable cardioverter defibrillator	LET	Liver function test
ICP	Intracranial pressure	LHRH	Luteinizing hormone-releasing hormone
ICS	Intercostal space, inhaled corticosteroid	LLE	Left lower extremity
ICU	Intensive-care unit	LLL	Left lower lobe
ID	Identification; infectious disease	LLQ	Left lower quadrant (abdomen)
IDDM	Insulin-dependent diabetes mellitus	LMD	Local medical doctor
IFN	Interferon	LMP	Last menstrual period
Ig	Immunoglobulin	LMWH	Low-molecular-weight heparin
IgA	Immunoglobulin A	LOS	Length of stay
IgD	Immunoglobulin D	LP	Lumbar puncture
IHD	Ischemic heart disease	LPN	Licensed Practical Nurse
IJ	Internal jugular	LPT	Licensed Physical Therapist
IM	Intramuscular; infectious mononucleosis	LR	Lactated Ringer's
INH	Isoniazid	LS	Lumbosacral
INR	International normalized ratio	LT_4	Levothyroxine
I/O	Intake and output	LUE	Left upper extremity
IOP	Intraocular pressure	LUL	Left upper lobe
IP	Intraperitoneal	LUQ	Left upper quadrant
IPG	Impedance plethysmography	LUTS	Lower urinary tract symptoms
IPN	Interstitial pneumonia	LV	Left ventricular
IRB	Institutional Review Board	LVH	Left ventricular hypertrophy
ISA	Intrinsic sympathomimetic activity	MAP	Mean arterial pressure
ISH	Isolated systolic hypertension	MAR	Medication administration record
IT	Intrathecal	MB-CK	A creatine kinase isoenzyme
ITP	Idiopathic thrombocytopenic purpura	mcg	Microgram
IU	International unit (this can be a dangerous abbreviation because it may be read as 'IV' for "intravenous")	MCH	Mean corpuscular hemoglobin
		MCHC	Mean corpuscular hemoglobin concentration
		MCV	Mean corpuscular volume
IUD	Intrauterine device	MD	Medical Doctor
IV	Intravenous; Roman numeral four; symbol for class 4 controlled substances	MDI	Metered-dose inhaler
		MDRD	Modification of diet in renal disease

MEFR	Maximum expiratory flow rate
mEq	Milliequivalent
mg	Milligram
MHC	Major histocompatibility complex
MI	Myocardial infarction; mitral insufficiency
MIC	Minimum inhibitory concentration
mL	Milliliter
MM	Multiple myeloma; an isoenzyme of creatine phosphokinase
MMR	Measles-mumps-rubella; midline malignant reticulosis
MOM	Milk of magnesia
MPV	Mean platelet volume
m/r/g	Murmur/rub/gallop
MRI	Magnetic resonance imaging
MRSA	Methicillin-resistant *Staphylococcus aureus*
MRSE	Methicillin-resistant *Staphylococcus epidermidis*
MS	Mental status; mitral stenosis; musculoskeletal; multiple sclerosis; morphine sulfate
MSE	Mental status exam
MSW	Master of Social Work
MTD	Maximum tolerated dose
MIX	Methotrexate
MVA	Motor vehicle accident
MVI	Multivitamin
MVR	Mitral valve replacement; mitral valve regurgitation
MVS	mitral valve stenosis; motor, vascular, and sensory
N&V	Nausea and vomiting
NAD	No acute (or apparent) distress
N/C	Noncontributory; nasal cannula
NG	Nasogastric
NGT	Nasogastric tube; normal glucose tolerance
NIDDM	Non-insulin-dependent diabetes mellitus
NIH	National Institutes of Health
NKA	No known allergies
NKDA	No known drug allergies
NHDA	Nonketotic hyperosmolar acidosis
NL	Normal
NOS	Not otherwise specified
NPN	Nonprotein nitrogen
NPO	Nothing by mouth (*nil per os*)
NS	Normal saline solution (0.9% sodium chloride solution); neurosurgery
NSAID	Nonsteroidal anti-inflammatory drug
NSR	Normal sinus rhythm
NSS	Normal saline solution
NSTE	Non-ST elevation
NTG	Nitroglycerin
NT/ND	Nontender, nondistended
NVD	Nausea/vomiting/diarrhea; neck vein distension; neovascularization of the disk; neurovesicle dysfunction; nonvalvular disease
N/V	Nausea and vomiting
NYHA	New York Heart Association
O&P	Ova and parasites

OA	Osteoarthritis
OB	Obstetrics
OCD	Obsessive-compulsive disorder
OD	Right eye (*oculus dexter*)
OGT	Oral glucose tolerance test
OPV	Oral poliovirus vaccine
OR	Operating room
OR×1	Oriented to time
OR×2	Oriented to time and place
OR×3	Oriented to time, place, and person
OS	Left eye (*oculus sinister*)
OSA	Obstructive sleep apnea
OT	Occupational therapy
OTC	Over the counter
OU	*Oculus uterque* (each eye)
P	Pulse; plan; percussion; pressure
P&A	Percussion and auscultation
P&T	Peak and trough
PA	Physician Assistant; posteroanterior; pulmonary artery
PAC	Premature atrial contraction
PaCO$_2$	Arterial carbon dioxide tension
PaO$_2$	Arterial oxygen tension
PAOP	Pulmonary artery occlusion pressure
PC	After meals (*post cibum*)
PCA	Patient-controlled analgesia
PCI	Percutaneous coronary intervention
PCKD	Polycystic kidney disease
PCN	Penicillin
PCP	*Pneumocystis carinii* pneumonia (also known as *Pneumocystis jirovecii* Pneumonia); pneumocystis pneumonia; primary care physician; phencyclidine
PCWP	Pulmonary capillary wedge pressure
PDE	Paroxysmal dyspnea on exertion
PE	Physical examination; pulmonary embolism
PEEP	Positive end-expiratory pressure
PEER	Peak expiratory flow rate
PEG	Percutaneous endoscopic gastrostomy; polyethylene glycol
Peg-IFN	Pegylated interferon
PERL	Pupils equal, react to light
PERRLA	Pupils equal, round, and reactive to light and accommodation
PERRRLA	Pupils equal, round, regular, and react to light and accommodation
PET	Positron-emission tomography
PFT	Pulmonary function test
pH	Hydrogen ion concentration
PH	Past history; personal history; pinhole; poor health; pubic hair; public health
PHx	Past history
PharmD	Doctor of Pharmacy
PID	Pelvic inflammatory disease
PJP	*Pneumocystis jirovecii* Pneumonia (also known as *Pneumocystis carinii* pneumonia)
PKU	Phenylketonuria
PMH	Past medical history

PMI	Past medical illness; point of maximal impulse
PMN	Polymorphonuclear leukocyte
PMS	Premenstrual syndrome
PND	Paroxysmal nocturnal dyspnea
PO	By mouth (*per os*)
PO$_2$	Partial pressure of oxygen
POAG	Primary open-angle glaucoma
POD	Postoperative day
PPBG	Postprandial blood glucose
ppd	Packs per day
PPD	Purified protein derivative (TB skin test)
PPN	Peripheral parenteral nutrition
PPI	Proton pump inhibitor
PPP	Chisholm-Burns *et al*/Pharmacotherapy Principles & Practice, 2nd ed.
Pr	Per rectum
PRBC	Packed red blood cells
PRERLA	Pupils round, equal, react to light and accommodation
PRN	When necessary; as needed (*pro re nata*)
PSA	Prostate-specific antigen
PSH	Past surgical history
PST	Paroxysmal supraventricular tachycardia
PSVT	Paroxysmal supraventricular tachycardia
Pt	Patient
PT	Prothrombin time; physical therapy; patient
PTA	Prior to admission; percutaneous transluminal angioplasty
PTCA	Percutaneous transluminal coronary angioplasty
PTE	Pulmonary thromboembolism
PTH	Parathyroid hormone
PTSD	Posttraumatic stress disorder
PTT	Partial thromboplastin time
PUD	Peptic ulcer disease
PVC	Premature ventricular contraction
PVD	Peripheral vascular disease
PVR	Peripheral vascular resistance
PVT	Paroxysmal ventricular tachycardia
q	Every (*quaque*)
QA	Quality assurance
qday	Every day
QI	Quality improvement
qid	Four times daily (*quater in die*)
QNS	Quantity not sufficient
qod	Every other day
QOL	Quality of life
QS	Quantity sufficient
QTc	Corrected QT interval
R&M	Routine and microscopic
R&R	Rate and rhythm
RA	Rheumatoid arthritis; right atrium
RAAS	Renin-angiotensin-aldosterone system
RBC	Red blood cell
RCA	Right coronary artery
RCM	Right costal margin
RDA	Recommended daily allowance
RDS	Respiratory distress syndrome
RDW	Red cell distribution width
REM	Rapid eye movement; recent event memory
RES	Reticuloendothelial system
RF	Rheumatoid factor; renal failure; rheumatic fever
Rh	Rhesus factor in blood
RHD	Rheumatic heart disease
RLE	Right lower extremity
RLL	Right lower lobe
RLQ	Right lower quadrant
RML	Right middle lobe
RN	Registered Nurse
RNA	Ribonucleic acid
R/O	Rule out
ROM	Range of motion
ROS	Review of systems
RPh	Registered Pharmacist
RR	Respiratory rate; recovery room
RRR	Regular rate and rhythm
RRT	Registered Respiratory Therapist
RSV	Respiratory syncytial virus
RT	Radiation therapy
RUE	Right upper extremity
RUL	Right upper lobe
RUQ	Right upper quadrant
RVH	Right ventricular hypertrophy
S$_1$	First heart sound
S$_2$	Second heart sound
S$_3$	Third heart sound (ventricular gallop)
S$_4$	Fourth heart sound (atrial gallop)
SA	Sinoatrial
SABA	Short-acting beta agonist
SAD	Seasonal affective disorder
SAH	Subarachnoid hemorrhage
SaO$_2$	Arterial oxygen percent saturation
SBE	Subacute bacterial endocarditis
SBFT	Small bowel follow-through
SBGM	Self blood glucose monitoring
SBO	Small bowel obstruction
SBP	Systolic blood pressure
SC	Subcutaneous; subclavian
SCr, sCr	Serum creatinine
SEM	Systolic ejection murmur
SG	Specific gravity
SGOT (AST)	Serum glutamic oxaloacetic transaminase (aspartate transaminase)
SGPT (ALT)	Serum glutamic pyruvic transaminase (alanine transaminase)
SH	Social history
SIADH	Syndrome of inappropriate antidiuretic hormone secretion
SIDS	Sudden infant death syndrome
SJS	Stevens-Johnson syndrome
SL	Sublingual
SLE	Systemic lupus erythematosus

SMA-6	Sequential multiplier analyzer for sodium, potassium, CO_2, chloride, glucose, and BUN
SMA-7	Sequential multiplier analyzer for sodium, potassium, CO_2, chloride, glucose, BUN, and creatinine
SMA-12	Sequential multiplier analyzer for glucose, BUN, uric acid, calcium, phosphorous, total protein, albumin, cholesterol, total bilirubin, alkaline phosphatase, SCOT, and LDH
SMA-23	Includes the entire SMA-12 plus sodium, potassium, CO_2, chloride, direct bilirubin, triglyceride, SGPT, indirect bilirubin, R fraction, and BUN/creatinine ratio
SMBG	Self-monitoring of blood glucose
SNF	Skilled nursing facility
SNS	Sympathetic nervous system
SOB	Shortness of breath; see order book; side of bed
S/P, s/p	Status post
SPF	Sun protection factor
SQ	Subcutaneous
s/s	Signs and symptoms
SSKI	Saturated solution of potassium iodide
SSRI	Selective serotonin reuptake inhibitor
STAT	Immediately, at once
STEMI	ST elevation myocardial infarction
STD	Sexually transmitted disease
SV	Stroke volume
SVC	Superior vena cava
SVRI	Systemic vascular resistance index
SVR	Supraventricular rhythm; systemic vascular resistance
SVT	Supraventricular tachycardia
SW	Social worker
Sx	Signs
T	Temperature
T_3	Triiodothyronine
T_4	Thyroxine
T&A	Tonsillectomy and adenoidectomy
T&C	Type and crossmatch
TB	Tuberculosis
TBG	Thyroid-binding globulin
TBI	Total-body irradiation, traumatic brain injury
TBW	Total body weight
T bili	Total bilirubin
TCA	Tricyclic antidepressant
TCN	Tetracycline
TDaP	Tetanus, diphtheria, acellular pertussis vaccine

TEE	Transesophageal echocardiogram
TFT	Thyroid function test
TG	Triglyceride
TIA	Transient ischemic attack
TIBC	Total iron-binding capacity
TID	Three times daily (*ter in die*)
TLC	Therapeutic lifestyle changes
TM	Tympanic membrane
TMJ	Temporomandibular joint
TMP-SMX	Trimethoprim-sulfamethoxazole
TNF	Tumor necrosis factor
TNTC	Too numerous to count
TOD	Target-organ damage
TPN	Total parenteral nutrition
TPR	Temperature, pulse, respiration
T PROT	Total protein
TSH	Thyroid-stimulating hormone
TURP	Transurethral resection of the prostate
Tx	Treat, treatment
UA	Urinalysis, uric acid
UC	Ulcerative colitis
UE	Upper extremity
UFH	Unfractionated heparin
UGI	Upper gastrointestinal
UOQ	Upper outer quadrant
UPT	Urine pregnancy test
URI	Upper respiratory infection
USP	United States Pharmacopeia
UTI	Urinary tract infection
UV	Ultraviolet
VF	Ventricular fibrillation
VLDL	Very low-density lipoprotein
VO	Verbal order
VOD	Veno-occlusive disease
V_A/Q	Ventilation-perfusion
VRE	Vancomycin-resistant *Enterococcus*
VS	Vital signs
VSS	Vital signs stable
VT	Ventricular tachycardia
VTE	Venous thromboembolism
WA	While awake
WBC	White blood cell (count)
W/C	Wheelchair
WDWN	Well-developed, well-nourished
WHO	World Health Organization
WNL	Within normal limits
W/U	Work-up
yo	Year-old
yr	Year

Ablation: Destruction of part or all of an organ or structure.

Abscess: A purulent (i.e., containing, discharging, or causing the production of pus) collection of fluid separated from surrounding tissue by a wall composed of inflammatory cells and adjacent organs. It usually contains necrotic debris, bacteria, and inflammatory cells.

Acanthosis nigricans: A skin condition characterized by dark, thickened, velvety patches, especially in the folds of skin in the armpits, groin, and back of the neck that is often associated with insulin resistance.

Acaricide: A chemical that kills mites and ticks.

Acetaldehyde: A by-product of alcohol metabolism.

Acetylcholinesterase: An enzyme that breaks down unused acetylcholine in the synaptic cleft. This enzyme is necessary to restore the synaptic cleft so it is ready to transmit the next nerve impulse

Achlorhydria: Low level or absence of gastric acid in the stomach.

Acidemia: An increase in the hydrogen ion concentration in the blood or a fall below normal in pH.

Acidosis: Any pathologic state that leads to acidemia.

Acromegaly: A pathologic condition characterized by excessive production of growth hormone during adulthood after epiphyseal (growth plate) fusions have completed.

Action potential: A rapid change in the polarity of the voltage of a cell membrane from negative to positive and back to negative. A wave of electrical discharge that travels across a cell membrane.

Acute chest syndrome: An acute respiratory complication of sickle cell disease characterized by chest pain, fever, and pulmonary infiltrates.

Acute coronary syndromes: Ischemic chest discomfort at rest most often accompanied by ST-segment elevation, ST-segment depression, or T-wave inversion on the 12-lead electrocardiogram; further, it is caused by plaque rupture and partial or complete occlusion of the coronary artery by thrombus. Acute coronary syndromes include myocardial infarction and unstable angina. Former terms used to describe types of acute coronary syndromes include Q-wave myocardial infarction, non-Q-wave myocardial infarction, and unstable angina.

Acute disorder: An acid-base disturbance that has been present for minutes to hours.

Acute kidney injury: Spectrum of acute changes in kidney function ranging from minor changes to those requiring renal replacement therapy.

Acute otitis media: Inflammation of the middle ear accompanied by fluid in the middle ear space and signs or symptoms of an acute ear infection.

Acute tubular necrosis: Form of acute kidney injury that results from toxic or ischemic injury to the cells in the proximal tubule of the kidney.

Addiction: A primary, chronic, neurobiologic disease, with genetic, psychosocial, and environmental factors influencing its development and manifestations. It is characterized by behaviors that include one or more of the following: impaired control over drug use, compulsive use, continued use despite harm, and craving.

Adenocarcinomas: Malignant tumor originating in glandular tissue.

Adenoma: A nonmalignant tumor of the epithelial tissue that is characterized by glandular structures.

Adenomatous polyposis coli (APC) gene: A tumor suppressor gene (see definition) that is one of the first genes mutated in the development of colon cancer. Patients with familial adenomatous polyposis (FAP) are born with this gene mutated.

Adjuvant chemotherapy: Treatment given after the primary surgical treatment and is designed to eliminate any remaining cancer cells that are undetectable with the goal of improving survival.

Adjuvant therapy: Therapy that supplements or follows primary therapy to prevent the risk of recurrence.

Adnexal: Adjacent or appending as the fallopian tubes and ovaries are to the uterus.

Adrenalectomy: Surgical removal of an adrenal gland.

Adrenocorticotropic hormone: A hormone secreted by the anterior pituitary that controls secretion of cortisol from the adrenal glands. Also referred to as corticotropin.

Adverse drug reaction (ADR): As defined by the American Society of Health-System Pharmacists, ADR is any unexpected, unintended, undesired, or excessive response to a medication that: requires discontinuing the medication; requires changing the medication; requires modifying the dose (except for minor dosage adjustments); necessitates admission to the hospital; prolongs stay in a health care facility; necessitates supportive treatment; significantly complicates diagnosis; negatively affects prognosis; or results in temporary or permanent harm, disability, or death.

Aeroallergen: An airborne substance that causes an allergic response.

Afterload: The force against which a ventricle contracts that is contributed to by vascular resistance, especially of the arteries, and by physical characteristics (mass and viscosity) of the blood.

Ageism: Discrimination against aged persons.

Air embolus: An obstruction in a small blood vessel caused by air that is introduced into a blood vessel and is carried through the circulation until it lodges in a smaller vessel.

Akathisia: Motor or subjective feelings of restlessness.

Akinesia: Lack of movement.

Alcohol dehydrogenase: An enzyme that degrades ethanol in the gut and liver.

Aldosterone: A hormone produced in and secreted by the zona glomerulosa of the adrenal cortex. Aldosterone acts on the kidneys to reabsorb sodium and excrete potassium. It is also a part of the renin-angiotensin-aldosterone system that regulates blood pressure and blood volume.

Alkalemia: A decrease in the hydrogen ion concentration of the blood or a rise above normal in pH.

Alkalosis: Any pathologic state that leads to alkalemia.

Allodynia: Pain that results from a stimulus that does not normally cause pain.

Allogeneic: In the setting of stem cell transplantation, the scenario in which the donor is a genetically similar but not identical to the recipient. The donor is frequently a sibling or a matched related donor. A matched unrelated donor may be used in the absence of a related donor.

Allograft: Tissue or organ transplanted from a donor of the same species but different genetic makeup; recipient's immune system must be suppressed to prevent rejection of the graft.

Allograft survival: After the transplant procedure, when the transplanted organ continues to have some degree of function, from excellent to poor.

Allorecognition: Recognition of the foreign antigens present on the transplant organ or the donor's antigen presenting cells.

Alopecia: Hair loss.

Amenorrhea: The absence or discontinuation of regular menstrual periods.

γ-Aminobutyric acid: An inhibitory amino acid found in the central nervous system.

Amotivation: Apathy, loss of effectiveness, and diminished capacity or willingness to carry out complex, long-term plans, endure frustration, concentrate for long periods, follow routines, or successfully master new material.

Amygdala: Part of the limbic system that mediates emotions and helps to coordinate the response to threatening or stressful situations.

Amylase: An enzyme that catalyzes the hydrolysis of starch into simpler compounds.

Amylin: A 37-amino acid polypeptide hormone that is secreted from the β-cells of the pancreas in response to nutrients. Mechanisms of action include slowing gastric emptying, suppressing postmeal glucagon secretion, and suppressing appetite.

Amyloid: Any of a group of chemically diverse proteins which are composed of linear nonbranching aggregated fibrils.

Anaphylactic/anaphylaxis: Immediate, severe, potentially fatal hypersensitivity reaction induced by an antigen.

Anaphylactoid: An anaphylactic-like reaction, similar in signs and symptoms but not mediated by IgE. The drug causing this reaction produces direct release of inflammatory mediators by a pharmacologic effect.

Anastomosis: The connection of two hollow organs to restore continuity after resection or to bypass disease process that is not resectable.

Anemia: A reduction below normal in the concentration of hemoglobin in the body that results in a reduction of the oxygen-carrying capacity of the blood.

Anemia of chronic kidney disease: A decline in red blood cell production caused by a decrease in erythropoietin production by the progenitor cells of the kidney. As kidney function declines in chronic kidney disease, erythropoietin production also declines, resulting in decreased red blood cell production. Other contributing factors include iron deficiency and decreased red blood cell lifespan, caused by uremia.

Anergy: A reduction or lack of an immune response to a specific antigen.

Aneuploidy: Abnormal number of chromosomes.

Angina: Discomfort in the chest or adjacent areas caused by decreased blood and oxygen supply to the myocardium (myocardial ischemia).

Angina pectoris: Severe constricting pain in the chest, often radiating from the precordium to a shoulder (usually left) and down the arm, due to ischemia of the heart muscle usually caused by a coronary disease.

Angioedema: Swelling similar to urticaria (hives), but the swelling occurs beneath the skin instead of on the surface. Angioedema is characterized by deep swelling around the eyes and lips and sometimes of the hands and feet. If it proceeds rapidly, it can lead to airway obstruction and suffocation, and it should therefore be treated as a medical emergency.

Angiogenesis: The formation of new blood vessels.

Anhedonia: Inability to experience pleasure.

Anorexia: An eating disorder generally characterized by distorted body image, fear of weight gain, unwillingness to eat, and restrictive diet; may also refer to loss of appetite and serious weight loss as a result of disease.

Anoxia: A lack of oxygen.

Anterograde amnesia: Memory loss affecting the transfer of new information or events to long-term storage.

Antiangiogenic: Preventing or inhibiting the formation and differentiation of blood vessels.

Anticoagulant: Any substance that inhibits, suppresses, or delays the formation of blood clots. These substances occur naturally and regulate the clotting cascade. Several anticoagulants have been identified in a variety of animal tissues and have been commercially developed for medicinal use.

Antimicrobial prophylaxis: Use of an antimicrobial to prevent an infection.

Antiproteinase: A substance that inhibits the enzymatic activity of a proteinase.

Antrectomy: A surgical excision of the wall of the antrum, the region of the stomach that produces the hormone gastrin.

Anuria: Urine output of less than 50 mL over 24 hours.

Anxiogenic: Something that promotes or causes anxiety.

Aphakia: The absence of a lens in the eye.

Aphasia: Impairment of language affecting the ability to speak and to understand speech.

Aphthous ulcer: A small superficial area of ulceration within the gastrointestinal mucosa, typically found in the oral cavity.

Apoptosis: Programmed cell death as signaled by the nuclei in normally functioning cells when age or state of cell health and condition dictates.

Arcuate scotoma: An arc-shaped area of blindness in the field of vision.

Arthralgia: Pain in joints.

Arthrocentesis: Puncture and aspiration of a joint. Certain drugs can be injected into the joint space for a local effect.

Arthus reaction: Local inflammatory response due to deposition of immune complexes in tissues.

Articular: Related to a joint or joints.

Ascites: Accumulation of fluid within the peritoneal cavity.

Asterixis: A flapping tremor of the arms and hands that is seen in patients with end-stage liver disease.

Astringent: A substance that causes tissues to constrict, resulting in a drying effect of the skin.

Ataxia: Defective muscular coordination, possibly manifested by a staggering gait.

Atelectasis: Decreased or absent air in a partial or entire lung, with resulting loss of lung volume.

Atherosclerosis: Accumulation of lipids, inflammatory cells, and cellular debris in the subendothelial space of the arterial wall.

Atopy: A genetic predisposition to develop type I hypersensitivity reactions against common environmental antigens. Commonly seen in patients with allergic rhinitis, asthma, and atopic dermatitis.

Atresia: Congenital absence of a normal opening or normally patent lumen.

Autograft: A tissue or organ grafted into a new position in or on the body of the same individual.

Autologous: In the setting of stem cell transplantation, the scenario in which the donor and recipient are the same person.

Automaticity: Ability of a cardiac fiber or tissue to spontaneously initiate depolarizations.

Autonomic (nervous system): The parasympathetic and sympathetic nerves that control involuntary actions in the body.

Azoospermic: Having no living spermatozoa in the semen, or failure of spermatogenesis.

Bacteriuria: Presence of bacteria in urine.

Barium enema: A diagnostic test using an x-ray examination to view the lower gastrointestinal tract (colon and rectum) after rectal administration of barium sulfate, a chalky liquid contrast medium.

Basal ganglia: Cluster of nerve cells deep in the brain that coordinate normal movement.

Bence-Jones proteins: Light-chained immunoglobulins found in the urine.

Bilateral: Pertaining to both sides.

Bilateral salpingo-oophorectomy: Surgical excision (removal) of both ovaries.

Bile acids: The organic acids in bile. Bile is the yellowish-brown or green fluid secreted by the liver and discharged into the duodenum where it aids in the emulsification of fats, increases peristalsis, and retards putrefaction; contains sodium glycocholate and sodium taurocholate, cholesterol, biliverdin and bilirubin, mucus, fat, lecithin, and cells and cellular debris.

Biliary sludge: A deposit of tiny stones or crystals made up of cholesterol, calcium bilirubinate, and other calcium salts. The cholesterol and calcium bilirubinate crystals in biliary sludge can lead to gallstone formation.

Bioavailability: The amount of agent that is absorbed orally relative to an equivalent dose administered intravenously.

Biopsy: A procedure that involves obtaining a tissue specimen for microscopic analysis to establish a precise diagnosis.

Blastopore: A fungal spore produced by budding.

Blood dyscrasias: Any abnormality in the blood or bone marrow's cellular components such as low white or red blood cell count or low platelets

Blood urea nitrogen (BUN): A waste product in the blood produced from the breakdown of dietary proteins. The kidneys filter blood to remove urea and maintain homeostasis; a decline in kidney function results in an increase in BUN.

Body mass index (BMI): A calculation utilized to correct weight changes for height and is a direct calculation regardless of gender. It is the result of the weight in kilograms divided by the height in meters squared. If nonmetric measurements are used, it is the result of the weight in pounds multiplied by 703 and then that quantity divided by the product of height in inches squared.

Bone and mineral disorders (BMMD): Altered bone turnover that results from sustained metabolic conditions that occur in chronic kidney disease, including secondary hyperparathyroidism, hyperphosphatemia, hypocalcemia, and vitamin D deficiency. The disease can be characterized by high bone turnover, low bone turnover or adynamic disease, or may be a mixed disorder.

Bone remodeling: The constant process of bone turnover involving bone resorption followed by bone formation.

Bouchard's nodes: Hard, bony enlargement of the proximal interphalangeal (middle) joint of a finger or toe.

Brachial plexus: Collection of nerves that arises from the spine at the base of the neck from nerves that supply parts of the shoulder, arm, forearm, and hand.

Brachytherapy: A procedure in which radioactive material sealed in needles, seeds, wires, or catheters is placed directly into or near a tumor. Also called internal radiation, implant radiation, or interstitial radiation therapy.

Bradykinesia: Slow movement.

Breakpoint: The concentration of the antimicrobial agent that can be achieved in serum after a normal or standard dose of that antimicrobial agent.

Bronchiectasis: Chronic condition of one or more bronchi or bronchioles marked by irreversible dilatation and destruction of the bronchial walls.

Bronchoalveolar lavage: Washing out of the lungs with saline or mucolytic agents for diagnostic or therapeutic purposes.

Bronchoscopy: An examination used for inspection of the interior of the tracheobronchial tree.

Bullectomy: Surgical removal of one or more bullae (air spaces in the lung measuring more than 1 cm in diameter in the distended state).

Bursitis: An inflammation of the bursa, the fluid-filled sac near the joint where tendons and muscles pass over bone.

Cachectic: Physical wasting with loss of weight and muscle mass caused by cancer.

Cachexia: Weight loss, wasting of muscle, loss of appetite, and general debility that can occur with cancer. Anorexia may or may not be present.

Capillary leak: Loss of intravascular volume into the interstitial space within the body.

Carcinoembryonic antigen (CEA): A protein normally seen during fetal development. When elevated in adults it suggests the presence of colorectal and other cancers. Normal range is less than 2.5 ng/mL (less than 2.5 mcg/L) in nonsmokers but can be elevated in smokers and other nonmalignant conditions such as pancreatitis.

Carcinogenesis: Production or origin of cancer.

Carcinoma: A malignant growth that arises from epithelium, found in skin or the lining of body organs. Carcinomas tend to infiltrate into adjacent tissue and spread to distant organs.

Carcinoma in situ: The cancer is limited to the epithelial cells of origin; it has not yet invaded the basement membrane.

Carcinomatosis: Condition of having widespread dissemination of carcinoma (cancer) in the body.

Cardiac cachexia: Physical wasting with loss of weight and muscle mass caused by cardiac disease. A wasting syndrome that causes weakness and a loss of weight, fat, and muscle.

Cardiac index: Cardiac output normalized for body surface area (cardiac index = cardiac output/body surface area).

Cardiac output: The volume of blood ejected from the left side of the heart per unit of time [cardiac output (L/min) = stroke volume × heart rate].

Cardiac remodeling: Genome expression resulting in molecular, cellular, and interstitial changes and manifested clinically as changes in size, shape, and function of the heart resulting from cardiac load or injury.

Carotid: The two main arteries in the neck.

Carotid bruit: Abnormal sound heard when auscultating a carotid artery caused by turbulent blood flow usually due to the presence of atherosclerotic plaques.

Carotid intima-media thickness: A measurement of the surface between the intima and media. This is a well-validated measure of the progression of atherosclerosis. Increasing measurements over time correlates with increasing atherosclerosis, whereas a decrease in the measurement is indicative of atherosclerotic regression.

Cataplexy: A sudden loss of muscle control with retention of clear consciousness that follows a strong emotional stimulus (as elation, surprise, or anger) and is a characteristic symptom of narcolepsy.

Causalgia: Persist entburning pain, allodynia, and hyperpathia following a traumatic nerve lesion.

Central pain: Pain that results from a lesion in or dysfunction of the central nervous system.

Cephalalgia: A term for head pain similar to headache.

Cervicitis: Inflammation of the cervix.

Chemoprevention: The use of drugs, vitamins, or other agents to reduce the risk, delay the development, or prevent the recurrence of cancer.

Chemoreceptor trigger zone (CTZ): Located in the area postrema of the fourth ventricle of the brain; it is exposed to cerebrospinal fluid and blood and is easily stimulated by circulating toxins to induce nausea and vomiting.

Chemosis: Edema of the conjunctiva.

Cheyne-Stokes respiration: Pattern of breathing with gradual increase in depth and sometimes in rate to a maximum, followed by a decrease resulting in apnea. The cycles ordinarily are 30 seconds to 2 minutes in duration, with 5 to 30 seconds of apnea.

Chimeric: Composed of parts from different origins.

Chloasma: Melasma characterized by irregularly shaped brown patches on the face and other areas of the skin, often seen during pregnancy or associated with the use of oral contraceptives.

Chlorpromazine equivalents: Dose of a first-generation antipsychotic approximately equivalent to 100 mg of chlorpromazine (relative potency).

Cholecystitis: Inflammation of the gallbladder.

Cholelithiasis: Also known as gallstones. Hard masses formed in the gallbladder or its passages that can block bile blow and cause severe upper right quadrant abdominal pain (sometimes radiating to the right shoulder).

Cholestasis: Reduced or lack of flow of bile, or obstruction of bile flow.

Cholesteatoma: A mass of keratinized epithelial cells and cholesterol resembling a tumor that forms in the middle ear or mastoid region.

Chorea: A type of dyskinesia with rhythmic dance-like movement. The increase in motor activity may be associated with fidgetiness, twitching, or flinging movements.

Chronic disorder: An acid–base disturbance that has been present for hours to days.

Chronic kidney disease (CKD): A progressive, irreversible decline in kidney function that occurs over a period of several months to years.

Chronic stable angina: Manifestation of ischemic heart disease (IHD) that typically results when an atherosclerotic plaque progresses to occlude at least 70% of a major coronary artery. Patients typically present with a sensation of chest pressure or heaviness that is evoked by exertion and relieved with rest or sublingual nitroglycerin.

Chronotropic: Referring to changes in the heart rate.

Chvostek's sign: Noted when a tap on the patient's facial nerve adjacent to the ear produces a brief contraction of the upper lip, nose, or side of the face.

Chylothorax: The presence of lymphatic fluid (chyle) in the pleural cavity.

Circadian: Events that occur over a 24-hour interval.

Circadian rhythm: 24-Hour cycles of behavior and physiology that are generated by endogenous biological clocks (pacemakers).

Circulatory shock: A condition wherein the circulatory system is inadequately supplying the oxygen and vital metabolic substrates to cells throughout the body.

Cirrhosis: Hepatic fibrosis and regenerative nodules that have destroyed the architecture of the liver, scarring the liver tissues.

Clinical cure: Resolution of signs and symptoms of a disease.

Clonal expansion: An immunological response in which lymphocytes stimulated by antigen proliferate and amplify the population of relevant cells.

Closed comedo: A plugged follicle of sebum, keratinocytes, and bacteria that remains beneath the surface of the skin. Also referred to as a "whitehead."

Clotting cascade: A series of enzymatic reactions by clotting factors leading to the formation of a blood clot. The clotting cascade is initiated by several thrombogenic substances. Each reaction in the cascade is triggered by the preceding one and the effect is amplified by positive feedback loops.

Clotting factor: Plasma proteins found in the blood that are essential to the formation of blood clots. Clotting factors circulate in inactive forms but are activated by their predecessor in the clotting cascade or a thrombogenic substance. Each clotting factor is designated by a roman numeral, e.g., Factor VII, and by the letter "a" when activated, e.g., Factor VIIa.

Clubbing: A deformity produced by proliferation of the soft tissues at the terminal phalanges of the fingers or toes.

Coalescence: Fusion of smaller lipid emulsion particles forming larger particles, resulting in destabilization of the emulsion.

Cognitive function: Executive function and mental processing such as understanding, perception, reasoning, language, and awareness. Executive function involves a long list of skills, which can be divided into four categories: organization, self-regulation, attention, and problem solving. For example, a patient may have trouble thinking quickly, making decisions, planning, and prioritizing tasks. These functions can be evaluated by various neuropsychological tests.

Coitus: Sexual intercourse.

Collateral damage: The development of resistance occurring in a patient's nontargeted flora that can cause secondary infections.

Colloids: Intravenous fluids composed of water and large-molecular weight molecules used to increase volume in patients with hypovolemic shock via increased intravascular oncotic pressure.

Colon cancer: A disease in which cells in the lining of the colon become malignant (cancer) and proliferate without control. Often referred to as colorectal cancer to include cancer cells found in the rectum.

Colonoscopy: A visual examination of the colon using a lighted, lens-equipped, flexible tube (colonoscope) inserted into the rectum.

Colony forming units: The number of microorganisms that form colonies when cultured and is indicative of the number of viable microorganisms in a sample.

Comedolytic: An agent that is able to break up or destroy a comedo.

Comorbidities: Multiple disease states occurring concurrently in one patient.

Compartment syndrome: The compression of nerves and blood vessels within an enclosed space.

Complex regimen: Taking medications three or more times per day, or 12 or more doses per day.

Complicated disorder: The presence of two or more distinct disorders.

Computed tomography: Radiographic imaging of anatomic information from a cross-sectional plane of the body.

Concreteness: Inability to think in abstract terms. It may be a primary developmental defect or secondary to organic mental disorder or schizophrenia.

Congenital adrenal hyperplasia: A rare inherited condition resulting from a deficiency in cortisol and aldosterone synthesis with resulting excess androgen production. The clinical presentation depends on the variant of the condition but typically manifests as abnormalities in sexual development and/or adrenal insufficiency.

Conidia: Propagating form (spores) of filamentous fungi that are released into soil and air currents. Inhalation of spores is the most common route of infections for endemic fungi and invasive molds.

Conjunctival injection: Erythema of the conjunctiva.

Conjunctivitis: Inflammation of the conjunctiva.

Conjunctivitis medicamentosa: A contact allergy to a topical medication.

Consolidation: A type of high-dose chemotherapy given as the second phase (after induction) of a treatment regimen for leukemia.

Contiguous: Describes two structures that are in close contact, or located next to each other.

Continuous positive airway pressure (CPAP): Therapy delivered using a nasal mask to improve the patency of the upper airway by maintaining sufficient air pressure to alleviate sleep-disordered breathing.

Contralateral: Pertaining to the opposite side of the body.

Convection: The movement of dissolved solutes across a semipermeable membrane by applying a pressure gradient to the fluid transport.

Convulsion: A violent involuntary contraction or series of contractions of voluntary muscles.

Copulation: Sexual union of male and female; coitus; sexual intercourse. Also, conjugation between two cells that do not fuse but separate after mutual fertilization.

Corneal arcus: Accumulation of lipid on the cornea.

Coronary Artery Bypass Graft (CABG) Surgery: Thoracic surgery where parts of a saphenous vein from a leg or internal mammary artery from the arm are placed as conduits to restore blood flow between the aorta and one or more coronary arteries to "bypass" the coronary artery stenosis (occlusion).

Coronary heart disease (CHD): Narrowing of one or more of the major coronary arteries, most commonly by atherosclerotic plaques. Also referred to as coronary artery disease.

Cor pulmonale: Right-sided heart failure, usually due to structural lung disease, e.g., pulmonary fibrosis, emphysema.

Corpus luteum: The small yellow endocrine structure that develops within a ruptured ovarian follicle and secretes progesterone and estrogen.

Corticotropin-releasing hormone: A hormone released by the hypothalamus that stimulates release of adrenocorticotropic hormone by the anterior pituitary gland.

Cortisol: An adrenal gland hormone responsible for maintaining homeostasis of carbohydrate, protein, and fat metabolism.

Cosyntropin: A synthetic version of adrenocorticotropic hormone.

Counterirritant: A substance that elicits a superficial inflammatory response with the objective of reducing inflammation in deeper, adjacent structures.

C-peptide levels: A peptide which is made when proinsulin is split into insulin and C-peptide. They split before proinsulin is released from endocytic vesicles within the pancreas—one C-peptide for each insulin molecule. C-peptide is the abbreviation for "connecting peptide." It is used to determine if a patient has type 1 or type 2 diabetes mellitus.

Creaming: Aggregation of lipid emulsion particles that then migrate to the surface of the emulsion; can be reversed with mild agitation.

Creatine kinase, Creatine kinase myocardial band: Creatine kinase (CK) enzymes are found in many isoforms, with varying concentrations depending on the type of tissue. CK is a general term used to describe the nonspecific total release of all types of CK, including that found in skeletal muscle (MM), brain (BB), and heart (MB). CK MB is released into the blood from necrotic myocytes in response to infarction and is a useful laboratory test for diagnosing myocardial infarction. If the total CK is elevated, then the relative index (RI), or fraction of the total that is composed of CK MB, is calculated as follows: RI equal to (CK MB/CK total) × 100. An RI greater than 2 is typically diagnostic of infarction.

Creatinine: A waste product in the blood produced from the breakdown of protein by-products generated by muscle in the body or ingested in the diet. The kidneys filter blood to remove creatinine and maintain homeostasis. A decline in kidney function results in an increase in creatinine.

Creatinine clearance: Rate at which creatinine is filtered across the glomerulus; estimate of glomerular filtration rate.

Cretinism: Obsolete term for congenital hypothyroidism.

Cross allergenicity: Sensitivity to one drug and then reacting to a different drug with a similar chemical structure.

CRP (C-reactive protein): A globulin produced by the liver that appears in the blood in certain acute inflammatory conditions, such as rheumatic fever and bacterial infections.

Crypt abscess: Neutrophilic infiltration of the intestinal glands (crypts of Lieberkuhn). A characteristic finding in patients with ulcerative colitis.

Crystalloids: Intravenous fluids composed of water and electrolytes, e.g., sodium, chloride, etc., used as intravascular volume expanders for patients with hypovolemic shock.

Culture-negative IE: Implies acute endocardial damage with negative blood cultures. It is common in patients treated with antibiotics before blood cultures are obtained.

Cutis laxis: Hyperflaccidity of the skin with loss of elasticity.

Cyanosis: Bluish discoloration of the skin and mucous membranes due to lack of oxygenation.

Cyclic citrullinated peptide (CCP): A circular peptide (a ring of amino acids) containing the amino acid citrulline. Autoantibodies directed against CCP provide the basis for a test of importance in rheumatoid arthritis.

Cyclooxygenase: An enzyme that catalyzes the conversion of arachidonic acid to prostaglandins and consists of two isoforms, generally referred to as COX-1 and COX-2.

Cystitis: Inflammation of urinary bladder.

Cyst: An abnormal membranous sac within the body that contains liquid or partially solid material.

Cystocele: Hernial protrusion of the bladder, usually through the vaginal wall.

Cytogenetic analysis: Laboratory identification of chromosomes that looks for mutational defects.

Cytokine: Regulatory proteins, such as interleukins and lymphokines, that are released by cells of the immune system and act as intercellular mediators in the generation of an immune response.

Dactylitis ("hand-foot syndrome"): Diffuse swelling of the hands and or feet often associated with pain and tenderness.

Deep vein thrombosis: A disorder of thrombus formation causing obstruction of a deep vein in the leg, pelvis, or abdomen.

Deescalation: Decreasing antimicrobial regimen spectrum of activity to provide coverage against specific antimicrobial-sensitive pathogens recovered from culture.

Delirium: Transient brain syndrome presenting as disordered attention, cognition, psychomotor behavior, and perception.

Dementia: An organic mental disorder characterized by a general loss of intellectual abilities involving impairment of memory, judgment, and abstract thinking as well as changes in personality.

Denervation: Loss of nerve impulse input, e.g., by severing a nerve during surgery or nerve impulse blockade farther up the nerve chain.

Dennie-Morgan line: A line or fold below the lower eyelids associated with atopy.

Dermatophytes: Any microscopic fungus that grows on the skin, scalp, nails, or mucosa but does not invade deeper tissues.

Desensitization: A method to reduce or eliminate an individual's negative reaction to a substance or stimulus.

Desquamation: Peeling or shedding of the epidermis (superficial layer of the skin) in scales or flakes.

Detumescence: The return of the penis to a flaccid state.

Diabetes insipidus: Polyuria due to the failure of renal tubules to reabsorb water in response to antidiuretic hormone.

Diabetic ketoacidosis: A reversible but life-threatening short-term complication primarily seen in patients with type 1 diabetes caused by the relative or absolute lack of insulin that results in marked ketosis and acidosis.

Dialysate: The physiologic solution used during dialysis to remove excess fluids and waste products from the blood.

Dialysis: The process of removing fluid and waste products from the blood across a semipermeable membrane to maintain fluid, electrolyte, and acid–base balance in patients with kidney failure.

Diaphoretic (diaphoresis): Sweating profusely.

Diarrhea: Loose, watery stools occurring more than three times in 1 day.

Diarthrodial joint: A freely moveable joint, e.g., knee, shoulder. Contrast with amphiarthrodial joint (a slightly movable joint, e.g., vertebral joint) and synarthrodial joint (an unmovable joint, e.g., fibrous joint).

Diastolic dysfunction: Abnormal filling of the ventricles during diastole.

Diphasic dyskinesia: Motor fluctuations occur while the plasma levodopa concentrations are rising and when they are falling. In each dosing interval, the patient may experience improvement, dyskinesia, and improvement (IDI) or dyskinesia, improvement, and dyskinesia (DID).

2,3-Diphosphoglycerate: A compound in red blood cells that affects oxygen binding to and release from hemoglobin.

Direct current cardioversion: The process of administering a synchronized electrical shock to the chest, the purpose of which is to simultaneously depolarize all of the myocardial cells, resulting in restoration of normal sinus rhythm.

Disease-free survival: Length of time after treatment during which no disease is found.

Disk diffusion test (D-test): A test performed in the microbiology laboratory to detect antibiotic sensitivity in bacteria.

Disseminated idiopathic skeletal hyperostosis (DISH): Excessive bone formation at skeletal sites subject to stress, generally where tendons and ligaments attach to bone.

DNA mismatch repair genes: Genes that identify and correct errors in DNA base pairs during DNA replication. Mutations in the genes can lead to cancer by allowing abnormal cells to continue to grow.

Dose intensity: Delivery of a predetermined dose per unit of time, i.e., $mg/m^2/week$.

Downregulation: The process of reducing or suppressing a response to a stimulus.

Drusen: Tiny yellow or white deposits of extracellular material in the eye.

Ductus arteriosus: Shunt connecting the pulmonary artery to the aortic arch that allows most of the blood from the right ventricle to bypass the fetus lungs.

Duodenal: The first of three parts of the small intestine.

Dysarthria: Difficult or defective speech, usually due to impairment of tongue movement or of other muscles essential to speech.

Dysentery: An illness involving severe diarrhea that is often associated with blood in the stool.

Dysesthesia: An unpleasant abnormal sensation.

Dysgeusia: Unpleasant taste in the mouth.

Dyskinesia: Abnormal involuntary movements, which include dystonia, chorea, and akathisia.

Dyslipidemia: Elevation of the total cholesterol, low-density lipoprotein cholesterol or triglyceride concentrations, or a decrease in high-density lipoprotein cholesterol concentration in the blood.

Dysmenorrhea: Crampy pelvic pain occurring with or just prior to menses. "Primary" dysmenorrhea implies pain in the setting of normal pelvic anatomy, while "secondary" dysmenorrhea is secondary to underlying pelvic pathology.

Dyspareunia: Pain during or after sexual intercourse.

Dysphagia: Painful or difficult swallowing, accompanied by a sensation of food being stuck in passage.

Dysphasic: An alteration in normal speech patterns or content.

Dysphonia: Impairment of the voice or difficulty speaking.

Dysphoria: A general mood of depression, dissatisfaction, and unrest.

Dyspnea: Shortness of breath or difficulty breathing.

Dyssynergic defecation: A lack of coordination between the pelvic floor muscles and the anal sphincter.

Dystonia: A type of dyskinesia. Movement is slow and twisting. It may be associated with painful muscle contractions or spasms.

Dysuria: Difficulty or pain related to urination

Ebstein's anomaly: Congenital heart defect in which the opening of the tricuspid valve is displaced toward the apex of the right ventricle of the heart.

Eburnation: A condition in which bone or cartilage becomes hardened and denser.

Ecchymoses: Passage of blood from ruptured blood vessels into subcutaneous tissue causing purple discoloration of the skin.

Ectopic pregnancy: Presence of a fertilized ovum outside of the uterine cavity.

Effector cells: Cells that become active in response to initiation of the immune response.

Ejection fraction: The fraction of the volume present at the end of diastole that is pushed into the aorta during systole.

Electrocardiogram: A noninvasive recording of the electrical activity of the heart.

Electroconvulsive therapy: Administration of electric current to the brain through electrodes placed on the head in order to induce seizure activity in the brain, used in the treatment of certain mental disorders.

Electroencephalogram (EEG): A recording of patterns of electrical impulses in the brain.

Electroencephalography: The recording of brain waves via electrodes placed on the scalp or cortex.

Embolectomy: Surgical removal of a clot or embolism.

Embolism: Sudden blockage of a vessel caused by a blood clot or foreign material which has been brought to the site by the flow of blood.

Embolization: The process by which a blood clot or foreign material dislodges from its site of origin, flows in the blood, and blocks a distant vessel.

Emesis: See vomiting.

End-stage liver disease: Liver failure that is usually accompanied by complications such as ascites or hepatic encephalopathy.

Endarterectomy: Removal of a thrombus from the carotid artery.

Endemic fungi: Fungi that are native or prevalent to a particular area or region.

Endocinch: An endoscopic sewing technique used to improve lower esophageal sphincter tone.

Endometritis: Inflammation of the endometrium.

Endoscopic evaluation: General term used to describe the visual inspection of the inside of hollow organs with an endoscope. Used mainly for diagnostic purposes. Refers to procedures such as gastroscopy, duodenoscopy, colonoscopy, sigmoidoscopy, and others.

Endoscopic retrograde cholangiopancreatography (ERCP): A technique in which an endoscope is passed through the mouth and stomach to the duodenum in order to examine abnormalities of the bile ducts, pancreas, and gallbladder.

Endoscopy: A procedure used to evaluate the interior surfaces of an organ by inserting a small scope into the body through which one can directly examine almost any part of the intestinal tract. Biopsies can be obtained, polyps removed, and clear images obtained.

Endothelial cell: A single layer of cell surrounding the lumen of arteries.

Engraftment: The process by which transplanted stem cells begin to grow and reproduce in the recipient to produce functioning leukocytes, erythrocytes, and platelets.

Enteral nutrition: Delivery of nutrients via the gastrointestinal tract, either by mouth or by feeding tube.

Enterobacteriaceae: A family of enteric Gram-negative bacilli, e.g., *Escherichia coli* or *Klebsiella pneumoniae.*

Enterocytes: Cells lining the small intestine.

Enuresis: Incontinence at night.

Enzyme-linked immunoabsorbent assay (ELISA): A solid phase in the form of a microtiter plate or bead to which HIV antigen is attached. The antigen may be either a preparation of lysed whole virus or a combination of recombinant viral antigens.

Epilepsy: A neurologic disorder characterized by recurring motor, sensory, or psychic malfunction with or without loss of consciousness or convulsive seizures.

Epistaxis: Nasal hemorrhage with blood drainage through the nostrils; a nosebleed.

Erectile dysfunction (ED): Condition defined as the inability to achieve or maintain an erection sufficient for sexual intercourse.

Erythema multiforme: A rash characterized by papular (small raised bump) or vesicular lesions (blisters), and reddening or discoloration of the skin often in concentric zones about the lesion.

Erythematous: Flushing of the skin caused by dilation of capillaries. Erythema is often a sign of inflammation and infection.

Erythrocyte sedimentation rate (ESR): A nonspecific inflammatory marker that may be elevated in some infections and inflammatory diseases; specifically, the ESR is obtained from a blood sample by measuring the distance that red blood cells precipitate after 1 hour.

Erythropoiesis stimulating agents (ESAs): Agents developed by recombinant DNA technology that have the same biological activity as endogenous erythropoietin to stimulate erythropoiesis (red blood cell production) in the bone marrow. The currently available agents in the United States are epoetin alfa and darbepoetin alfa.

Erythropoietin: A hormone primarily produced by the progenitor cells of the kidney that stimulates red blood cell (RBC) production in the bone marrow. Lack of this hormone leads to anemia.

Esophageal varices: Dilated blood vessels in the esophagus.

Esophagitis: Inflammation of the esophagus that occurs when the esophagus is repeatedly exposed to refluxed material for prolonged periods of time.

Essential fatty acid deficiency: Deficiency of linoleic acid, linolenic acid, and/or arachidonic acid, characterized by hair loss, thinning of skin, and skin desquamation. Long-chain fatty acids include trienes (containing three double-bonds, e.g., 5,8,11-eicosatrienoic (or Mead) acid, trienoic acids,) and tetraenes (containing four double bonds, e.g., arachidonic acid). Biochemical evidence of essential fatty acid deficiency includes atriene:tetraene greater than 0.2 and low linoleic or arachidonic acid plasma concentrations.

Euthymia: Normal mood.

Euthyroid: State of normal thyroid function or hormone activity.

Event-free survival: This term refers to the length of time after treatment that a person remains free of certain negative events.

Evoked potential testing: A procedure in which sensory nerve pathways are stimulated, and the time lapse to electrical response in the corresponding area of the brain is measured.

Exanthem: Skin eruption.

Exfoliative dermatitis: Severe inflammation of the entire skin surface due to a reaction to certain drugs.

Exophthalmos: Abnormal protrusion of the eyeball, seen in Grave's disease.

Exploratory laparotomy: Surgical incision into the abdominal cavity, performed to examine the abdominal organs and cavity in search of an abnormality and diagnosis.

External beam radiotherapy: Treatment by radiation emitted from a source located at a distance from the body. Also called beam therapy and external beam therapy.

Extra-abdominal: Outside of the abdominal cavity.

Extraction ratio: Fraction of the drug entering the liver in the blood which is irreversibly removed.

Extrapyramidal reaction: A combination of neurologic effects which includes tremor, chorea, athetosis, and dystonia; a common side effect of antipsychotic agents.

Extrapyramidal symptoms: Adverse effects of medications such as antipsychotics. They include dystonia (involuntary muscle contractions), tardive dyskinesia (repetitive, involuntary movements), parkinsonian symptoms (akinesia, rigidity, and tremors), and akathisia (motor or subjective restlessness).

Extravasation: Movement of fluid from inside a blood vessel into the surrounding tissues.

Facultative: Biologically capable but not restricted to a particular function or mode of life, e.g., survival within macrophages.

Facultative anaerobe: An organism that makes ATP by aerobic respiration if oxygen is present, but switches to fermentation under anaerobic conditions.

Felty's syndrome: An extra-articular manifestation of rheumatoid arthritis associated with splenomegaly and neutropenia.

Festination: Walking with short, rapid, shuffling steps.

Fibrin: An insoluble protein that is one of the principal ingredients of a blood clot. Fibrin strands bind to one another to form a fibrin mesh. The fibrin mesh often traps platelets and other blood cells.

Fibrinolysis: A normal ongoing process that dissolves fibrin and results in the removal of small blood clots; hydrolysis of fibrin.

Fibroadenoma: A benign neoplasm which commonly occurs in breast tissue and is derived from glandular epithelium.

Fibrosis: Formation of tissue containing connective tissues formed by fibroblasts as part of tissue repair or as a reactive process.

Fistula: Abnormal connection between two internal organs (e.g., arteriovenous fistula, a connection between an artery and a vein) or between an internal organ and the exterior or skin (e.g., enterocutaneous fistula, a connection between the intestine and the skin); often seen in severe cases of Crohn's disease.

Flight of ideas: A nearly continuous flow of rapid speech and thought that jumps from topic to topic, usually loosely connected.

Floppy iris syndrome: Disorder associated with excessive relaxation of the iris dilator muscle, which results in a flaccid iris.

Flow cytometry: Technology used to study characteristics of individual cells in a suspension.

Fluorescence *in situ* hybridization (FISH): A laboratory technique used to look at genes or chromosomes in cells and tissues. Pieces of DNA that contain a fluorescent dye are made in the laboratory and added to cells or tissues on a glass slide. When these pieces of DNA bind to specific genes or areas of chromosomes on the slide, they light up when viewed under a microscope with a special light.

Foam cell: Lipid-laden white blood cells.

Forced expiratory volume in 1 second: The volume of air that a patient can forcibly blow out in the first second of forced exhalation after taking a maximal breath.

Forced vital capacity: The maximum volume of air that can be forcibly exhaled after taking a maximal breath.

Fragility fracture: Fracture resulting from a fall from standing height or less amount of trauma.

Frailty: Excess demand imposed upon reduced capacity; a common biological syndrome in the elderly.

Frank-Starling mechanism: One of the mechanisms by which the heart can increase cardiac output.

Freelite assay: A highly sensitive assay that determines the ratio of serum-free light chain kappa to lambda.

Friable: Easily crumbled, pulverized, or reduced to powder.

Friction: Risk factor for pressure ulcers that is created when a patient is dragged across a surface, which can lead to superficial skin damage.

Fronto-temporal: Located to the front or side of the head.

Fructooligosaccharides: Polymers of fructose that reach the colon undigested and are broken down there to short-chain fatty acids by bacterial enzymes.

Functional gastrointestinal disorder: A term used to describe symptoms occurring in the gastrointestinal tract in the absence of a demonstrated pathologic condition. The clinical product of psychosocial factors and altered intestinal physiology involving the brain–gut interrelationship.

Gadolinium: An intravenous contrast agent used with magnetic resonance imaging.

Galactorrhea: Inappropriate breast milk production and secretion.

Gallstone (cholelithiasis): A solid formation in the gallbladder or bile duct (choledocholithiasis if in the bile duct) composed of cholesterol and bile salts.

Gamma knife: A device which uses multiple converging beams of γ-radiation from cobalt-60 to highly focus radiation on small tumors within the brain.

Gastric bypass: A surgical procedure for weight loss that elicits its effectiveness through malabsorption and volume limitation. The procedure involves full partitioning of the proximal gastric segment into a jejunal loop.

Gastritis: Acute or chronic inflammation of the lining of the stomach.

Gastroenteritis: Inflammation of the gastrointestinal tract causing nausea, vomiting, diarrhea, and fever; sometimes referred to as the stomach flu although not related to influenza.

Gastroesophageal reflux disease: Troublesome symptoms and/or complications caused by refluxing the stomach contents into the esophagus. These troublesome symptoms adversely affect the well-being of the patient.

Gastroparesis: A form of autonomic neuropathy involving nerves of the stomach. It may include nausea, vomiting, feeling full, bloating, and lack of appetite. It may cause wide fluctuations in blood sugars due to insulin action and nutrient delivery not occurring at the same time.

Gastroplasty: A surgical procedure for weight loss that elicits its effectiveness through gastric volume limitation. The procedure involves partial partitioning at the proximal gastric segment with the placement of a gastric outlet stoma of fixed diameter.

Gastroschisis: Inherited congenital abdominal wall defect in which the intestines and sometimes other organs develop outside the fetal abdomen through an opening in the abdominal wall.

Gastrostomy: Operative placement of a new opening into the stomach, usually associated with feeding tube placement.

Geniculate nucleus: The portion of the brain that processes visual information from the optic nerve and relays it to the cerebral cortex.

Genotype: The genetic constitution of an individual.

Geriatric syndrome: Age-specific presentations or differential diagnoses, including visual and hearing impairment, malnutrition and weight loss, urinary incontinence, gait impairment and falls, osteoporosis, dementia, delirium, sleep problems, and pressure ulcers. Commonly seen conditions in elder patients.

Gestational diabetes: Diabetes that occurs during pregnancy which may or may not end at delivery.

Gigantism: A condition of abnormal size or overgrowth of the entire body or any of its parts. Characteristic of growth hormone excess that manifests prior to closure of epiphyseal plates.

Glasgow Coma Scale (GCS): A scale for evaluating level of consciousness after central nervous system injury (evaluates eye opening and verbal and motor responsiveness).

Glomerular filtration rate (GFR): The volume of plasma that is filtered by the glomerulus per unit time, usually expressed as mL/min or mL/min/1.73 m², which adjusts the value for body surface area. This is the primary index used to describe overall renal function.

Glomerulonephritis: Glomerular lesions that are characterized by inflammation of the capillary loops of the glomerulus. These lesions are generally caused by immunologic, vascular, or other idiopathic diseases.

Glucagon: Hormone involved in carbohydrate metabolism that is produced by the pancreas and released when glucose levels in the blood are low. When blood glucose levels decrease, the liver converts stored glycogen into glucose, which is released into the bloodstream. The action of glucagon is opposite to that of insulin.

Gluconeogenesis: Formation of glucose from precursors other than carbohydrates especially by the liver and kidney using amino acids from proteins, glycerol from fats, or lactate produced by muscle during anaerobic glycolysis.

Glucuronidation: A metabolic pathway in the body that combines a drug (or other compound) that possesses a phenol, alcohol, or carboxyl group with glucuronic acid.

Glutamate: An excitatory amino acid found in the central nervous system.

Glycogenolysis: The process by which glycogen is broken down into glucose in body tissues.

Goiter: An enlargement of the thyroid gland, causing a swelling in the front part of the neck.

Gonioscopy: Examination of the anterior chamber angle. A gonioprism or Goldman lens is used to perform gonioscopic evaluation.

Gout: A group of disorders of purine metabolism, manifested by various combinations of (1) hyperuricemia; (2) recurrent acute inflammatory arthritis induced by crystals of monosodium urate monohydrate; (3) tophaceous deposits of these crystals in and around the joints of the extremities, which may lead to crippling destruction of joints; and (4) uric acid urolithiasis.

Graft-versus-host disease: The phenomenon by which transplanted donor T cells recognize normal host tissues as foreign and attack these tissues, resulting in increased morbidity and mortality in allogeneic transplant patients.

Graft-versus-tumor effect: The phenomenon by which transplanted donor cells recognize host malignant cells as foreign and eradicate the malignant cells through immunologic mechanisms.

Grandiosity: Exaggerated sense of self-importance, ideas, plans, or abilities.

Granulomas: Masses of chronically inflamed tissues with granulations.

Gummatous: A tumor of rubbery consistency that is characteristic of the tertiary stage of syphilis.

Gut-associated lymphoid tissue: Lymphoid tissue, including Peyer's patches, found in the gut that are important for providing localized immunity to pathogens.

Hallucinosis: Auditory hallucinations that occur during a clear sensorium.

Haptenation: The process where a drug, usually of low molecular weight, is bound to a carrier protein or cell and becomes immunogenic.

Health literacy: Degree to which individuals have the capacity to obtain, process, and understand basic health information and services needed to make appropriate health decisions.

Heberden's nodes: Hard, bony enlargement of the distal interphalangeal (terminal) joint of a finger or toe.

Hemarthrosis: Blood in the joint space.

Hematemesis: The vomiting of blood.

Hematochezia: Passage of stool that is bright red or maroon, usually because of bleeding from the lower gastrointestinal tract.

Hematogenous: Spread through the blood.

Hematuria: Presence of blood or red blood cells in urine.

Hemiballismus: A rare movement disorder that can be life threatening. Patients with hemiballismus have a dismal prognosis, with physical exhaustion, injuries, and medical complications often leading to death.

Hemiparesis: Weakness or slight paralysis involving one side of the body.

Hemisensory deficit: Loss of sensation on one side of the body.

Hemithorax: A single side of the trunk between the neck and the abdomen in which the heart and lungs are situated.

Hemolytic uremic syndrome: A disease characterized by microangiopathic hemolytic anemia, acute renal failure, and a low platelet count (thrombocytopenia).

Hemoptysis: The expectoration of blood or blood-tinged sputum from the larynx, trachea, bronchi, or lungs.

Hemorrhagic conversion: Conversion of an ischemic stroke into a hemorrhagic stroke.

Hemostasis: Cessation of bleeding through natural (clot formation or construction of blood vessels), artificial (compression or ligation), or surgical means.

Heparin-induced thrombocytopenia: A clinical syndrome of IgG antibody production against the heparin-platelet factor 4 complex occurring in approximately 1% to 5% of patients exposed to either heparin or low-molecular-weight heparin. Heparin-induced thrombocytopenia results in excess production of thrombin, platelet aggregation, and thrombocytopenia (due to platelet clumping), often leading to venous and arterial thrombosis, amputation of extremities, and death.

Hepatic encephalopathy: Confusion and disorientation that a patient with advanced liver disease experiences due to accumulation of ammonia levels.

Hepatic steatosis: Accumulation of fat in the liver.

Hepatocellular carcinoma (HCC): Cancer of the liver.

Hepatojugular reflex: Distention of the jugular vein induced by pressure over the liver; suggestive of insufficiency of the right heart.

Hepatosplenomegaly: An enlarged liver and spleen secondary to leukemic infiltration.

Hepatotoxicity: Toxicity to the liver causing damage to liver cells.

Herniation: Protrusion of the brain through the cranial wall.

Hesitancy: Difficulty with initiating micturition.

Heterotopic: Placing a transplanted organ into an abnormal anatomic location.

Heterozygous: Having different alleles at a gene locus.

Hirsutism: Excess body hair, especially appearing on the lower abdomen, around the nipples, around the chin and upper lip, between the breasts, and on the lower back.

Histocompatibility: The examination of human leukocyte antigen (HLA) differences between a donor and a recipient in order to determine if the recipient is more likely to accept, rather than reject, a graft from that particular donor.

HIV genotype: A type of resistance testing for HIV in which a patient's blood sample is obtained, the HIV RNA is sequenced, and mutations that may confer resistance to antiretrovirals are reported.

HIV phenotype: A type of resistance testing for HIV in which a patient's blood sample is obtained and the patient's HIV genes that encode for reverse transcriptase and protease are removed and placed in an HIV viral vector. This viral vector is replicated in a cell culture system with varying concentrations of antiretrovirals. A drug concentration-viral inhibition curve is developed and the concentration needed to inhibit 50% of the patient's virus is reported. This is used to predict resistance versus susceptibility.

HIV virtual phenotype: A database of matching HIV genotypes and phenotypes is developed. When an HIV genotype for a patient is obtained, the database is used to predict the patient's phenotype based on their actual genotype using matches that occur in the database.

Homeostenosis: Impaired capability to withstand stressors and decreased ability to maintain physiological and psychosocial homeostasis; a state commonly found in the elderly.

Homonymous: Pertaining to the same side.

Homozygous: Having identical alleles at a gene locus.

Hospice: The provision of palliative care during the last 6 months of life as defined by federal guidelines.

Hot flashes: A feeling of warmth that is commonly accompanied by skin flushing and mild to severe perspiration.

Human leukocyte antigens (HLA): Groups of genes found on the major histocompatibility complex, which contain cell-surface antigen presenting proteins. The body uses HLA to distinguish between self cells and nonself cells.

Humoral: Products secreted into the blood or body fluids.

Hydramnios: Increased amniotic fluid.

Hydronephrosis: Distention of the pelvis and kidney with urine resulting from obstruction of the ureter.

β-Hydroxybutyric acid: A ketone body that is elevated in ketosis, is synthesized in the liver from acetyl-CoA, and can be used as an energy source by the brain when blood glucose is low.

Hyperalgesia: An exaggerated intensity of pain sensation.

Hypercalcemia: Excessive amount of calcium in the blood.

Hypercalciuria: Excessive amount of calcium in the urine.

Hypercapnia: Abnormally high concentration of carbon dioxide in the blood.

Hypercoagulable state: A disorder or state of excessive or frequent thrombus formation; also known as thrombophilia.

Hyperemesis gravidarum: A rare disorder of severe and persistent nausea and vomiting during pregnancy that can result in dehydration, malnutrition, weight loss, and hospitalization.

Hyperglycemic hyperosmolar nonketotic syndrome: Severe increase in serum glucose concentration without the production of ketones, leading to an increase in serum osmolality and symptoms such as increased thirst, increased urination, weakness, fatigue, confusion, and in severe cases convulsions and/or coma.

Hyperopia: Farsightedness.

Hyperosmolar hyperglycemic state: Blood glucose levels greater than 600 mg/dL without significant ketones where extreme dehydration, insulin deficiency, hyperosmolarity, and electrolyte deficiency are common.

Hyperpathia: A painful syndrome, characterized by increased reaction to a stimulus, especially a repetitive stimulus, as well as an increased threshold.

Hyperpigmentation: A common darkening of the skin that occurs when an excess of melanin forms deposits in the skin.

Hyperplasia: An abnormal or unusual increase in the cells of a body part.

Hyperprolactinemia: A medical condition of elevated serum prolactin characterized by prolactin serum concentrations greater than 20 ng/mL (20 mcg/L) in men or 25 ng/mL (25 mcg/L) in women.

Hypersomnia: Sleeping for unusually prolonged periods of time.

Hyperthermia: An unusually high body temperature.

Hyperthyroidism: State caused by excess production of thyroid hormone.

Hypertrichosis: Excessive growth of hair.

Hypertrophy: An increase in the size of the cells in a tissue or organ.

Hyperuricemia: Elevated serum uric acid concentration, defined as a level greater than 7.0 mg/dL (416 μmol/L); it is a prerequisite for the development of gout and may lead to renal disease.

Hypervigilance: The state of being extremely alert and watchful, possibly to avoid danger or harm.

Hypochlorhydria: Hypoacidity. Decreased hydrochloric acid secretion by the stomach.

Hypocretin: A wake-promoting hypothalamic neuropeptide whose deficiency is involved in the pathophysiology of narcolepsy.

Hypogammaglobinemia: Reduced levels of antibodies.

Hypogonadism: A syndrome associated with testosterone deficiency resulting from either testicular or pituitary/hypothalamic diseases. Presenting symptoms differ according to the timing of disease onset in relation to puberty.

Hypomania: Abnormal mood elevation that does not meet criteria for mania.

Hypopituitarism: A clinical disorder characterized by complete or partial deficiency in pituitary hormone production.

Hypothalamic-pituitary-adrenal axis: A neuroendocrine feedback loop that controls response to stress.

Hypothermia: An unusually low body temperature.

Hypothyroidism: State caused by inadequate production of thyroid hormone.

Hypovolemic shock: Circulatory shock caused by severe loss of blood volume and/or body water.

Hypoxemia: Deficiency of oxygen in the blood.

Hypoxia: Deficiency of oxygen.

Hysterectomy: Excision of the uterus.

Immunocompromised: A condition in which the immune system is not functioning normally. This condition is seen in very young, very old, HIV infected individuals, or in transplant patients.

Immunogenicity: The property that gives a substance the ability to provoke an immune response.

Immunoglobulin G index: The ratio of immunoglobulin G to protein in the serum or cerebrospinal fluid.

Immunophenotype: The process of identification and quantitation of cellular antigens through fluorochrome-labeled monoclonal antibodies.

Immunotherapy: Treatment of a disease by stimulating the body's own immune system.

Impedance monitoring: A diagnostic technique used to evaluate esophageal bolus transit. When combined with pH monitoring, impedance monitoring helps identify both acidic and weakly acidic reflux episodes.

Implantable cardioverter-defibrillator: A device implanted into the heart transvenously with a generator implanted subcutaneously in the pectoral area that provides internal electrical cardioversion of ventricular tachycardia or defibrillation of ventricular fibrillation.

Incretin effect: A greater insulin stimulatory effect after an oral glucose load than that caused by an intravenous glucose infusion. The majority of the effect is thought to be due to glucose-dependent insulinotropic peptide (GIP) and glucagon like peptide-1 (GLP-1). Patients with type 2 diabetes have a significant reduction of the incretin effect, implying that these patients either have decreased concentration of the incretin hormones, or a resistance to their effects. GLP-1 concentrations are reduced in patients with type 2 diabetes in response to a meal, while GIP concentrations are either normal or increased, suggesting a resistance to the actions of GIP, thus making GLP-1 a more logical target for therapeutic intervention.

Index patient: The patient originally diagnosed with a disease.

Indirect immunofluorescence assay (IFA): HIV-infected T-lymphocytes are fixed onto a microscope slide, covered with the blood sample to be tested, incubated under heat, and washed. If antibodies to HIV are bound to the fixed viral antigens, they will remain on the slide. FITC-conjugated antihuman globulin is then added, incubated, and washed. If the sample contains antibodies to HIV, the cells will show a bright, fluorescent membrane under the microscope.

Induction: Treatment designed to be used as the first step in eliminating the leukemic burden.

Infarction: The formation of an infarct, an area of tissue death due to a local lack of oxygen.

Infective endocarditis (IE): Historically referred to as bacterial endocarditis, IE is an infection, either acute or subacute, that primarily affects the heart valves, but may extend into other surrounding areas of the heart.

Inotropic: Pertaining to the force of contraction of the heart muscle, or relating to or influencing the force of muscular contractions.

Insulin-like growth factor-I: An anabolic peptide that acts as a direct stimulator of cell proliferation and growth in all body cells.

Insulin resistance: A decreased response to insulin found before or early in the diagnosis of type 2 diabetes mellitus.

International normalized ratio (INR): The ratio of the patient's clotting time to the clinical laboratory's mean reference value; normalized by raising it to the international sensitivity index (ISI) power to account for differences in thromboplastin reagents. Thus, INR = (patient's prothrombin time/laboratory's mean normal prothrombin time)^{ISI}.

Intima: The inner layer of the wall of an artery or vein.

Intra-abdominal: Within the abdominal cavity.

Intra-articular: Administered to or occurring in the space within joints. Intraperitoneal: Within the peritoneal cavity.

Intrathecal: Within the meninges of the spinal cord.

Intravesicular: Administration directly into the bladder through the urethra.

Intussusception: Infolding, like the closing of a telescope, of a segment of the small intestine into the adjacent but more distal segment of the intestine, reducing blood supply to the affected part of the intestine and eventually causing intestinal obstruction.

Iontophoresis: Introduction of a medication into tissue through use of an electric current.

Ipsilateral: Pertaining to the same side of the body.

Ischemic heart disease (IHD): Imbalance between myocardial oxygen supply and oxygen demand.

Jejunal: A section of the small intestine connecting the duodenum to the ileum.

Jejunostomy: Operative placement of a new opening into the jejunum, usually associated with feeding tube placement.

Kegel exercises: Specific exercises that strengthen the pelvic floor muscles and help to prevent and treat stress incontinence.

Keratinization: The sloughing of epithelial cells in the hair follicle.

Keratinocyte: The epidermal cell that synthesizes keratin; making up 95% of all epidermal cells; commonly called "skin cells."

Keratitis: Infection of the cornea.

Keratoconjunctivitis sicca: Also known as Sjogren's syndrome or dry eye syndrome.

Keratotic: Pertaining to any horny growth such as a wart or callus.

Ketosis: An abnormal increase of ketone bodies present in conditions of reduced or disturbed carbohydrate metabolism.

Kindling: Repeated application of electrical stimulation to specific areas of the brain that leads to an alteration in the seizure threshold and the development of epilepsy. This process is used only in animal experimental models, but a similar phenomenon is thought to occur in humans.

Koebner's phenomenon: The occurrence of psoriatic lesions due to skin trauma.

Korotkoff sounds: The noise heard over an artery by auscultation when pressure over the artery is reduced below the systolic arterial pressure.

Korsakoff's syndrome: May occur as a sequel to chronic alcohol use. Characterized by psychosis, polyneuritis, disorientation, insomnia, delirium, hallucinations. Bilateral foot or wrist drop may also occur, possibly accompanied by pain.

Kyphosis: Abnormal curvature of the spine resulting in protrusion of the upper back; hunchback.

Lacrimation: Tearing and discharge of tears from the eyes.

β-Lactam allergy: Allergy to the (β-lactam family, namely penicillins and cephalosporins, but may also include carbapenems.

Lactose intolerance: An inability to digest milk and some dairy products, resulting in abnormal bloating, cramping, and diarrhea; caused by enzymatic lactase deficiency.

Lag-ophthalmos: Poor closure of the upper eyelid.

Lamina cribrosa: A series of perforated sheets of connective tissue that the optic nerve passes through as it exits the eye.

Laminectomy: Excision of the posterior arch of a vertebra to relieve pressure on the spinal cord.

Laparoscopic: Abdominal exploration or surgery employing a type of endoscope called laparoscope.

Laparotomy: Surgical opening of the abdominal cavity.

Latent autoimmune diabetes in adults (LADA): A slow, progressive form of type 1 diabetes mellitus in which a patient does not require insulin for a number of years. In its early stages, LADA typically presents as type 2 diabetes mellitus and is often misdiagnosed as such. However, LADA more closely resembles type 1 diabetes mellitus and shares common physiological characteristics of type 1 diabetes mellitus for metabolic dysfunction, genetics, and autoimmune features. LADA does not affect children and is classified distinctly as being separate from juvenile diabetes.

Lentigines: Plural of lentigo. A small, flat, tan to dark brown or black, macular melanosis on the skin, which looks like a freckle but is histologically distinct. Lentigines do not darken on exposure to sunlight, freckles do.

Leukemoid reaction: An elevated white blood cell count, or leukocytosis, that is a physiologic response to stress or infection (as opposed to a primary blood malignancy, such as leukemia).

Leukocytoclastic: The breaking up of white blood cells.

Leukopenia: A condition where the number of circulating white blood cells are abnormally low due to decreased production of new cells, possibly in conjunction with medication toxicities.

Leukostasis: An abnormal intravascular leukocyte aggregation and clumping seen in leukemia patients. The brain and the lungs are the two most frequent organs involved.

Lewy bodies: Abnormal masses inside some nerve cells. They occur in a variety of locations, and their structure and composition vary depending on location.

Lhermitte's sign: Tingling or shock-like sensation passing down the arms or trunk when the neck is flexed.

Libido: Conscious or unconscious sexual desire.

Ligament of Treitz: Landmark in the proximal portion of the jejunum beyond which it is preferred that postpyloric feedings be delivered for minimization of aspiration.

Linear accelerator: A device that uses microwave technology to accelerate electrons in a highly focused beam to deliver targeted radiation to tumor sites.

Lipase: Any one of a group of lipolytic enzymes that cleave a fatty acid residue from the glycerol residue in a neutral fat or a phospholipid.

Lipophilic: Having an affinity for fatty substances.

Lipoprotein lipase: Enzyme located in the capillary endothelium involved in the breakdown of intravenous lipid emulsion particles.

Liver biopsy: A procedure whereby tissue is removed from the liver and is used to determine the severity of liver damage.

Locus ceruleus: Nucleus of norepinephrine containing neurons located in the brainstem which is responsible for physiologic response to stress and panic.

Luteolysis: Death of the corpus luteum.

Lymphadenectomy: Surgical excision of lymph nodes.

Lymphadenitis: Inflammation of the lymph nodes, which become swollen, painful, and tender.

Lymphangitis: Inflammation of lymphatic channels.

Lymphatic: The network of vessels carrying tissue fluids.

Lymphoproliferative: Of or related to the growth of lymphoid tissue.

Maceration: The softening or breaking down of a solid by leaving it immersed in a liquid.

Macrophages: A large scavenger cell.

Macrovascular complications: Vascular complications that are contributed to by diabetes and include heart attacks, strokes, or peripheral vascular disease.

Macula: The central portion of the retina.

Maculopapular: A rash that contains both macules and papules. A macule is a flat discolored area of the skin, and a papule is a small raised bump. A maculopapular rash is usually a large area that is red and has small confluent bumps.

Magnetic resonance imaging: Method of body imaging that uses a magnetic field and radio waves to create cross-sectional images of one's body, which provides detailed pictures of organs and tissues.

Major malformation: A defect that has either cosmetic or functional significance.

Mastalgia: Tenderness of the breast.

Matrix metalloproteinases: Enzymes responsible for the degradation of connective tissue, normally located in the extracellular space of tissue, that break down proteins (e.g., collagen) and require zinc or calcium atoms as cofactors for enzymatic activity.

Meconium: The first intestinal discharge or "stool" of a newborn infant, usually green in color and consisting of epithelial cells, mucus, and bile.

Media: The middle layer of the wall of an artery or vein.

Mediastinum: The space in the thoracic cavity between the pleural sacs and behind the sternum.

Melanosis: Excessive pigmentation of the skin due to a disturbance in melanin pigmentation; called also melanism.

Melasma: Patchy skin pigmentation, often seen during pregnancy.

Melena: Tarry stools.

Menarche: The onset of cyclic menstrual periods in a woman.

Meningeal: Membranes that surround the brain and spinal cord.

Meninges: Covering of the brain consisting of three layers.

Menopause: Permanent cessation of menstruation.

Menorrhagia: Menstrual blood loss of greater than 80 mL per cycle; a more practical definition is heavy menstrual flow associated with problems of containment of flow, unpredictably heavy flow days, or other associated symptoms.

Mesocortical: A neural pathway that connects the ventral tegmentum to the cortex, particularly the frontal lobes. It is one of the major dopamine pathways in the brain.

Mesocorticolimbic pathway: A neural pathway that loops between the midbrain, the cortex, and limbic areas of the brain. An integral part of the brain reward system.

Mesothelioma: A benign or malignant tumor affecting the lining of the chest or abdomen. Commonly caused by exposure to asbestos fibers.

Metabolic acidosis: A condition in the blood and tissues that is a consequence of an accumulation of lactic acid resulting from tissue hypoxia and anaerobic metabolism.

Metabolic alkalosis: Alkalosis that is caused by an increase in the concentration of alkaline compounds (typically bicarbonate).

Metabolic syndrome: Constellation of cardiovascular risk factors related to hypertension, abdominal obesity, dyslipidemia, and insulin resistance diagnosed by the presence of at least three of the following criteria: increased waist circumference, elevated triglyceride concentrations, decreased high-density lipoprotein (HDL) cholesterol or active treatment to raise HDL cholesterol, elevated blood pressure or active treatment with antihypertensive therapy, or elevated fasting glucose or active treatment for diabetes.

Metastasis: Pleural is metastases. Cancer that has spread from the original site of the tumor.

Micelle: A microscopic particle of digested fat and cholesterol.

Microalbuminuria: Loss of small amounts of protein in the urine. An albumin excretion ratio of 30 to 300 mg/24 hour, which is a sign of chronic kidney disease. The normal mean value for urine albumin excretion in adults is 10 mg/day.

Microdialysis: A brain research technique whereby very small probes are inserted into the brain, and the concentration of brain chemicals, such as neurotransmitters, can be measured.

β_2 Microglobulin: A low-molecular-weight protein that may be elevated in multiple myeloma.

Micrognathia: Abnormal smallness of the jaws, especially of the mandible.

Microvascular complications: Vascular complications contributed to by diabetes that include retinopathy, neuropathy, and nephropathy.

Microvascular pulmonary emboli: An obstruction in the small blood vessels in the lung caused by material (e.g., blood clot, fat, air, and foreign body) that is carried through the circulation until it lodges in another small vessel.

Micturition: Voiding, urination.

Migraineur: A person who suffers from migraine headaches.

Migrographia: Small handwriting, often seen in patients with Parkinson's disease.

Minimal residual disease: A quantitative assessment of subclinical remnant of leukemic burden remaining at the end of the initial phase of treatment (induction) when a patient may appear to be in a complete morphologic remission.

Minimum inhibitory concentration: The lowest concentration of an antimicrobial agent that inhibits visible bacterial growth after approximately 24 hours.

Minor malformation: A defect that occurs infrequently (less than 4% of the population) but that has neither cosmetic nor functional significance to the child.

Miosis: Pupillary constriction, "pinpoint" pupils.

Mitogenicity: Producing or stimulating mitosis (a process that takes place in the nucleus of a dividing cell resulting in the formation of two new nuclei, each having the same number of chromosomes as the parent nucleus).

Mixed disorder: The presence of two or more distinct disorders. See also Complicated disorder.

Mixed mood episodes: Symptoms of mania and depression occurring simultaneously or in close juxtaposition.

Mobilization: The release of stem cells into the peripheral blood from the bone marrow compartment for the purpose of collecting these stem cells in anticipation of stem cell transplantation.

Mobitz type I: A type of second-degree AV nodal blockade.

Mobitz type II: A type of second-degree AV nodal blockade.

Moebius (also Möbius) syndrome: An extremely rare congenital neurologic disorder which is characterized by facial paralysis and the inability to move the eyes from side to side.

Monocytes: A variety of white blood cells.

Monoparesis: Slight or incomplete paralysis affecting a single extremity or part of one.

Monosodium urate: A crystallized form of uric acid that can deposit in joints leading to an inflammatory reaction and the symptoms of gout.

Mood lability: Unstable or changeable moods.

Morphology: The science of structure and form of cells without regard to function.

Motor tics: Involuntary brief spasmodic muscular movement or contraction, usually of the face or extremities.

Mu receptors: One of the three major classes of endogenous opioid receptors in the body. Mu receptors appear to be responsible for the majority of both the analgesic and rewarding properties of opioids.

Mucositis: Inflammation of mucous membranes, typically within the oral and esophageal mucosa. Usually associated with certain chemotherapy agents and radiation therapy involving mucosal areas.

Mucous colitis: A condition of the mucous membrane of the colon characterized by pain, constipation or diarrhea (sometimes alternating), and passage of mucus or mucous shreds.

Multiparity: Condition of having given birth to multiple children.

Mydriasis: Pronounced or abnormal dilation of the pupils.

Myelin: A protein and phospholipid sheath that surrounds the axons of certain neurons. Myelinated nerves conduct impulses more rapidly than nonmyelinated nerves.

Myeloablative preparative regimen: Radiation and/or chemotherapy that destroys bone marrow activity in preparation for a stem cell transplant. Patients will not likely recover bone marrow function without an infusion of "rescue" autologous or allogeneic stem cells.

Myelodysplastic syndrome: A disease in which bone marrow does not function properly.

Myeloproliferative disorder: A group of diseases of bone marrow in which excess cells, usually lymphocytes, are produced.

Myelosuppression: Reduction in white blood cells, red blood cells, and platelets.

Myocarditis: Inflammation of the muscular wall of the heart.

Myoclonus: A sudden, involuntary jerking of a muscle or group of muscles.

Myoglobinuria: The presence of myoglobin in urine.

Myonecrosis: Necrotic damage to muscle tissue.

Myopathy: Any disease of the muscle causing weakness, pain, and tenderness.

Myringotomy: A surgical incision in the tympanic membrane to relieve pressure and drain fluid from the middle ear.

Myxedema: Relatively hard edema associated with hypothyroidism.

Nasal scotoma: An area of blindness in the nasal portion of peripheral vision.

Nascent: Immature.

Nasolacrimal occlusion: The closing of the tear duct to decrease systemic absorption of a drug.

Nausea: The subjective feeling of a need to vomit.

Necrotizing enterocolitis: Medical condition primarily seen in premature infants, where portions of the bowel undergo necrosis.

Nelson's syndrome: A condition characterized by the aggressive growth of a pituitary tumor and hyperpigmentation of the skin.

Neoadjuvant therapy: Chemotherapy or radiation therapy given prior to primary surgical treatment. In cancer, it is often used to downstage the tumor to a resectable stage.

Neovascular maculopathy: Proliferation of blood vessels in the macula.

Neovascularization: New blood vessel formation (vascularization) especially in abnormal quantity (some conditions of the retina) or in abnormal tissue (tumor).

Nephrolithiasis: A condition marked by the presence of renal calculi (stones) in the kidney or urinary system.

Nephron: The working unit of the kidney that filters blood to remove fluid, toxins, and drugs. Each kidney contains approximately 1 million nephrons.

Nephrostomy: Insertion of a catheter through the skin into the renal pelvis to bypass ureteral obstruction and facilitate urine drainage.

Neuralgia: Pain which extends along the course of one or more nerves.

Neuritic (senile) plaque: An abnormal cluster of dead and dying nerve cells, other brain cells, and protein. One of the structural abnormalities found in the brains of patients with Alzheimer's disease.

Neuritis: Inflammation of a nerve.

Neurofibrillary tangle: An accumulation of twisted protein fragments inside nerve cells; one of the structural abnormalities found in the brains of patients with Alzheimer's disease.

Neuroimaging: Radiologic studies of the brain, usually referring to computerized tomography (CT) or magnetic resonance imaging (MRI).

Neurologic focality: Symptomatic sensory or motor deficits that point to specific lesions or dysfunction in the brain.

Neuropathic pain: Pain resulting from a lesion or dysfunction of the nervous system.

Neuropathy: An abnormal and usually degenerative state of the nervous system or nerves.

Neurotransmitters: Chemicals in the brain that allow the passage of a message between neurons or nerve cells.

Neutralizing antibodies: Antibodies that develop in response to a therapeutic agent that decrease the efficacy of the agent.

Nf-κB: Nuclear factor kappa B regulates cytokine production.

Nidus: A central point or focus consisting of a fibrin matrix (in the case of infective endocarditis), where bacteria are able to accumulate and multiply, allowing for formation of an infected vegetation.

Nitric oxide: An endogenous vasodilator.

Nociception: The perception of pain.

Nociceptors: Receptors for pain caused by injury from physical stimuli (mechanical, electrical, or thermal) or chemical stimuli (toxins); located in the skin, muscles, or in the walls of the viscera.

Nocturia: Micturition at night. Usually characterized by excessive urination at night.

Nocturnal polysomnography: Visual and electrophysiologic assessment of human sleep minimally composed of electroencephalogram, electrooculogram, and electromyogram that allows determination of sleep stage, breathing events, and muscle movements.

Nodules: When seen in rheumatoid arthritis, nodules are subcutaneous knobs over bony prominences or extensor surfaces.

Nonbacterial thrombotic endocarditis (NBTE): Endocarditis caused by noninfectious vegetations.

Nonmyeloablative preparative regimen: Radiation and/or chemotherapy that does not completely eradicate host bone marrow activity. Host bone marrow activity is suppressed but may recover after approximately 4 weeks even in the absence of "rescue" allogeneic stem cells.

Nonnucleoside reverse transcriptase inhibitor (NNRTI): A noncompetitive inhibitor of the viral reverse transcriptase enzyme by binding to the active site of the enzyme itself, rather than by terminating the enzymatic product. NNRTIs are only active against HIV-1.

Nonpolyposis: Absence of polyps.

Nonprotein kilocalorie-to-nitrogen ratio: Numerical value derived from dividing kilocalories from carbohydrate plus fat by the number of grams of nitrogen in the diet.

Non-REM sleep: A state of usually dreamless sleep that occurs regularly during a normal period of sleep with intervening periods of REM sleep and that consists of four distinct substages and low levels of autonomic physiological activity.

Non-ST-segment elevation: A type of myocardial infarction that is limited to the subendocardial myocardium and is smaller and less extensive than an ST-segment MI. Usually there is no pathologic Q wave on the ECG.

Normal flora: Normal colonizing bacteria of a human host.

Normochromic: Being normal in color; especially referring to red blood cells.

Normocytic: Normal size especially referring to red blood cells.

Nosocomial: An infection acquired within the health care system, e.g., hospital. Generally, symptoms of infection must occur after at least 48 hours of care to be considered nosocomial.

Nuchal rigidity: Neck stiffness.

Nuclear medicine scan: Method of body imaging that uses a radioactive tracer material (e.g., technetium and gallium) to produce body images. For example, bone scans detect uptake and cellular activity in areas of inflammation.

Nucleoside reverse transcriptase inhibitor (NRTI)/nucleotide reverse transcriptase inhibitor (NtRI): A modified version of a naturally occurring nucleoside or nucleotide that prevents HIV replication by interfering with the function of the viral reverse transcriptase enzyme. The nucleoside/nucleotide analog causes early termination of the proviral DNA chain. For activity, an NRTI requires three phosphorylation steps once inside the cell, whereas an NtRIs has a phosphate group attached and needs only two phosphorylation steps inside the cell for activity.

Nucleus accumbens: One of three nuclei that comprise the striatum (part of the basal ganglia). It receives dopaminergic input from the ventral tegmental area and is part of the limbic loop that plays a part in the motivational regulation of behavior and emotions.

Nulliparity: Not having given birth to a child.

Nystagmus: Rapid, involuntary movement of the eyes.

Obliterative bronchiolitis: Inflammation of the bronchioles (the small elements of the tracheobronchial tree) characterized by obliteration and/or permanent narrowing of the airways.

Off-label use: Use of a medication outside the scope of its approved, labeled use.

Offloading: Modalities, such as orthotics, that help off-weight/load an area of pressure, giving tissues time to heal without repetitive stress, which delays wound healing.

Oiling out: Continued coalescence of lipid emulsion particles, resulting in irreversible separation of the emulsion (or "breaking" of the emulsion).

Olfactory tubercle: Both the olfactory tubercle and the amygdala receive direct input from the olfactory bulb, and together they appear to help regulate the emotional, endocrine, and visceral consequences of odors.

Oligoanovulation: The condition of having few to no ovulatory menstrual cycles.

Oligoclonal bands: Small discrete bands in the γ-globulin region of fluid electrophoresis.

Oligohydramnios: Decreased amniotic fluid.

Oligomenorrhea: Abnormally light or infrequent menstruation.

Oliguria: Reduced urine output. Usually defined as less than 400 mL in 24 hours or less than 0.5 mL/kg/h.

Omentumectomy: Excision of the double fold of peritoneum attached to the stomach and connecting it with abdominal viscera (omentum).

Oncogene: Genes that cause transformation of normal cells into cancer cells by promoting uncontrolled cell growth and multiplication leading to tumor formation.

Oophorectomy: Surgery to remove the ovaries.

Open comedo: A plugged follicle of sebum, keratinocytes, and bacteria that protrudes from the surface of the skin and appears black or brown in color. Also referred to as a "blackhead."

Opsonization: The process by which an antigen is altered so as to become more readily and more efficiently engulfed by phagocytes.

Optic neuritis: Usually monocular central visual acuity loss and ocular/periorbital pain caused by demyelination of the optic nerve.

Orbital/supraorbital: Pertaining to the eye socket and the area directly above it.

Orchiectomy: The surgical removal of the testicles.

Organification: Binding of iodine to tyrosine residues of thyroglobulin.

Orthopnea: Difficulty in breathing that occurs when lying down and is relieved upon changing to an upright position.

Orthostasis: Characterized by a drop in blood pressure when standing up from sitting or lying down, often causing lightheadedness and dizziness.

Orthotopic transplant: Placing a transplanted organ into the normal anatomic location.

Osmolality: A measure of the number of osmotically active particles per unit solution, independent of the weight or nature of the particle.

Osmolar gap: The difference between the measured serum osmolality and the calculated serum osmolality.

Osmophobia: A fear of strong odors and unpleasant smells; also called olfactophobia.

Osteoblasts: Cells involved in bone formation; "builders of bone."

Osteoclasts: Cells involved in bone resorption; "creators of cavities."

Osteomalacia: Softening of the bones.

Osteonecrosis: Death of bone tissue.

Osteopenia: Low bone density, which can lead to osteoporosis.

Osteophytes: Bony outgrowths (bone spurs) into the joint space.

Osteoporosis: Disease of the bones characterized by a loss of bone tissue, resulting in brittle, weak bones that are susceptible to fracture (porous bones).

Ostomy: Surgical operation where part of the abdominal wall is opened and part of the intestine is connected to the opening for intestinal draining, e.g., colostomy, ileostomy.

Otitis media with effusion: Fluid in the middle ear space with no signs or symptoms of an acute infection.

Ovulation: Periodic ripening and rupture of mature follicle and the discharge of ovum from the cortex of the ovary.

Oxygen desaturation: A decrease in the oxygen saturation of the blood. Oxygen saturation is described as the oxygen content of blood divided by oxygen capacity and expressed in volume percent.

Pacemaker: A mass of fibers that possess actual or potential automaticity, which initiates and determines the rate of spontaneous depolarizations.

Palliative care: According to the World Health Organization, the active, total care of patients whose disease is not responsive to curative treatment.

Palmar-plantar erythrodysesthesia (PPE): Syndrome characterized by numbness, tingling or burning sensations with edema, and redness of the hands and feet often resulting in cracked skin and blisters with marked peeling of skin.

Pancolitis: Inflammation that involves the majority of the colon in patients with inflammatory bowel disease.

Pancreatitis: Inflammation of the pancreas.

Panhypopituitarism: A clinical disorder characterized by complete deficiency in pituitary hormone production.

Pannus: Inflamed synovial tissue that invades and destroys articular structures.

Papilledema: Edema of the optic disc typically associated with increased intracranial pressure. Also called a choked disc.

Paracentral scotoma: Blind spots near the center of the visual field.

Parasomnia: Undesirable physical or behavioral phenomena (e.g., sleep walking, bruxism, enuresis, sleep talking, and REM behavior disorder) that occur predominantly during sleep.

Parenchyma: Specific cells or tissues of an organ.

Parenteral nutrition: Delivery of nutrients via the intravenous route.

Paresthesia: An abnormal touch sensation, such as burning or prickling, often in the absence of external stimulus.

Parieto-occipital: Located at the top and back of the head.

Paroxysmal: Intermittent occurrence, initiating suddenly and spontaneously, lasting minutes to hours, and terminating suddenly and spontaneously.

Pars reticulate: Dopaminergic cell bodies located in the substantia nigra that project to the thalamus and cortex. Considered one of the basal ganglia pathways; involved not only with movement but also with emotions, motivations, and cognition that drive movement.

Peak expiratory flow: The maximum flow rate of air leaving the lungs upon forced exhalation.

Pelvic inflammatory disease: Inflammation of the endometrium, uterine tubes, and pelvic peritoneum; often due to a sexually transmitted infection.

Percutaneous coronary intervention (PCI): A minimally invasive procedure whereby access to the coronary arteries is obtained through the femoral artery up the aorta to the coronary os. Contrast media is used to visualize the coronary artery stenosis using a coronary angiogram. A guidewire is used to cross the stenosis and a small balloon is inflated and/or stent is deployed to break up atherosclerotic plaque and restore coronary artery blood flow. The stent is left in place to prevent acute closure and restenosis of the coronary artery. Newer stents are coated with antiproliferative drugs, such as paclitaxel and sirolimus, which further reduce the risk of restenosis of the coronary artery.

Percutaneous endoscopic gastrostomy: Gastric feeding tube placed via endoscopic technique.

Percutaneous endoscopic jejunostomy: Jejunal feeding tube placed via endoscopic technique.

Perihilar: The area surrounding the depression in the medial surface of a lung that forms the opening through which the bronchus, blood vessels, and nerves pass.

Perimenopause: Also known as the climacteric, is the period of time prior to menopause when hormonal and biological changes and physical symptoms begin to occur and usually lasts for 1 year after the last menstrual period. The perimenopausal period may last for an average of 3 to 5 years.

Perimetry: Measurement of the field of vision.

Peripheral artery disease: Atherosclerosis of the peripheral arteries.

Peripheral resistance: The sum of resistance to blood flow offered by systemic blood vessels.

Peritonitis: An acute inflammatory reaction of the peritoneal lining to microorganisms or chemical irritation.

PET scan: A scan that produces images of the body after the injection of a radiolabeled form of glucose. A PET scan is often used to detect cancer or follow response to treatment since tumors use more sugar than normal cells.

Petechiae: Tiny localized hemorrhages from the small blood vessels just beneath the surface of the skin

Phagocytic cell: A cell that absorbs waste material, harmful microorganisms, or other foreign bodies in the bloodstream and tissues.

Phagocytosis: The process of engulfing and ingesting an antigen by phagocytes.

Pharmacodynamics: Describing the actions of a drug on the body or a part of the body, e.g., a receptor or organ.

Pharmacogenomic: The influence of genetic variation on drug response in patients, used to correlate gene expression with a drug's efficacy or toxicity.

Pharmacokinetics: Refers to a mathematical method of describing a patient's drug exposure *in vivo* in terms of absorption, distribution, metabolism, and elimination.

Pharyngitis: Inflammation and/or infection of the pharynx that causes throat pain.

Phenotype: The visible properties of an organism that are produced by the interaction of the genotype and the environment.

Pheochromocytoma: A tumor arising from chromaffin cells, most commonly found in the adrenal medulla. The tumor causes the adrenal medulla to hypersecrete epinephrine and norepinephrine resulting in hypertension and other signs and symptoms of excessive sympathetic nervous system activity. The tumor is usually benign but may occasionally be cancerous.

Phlebitis: Inflammation of a blood vessel, e.g., vein.

Phonophobia: A fear of sounds, loud noises, and even one's own voice.

Photochemotherapy: The use of phototherapy together with topical or systemic drugs in the treatment of psoriasis.

Photodynamic therapy: Cancer treatment that uses interaction between laser light and a substance that makes the cells more sensitive to light. When light is applied to cells that have been treated with this substance, a chemical reaction occurs and destroys cancer cells.

Photophobia: An abnormal sensitivity to or intolerance of light.

Phototherapy: The use of ultraviolet light applied to the skin, e.g., in treating psoriasis or neonatal hyperbilirubinemia.

Physical dependence: A state of adaptation that is manifested by a drug-class specific withdrawal syndrome that can be produced by abrupt cessation, rapid dose reduction, decreasing blood level of the drug, and/or administration of an antagonist.

Piloerection: Erection of hairs, due to stimulation or contraction of the arrector pili muscles, also described as "gooseflesh."

Pilosebaceous unit: A hair follicle and the surrounding sebaceous glands.

Plasma cell: Antibody producing cells.

Plasmapheresis: The process of separating blood cells from plasma. This process is used to remove the monoclonal antibodies from the blood.

Pleocytosis: A transient increase in the number of leukocytes in a body fluid.

Pleuritis: Inflammation of the lining around the lungs.

Pneumatic otoscopy: A diagnostic technique involving visualization of the tympanic membrane for transparency, position, and color, and its response to positive and negative air pressure to assess mobility.

Pneumothorax: The presence of air in the pleural cavity, often causing part of the lung to collapse.

Polycythemia: An abnormal increase in the number of erythrocytes in the blood.

Polydipsia: Excessive thirst.

Polymorphic metabolism: Genetically determined rates of metabolism (fast versus slow) by selected isozymes of cytochrome P450 drug-metabolizing enzymes.

Polymorphisms: Interindividual variations in the genetic code at the level of one nucleotide.

Polymorphonuclear leukocyte: A subgroup of white blood cells, filled with granules of toxic chemicals that enable them to digest microorganisms by phagocytosis.

Polyphagia: Eating excessively large amounts of food at a meal.

Polypharmacy: Taking multiple medications concurrently.

Polyp: A growth from a mucous membrane commonly found in organs such as the colon, rectum, and the nose. Usually not malignant, these can develop into cancer and require removal once found.

Polyuria: Excessive excretion of urine resulting in profuse micturition.

Portal hypertension: Increased blood pressure within the portal vein that supplies the liver.

Postpyloric feeding: Delivery of nutrients via a tube placed with its tip past the pyloric sphincter separating the stomach from the duodenum.

Prader-Willi syndrome: A genetic disorder characterized by short stature, mental retardation, low muscle tone, abnormally small hands and feet, hypogonadism, and excessive eating leading to extreme obesity.

Prediabetes: An asymptomatic but abnormal state that precedes the development of clinically evident diabetes.

Preload: The stretched condition of the heart muscle at the end of diastole just before contraction. Volume in the left ventricle at the end of diastole estimated by the pulmonary artery occlusion pressure (also known as the pulmonary artery wedge pressure or pulmonary capillary wedge pressure).

Preparative regimen (conditioning regimen): Radiation and/ or chemotherapy given to stem cell transplant patients in order to kill malignant cells, create space in the bone marrow compartment, and suppress the immune system of the host in order to prevent graft rejection.

Priapism: A prolonged, painful erection lasting more than 4 hours. Considered a medical emergency.

Primary amenorrhea: Absence of menses by age 16 in the presence of normal secondary sexual development or absence of menses by age 14 in the absence of normal secondary sexual development.

Primary prevention: The removal or reduction of risk factors before the development of disease.

Prinzmetal angina: Vasospasm or contraction of the coronary arteries in the absence of significant atherosclerosis. Also referred to as variant angina.

Probiotics: Dietary supplements containing potentially beneficial bacteria that promote health by stimulating optimal mucosal immune responses.

Proctitis: Inflammation confined to the rectum in patients with inflammatory bowel disease.

Prodrome: Early symptom(s) indicating the onset of an attack or a disease.

Progenitor: A primitive cell.

Prolapse: Protrusion of an organ or part of an organ through an opening, e.g., uterine prolapse occurs when the uterus is displaced downward such that the cervix is within the vaginal opening (first degree), the cervix is outside the opening (second degree), or the entire uterus is outside the opening (third degree).

Proptosis: Forward displacement of the eyeball.

Prostaglandin: Any of a large group of biologically active, carbon-20, unsaturated fatty acids that are produced by the metabolism of arachidonic acid through the cyclooxygenase pathway.

Prostate specific antigen: This secretion of prostatic epithelial cells is used as a tumor marker for prostate cancer. It is not specific for prostate cancer. Thus, serum prostate-specific antigen concentrations may be increased in the face of any inflammatory or infectious disorder of the prostate, benign prostatic hyperplasia, or because of instrumentation of the prostate.

Prostatectomy: Surgical removal of the prostate, which can be performed transurethrally, suprapubically, or retropubically. There are two main types: transurethral prostatectomy (TURP) and radical prostatectomy. TURP removes part of the tissue surrounding the urethra, which may be blocking the flow of urine. Radical prostatectomy removes all of the prostate and the seminal vesicles.

Prostatic hyperplasia: Enlargement of the prostate.

Prosthetic-valve endocarditis (PVE): Endocarditis that occurs in patients with bioprosthetic or synthetic implanted heart valves.

Protease: Any one of various enzymes, including proteinases and peptidases, that catalyze the hydrolytic breakdown of proteins.

Protease inhibitor (PI): A drug that acts by inhibiting the viral protease enzyme, which prevents long strands of protein from being cleaved into the smaller proteins the virus requires for assembly.

Protectant: An agent that forms an occlusive barrier between the skin and surrounding moisture.

Protected specimen brush: Used in bronchoscopy, a brush in the lumen of a tube inside the bronchoscope. The brush is extended into the lung to obtain a sample, then retracted back into the tube for removal from the lung.

Proteinase: Any of numerous enzymes that catalyze the breakdown of proteins. Also called protease.

Proteinuria: The presence of measurable amounts of protein (greater than 150 mg/day) in the urine, which is often indicative of glomerular or tubular damage in the kidney.

Proteoglycan: Any one of a class of glycoproteins of high molecular weight that are found in the extracellular matrix of connective tissue. They are made up mostly of carbohydrate consisting of various polysaccharide side chains linked to a protein and resemble polysaccharides rather than proteins with regard to their properties.

Proteolysis: The hydrolysis of proteins, usually by enzyme action, into simpler substances.

Proteosome: An enzyme complex that degrades intracellular proteins.

Prothrombin: A clotting factor that is converted to thrombin. Also known as Factor II.

Prothrombin time: A measure of coagulation representing the amount of time required to form a blood clot after the addition of thromboplastin to the blood sample. Also known as Quick test.

Prothrombotic state: A state of high coagulation of the blood.

Pruritis: Localized or generalized itching due to irritation of sensory nerve endings.

Pseudoaddiction: A term used to describe patient behaviors (e.g., "drug-seeking," "clock watching," or illicit drug use) that may occur when pain is undertreated. Pseudoaddiction can be distinguished from true addiction in that the behaviors resolve when pain is effectively treated.

Pseudohyphae: Elongated forms created by replicating yeast that form buds but do not detach from one another.

Pseudophakia: Refers to presence of a lens after cataract extraction.

Pseudopolyps: An area of hypertrophied gastrointestinal mucosa that resembles a polyp and contains nonmalignant cells.

Pseudoseizure: Convulsions or seizure-like activity that results from causes other than abnormal electrical activity in the brain.

Psychodynamic: The explanation or interpretation of behavior or mood in terms of mental or emotional forces or processes.

Psychomotor retardation: A slowness of thought and physical movement that is primarily due to the psychological state.

Psychosocial: The interface between psychological and social functioning.

Pulmonary artery catheter: An invasive device used to measure hemodynamic parameters directly, including cardiac output and pulmonary artery occlusion pressure. Calculated parameters include stroke volume and systemic vascular resistance.

Pulmonary artery occlusion pressure: A hemodynamic measurement obtained via a catheter placed into the pulmonary artery used to evaluate patient volume status within the circulation.

Pulmonary embolism: A disorder of thrombus formation causing obstruction of a pulmonary artery or one of its branches and resulting in pulmonary infarction.

Pulsus paradoxus: A large fall in systolic blood pressure and pulse volume during inspiration or an abnormal variation in pulse volume during respiration in which the pulse becomes weaker with inspiration and stronger with expiration.

Purkinje fibers: Specialized myocardial fibers that conduct impulses from the AV node to the ventricles.

Purpura: A small hemorrhage of the skin, mucous membrane, or serosal surface.

Purulent: Containing, consisting of, or being pus.

Pyelonephritis: Inflammation of a kidney.

Pyloroplasty: A surgical procedure for enlarging the opening of the stomach to the duodenum.

Pyuria: Presence of pus in urine when voided.

Quality indicators: A list of indicators used by long-term care facility administrators and government overseers to identify potential problems in patient care.

Quality of Life: According the National Center for Chronic Disease Prevention and Health Promotion, the perceived physical and mental health over time.

Radiofrequency catheter ablation: Procedure during which radiofrequency energy is delivered through a catheter positioned at the atrioventricular node for the purpose of destroying one pathway of a reentrant circuit.

Raphe nuclei: Bed of serotonin containing neurons that extend to the hypothalamus, septum, hippocampus, and cingulated gyrus.

Recombinant activated factor VII: A clotting factor manufactured via recombinant technology used off-label (non-FDA approved) to foster clotting in hemorrhagic shock patients with massive hemorrhage refractory to conventional therapies such as fresh frozen plasma.

Rectal prolapse: Sinking of the rectum through the anal sphincter so that it is visible externally.

Recurrence: A relapse that occurs after a clear-cut recovery.

5α-Reductase: Intracellular enzyme in some target cells which activates testosterone to dihydrotestosterone. In these androgen-dependent target cells, dihydrotestosterone is more potent than testosterone.

Reentry: Circular movement of electrical impulses, a mechanism of many arrhythmias.

Refractory periods: The period of time after an impulse is initiated and conducted during which cells cannot be depolarized again.

Regurgitation: A passive process without involvement of the abdominal wall and the diaphragm wherein gastric or esophageal contents move into the mouth.

Relapse: The return of symptoms, satisfying the full syndrome criteria, after a patient has responded, but prior to recovery.

REM sleep: A state of sleep that recurs cyclically several times during a normal period of sleep and that is characterized by increased neuronal activity of the forebrain and midbrain, by depressed muscle tone, and by dreaming, rapid eye movements, and vascular congestion of the sex organs.

Remission: Relief of symptoms and return to full functioning in all areas of life.

Renin-angiotensin-aldosterone system: The hormonal system controlled mainly by the kidneys and adrenal glands that regulates blood pressure, blood volume, and electrolyte balance.

Replication capacity: This term is often used interchangeably with the term "viral fitness" and refers to how quickly an HIV reproduces or replicates. The slower HIV replicates, the less likely a patient is to have disease progression. A replication capacity may be reported on a resistance test. It is reported as a percentage of the median replication rate for drug-sensitive (wild-type) HIV strains.

Resorption: The process of bone breakdown by osteoclasts.

Respiratory acidosis: Acidosis that is caused by an accumulation of carbon dioxide.

Respiratory alkalosis: Alkalosis that is caused by a loss of carbon dioxide.

Respiratory disturbance index: A summary measure that quantifies the number of apneas, hypopneas, and respiratory effort-related arousals per hour of sleep.

Response: Refers to a predefined reduction of symptoms from baseline that generally results in significant functional improvement.

Response inhibition: Ability to stay on task.

Restenosis: Renarrowing of the coronary artery after a percutaneous intervention to improve coronary blood flow.

Retching: A process that follows nausea and consists of diaphragm, abdominal wall, and chest wall contractions and spasmodic breathing against a closed glottis.

Reticulocytes: Immature blood cells that mature into erythrocytes.

Reticuloendothelial system: Phagocytic cells excluding granulocytes; widely distributed throughout the body.

Retinopathy: The leading cause of blindness in people aged 20 to 74; occurs when the microvasculature nerve layer that provides blood and nutrients to the retina are damaged.

Retrograde ejaculation: Disorder in which semen flows in a backward fashion up the urethra and into the bladder during climax. The patient will complain of dry sex or no ejaculation during sexual intercourse, which may be worrisome to the patient.

Retroperitoneal fibrosis: An accumulation of fibrotic tissues located behind the organs contained in the abdominal sac.

Reye's syndrome: A sudden, sometimes fatal, syndrome characterized by encephalopathy and liver degeneration, which occurs in children after viral infection and is also associated with aspirin use.

Rhabdomyolysis: A rapid lysis or destruction of skeletal muscles that can be associated with renal failure and death.

Rheumatic fever: An acute inflammatory disease involving the joints, heart, skin, brain, and other tissues caused by an immune response to streptococcal infection in genetically susceptible people, particularly in children.

Rheumatoid factors: Antibodies reactive with the Fc region of IgG.

Rhinorrhea: Nasal secretions; a runny nose.

Rhinosinusitis: Inflammation of the mucous membranes in the nose and sinuses.

Rhonchi: Abnormal, rumbling sounds heard on auscultation of an obstructed airway. They are more prominent during expiration and may clear somewhat on coughing.

Rouleaux formation: The stacking of red blood cells on a peripheral smear when diluted.

Rubefacient: A substance that produces redness of the skin.

Rule of six: A previously used weight-based guideline for calculating intravenous continuous infusions by multiplying body weight (kg) by six and adding this amount of drug to 100 mL of fluid, resulting in a concentration and infusion rate of 1 mcg/kg/min and 1 mL/h.

Salicylism: A toxic syndrome caused by excessive doses of acetylsalicylic acid (aspirin), salicylic acid, or any other salicylate product. Signs and symptoms may include severe headache, nausea, vomiting, tinnitus (ringing in the ears), confusion, increased pulse, and increased respiratory rate.

Scarlatiniform rash: Bright, scarlet-colored skin eruption that occurs in patches over the entire body with eventual peeling as a result of streptococcal infection.

Scleral icterus: Jaundice of the outer layer of the eyeball.

Scleritis: Inflammation of the outer layer of the eyeball.

Scoliosis: A congenital lateral curvature of the spine.

Scotoma: Referring to a partial loss of vision.

Secondary amenorrhea: Absence of menses for three cycles or 6 months in a previously menstruating woman.

Secondary hyperparathyroidism (sHPT): Increased secretion of parathyroid hormone from the parathyroid glands caused by hyperphosphatemia, hypocalcemia, and vitamin D deficiency that result from decreased kidney function. Secondary hyperparathyroidism can lead to bone disease (bone and mineral metabolism disorders).

Secondary prevention: Early detection of the premalignant condition or cancer, leading to earlier intervention.

Secondary transmission: Transferring a disease from the primary source to another person.

Seizure: A sudden attack due to involuntary electrical activity in the brain. It is caused by an uncontrolled burst of electrical activity in the brain that can result in a wide variety of clinical manifestation such as: muscle jerks or twitches, staring, tongue biting, loss of consciousness, and total body shaking.

Semiology: The clinical appearance or symptoms of a seizure.

Sentinel lymph node: The first lymph node to receive lymph draining from a tumor.

Sepsis: A syndrome characterized by a systemic inflammatory response (abnormal increases in body temperature, heart rate, respiratory rate, and/or white blood cell concentration) caused by infection.

Sera: Pertaining to human serum.

Serosa: An enclosing serous membrane of the pericardium, pleura, and peritoneum.

Serum ferritin: Quantifies the iron-binding capacity of transferring.

Serum sickness: A group of symptoms caused by a delayed immune response to certain medications. Arthralgias, fever, malaise, and urticaria may develop usually 7 to 14 days after exposure to the causative antigen.

Shear stress: Risk factor for pressure ulcers that is generated when the head of a patient's bed is elevated and can cause deeper blood vessels to crimp, leading to ischemia.

Sialorrhea: Drooling.

Sick sinus syndrome: Idiopathic sinus node dysfunction leading to symptomatic sinus bradycardia.

Sickle cell anemia: Genetic disorder in which the red blood cells become crescent shaped.

Sickle cell syndrome: Describes a group of autosomal recessive genetic disorders that are characterized by the presence of at least one sickle hemoglobin gene.

Sickle hemoglobin: A defective form of hemoglobin produced as a result of a single substitution of the amino acid valine for glutamic acid at position 6 of the β-polypeptide chain.

Sigmoidoscopy: A visual inspection of the sigmoid colon and rectum with a flexible tube called a sigmoidoscope.

Simple disorder: The presence of a single acid–base disorder, with or without compensation.

Sjogren's syndrome: An autoimmune disorder that causes inflammation of the salivary glands; decreasing the production of saliva, which is a buffer against esophageal erosions.

Sleep apnea: The temporary stopping of breathing during sleep; can be caused by narrowing of the airways resulting from swelling of soft tissue.

Sleep latency: The amount of time it takes to fall asleep.

Sliding scale insulin: An increase or decrease in the number of units of insulin administered to correct a blood glucose level at a particular point in time that does not prevent the problem from occurring and does not take into account differing total daily insulin requirements of patients.

Slit lamp biomicroscope: An instrument that allows for the microscopic examination of the cornea, anterior chamber lens, and posterior chamber.

Somatic hypermutation: The occurrence of multiple point mutations.

Somatotrope: Growth hormone producing cells in the anterior pituitary.

Somnolence: Prolonged drowsiness or sleepiness.

Source control: Removal of the primary cause of an infection such as contaminated prosthetic materials (e.g., catheters), necrotic tissue, or drainage of an abscess. Antimicrobials are unlikely to be effective if the process or source that led to the infection is not controlled.

Spastic colon: A synonym for irritable bowel syndrome.

Spasticity: A motor disorder characterized by an increase in muscle tone with exaggerated tendon jerks, resulting from hyperexcitability of the stretch reflex.

Spectrum of activity: A qualitative term that describes the number of different bacterial species that are susceptible to an antimicrobial regimen. Generally, broad-spectrum activity refers to regimens that possess activity against many bacterial species, whereas narrow-spectrum therapy refers to activity against a few bacterial species.

Sphincter of Oddi: Structure through which the common bile duct empties bile and pancreatic secretions into the duodenum.

Spirometry: Measurement by means of a spirometer of the air entering and leaving the lungs.

Splenomegaly: An enlarged spleen secondary to leukemic infiltration.

Spontaneous bacterial peritonitis: Bacterial infection of the peritoneal fluid without abdominal source.

Sprain: An overstretching of supporting ligaments that results in a partial or complete tear of the ligament.

Status epilepticus: Any seizure lasting more than 30 minutes, with or without a loss of consciousness; or having recurrent seizures without regaining consciousness between seizure episodes.

Steatohepatitis: A severe form of liver disease caused by fat deposition in the liver, characterized by hepatic inflammation that may rapidly progress to liver fibrosis and cirrhosis.

Steatorrhea: Excessive loss of fat in stool.

Steatosis: Excessive fat accumulation.

Stenosis: Blockage of an artery.

Stenting: Placement of a stent to allow blood flow through an artery.

Stereotactic radiosurgery: Radiation technique that uses a large number of narrow, precisely aimed, highly focused beams of ionizing radiation. The beams are aimed from many directions circling the head and meet at a specific point.

Stereotyped behavior: Behavior that is associated with repetitive postures or movements without meaning.

Stevens-Johnson syndrome: A severe expression of erythema multiforme (also known as erythema multiforme major). It typically involves the skin and the mucous membranes with the potential for severe morbidity and even death.

Stimulant: Any amphetamine or amphetamine-like substance (methylphenidate) that causes an increase in dopaminergic and norepinephrine activity in the brain resulting in lessening of hyperactivity, impulsiveness and/ or inattentiveness.

Stomatitis: Inflammation of mucous membranes in the mouth.

Strain: Damage to the muscle fibers or muscle sheath without tearing of the ligament.

Stretta procedure: Application of radiofrequency to increase lower esophageal sphincter tone.

Striae: Linear, atrophic, pinkish or purplish, scar-like lesions that later become white (striae albicantes, lineae albicantes), which may occur on the abdomen, breasts, buttocks, and thighs. They are due to weakening of the elastic tissues; commonly called stretch marks.

Stricture: Abnormal narrowing of a tubular structure in the body. An area of narrowing or constriction in the gastrointestinal tract due to buildup of fibrotic tissue, often a result of longstanding inflammation.

Stroke volume: The amount of blood ejected from the heart during systole.

ST-segment elevation: A type of myocardial infarction that typically results in an injury that transects the thickness of the myocardial wall. Following an ST-elevation MI, pathologic Q waves are frequently seen on the ECG, indicating transmural myocardial infarction.

Subchondral: Situated beneath and supporting cartilage.

Substantia nigra: The area in the brainstem with highly pigmented cells that make dopamine.

Surgical margins: An area of tissue surrounding a tumor when it is removed by surgery.

Surgical site infection: Infections occurring at or near the surgical incision within 30 days of the operation; up to 1 year if a prosthesis is implanted.

Suspending agent: An additive used in the compounding of oral liquid medications to suspend drug particles throughout a liquid and enables resuspension of particles by agitation (shaking well).

Synechia: Adhesions or the abnormal attachment of the iris to another structure. Peripheral anterior synechia refers to occurrence of synechia with the trabecular meshwork.

Synovitis: Inflammation of the synovial membrane, often in combination with pain and swelling of the affected joint.

Synovium: Membrane lining the internal surfaces of the joint.

Systolic dysfunction: An abnormal contraction of the ventricles during systole.

Tachycardia: Abnormally fast heart rate.

Tachyphylaxis: Rapid decreasing response to a drug or other physiologically active agent after a few doses.

Tachypnea: Abnormally fast respiratory rate.

Tangentiality: Abandoning one's ideational objective in pursuit of thoughts peripheral to the original goal. Used to describe a thought and speech pattern wherein the individual never gets to the point or answers the question.

Tardive dyskinesia: A chronic disorder of the nervous system characterized by involuntary jerky or writhing movements of the face, tongue, jaws, trunk, and limbs, usually developing as a late side effect of prolonged treatment with antipsychotic drugs.

Telangiectasia: Permanent dilation of preexisting small blood vessels (capillaries, arterioles, and venules), usually in the skin or mucous membranes which presents as a coarse or fine red line.

Tendonitis: Inflammation of the tendon.

Tenesmus: Refers to straining, especially painful, or ineffectual straining with a bowel movement or straining on defecation owing to spasms of an inflamed rectal sphincter as occurs in shigellosis.

Tenosynovitis: Inflammation of the tendon sheath.

Teratogen: An exogenous agent or substance that can modify normal embryonic or fetal development. The manifestation of teratogenicity can include structural anomalies, functional deficit, cancer, growth retardation, and death (spontaneous abortion, stillbirth).

Teratogenic potential: The ability of an agent to cause harm or malformations to a fetus or embryo. Medications are assigned pregnancy categories based on their teratogenic potential.

Teratogenicity: The property of causing malformations in the developing fetus.

Terminal secretions: The noise produced by the oscillatory movements of secretions in the upper airways in association with the inspiratory and expiratory phases of respiration. Also known as "death rattle."

Tetany: Hyperexcitability of nerves and muscles characterized by muscular twitching and cramps, laryngospasm with inspiratory stridor, and hyperreflexia.

Third spacing: Fluid accumulation in the interstitial space disproportionate to the intracellular and extracellular fluid spaces.

Thoracentesis: Removal of fluid that is present in the pleural space. Common procedure to determine cause of the fluid accumulation.

Thrombin: The enzyme formed from prothrombin, which converts fibrinogen to fibrin. It is the principal driving force in the clotting cascade.

Thrombocytopenia: Decrease in platelet concentration in the blood.

Thrombocytosis: Increased number of platelets in the blood.

Thrombogenesis: The process of forming a blood clot.

Thrombolysis: The process of enzymatically dissolving or breaking apart a blood clot.

Thrombolytic: An enzyme that dissolves or breaks apart blood clots.

Thrombophlebitis: Inflammation of a blood vessel (e.g., a vein) associated with the stimulations of clotting and formation of a thrombus (or blood clot).

Thromboplastin: A substance that triggers the coagulation cascade. Tissue factor is a naturally occurring thromboplastin and is used in the prothrombin time test.

Thrombosis: The process of forming a thrombus.

Thrombotic thrombocytopenic purpura: Condition characterized by formation of small clots within the circulation resulting in the consumption of platelets and a low platelet count.

Thrombus: Blood clot attached to the vessel wall and consisting of platelets, fibrin and clotting factors. A thrombus may partially or completely occlude the lumen of a blood vessel compromising blood flow and oxygen delivery to distal tissue.

Thymoma: A tumor derived from the epithelial or lymphoid elements of the thymus.

Thyroglobulin: A thyroid hormone-containing protein, usually stored in the colloid within the thyroid follicles.

Thyroid peroxidase: Enzyme that catalyzes the organification and coupling steps of thyroid hormone synthesis.

Thyroiditis: Inflammation of the thyroid gland.

Thyrotoxicosis: State caused by excess amount of thyroid hormone.

Tocolytic: Medication used to suppress premature labor.

Tolerance: A state of adaptation in which exposure to a drug induces changes that result in a diminution of one or more of the drug's effects over time.

Tonometry: A method by which the cornea is indented or flattened by an instrument. The pressure required to achieve corneal indentation or flattening is a measure of intraocular pressure.

Tophi: Chalky deposits of sodium urate occurring in gout; tophi form most often around joints in cartilage, bone, bursae, and subcutaneous tissue and in the external ear, producing a chronic, foreign-body inflammatory response. If untreated, tophi can lead to joint deformity or destruction.

Topoisomerase: Enzyme that temporarily alters supercoiled DNA by cutting the DNA causing the DNA to relax the supercoil during DNA replication. Topoisomerase inhibitors prevent the DNA from sealing the cut which causes DNA strand breakage.

Torsade de pointes: Very rapid ventricular tachycardia characterized by a gradually changing QRS complex in the ECG; may change into ventricular fibrillation.

Toxic epidermal necrolysis: A life-threatening skin disorder characterized by blistering and peeling of the top layer of skin.

Toxoid: A modified bacterial exotoxin that has lost toxicity.

Tracheal aspirate: Suctioning of secretions from the trachea.

Transaminases: Hepatocellular enzymes that are released into the bloodstream after hepatic damage.

Transesophageal echocardiogram: Procedure used to generate an image of the heart via sound waves, via a probe introduced into the esophagus (rather than the traditional transthoracic view) in order to obtain a better image of the left atrium.

Transferrin saturation: Indicates the amount of transferrin that is bound with iron.

Transient ischemic attack: Focal neurologic deficit lasting less than 24 hours in which symptoms resolve completely.

Translocation: Movement of bacteria and endotoxin from the intestinal lumen through the gut mucosa and into the lymphatic and systemic circulation.

Transmural: Across the wall of an organ or structure. In Crohn's disease, inflammation may extend through all four layers of the intestinal wall.

Transsphenoidal pituitary microsurgery: Surgery through the nasal cavity to access the pituitary gland through the sphenoid bone.

Transvenous pacing: Insertion of a pacemaker into the heart via venous access for the purpose of pacing.

Traveler's diarrhea: An acute infectious diarrhea that afflicts travelers during or immediately upon return from visits to other countries. The presence of at least three loose stools within 24 hours that are associated with nausea, vomiting, abdominal pain, fecal urgency, or dysentery.

Tremulousness: Exhibiting trembling or shaking.

Trigeminal neuralgia: A disorder of the fifth cranial (trigeminal) nerve characterized by excruciating paroxysms of pain in the face.

Trigeminovascular: The complex of vascular supply to and from the trigeminal nerve. The trigeminal nerve is the fifth cranial nerve responsible for pain perception in the head and face.

Trophic: Stimulatory effect.

Troponins T or I: Proteins found predominately in cardiac and not skeletal muscle which regulates calcium-mediated interaction of actin and myosin. Troponin I and T are released into the blood from the myocytes at the time of myocardial cell necrosis secondary to infarction. These biochemical markers become elevated and are used in the diagnosis of myocardial infarction. Troponin I and T are more sensitive and specific for infarction than creatine kinase, which is found in both skeletal and myocardial cells. The exact value of troponin I or T, which is diagnostic of infarction, differs based upon assay.

Tubal ligation: Surgical process of tying up the fallopian tubes to prevent passage of ova from the ovaries to the uterus.

Tuberoeruptive xanthomas: Small yellow–red raised papules usually presenting on the elbows, knees, back, and buttocks.

Tubulointerstitial: Involving the tubules or interstitial tissue of the kidneys.

Tumor lysis syndrome: A syndrome resulting from cytotoxic therapy, occurring generally in aggressive, rapidly proliferating lymphoproliferative disorders. It is characterized by combinations of hyperuricemia, lactic acidosis, hyperkalemia, hyperphosphatemia, and hypocalcemia.

Tumor suppressor gene: A gene that suppresses growth of cancer cells.

T2-weighted magnetic resonance imaging: A setting of the magnetic resonance imaging machine that shows water as a bright signal.

Tympanocentesis: Puncture of the tympanic membrane with a needle to aspirate middle ear fluid.

Tympanostomy tube: Small plastic or metal tube inserted into the eardrum to keep the middle ear aerated and improve hearing in patients with chronic middle ear effusion.

Uhthoff's phenomenon: Acute worsening of multiple sclerosis symptoms on exposure to heat because high body temperatures may exceed the capacitance of the demyelinated nerve and conduction may fail.

Ulceration: A suppurative or nonhealing lesion on a surface such as skin, cornea, or mucous membrane.

Ultrafiltration: The movement of plasma water across a semipermeable membrane.

Ultrasound: Noninvasive imaging of organ or tissue to detect fluid, masses, or cyst.

Uncomplicated disorder: The presence of a single acid–base disorder, with or without compensation. See also Simple disorder.

Unilateral: Pertaining to one side.

Uremia: A condition that results from accumulation of metabolic waste products and endogenous toxins in the body resulting from impaired kidney function. Symptoms of uremia include nausea, vomiting, weakness, loss of appetite and mental confusion.

Uric acid: A by-product of purine metabolism in mammals, including humans. A high serum uric acid concentration is a major risk factor for gout.

Uricosuric: Pertaining to, characterized by, or promoting renal secretion of uric acid.

Urosepsis: Sepsis resulting from a urinary source.

Urticaria: Itchy, raised, swollen areas on the skin. Also known as hives.

Uveitis: An inflammation of the uvea, including the iris, ciliary body or choroid.

Vagal maneuvers: Stimulate the activity of the parasympathetic nervous system, which inhibits AV nodal conduction. Examples of vagal maneuvers include cough, carotid sinus massage, and Valsalva.

Vagotomy: A surgical procedure that blocks vagal (cholinergic) stimulation to the stomach.

Valsalva maneuver: Vagal maneuver; patient bears down against a closed glottis, as if they were having a bowel movement.

Variceal bleeding: Gastric, esophageal, or rectal bleeding from collateral vessels (varices).

Vasculitis: Inflammation of the walls of blood vessels.

Vasopressors: Medications that cause constriction of blood vessels, increase in vascular resistance, and increase in blood pressure.

Vasospasm: Narrowing (constriction) of a blood vessel causing a reduction in blood flow.

Ventilation/perfusion ratio (Va/Q): A comparison of the proportion of lung tissue being ventilated by inhaled air to the rate of oxygenation of pulmonary blood.

Ventral tegmental area: Part of the basal ganglia, containing dopamine neurons that project to the striatum, specifically the nucleus accumbens. This is part of the reward pathway in the brain.

Ventricular depolarization: Change in the membrane potential of a ventricular myocyte, resulting in loss of polarization. Under normal conditions, depolarization of ventricular myocytes is followed by ventricular contraction.

Vertigo: Sensation of spinning or feeling out of balance.

Vesicants: Chemotherapy drugs that cause significant tissue damage if extravasation occurs.

Virilization: Production or acquisition of virilism or the possession of masculine characteristics.

Volvulus: Twisting of the intestine causing obstruction and possible necrosis.

Vomiting: A reflexive rapid and forceful oral expulsion of upper gastrointestinal contents due to powerful and sustained contractions in the abdominal and thoracic musculature.

Waist circumference: A practical tool to measure the abdominal fat in patients with a BMI of less than 35.

Wernicke's syndrome: A syndrome that can be associated with chronic alcohol use, characterized by loss of memory, disorientation, and confabulation.

Western blot (WB): "Gold standard" for HIV diagnostic testing. Disrupted virus is purified, gel electrophoresed to separate by molecular weight to form bands corresponding to the nine HIV antigens, and blotted onto a membrane support. HIV serum antibodies from the patient are allowed to bind to proteins in the membrane support. If HIV antibodies from the patient are bound, the bands will change color. The test is considered reactive if two of the three major bands (p24, gp41, and/or gp120/160) change color. The test is nonreactive if no viral bands are visible.

Wheeze: A high pitched whistling sound caused by air moving through narrowed airways. Wheezes are usually heard at the end of expiration but may be heard during inspiration and expiration in acute severe asthma.

White coat hypertension: A persistently elevated average office blood pressure of greater than 140/90 mm Hg and an average awake ambulatory reading of less than 135/85 mm Hg.

Wilson's disease: A disorder of copper metabolism, characterized by cirrhosis of the liver and neurologic manifestations.

Xanthoma: Firm, raised nodules composed of lipid-containing histiocytes.

Xerostomia: Dryness of the mouth resulting from diminished or arrested salivary secretion.

ZAP-70 expression: An intracellular tyrosine kinase found in CLL B-cells.

Appendix E: Example Careplans

Six pharmacotherapy careplans based on cases in the book have been provided so the student will have a better understanding of the structure and content of typical careplans. Note that some information has been left out of these examples so you will not have all the 'answers' for your own workup of these cases. As discussed in Chapter 1, the careplan forms are meant to be a guide in structuring your thoughts and information, and there is no single correct way to do it. As you gain more experience, developing the elements of the care plan will become more intuitive. Remember, your most important job is to provide the best possible drug therapy for the patient.

26 Euvolemic Hyponatremia: Example Careplan with Missing Data

Mark A. Malesker   Cara Olsen   Lee E. Morrow

PATIENT DATABASE FORM

Patient Name: Albert Buterol	**Patient ID:** 09921234	**Location:** ICU
Physician: Dr. Pepper	**Pharmacy:**	
Age (or Date of Birth): 89 yo	**Race:** Caucasian	**Sex:** Male
Height: 71 in. (180 cm)	**Weight:** 155.5 lb (70.7 kg)	
Date of Admission/Initial Visit: 6/15/2009	**Occupation:** Retired Factory Worker	

Allergies/Intolerances/ADRs

❏ No known drug allergies/ADRs

❏ Not known/inadequate information

Drug:	Reaction:
Antihistamines	Unknown
Sulfa	Unknown
Tramadol	Unknown
Amitriptyline	Unknown

HPI, PMH, FH, SH, etc...

MI, post-PCI

Pacemaker for bradycardia

HTN

Enlarged prostate with frequent UTIs

Quit smoking 10 yr ago

Denies alcohol and illicit drug use

Medications prior to admission:

HCTZ 50 mg PO daily

Celecoxib 200 mg PO daily

Finasteride 5 mg PO daily

Pantoprazole 40 mg PO daily

Cotrimoxazole PO twice daily

Lorazepam 1 mg PO q 8 h PRN anxiety

Latanoprost eyedrops both eyes at bedtime

Prioritized Medical Problem List	Medication Profile
Intracranial pressure	Nicardipine IV infusion to keep systolic BP <160 mmHg
	Codeine 15–30 mg IV q 8 h as needed for cough
Euvolemic hyponatremia	3% NaCl initiate at 15 mL/h
_____	Piperacillin–tazobactam 3.375 g IV q 6 h
	Levofloxacin 500 mg IV q 24 h
	Vancomycin 1 g IV q 24 h
HTN	Nicardipine IV drip to keep BP <160 mmHg
History of GERD/stress ulcer prophylaxis	Pantoprazole 40 mg IV daily
Nausea/vomiting	Metoclopramide 10 mg IV q 6 h as needed
Verification of medication allergies, intolerances	

The form is from *ASHP National Clinical Skills Competition Case Documents*, Copyright 2009. American Society of Health-System Pharmacists, Bethesda, MD (www.ashp.org). Adapted with permission.

Vital Signs, Laboratory Data, and Diagnostic Test Results			
Date	6/16/2009 at 0600	6/16/2009 at 2000	6/17/2009 at 0745
Weight (lb/kg)	155.5 (70.7)		
Temperature (°C)	37.4	36.5	
Blood pressure (mm Hg)	148/83	147/60	
Pulse	120	71	
Respiratory rate	19	20	
Na 135–145 mEq/L (135–145 mmol/L)	119	125	129
K 3.3–4.9 mEq/L (3.3–4.9 mmol/L)	3.7	3.6	4.1
Cl 97–110 mEq/L (97–110 mmol/L)	84	84	87
CO_2/HCO_3 22–26 mEq/L (22–26 mmol/L)	27	27	23
BUN 8–25 mg/dL (2.9–8.9 mmol/L)	16 (5.7)	26 (9.3)	20 (7.1)
Creatinine (adult) Male 0.7–1.3 mg/dL; female 0.6–1.1 mg/dL (male 62–115 μmol/L; female 53–97 μmol/L)	1.0 (88)	1.0 (88)	1.3 (115)
Creatinine clearance (adult) 85–135 mL/min (1.42–2.25 mL/s)			
Glucose (fasting) 65–109 mg/dL (3.6–6.0 mmol/L)	186 (10.3)	171(9.5)	160 (8.9)
Total Ca 8.6–10.3 mg/dL (2.15–2.58 mmol/L)	8.3 (2.08)	8.5 (2.13)	8.6 (2.15)
Mg 1.3–2.2 mEq/L (0.65–1.10 mmol/L)			
PO_4 2.5–4.5 mg/dL (0.81–1.45 mmol/L)			
Hemoglobin Male 13.8–17.2 g/dL; female 12.1–15.1 g/dL (male 138–172 g/L; female 121–151 g/L; male 8.57–10.68 mmol/L; female 7.51–9.38 mmol/L)	12.9 (129; 8.01)		
Hematocrit Male 40.7–50.3%; female 36.1–44.3% (male 0.407–0.503; female 0.361–0.443)	31.2 (0.312)		
MCV 80.0–97.6 μm³ (80.0–97.6 fL)			
WBC 4–10 × 10³/mm³ (4–10 × 10⁹/L)	12.9		
Differential			
Platelet 140–440 × 10³/mm³ (140–440 × 10⁹/L)	182		
Albumin 3.5–5.0 g/dL (35–50 g/L)			
Total bilirubin 0.3–1.1 mg/dL (5.1–18.8 μmol/L)			
Direct bilirubin 0–0.3 mg/dL (0–5.1 μmol/L)			
AST 11–47 IU/L (0.18–0.78 μkat/L)			
ALT 7–53 IU/L (0.12–0.88 μkat/L)			
Alk phos (adult) 38–126 IU/L (0.63–2.10 μkat/L)			

Vital Signs, Laboratory Data, and Diagnostic Test Results			
Plasma osmolality 273–300 mOsm/kg (273–300 mmol/kg)		265	
Urine osmolality 250–900 mOsm/kg (250–900 mmol/kg)	475		
Urine sodium 20–250 mEq/L (20–250 mmol/L)	<20		

Notes

DRUG THERAPY PROBLEM WORKSHEET

Type of Problem	Possible Causes	Problem List	Notes
Correlation between drug therapy and medical problems	Drugs without obvious medical indications	Home medications latanoprost, celecoxib, pantoprazole, lorazepam	
	Medications unidentified		
	Untreated medical conditions		
Need for additional drug therapy	New medical condition requiring new drug therapy	Hyponatremia	
	Chronic disorder requiring continued drug therapy		
	Condition best treated with combination drug therapy		
	May develop new medical condition without prophylactic or preventative therapy or premedication		
Unnecessary drug therapy	Medication with no valid indication		
	Condition caused by accidental or intentional ingestion of toxic amount of drug or chemical		
	Medical problem(s) associated with use of or withdrawal from alcohol, drug, or tobacco		
	Condition is better treated with nondrug therapy		
	Taking multiple drugs when single agent as effective		
	Taking drug(s) to treat an avoidable adverse reaction from another medication		
Appropriate drug selection	Current regimen not usually as effective as other choices		
	Current regimen not usually as safe as other choices		
	Therapy not individualized to patient		
Wrong drug	Medical problem for which drug is not effective		
	Patient has risk factors that contraindicate use of drug		
	Patient has infection with organisms resistant to drug		
	Patient refractory to current drug therapy		
	Taking combination product when single agent appropriate		
	Dosage form inappropriate		
	Medication error		
Drug regimen	PRN use not appropriate for condition		
	Route of administration/dosage form/mode of administration not appropriate for current condition		
	Length or course of therapy not appropriate		
	Drug therapy altered without adequate therapeutic trial		
	Dose or interval flexibility not appropriate		
Dose too low	Dose or frequency too low to produce desired response in this patient		
	Serum drug level below desired therapeutic range		
	Timing of antimicrobial prophylaxis not appropriate		
	Medication not stored properly		
	Medication error		
Dose too high	Dose or frequency too high for this patient		
	Serum drug level above the desired therapeutic range		
	Dose escalated too quickly		
	Dose or interval flexibility not appropriate for this patient		
	Medication error		

DRUG THERAPY PROBLEM WORKSHEET

Type of Problem	Possible Causes	Problem List	Notes
Therapeutic duplication	Receiving multiple agents without added benefit		
Drug allergy/ adverse drug events	History of allergy or ADE to current (or chemically related) agents	Sulfa allergy—verify celecoxib and HCTZ	
	Allergy or ADE history not in medical records		
	Patient not using alert for severe allergy or ADE		
	Symptoms or medical problems that may be drug induced		
	Drug administered too rapidly		
	Medication error, actual or potential		
Interactions (drug–drug, drug–disease, drug–nutrient, drug–laboratory test)	Effect of drug altered due to enzyme induction/ inhibition from another drug patient is taking		
	Effect of drug altered due to protein-binding alterations from another drug patient is taking		
	Effect of drug altered due to pharmacodynamic change from another drug patient is taking		
	Bioavailability of drug altered due to interaction with another drug or food		
	Effect of drug altered due to substance in food		
	Patient's laboratory test altered due to interference from a drug the patient is taking		
Failure to receive therapy	Patient did not adhere with the drug regimen		
	Drug not given due to medication error		
	Patient did not take due to high drug cost/lack of insurance		
	Patient unable to take oral medication		
	Patient has no IV access for IV medication		
	Drug product not available		
Financial impact	The current regimen is not the most cost-effective		
	Patient unable to purchase medications/no insurance	Unknown	
Patient knowledge of drug therapy	Patient does not understand the purpose, directions, or potential side effects of the drug regimen	Patient unresponsive	
	Current regimen not consistent with the patient's health beliefs	Unknown	

PHARMACOTHERAPY CARE PLAN

Medical Problem List	Current Drug Regimen	Drug Therapy Problems	Therapy Goals, Desired Endpoints	Therapeutic Recommendations	Rationale	Therapeutic Alternatives	Monitoring
Euvolemic hyponatremia	————	May be due to ————	Return sodium to within normal limits; no further increase in ICP; correct serum Na no faster than 0.5 mEq/L/h (0.5 mmol/L/h) since hyponatremia	———— After the patient recovers from head trauma, investigate the cause of euvolemic hyponatremia and treat accordingly	Need for acute management due to compromised neurostatus; 1 L of 3% sodium chloride will correct the sodium by about 9 mEq (9 mmol) in this patient; avoid too-rapid correction and risk of osmotic myelinolysis syndrome	———— Conivaptan IV, but unclear safety and efficacy in neurotrauma patient	Monitor electrolytes q 2–4 h to ensure you do not correct the sodium by more than 12 mEq (12 mmol) q 24 h
Hypokalemia	————	May be due to HCTZ	Serum K >4.0 mEq/L (>4.0 mmol/L) in critically ill patients	————	Unable to give PO; risk of hypokalemia-related complications in critically ill patients	K phosphate, K acetate if hypophosphatemic or acidotic	————
Pneumonia	————		Cure infection	————	Broad coverage since critically ill, pneumonia; history not clear	Carbapenem, third-generation cephalosporin	CBC, CXR q 24 h; ABGs q 6 h
HTN	HCTZ		————	Nicardipine IV infusion When recovered from head trauma, reassess HTN regimen	Improves cerebral perfusion	————	BP, neurochecks q 1 h
Nausea/ vomiting			Prevent vomiting-related increased ICP	Metoclopramide 10 mg IV q 6 h PRN		————	————
Hx GERD/ stress ulcer prophylaxis	————		No stress ulcer bleeding	Pantoprazole 40 mg q 24 h	Stress ulcer prophylaxis indicated in head trauma, mechanical ventilation	————	CBC; hemoccult; NG suction fluid

PATIENT EDUCATION SUMMARY	
Notes	
• Patient is unresponsive at this time.	

33 Parkinson's Disease: Example Careplan with Missing Data

Jack J. Chen

PATIENT DATABASE FORM

Patient Name: Oliver Covey	**Patient ID:** 01892500	**Location:** Neurologist's Office
Physician:	**Pharmacy:**	
Age (or Date of Birth): 62 yo	**Race:** Caucasian	**Sex:** Male
Height: 71 in. (180 cm)	**Weight:** 180 lb (81.8 kg)	
Date of Admission/Initial Visit: 10/20/2009	**Occupation:** Agricultural Irrigation Consultant	

Allergies/Intolerances/ADRs

❏ No known drug allergies/ADRs

❏ Not known/inadequate information

Drug:	Reaction:
Sulfonamides	Rash

HPI, PMH, FH, SH, etc...

BPH × 1 yr

GERD × 1 yr

Hyperlipidemia × 5 yr

Nephrolithiasis in the past

Tonsillectomy

Tennis player

Prioritized Medical Problem List	Medication Profile
Parkinson's disease	
BPH	Silodosin 8 mg PO q 24 h
GERD	Omeprazole 20 mg PO q 24 h
_____	Simvastatin 20 mg PO q 24 h
	Multivitamin one tablet PO q 24 h

Vital Signs, Laboratory Data, and Diagnostic Test Results			
Date	09/20/2009		
Weight (lb/kg)	178 (80.9)		
Temperature (°C)	36.2		
Blood pressure (mm Hg)	126/74		
Pulse	77		
Respiratory rate	15		
Na 135–145 mEq/L (135–145 mmol/L)	140		
K 3.3–4.9 mEq/L (3.3–4.9 mmol/L)	4.0		
Cl 97–110 mEq/L (97–110 mmol/L)	99		
CO_2/HCO_3 22–26 mEq/L (22–26 mmol/L)	29		
BUN 8–25 mg/dL (2.9–8.9 mmol/L)	14 (5.0)		
Creatinine (adult) Male 0.7–1.3 mg/dL; female 0.6–1.1 mg/dL (male 62–115 µmol/L; female 53–97 µmol/L)	1 (88)		
Creatinine clearance (adult) 85–135 mL/min (1.42–2.25 mL/s)	81.6 (1.36)		
Glucose (fasting) 65–109 mg/dL (3.6–6.0 mmol/L)	90 (5.0)		
Total Ca 8.6–10.3 mg/dL (2.15-2.58 mmol/L)	9.5 (2.38)		
Mg 1.3–2.2 mEq/L (0.65–1.10 mmol/L)	2.2 (1.10)		
PO_4 2.5–4.5 mg/dL (0.81–1.45 mmol/L)	3.5 (1.13)		
Hemoglobin Male 13.8–17.2 g/dL; female 12.1–15.1 g/dL (male 138–172 g/L; female 121–151 g/L; male 8.57–10.68 mmol/L; female 7.51–9.38 mmol/L)	16.4 (164; 10.18)		
Hematocrit Male 40.7–50.3%; female 36.1–44.3% (male 0.407–0.503; female 0.361–0.443)	48.7 (0.487)		
MCV 80.0–97.6 µm³ (80.0–97.6 fL)	86.4		
WBC $4–10 \times 10^3/mm^3$ ($4–10 \times 10^9/L$)	8.5		
Differential			
Platelet $140–440 \times 10^3/mm^3$ ($140–440 \times 10^9/L$)	300		
Albumin 3.5–5.0 g/dL (35–50 g/L)	3.7 (37)		
Total bilirubin 0.3–1.1 mg/dL (5.1–18.8 µmol/L)			
Direct bilirubin 0–0.3 mg/dL (0–5.1 µmol/L)			
AST 11–47 IU/L (0.18–0.78 µkat/L)			
ALT 7–53 IU/L (0.12–0.88 µkat/L)			
Alk phos (adult) 38–126 IU/L (0.63–2.10 µkat/L)			

Vital Signs, Laboratory Data, and Diagnostic Test Results			
Total cholesterol <200 mg/dL (<5.17 mmol/L)	180 (4.65)		
LDL cholesterol <130 mg/dL (<3.36 mmol/L)	100 (2.59)		
HDL cholesterol >35 mg/dL (>0.91 mmol/L)	38 (0.98)		

Notes

DRUG THERAPY PROBLEM WORKSHEET

Type of Problem	Possible Causes	Problem List	Notes
Correlation between drug therapy and medical problems	Drugs without obvious medical indications		
	Medications unidentified		
	Untreated medical conditions		
Need for additional drug therapy	New medical condition requiring new drug therapy	Parkinson's disease	
	Chronic disorder requiring continued drug therapy		
	Condition best treated with combination drug therapy		
	May develop new medical condition without prophylactic or preventative therapy or premedication		
Unnecessary drug therapy	Medication with no valid indication		
	Condition caused by accidental or intentional ingestion of toxic amount of drug or chemical		
	Medical problem(s) associated with use of or withdrawal from alcohol, drug, or tobacco		
	Condition is better treated with nondrug therapy		
	Taking multiple drugs when single agent as effective		
	Taking drug(s) to treat an avoidable adverse reaction from another medication		
Appropriate drug selection	Current regimen not usually as effective as other choices		
	Current regimen not usually as safe as other choices		
	Therapy not individualized to patient		
Wrong drug	Medical problem for which drug is not effective		
	Patient has risk factors that contraindicate use of drug		
	Patient has infection with organisms resistant to drug		
	Patient refractory to current drug therapy		
	Taking combination product when single agent appropriate		
	Dosage form inappropriate		
	Medication error		
Drug regimen	PRN use not appropriate for condition		
	Route of administration/dosage form/mode of administration not appropriate for current condition		
	Length or course of therapy not appropriate		
	Drug therapy altered without adequate therapeutic trial		
	Dose or interval flexibility not appropriate		
Dose too low	Dose or frequency too low to produce desired response in this patient		
	Serum drug level below desired therapeutic range		
	Timing of antimicrobial prophylaxis not appropriate		
	Medication not stored properly		
	Medication error		
Dose too high	Dose or frequency too high for this patient		
	Serum drug level above the desired therapeutic range		
	Dose escalated too quickly		
	Dose or interval flexibility not appropriate for this patient		
	Medication error		

DRUG THERAPY PROBLEM WORKSHEET

Type of Problem	Possible Causes	Problem List	Notes
Therapeutic duplication	Receiving multiple agents without added benefit		
Drug allergy/ adverse drug events	History of allergy or ADE to current (or chemically related) agents		
	Allergy or ADE history not in medical records	Any allergies or ADEs other than sulfonamides?	
	Patient not using alert for severe allergy or ADE		
	Symptoms or medical problems that may be drug induced	Any previous use of neuroleptics, metoclopramide, or other dopamine receptor-blocking agents?	
	Drug administered too rapidly		
	Medication error, actual or potential		
Interactions (drug–drug, drug–disease, drug–nutrient, drug–laboratory test)	Effect of drug altered due to enzyme induction/ inhibition from another drug patient is taking		
	Effect of drug altered due to protein-binding alterations from another drug patient is taking		
	Effect of drug altered due to pharmacodynamic change from another drug patient is taking		
	Bioavailability of drug altered due to interaction with another drug or food	Multivitamin may contain Fe^{++}. If carbidopa/levodopa is initiated, Fe^{++} will reduce levodopa bioavailability by 50%	If carbidopa/levodopa therapy is selected, make sure the patient is educated about proper times to administer
	Effect of drug altered due to substance in food		
	Patient's laboratory test altered due to interference from a drug the patient is taking		
Failure to receive therapy	Patient did not adhere with the drug regimen		
	Drug not given due to medication error		
	Patient did not take due to high drug cost/lack of insurance		
	Patient unable to take oral medication		
	Patient has no IV access for IV medication		
	Drug product not available		
Financial impact	The current regimen is not the most cost-effective		
	Patient unable to purchase medications/no insurance	Insurance coverage not known	If a branded drug is initiated, can provide drug samples to see if the drug is effective and tolerated
Patient knowledge of drug therapy	Patient does not understand the purpose, directions, or potential side effects of the drug regimen	Patient's background understanding of anti-PD medications unknown	Educate the patient and caregiver about purpose, directions, and potential side effects of drug regimen
	Current regimen not consistent with the patient's health beliefs	Cultural beliefs not known	

PHARMACOTHERAPY CARE PLAN

Medical Problem List	Current Drug Regimen	Drug Therapy Problems	Therapy Goals, Desired Endpoints	Therapeutic Recommendations	Rationale	Therapeutic Alternatives	Monitoring
PD	_____	_____	Improve motor symptoms (tremor, rigidity, slowness). Allow the patient to continue to enjoy his tennis game	_____ _____ Avoid medications that may worsen symptoms (dopamine blockers)	Appropriate for mild-severity PD. Well-tolerated and once-daily administration No anticholinergic due to BPH	Dopamine agonist such as pramipexole or ropinirole. Titrated to maintenance dose as per package insert. Ropinirole immediate release is generic, so may be more cost-effective	Rasagiline is well tolerated. Monitor for nausea. Self-monitor symptoms (tennis game); return to neurologist 2 mo If dopamine agonist, monitor for: _____ _____
BPH	Silodosin 8 mg PO q 24 h	_____	Improve urinary voiding dysfunction	_____ _____	_____ _____	Other α_1-receptor blockers, 5α- reductase inhibitors, combination therapy	Monitor for side effects such as dizziness, orthostatic hypotension, sexual dysfunction
GERD	Omeprazole 20 mg PO q 24 h		No GERD symptoms	_____ _____	_____ _____	_____ _____	_____ _____
_____	Simvastatin 20 mg PO q 24 h		_____ _____	Continue with current regimen. Provide healthy lifestyle (diet, exercise) recommendations	LDL and HDL are at goal	_____ _____	Recheck lipid panel in 3 mo

PATIENT EDUCATION SUMMARY

Notes

Parkinson's Disease

- The reason for taking this medication called rasagiline is to replace or enhance the dopamine that your brain is not producing in adequate amounts. In doing so, your movement should get better.
- Take this medication once a day as your physician directed.
- If you experience stomach upset or nausea while taking this medication, take it with _____.
- If you miss a dose, _____.
- You should begin to feel better within _____ wk of starting this medication, maybe sooner.
- This is a very well-tolerated medication, and these problems will not occur if you take the medication as directed.
- Call your physician immediately if you experience any effects that you believe might be a side effect.
- Since there is no cure for Parkinson's disease, you will likely need to take this medication indefinitely.

Benign Prostatic Hypertrophy

- Continue with your drug regimen as long as it is controlling your symptoms. If you have any questions, consult with your primary care physician.

Gastroesophageal Reflux Disease

- Continue with your drug regimen as long as it is controlling your symptoms. If you have any questions, consult with your primary care physician.

Hyperlipidemia

- Your total cholesterol and LDL (the "bad") cholesterol is in control. Your HDL (the "good") cholesterol is adequate. You will need periodic blood tests to make sure your lipid levels are still controlled and to assess for side effects.
- If you notice any muscle pains not explained by exercise, notify your physician.
- Continue with your drug regimen and remember to keep a healthy diet, keep exercising, and avoid using tobacco, and consume alcohol in moderation.
- If you have questions, consult with your primary care physician.

42   Anxiety: Example Careplan with Missing Data

Sheila Botts

PATIENT DATABASE FORM

Patient Name: Angela Brown	**Patient ID:** 00869702	**Location:** Physician's Office
Physician:	**Pharmacy:** Wal-Mart	
Age (or Date of Birth): 32 yo	**Race:** Caucasian	**Sex:** Female
Height: 65 in. (165 cm)	**Weight:** 145 lb (65.9 kg)	
Date of Admission/Initial Visit: 12/2/2009	**Occupation:** Art Teacher	

Allergies/Intolerances/ADRs

❑ No known drug allergies/ADRs
❑ Not known/inadequate information

Drug:	Reaction:
Fluoxetine	Agitation and anxiety

HPI, PMH, FH, SH, etc…

Depression 3 yr ago after death of father
Migraine headache diagnosed 5 yr ago
Sibling treated for anxiety with citalopram

Prioritized Medical Problem List

Panic disorder with agoraphobia
Depressive symptoms
Migraine headaches
EtOH use
Muscle aches, ? Due to anxiety
Tachycardia, ? Due to anxiety

Medication Profile

Diazepam 5 mg PO PRN
Zolmitriptan 2.5 mg PO PRN
Ibuprofen 400 mg PO PRN

The form is from *ASHP National Clinical Skills Competition Case Documents*, Copyright 2009, American Society of Health-System Pharmacists, Bethesda, MD (www.ashp.org). Adapted with permission.

Vital Signs, Laboratory Data, and Diagnostic Test Results			
Date	12/1/2009		
Weight (lb/kg)	145 (65.9)		
Temperature (°C)	37.1		
Blood pressure (mm Hg)	118/76		
Pulse	88		
Respiratory rate	18		
Na 135–145 mEq/L (135–145 mmol/L)	142		
K 3.3–4.9 mEq/L (3.3–4.9 mmol/L)	4.1		
Cl 97–110 mEq/L (97–110 mmol/L)	100		
CO_2/HCO_3 22–26 mEq/L (22–26 mmol/L)	24		
BUN 8–25 mg/dL (2.9–8.9 mmol/L)	10 (3.6)		
Creatinine (adult) Male 0.7–1.3 mg/dL; female 0.6–1.1 mg/dL (male 62–115 μmol/L; female 53–97 μmol/L)	0.7 (62)		
Creatinine clearance (adult) 85–135 mL/min (1.42–2.25 mL/s)			
Glucose (fasting) 65–109 mg/dL (3.6–6.0 mmol/L)	98 (5.4)		
Total Ca 8.6–10.3 mg/dL (2.15–2.58 mmol/L)			
Mg 1.3–2.2 mEq/L (0.65–1.10 mmol/L)			
PO_4 2.5–4.5 mg/dL (0.81–1.45 mmol/L)			

Hemoglobin
Male 13.8–17.2 g/dL; female 12.1–15.1 g/dL (male 138–172 g/L;
  female 121–151 g/L; male 8.57–10.68 mmol/L;
  female 7.51–9.38 mmol/L)
	14.5 (145; 9.00)		

Hematocrit Male 40.7–50.3%; female 36.1–44.3% (male 0.407–0.503; female 0.361–0.443)	42 (0.42)		
MCV 80.0–97.6 μm³ (80.0–97.6 fL)			
WBC 4–10 × 10³/mm³ (4–10 × 10⁹/L)	6.8		
Differential			
Platelet 140–440 × 10³/mm³ (140–440 × 10⁹/L)			
Albumin 3.5–5.0 g/dL (35–50 g/L)			
Total bilirubin 0.3–1.1 mg/dL (5.1–18.8 μmol/L)			
Direct bilirubin 0–0.3 mg/dL (0–5.1 μmol/L)			
AST 11–47 IU/L (0.18–0.78 μkat/L)	22 (0.37)		
ALT 7–53 IU/L (0.12–0.88 μkat/L)	28 (0.47)		
Alk phos (adult) 38–126 IU/L (0.63–2.10 μkat/L)	40 (0.67)		

Vital Signs, Laboratory Data, and Diagnostic Test Results			
TSH 0.35–6.20 µU/mL (0.35–6.20 mU/L)	1.2		
Total cholesterol <200 mg/dL (<5.17 mmol/L)	178 (4.60)		
LDL cholesterol <130 mg/dL (<3.36 mmol/L)	89 (2.30)		
HDL cholesterol >35 mg/dL (>0.91 mmol/L)	36 (0.93)		

Notes
Urine drug screen: (+) benzodiazepines
Urine pregnancy test (−)
ECG report from ER noted sinus tachycardia, otherwise no significant findings

DRUG THERAPY PROBLEM WORKSHEET

Type of Problem	Possible Causes	Problem List	Notes
Correlation between drug therapy and medical problems	Drugs without obvious medical indications		
	Medications unidentified	Supplement use?; other analgesics	
	Untreated medical conditions		
Need for additional drug therapy	New medical condition requiring new drug therapy	Panic disorder	Currently receiving diazepam PRN
	Chronic disorder requiring continued drug therapy	? Migraine	
	Condition best treated with combination drug therapy		
	May develop new medical condition without prophylactic or preventative therapy or premedication		
Unnecessary drug therapy	Medication with no valid indication		
	Condition caused by accidental or intentional ingestion of toxic amount of drug or chemical		
	Medical problem(s) associated with use of or withdrawal from alcohol, drug, or tobacco	EtOH use increased to control anxiety; may increase depressive symptoms also	
	Condition is better treated with nondrug therapy		
	Taking multiple drugs when single agent as effective		
	Taking drug(s) to treat an avoidable adverse reaction from another medication		
Appropriate drug selection	Current regimen not usually as effective as other choices		
	Current regimen not usually as safe as other choices		
	Therapy not individualized to patient		
Wrong drug	Medical problem for which drug is not effective		
	Patient has risk factors that contraindicate use of drug		
	Patient has infection with organisms resistant to drug		
	Patient refractory to current drug therapy		
	Taking combination product when single agent appropriate		
	Dosage form inappropriate		
	Medication error		
Drug regimen	PRN use not appropriate for condition	Panic disorder	
	Route of administration/dosage form/mode of administration not appropriate for current condition		
	Length or course of therapy not appropriate		
	Drug therapy altered without adequate therapeutic trial		
	Dose or interval flexibility not appropriate		
Dose too low	Dose or frequency too low to produce desired response in this patient		
	Serum drug level below desired therapeutic range		
	Timing of antimicrobial prophylaxis not appropriate		
	Medication not stored properly		
	Medication error		

DRUG THERAPY PROBLEM WORKSHEET

Type of Problem	Possible Causes	Problem List	Notes
Dose too high	Dose or frequency too high for this patient		
	Serum drug level above the desired therapeutic range		
	Dose escalated too quickly		
	Dose or interval flexibility not appropriate for this patient		
	Medication error		
Therapeutic duplication	Receiving multiple agents without added benefit		
Drug allergy/ adverse drug events	History of allergy or ADE to current (or chemically related) agents	Fluoxetine	Did not tolerate— starting dose too high, experienced agitation, and anxiety
	Allergy or ADE history not in medical records	Other allergies or medication intolerance?	
	Patient not using alert for severe allergy or ADE		
	Symptoms or medical problems that may be drug induced		
	Drug administered too rapidly		
	Medication error, actual or potential		
Interactions (drug–drug, drug–disease, drug–nutrient, drug–laboratory test)	Effect of drug altered due to enzyme induction/ inhibition from another drug patient is taking		
	Effect of drug altered due to protein-binding alterations from another drug patient is taking		
	Effect of drug altered due to pharmacodynamic change from another drug patient is taking	Diazepam use with EtOH will increase CNS depression; potential SSRI/ triptan interaction	Diazepam not recommended
	Bioavailability of drug altered due to interaction with another drug or food		
	Effect of drug altered due to substance in food		
	Patient's laboratory test altered due to interference from a drug the patient is taking		
Failure to receive therapy	Patient did not adhere with the drug regimen		
	Drug not given due to medication error		
	Patient did not take due to high drug cost/lack of insurance		
	Patient unable to take oral medication		
	Patient has no IV access for IV medication		
	Drug product not available		
Financial impact	The current regimen is not the most cost-effective		
	Patient unable to purchase medications/no insurance	No information on insurance status	
Patient knowledge of drug therapy	Patient does not understand the purpose, directions, or potential side effects of the drug regimen		
	Current regimen not consistent with the patient's health beliefs	Health beliefs not known	Discuss treatment preference (pharmacologic vs. nonpharmacologic) with the patient

Medical Problem List	Current Drug Regimen	Drug Therapy Problems	Therapy Goals, Desired Endpoints	Therapeutic Recommendations	Rationale	Therapeutic Alternatives	Monitoring
Panic disorder	___ ___	EtOH and benzodiazepine use; PRN treatment not best	Reduce panic attack frequency and severity; reduce anticipatory anxiety; reduce agoraphobic avoidance	___ ___ ___	Antidepressant therapy preferred for chronic treatment; starting dose low to avoid drug-induced anxiety and panic	Switch to another SSRI, SNRI (e.g., venlafaxine), or cognitive behavioral therapy (CBT). May also augment medication with CBT if some benefit with initial medication	Monitor weekly during first month for ADEs (GI, altered sleep, HA, etc.) and improvement in panic symptoms; if patient without considerable reduction in anxiety symptoms at 6–8 wk, consider changing antidepressant or augmentation
Depressive symptoms		___ ___ ___	No signs or symptoms of depression	___ ___	Antidepressant therapy indicated with comorbid panic disorder and depression; unclear if this patient has major depression, but symptoms expected to improve with treatment	As per panic disorder Plan	Assess depressive symptoms at the same time as anxiety symptoms
Migraine Headaches	Zolmitriptan 2.5 mg PO PRN	Frequency of use unknown; responsiveness to ibuprofen? Risk of serotonin syndrome, triptan, SSRI	___ ___ ___	Migraine frequency and severity may improve with SSRI treatment of anxiety disorder	___ ___ ___ ___	If frequency of headaches increases to warrant prophylactic treatment, consider first-line agent such as propranolol, topiramate, or divalproex	Headache frequency and intensity; signs and symptoms of serotonin syndrome with SSRI and triptan use

PHARMACOTHERAPY CARE PLAN

Medical Problem List	Current Drug Regimen	Drug Therapy Problems	Therapy Goals, Desired Endpoints	Therapeutic Recommendations	Rationale	Therapeutic Alternatives	Monitoring
EtOH use			———— ———— ———— ————	EtOH use likely to decrease anxiety symptoms improve and sleep restored		If EtOH use continues or increases, refer to substance-abuse counseling/ program	———— ———— ———— ————
Muscle aches	———— ————		———— ————	Continue PRN use as needed; shoulder aches likely to improve with anxiety treatment; nondrug therapy (exercise, yoga, hot baths, massage)	Muscle aches commonly accompany tension associated with severe anxiety	———— ————	———— ————
Tachycardia	None		———— ————	Likely to improve with reduction of anxiety symptoms; if continues to worsen, refer for workup	———— ————	If not severe and ECG normal, no treatment recommended	Reassess at the next clinic visit along with anxiety symptoms; self-monitoring

PATIENT EDUCATION SUMMARY

Notes

Panic Disorder

- This medication is being used to reduce your anxiety, fears, and panic attacks. Over time it will also help with worry about having future panic attacks and avoiding places or situations due to anxiety.
- Take this medication once daily as your health care provider directed.
- If you miss a dose, _____.
- You should begin to feel better within _____ weeks of starting this medication, but it may take up to _____ wk for the full benefit. You will initially notice an improvement in your anxiety and sleep. Mood and panic attack reduction may take longer.
- This medication may cause _____. The side effects often go away as the treatment continues. If you experience suicidal thoughts or extreme irritability, you should stop the medication and call your health care provider.
- Do not abruptly discontinue this medication, unless instructed by your health care provider. Abrupt discontinuation can lead to an increase in anxiety symptoms, stomach upset, nausea, diarrhea, and body aches.
- It is very important to keep regular appointments with your health care provider to monitor your therapy so that you can gain the full benefit of this therapy while avoiding potential side effects.

Migraine Headaches

- Your migraine headaches may improve with the treatment of your anxiety disorder; however, if your headaches increase, you should inform your health care provider immediately.
- Your antimigraine medication in combination with your anxiety mediaction can result in a rare adverse reaction called serotonin syndrome. Serotonin syndrome occurs rapidly and causes symptoms of _____ _____. If you notice any of these symptoms, you should seek immediate care.

Depression

- Your depressive symptoms may be worsened by your alcohol use. Reduction in your daily alcohol consumption to one drink or less may improve your mood. Also, the medication prescribed for your anxiety will also help with depression.
- If your mood worsens or you begin to have suicidal thoughts after starting the medication, you should inform your health care provider immediately.

EtOH Use

- Your current alcohol consumption, in response to your anxiety, may worsen your sleep and increase your depression. This amount of alcohol use over time may also put you at risk for other chronic health conditions.
- You are being prescribed medication to reduce your anxiety, which may take a few weeks to work.
- If you are unable to reduce your alcohol use on your own, your provider will help you with other treatment options.

Muscle Aches

- Your muscle aches in your shoulders may improve as your anxiety improves.
- Regular exercise, stretching, yoga, massage, and hot baths may also be helpful.

Tachycardia

- Your rapid heart rate should improve as your anxiety is reduced.
- Rapid increases in your heart rate may also be a sign of other medical problems or drug interactions and should be reported to your health care provider.
- Relaxation exercises, deep breathing, and meditation may also be helpful.

48 Hypothyroidism: Example Careplan with Missing Data

Michael D. Katz

Patient Name: Yi-Ling Wang	**Patient ID:** 01892487	**Location:** Physician's Office
Physician:	**Pharmacy:**	**Sex:** Female
Age (or Date of Birth): 49 yo	**Race:** Chinese	
Height: 62 in (157.5 cm)	**Weight:** 127.6 lb (58 kg)	
Date of Admission/Initial Visit: 04/29/2009	**Occupation:**	

Allergies/Intolerances/ADRs

❏ No known drug allergies/ADRs

❏ Not known/inadequate information

Drug:	Reaction:
Penicillin	Rash

HPI, PMH, FH, SH, etc…

Iron-deficiency anemia diagnosed 6 mo ago

Depression for 6 mo

Menorrhagia diagnosed 6 mo ago

Osteopenia for 1 yr

Prioritized Medical Problem List	Medication Profile
Hypothyroidism	
_____ vs. hypothyroid symptoms	Sertraline 50 mg PO q 24 h
Dyslipidemia, ? due to hypothyroidism	
Osteopenia	Calcium carbonate 1,000 mg PO q 12 h
	Alendronate 35 mg PO weekly
Constipation, ? due to hypothyroidism, medications (Fe^{++}, Ca^{++})	MOM 30 mL PO q 24 h PRN
	Chinese herb PRN
_____, now resolved	FeSO$_4$ 30 mg PO q 24 h
_____, now resolved	Ortho Tri-Cyclen-28 PO q 24 h
	Acetaminophen 650 mg PO PRN HA, body aches

Vital Signs, Laboratory Data, and Diagnostic Test Results			
Date	04/29/2009		
Weight (lb/kg)	127.6 (58)		
Temperature (°C)	36.2		
Blood pressure (mm Hg)	112/76		
Pulse	64		
Respiratory rate	12		
Na 135–145 mEq/L (135–145 mmol/L)	142		
K 3.3–4.9 mEq/L (3.3–4.9 mmol/L)	4.1		
Cl 97–110 mEq/L (97–110 mmol/L)	100		
CO_2/HCO_3 22–26 mEq/L (22–26 mmol/L)	24		
BUN 8–25 mg/dL (2.9–8.9 mmol/L)	7 (2.5)		
Creatinine (adult) Male 0.7–1.3 mg/dL; female 0.6–1.1 mg/dL (male 62–115 μmol/L; female 53–97 μmol/L)	0.7 (62)		
Creatinine clearance (adult) 85–135 mL/min (1.42–2.25 mL/s)	96 (1.60)		
Glucose (fasting) 65–109 mg/dL (3.6–6.0 mmol/L)	104 (5.8)		
Total Ca 8.6–10.3 mg/dL (2.15–2.58 mmol/L)	9.4 (2.35)		
Mg 1.3–2.2 mEq/L (0.65–1.10 mmol/L)	1.8 (0.90)		
PO_4 2.5–4.5 mg/dL (0.81–1.45 mmol/L)	3.8 (1.23)		
Hemoglobin Male 13.8–17.2 g/dL; female 12.1–15.1 g/dL (male 138–172 g/L; female 121–151 g/L; male 8.57–10.68 mmol/L; female 7.51–9.38 mmol/L)	13.5 (135; 8.38)		
Hematocrit Male 40.7–50.3%; female 36.1–44.3% (male 0.407–0.503; female 0.361–0.443)	39.7 (0.397)		
MCV 80.0–97.6 μm³ (80.0–97.6 fL)	83.0		
WBC 4–10 × 10³/mm³ (4–10 × 10⁹/L)	7.6 (7.6)		
Differential			
Platelet 140–440 × 10³/mm³ (140–440 × 10⁹/L)			
Albumin 3.5–5.0 g/dL (35–50 g/L)	3.8 (38)		
Total bilirubin 0.3–1.1 mg/dL (5.1–18.8 μmol/L)			
Direct bilirubin 0–0.3 mg/dL (0–5.1 μmol/L)			
AST 11–47 IU/L (0.18–0.78 μkat/L)			
ALT 7–53 IU/L (0.12–0.88 μkat/L)			
Alk phos (adult) 38–126 IU/L (0.63–2.10 μkat/L)			

Vital Signs, Laboratory Data, and Diagnostic Test Results			
TSH 0.35–6.20 μU/mL (0.35–6.20 mU/L)	12.8		
Free T$_4$ 0.7–1.9 ng/dL (9.0–24.5 pmol/L)	0.71 (9.1)		
Anti-TPO antibody	+		
Total cholesterol <200 mg/dL (<5.18 mmol/L)	268 (6.93)		
LDL cholesterol <130 mg/dL (<3.36 mmol/L)	142 (3.67)		
HDL cholesterol >35 mg/dL (>0.91 mmol/L)	36 (0.93)		

Notes

DRUG THERAPY PROBLEM WORKSHEET

Type of Problem	Possible Causes	Problem List	Notes
Correlation between drug therapy and medical problems	Drugs without obvious medical indications		
	Medications unidentified	Chinese herbal product	Identify ingredients
	Untreated medical conditions		
Need for additional drug therapy	New medical condition requiring new drug therapy	Overt hypothyroidism	
	Chronic disorder requiring continued drug therapy		
	Condition best treated with combination drug therapy		
	May develop new medical condition without prophylactic or preventative therapy or premedication		
Unnecessary drug therapy	Medication with no valid indication		
	Condition caused by accidental or intentional ingestion of toxic amount of drug or chemical		
	Medical problem(s) associated with use of or withdrawal from alcohol, drug, or tobacco		
	Condition is better treated with nondrug therapy		
	Taking multiple drugs when single agent as effective		
	Taking drug(s) to treat an avoidable adverse reaction from another medication		
Appropriate drug selection	Current regimen not usually as effective as other choices		
	Current regimen not usually as safe as other choices		
	Therapy not individualized to patient		
Wrong drug	Medical problem for which drug is not effective		
	Patient has risk factors that contraindicate use of drug		
	Patient has infection with organisms resistant to drug		
	Patient refractory to current drug therapy		
	Taking combination product when single agent appropriate		
	Dosage form inappropriate		
	Medication error		
Drug regimen	PRN use not appropriate for condition		
	Route of administration/dosage form/mode of administration not appropriate for current condition		
	Length or course of therapy not appropriate		
	Drug therapy altered without adequate therapeutic trial		
	Dose or interval flexibility not appropriate		
Dose too low	Dose or frequency too low to produce desired response in this patient		
	Serum drug level below desired therapeutic range		
	Timing of antimicrobial prophylaxis not appropriate		
	Medication not stored properly		
	Medication error		
Dose too high	Dose or frequency too high for this patient		
	Serum drug level above the desired therapeutic range		
	Dose escalated too quickly		
	Dose or interval flexibility not appropriate for this patient		
	Medication error		

DRUG THERAPY PROBLEM WORKSHEET

Type of Problem	Possible Causes	Problem List	Notes
Therapeutic duplication	Receiving multiple agents without added benefit		
Drug allergy/ adverse drug events	History of allergy or ADE to current (or chemically related) agents		
	Allergy or ADE history not in medical records	Any allergies or ADEs other than penicillin?	
	Patient not using alert for severe allergy or ADE		
	Symptoms or medical problems that may be drug induced	Constipation due to or worsened by Fe^{++} or Ca^{++}	
	Drug administered too rapidly		
	Medication error, actual or potential		
Interactions (drug–drug, drug–disease, drug–nutrient, drug–laboratory test)	Effect of drug altered due to enzyme induction/ inhibition from another drug patient is taking		
	Effect of drug altered due to protein-binding alterations from another drug patient is taking		
	Effect of drug altered due to pharmacodynamic change from another drug patient is taking		
	Bioavailability of drug altered due to interaction with another drug or food	_____	Make sure the patient is educated about proper times to administer
	Effect of drug altered due to substance in food		
	Patient's laboratory test altered due to interference from a drug the patient is taking		
Failure to receive therapy	Patient did not adhere with the drug regimen	Patient's prior adherence not known	
	Drug not given due to medication error		
	Patient did not take due to high drug cost/lack of insurance		
	Patient unable to take oral medication		
	Patient has no IV access for IV medication		
	Drug product not available		
Financial impact	The current regimen is not the most cost-effective		
	Patient unable to purchase medications/no insurance	_____	
Patient knowledge of drug therapy	Patient does not understand the purpose, directions, or potential side effects of the drug regimen		
	Current regimen not consistent with the patient's health beliefs	Cultural beliefs not known	

Medical Problem List	Current Drug Regimen	Drug Therapy Problems	Therapy Goals, Desired Endpoints	Therapeutic Recommendations	Rationale	Therapeutic Alternatives	Monitoring
Hypothyroidism	None	Ca, Fe will be an issue with LT_4	Relieve symptoms (fatigue, cognition, dry skin, constipation); euthyroid state with TSH in target range [0.5–2.5 μU/mL (0.5–2.5 mU/L)]	———— ———— ———— ————	Drug of choice; most physiologic treatment; brand name to assure the same product with each refill; less-than-full replacement dose since hypothyroidism state not severe	———— ———— ———— ————	Patient to self-monitor s/s daily; repeat TSH in 6 wk; if TSH not in target range, recheck TSH 6–8 wk after each dose change; once LT_4 dose stable, check TSH q 6–12 mo, or if clinical status changes; monitor for ADEs
————	Sertraline 50 mg q 24 h		No signs or symptoms of depression	———— ———— ————	Not clear if the patient has major depression based on information provided	If major depression and not responding to sertraline and LT_4, consider changing to alternative antidepressant (venlafaxine, bupropion, etc.)	———— ———— ———— ————
Dyslipidemia	None		———— ———— ————	LDL likely to reach target when euthyroid, so no lipid-lowering drugs at this point; provide healthy lifestyle (diet, exercise) recommendations	LDL will be reduced with LT_4 therapy	If LDL does not reach target after TSH at target, initiate simvastatin 10 mg q HS	———— ———— ———— ————
Osteopenia	———— ————	Ca may interfere with LT_4 absorption	———— ———— ————	Continue current therapy; take LT_4 at least 2 h apart from Ca	Effective treatment; weekly bisphosphonate more convenient than daily	———— ————	BMD q 2 yr; self-monitor for ADEs

Medical Problem List	Current Drug Regimen	Drug Therapy Problems	Therapy Goals, Desired Endpoints	Therapeutic Recommendations	Rationale	Therapeutic Alternatives	Monitoring
Constipation	Milk of Magnesia 30 mL q 24 h PRN	Not sure what is in Chinese herb; may be due to or worsened by Ca, Fe	Normal bowel movements	———— ———— ———— ————	———— ———— ———— ————	If not better, add senna two tablets PO bid	———— ———— ———— ————
	Chinese herb						
————	FeSO$_4$ 300 mg q 24 h	May be worsening constipation; problem may be resolved since menorrhagia improved; Fe may reduce LT$_4$ absorption	———— ———— ———— ————	Consider DC Fe	May no longer need Fe since the underlying problem resolved		Self-monitor menses; CBC q 6 mo
————	Ortho Tri-Cyclen-28 q 24 h		Normal menses; prevent Fe deficiency	———— ———— ———— ————	———— ———— ———— ————	If not effective or ADE develops, alter estrogen and/or progestin component	———— ———— ———— ————

PATIENT EDUCATION SUMMARY

Notes

Hypothyroidism

- The reason for taking this medication (levothyroxine, LT$_4$) is to replace the hormone that your thyroid gland is not producing in adequate amounts. In doing so, your symptoms should disappear and your abnormal laboratory values should return to normal.
- Make sure you receive the same brand of this medication each time the prescription is filled. _____
_____.
- Take this medication once a day exactly as your physician directed.
- Space this medicine from your iron and calcium tablets by _____ h. The iron and calcium tablets may _____
_____.
- Although taking this medication with food can decrease the absorption, it is more important to take this medication in a consistent manner in regard to food intake and time of day.
- If you miss a dose, _____
_____.
- You should begin to feel better within 2–3 wk of starting this medication. You will initially notice an improvement in your energy and mood. Other symptoms, such as dry skin, may take longer to disappear.
- Blood tests will need to be checked periodically (every _____ wk) until your physician determines the best dose for you. After that, you will need to have a blood test only once or twice a year unless there is a change in your condition or if the brand of medication is changed.
- If the dose of your medication is too high, you may experience _____. Call your physician if you notice these side effects. Over a long period of time, taking too much of this medication can cause problems with your bones and heart.
- Taking too little of the medication can make you have the same symptoms you started with, plus you can develop hypertension, high cholesterol levels and an increased risk of heart disease. This is a very safe medication, and these problems will not occur if you take the medication as directed and if your thyroid blood tests are checked periodically and stay in the desired range.
- Call your physician immediately if you experience any _____.
- Because your thyroid gland is not producing enough thyroid hormone, you will likely need to take this medication for the rest of your life.
- It is very important to keep regular appointments with your physician to monitor your therapy so that you can gain the full benefit of this therapy while avoiding potential side effects.

Depression

- Your depression symptoms may be due to your hypothyroidism. If so, those symptoms should improve as your thyroid condition improves with LT$_4$ therapy. The sertraline should be continued until you are instructed to stop taking it.

Dyslipidemia

- _____.
- You should adopt a healthy lifestyle by improving your diet, exercising, not using tobacco, and using alcohol in moderation.

Osteopenia

- Take your calcium at least _____ h before or after your LT$_4$ dose.
- Make sure you follow the instructions provided for your alendronate therapy (_____).
- Make sure you participate in weight-bearing exercise at least _____ d/wk.

Constipation

- Your constipation may improve as your hypothyroidism improves and if your iron tablets are stopped.
- Drinking adequate amounts of liquids and exercise can also help constipation.
- Do not use other laxatives or enemas unless you talk to your physician or pharmacist first.

History of Fe-Deficiency Anemia

- Since your anemia has resolved and your periods are now normal, you no longer need to take iron.

Menorrhagia

- _____.
- Do not use tobacco since that could increase your risk of heart attacks.
- If you develop sudden shortness of breath, leg pain, chest pain, loss of vision, severe headache, or abdominal pain, please call your physician immediately.

50 Pregnancy: Example Careplan with Missing Data

Ema Ferreira   Caroline Morin   Évelyne Rey

PATIENT DATABASE FORM

Patient Name: Loretta Baldwin	**Patient ID:** 467788	**Location:** Physician's Office
Physician: Dr. J. Brown (Medical Clinic)	**Pharmacy:** Unknown	
Age (or Date of Birth): 26 yo	**Race:** Caucasian	**Sex:** Female
Height: 67 in (170 cm)	**Weight:** 207.2 lb (94.2 kg)	
Date of Admission/Initial Visit: 09/01/2009	**Occupation:** Clerk	

Allergies/Intolerances/ADRs

☐ No known drug allergies/ADRs

☒ Not known/inadequate information

Drug:	Reaction:
Phenytoin	Unknown reaction at the age of 13

HPI, PMH, FH, SH, etc...

HPI: Pregnancy

PMH: Epilepsy, obesity, chronic headaches, occasional constipation, light nausea

FMH: DM, HTN, obesity, hypothyroidism

Prioritized Medical Problem List	Medication Profile
Epilepsy	Lamotrigine 200 mg PO twice daily; stopped yesterday
	Carbamazepine CR 400 mg PO twice daily; stopped yesterday
Pregnancy	No folic acid or multivitamins
Chronic headaches	Feverfew herbal tea two to five times a week
	Ibuprofen 400 mg PO PRN headache; twice weekly in the last month
Light nausea	No medication
Constipation	Milk of Magnesia 30 mL PO once daily as needed
Obesity	No medication; poor diet

The form is from *ASHP National Clinical Skills Competition Case Documents*, Copyright 2009, American Society of Health-System Pharmacists, Bethesda, MD (www.ashp.org). Adapted with permission.

Vital Signs, Laboratory Data, and Diagnostic Test Results			
Date	09/01/2009		
Weight (lb/kg)	207.2 (94.2)		
Temperature (°C)	36.2		
Blood pressure (mm Hg)	112/76		
Pulse	89		
Respiratory rate	12		
Na 135–145 mEq/L (135–145 mmol/L)			
K 3.3–4.9 mEq/L (3.3–4.9 mmol/L)			
Cl 97–110 mEq/L (97–110 mmol/L)			
CO_2/HCO_3 22–26 mEq/L (22–26 mmol/L)			
BUN 8–25 mg/dL (2.9–8.9 mmol/L)			
Creatinine (adult) Male 0.7–1.3 mg/dL; female 0.6–1.1 mg/dL (male 62–115 µmol/L; female 53–97 µmol/L)	0.63 (56)		
Creatinine clearance (adult) 85–135 mL/min (1.42–2.25 mL/s)			
Glucose (fasting) 65–109 mg/dL (3.6–6.0 mmol/L)	100.9 (5.6)		
Total Ca 8.6–10.3 mg/dL (2.15–2.58 mmol/L)			
Mg 1.3–2.2 mEq/L (0.65–1.10 mmol/L)			
PO_4 2.5–4.5 mg/dL (0.81–1.45 mmol/L)			
Hemoglobin Male 13.8–17.2 g/dL; female 12.1–15.1 g/dL (male 138–172 g/L; female 121–151 g/L; male 8.57–10.68 mmol/L; female 7.51–9.38 mmol/L)	12.3 (123; 7.63)		
Hematocrit Male 40.7–50.3%; female 36.1–44.3% (male 0.407–0.503; female 0.361–0.443)	37.8 (0.378)		
MCV 80.0–97.6 µm³ (80.0–97.6 fL)	82		
WBC 4–10 × 10³/mm³ (4–10 × 10⁹/L)	5.4		
Differential			
Platelet 140–440 × 10³/mm³ (140–440 × 10⁹/L)	203		
Albumin 3.5–5.0 g/dL (35–50 g/L)			
Total bilirubin 0.3–1.1 mg/dL (5.1–18.8 µmol/L)			
Direct bilirubin 0–0.3 mg/dL (0–5.1 µmol/L)			
AST 11–47 IU/L (0.18–0.78 µkat/L)			
ALT 7–53 IU/L (0.12–0.88 µkat/L)			

Vital Signs, Laboratory Data, and Diagnostic Test Results			
Alk phos (adult) 38–126 IU/L (0.63–2.10 μkat/L)			
Urine pregnancy test	+		
Blood group/Rhesus type	O⁺		
Urinalysis	Normal		
Urine culture	−		
Rubella antibody	+		
Hepatitis B surface antigen	−		
HIV antibody	−		
Vaginal culture	−		
Lamotrigine level	Not done		
Carbamazepine level 4–10 mcg/L (17–42 μmol/L)	4.2 (18)		

Notes

DRUG THERAPY PROBLEM WORKSHEET

Type of Problem	Possible Causes	Problem List	Notes
Correlation between drug therapy and medical problems	Drugs without obvious medical indications	Feverfew	
	Medications unidentified		
	Untreated medical conditions	Obesity	Dietitian consult required; no drug therapy recommended
		Mild nausea	To evaluate if treatment required
Need for additional drug therapy	New medical condition requiring new drug therapy	Pregnancy	Folic acid required
		Mild nausea	To evaluate if treatment required
	Chronic disorder requiring continued drug therapy	Epilepsy	To continue treatment
	Condition best treated with combination drug therapy		
	May develop new medical condition without prophylactic or preventative therapy or premedication	Pregnancy— prevention of congenital anomalies	Folic acid required
Unnecessary drug therapy	Medication with no valid indication	Feverfew herbal tea	No proven efficacy; no safety data available
	Condition caused by accidental or intentional ingestion of toxic amount of drug or chemical		
	Medical problem(s) associated with use of or withdrawal from alcohol, drug, or tobacco		
	Condition is better treated with nondrug therapy	Mild nausea Constipation Obesity	
	Taking multiple drugs when single agent as effective	Lamotrigine and carbamazepine	To evaluate if single therapy can be used
	Taking drug(s) to treat an avoidable adverse reaction from another medication		
Appropriate drug selection	Current regimen not usually as effective as other choices		
	Current regimen not usually as safe as other choices	_____	Should be stopped at 26 wk Acetaminophen first choice during pregnancy
	Therapy not individualized to patient		
Wrong drug	Medical problem for which drug is not effective	Feverfew herbal tea	No proven efficacy
	Patient has risk factors that contraindicate use of drug		
	Patient has infection with organisms resistant to drug		
	Patient refractory to current drug therapy		
	Taking combination product when single agent appropriate		
	Dosage form inappropriate	Feverfew	Formulation and dosage not effective
	Medication error		
Drug regimen	PRN use not appropriate for condition	Milk of Magnesia PRN	PRN laxative might not be effective for chronic constipation
	Route of administration/dosage form/mode of administration not appropriate for current condition		
	Length or course of therapy not appropriate		
	Drug therapy altered without adequate therapeutic trial		
	Dose or interval flexibility not appropriate		

DRUG THERAPY PROBLEM WORKSHEET

Type of Problem	Possible Causes	Problem List	Notes
Dose too low	Dose or frequency too low to produce desired response in this patient		
	Serum drug level below desired therapeutic range	_____	Obtain levels if possible
	Timing of antimicrobial prophylaxis not appropriate		
	Medication not stored properly		
	Medication error		
Dose too high	Dose or frequency too high for this patient		
	Serum drug level above the desired therapeutic range		
	Dose escalated too quickly		
	Dose or interval flexibility not appropriate for this patient		
	Medication error		
Therapeutic duplication	Receiving multiple agents without added benefit		
Drug allergy/ adverse drug events	History of allergy or ADE to current (or chemically related) agents		
	Allergy or ADE history not in medical records		
	Patient not using alert for severe allergy or ADE		
	Symptoms or medical problems that may be drug induced		
	Drug administered too rapidly		
	Medication error, actual or potential		
Interactions (drug–drug, drug–disease, drug–nutrient, drug–laboratory test)	Effect of drug altered due to enzyme induction/inhibition from another drug patient is taking	Interaction between lamotrigine and carbamazepine	_____ _____
	Effect of drug altered due to protein-binding alterations from another drug patient is taking		
	Effect of drug altered due to pharmacodynamic change from another drug patient is taking		
	Bioavailability of drug altered due to interaction with another drug or food		
	Effect of drug altered due to substance in food		
	Patient's laboratory test altered due to interference from a drug the patient is taking		
Failure to receive therapy	Patient did not adhere with the drug regimen	Patient stopped her anticonvulsants	
	Drug not given due to medication error		
	Patient did not take due to high drug cost/lack of insurance		
	Patient unable to take oral medication		
	Patient has no IV access for IV medication		
	Drug product not available		
Financial impact	The current regimen is not the most cost-effective		
	Patient unable to purchase medications/no insurance		
Patient knowledge of drug therapy	Patient does not understand the purpose, directions, or potential side effects of the drug regimen	Patient does not understand the risk of stopping anticonvulsants	
	Current regimen not consistent with the patient's health beliefs	Patient does not know risks of anticonvulsant therapy during pregnancy	

Medical Problem List	Current Drug Regimen	Drug Therapy Problems	Therapy Goals, Desired Endpoints	Therapeutic Recommendations	Rationale	Therapeutic Alternatives	Monitoring
____	Carbamazepine 400 mg CR PO twice daily (stopped yesterday) Lamotrigine 200 mg PO twice daily (stopped yesterday)	Medication stopped	Prevent seizures Prevent pregnancy complication due to seizures	____ ____ ____	Seizure control is important during pregnancy Use treatment that controls seizure in this patient	____ ____ ____	Seizures Aura Drugs levels every trimester if dose is changed or if clinical condition warrants it
Pregnancy	None	No prevention of congenital anomalies	Prevent neural tube defects and other congenital anomalies	Start folic acid 4 mg once daily ASAP and continue throughout first trimester	Folic acid reduces the risk of neural tube defects and other congenital anomalies	None	
Pregnancy	None	Patient does not understand the risks of disease and drugs	Promote drug compliance and optimal treatment		Proper counseling will encourage compliance to anticonvulsants		Interview the patient at follow-up
Nausea	None	____	Relief of nausea Ensure absorption of other treatments	Nonpharmacologic methods (i.e., small meals, etc.) Doxylamine and pyridoxine if necessary ____	____ ____ ____	____ ____ ____	____ ____ ____
Constipation	Milk of Magnesia 30 mL once daily as needed	Constipation treatment is not optimal	Normal bowel movements Prevention of hemorrhoids	____ ____ ____	____ ____	Add docusate sodium if constipation persists or ____ ____	Self-monitor daily

Medical Problem List	Current Drug Regimen	Drug Therapy Problems	Therapy Goals, Desired Endpoints	Therapeutic Recommendations	Rationale	Therapeutic Alternatives	Monitoring
Chronic headaches	Ibuprofen 400 mg orally as needed Feverfew herbal tea as needed	Ibuprofen is not an optimal treatment during pregnancy Herbal product has no proven efficacy	___ ___ ___	Acetaminophen 500–1,000 mg PO q 6 h as needed (maximum 4 g/24 h) Ibuprofen sporadically as needed (maximum for 48 h and stop at 26 wk pregnancy) Stop feverfew herbal tea	Ibuprofen is associated with: ___ ___ ___ Feverfew should be discontinued since: ___ ___	Encourage lifestyle changes (rest, avoidance of triggers, etc.) If acetaminophen is not sufficient and if severe headaches, consider adding an opiate (e.g., codeine)	___ ___ ___ ___
Obesity	___		Healthy diet Healthy weight gain during pregnancy	Dietitian consultation Add vitamin supplements if necessary. Mild-to-moderate exercise	Healthy diet is important during pregnancy for fetal growth Use of drugs to promote weight loss is not recommended during pregnancy		Weight at each prenatal visit Monitor for anemia Evaluation by dietitian

PATIENT EDUCATION SUMMARY

Notes

Epilepsy

- Seizure control during pregnancy is important.
- Drug compliance is essential.
- Risk of congenital malformations is of 2–3% in the general population and is increased to approximately 5% with these anticonvulsants (95% chance of having a healthy baby).
- You will have drug levels measured regularly to ensure that drugs are at optimal levels.

Pregnancy and Folic Acid

- Folic acid will _____.
- You will need to take a folic acid supplement until at least the end of the _____ trimester.

Constipation

- Your constipation is worsened by pregnancy.
- It is important to eat a diet _____ in fiber.
- Drinking adequate amounts of liquids and exercise can also help constipation. Some medication are useful and safe during pregnancy.
- Treating and preventing constipation will prevent hemorrhoids that are also common during pregnancy.
- _____ use other laxatives or enemas unless you talk to your health care provider.

Chronic Headaches

- Regular ibuprofen is not the first choice throughout pregnancy since it can affect _____.
- Regular rest and avoidance of too much caffeine or other triggers is helpful to prevent headaches.
- Use acetaminophen, which is safe throughout pregnancy.
- Talk to your physician or pharmacist if headaches persist despite the use of acetaminophen. (Other treatments are available.)

Obesity

- A healthy diet during pregnancy is important.
- A dietitian can evaluate your diet and recommend a program to promote healthy habits.
- You might have to take calcium and iron supplements.
- Healthy weight gain is approximately _____.
- Dieting (with or without drugs) is not recommended during pregnancy.

Nausea

- _____.
- _____.

86 Acute Osteomyelitis: Example Careplan with Missing Data

Melinda M. Neuhauser   Susan L. Pendland

PATIENT DATABASE FORM

Patient Name: Sam Cole	Patient ID:	Location: ED
Physician:	Pharmacy:	
Age (or Date of Birth): 18 yo	Race: Caucasian	Sex: Male
Height: 69 in. (175.3 cm)	Weight: 162.8 lb (74 kg)	
Date of Admission/Initial Visit: 08/03/2010	Occupation: Full-time student; part-time job at movie theater	

Allergies/Intolerances/ADRs

❏ No known drug allergies/ADRs

❏ Not known/inadequate information

Drug:	Reaction:
Benadryl	Jittery

HPI, PMH, FH, SH, etc...

Fractured proximal humerus (7 d ago)

Asthma

Allergic rhinitis

Prioritized Medical Problem List	Medication Profile
Acute osteomyelitis	Vancomycin 20 mg/kg infusion q 12 h (or student may have selected or calculated different dosage regimen)
_____	Cephalexin 500 mg one capsule PO q 6 h for 7 d
	Ibuprofen 400 mg one tablet PO q 6 h PRN mild-to-moderate arm pain
	Hydrocodone/acetaminophen 5/500 mg one tablet PO q 4 h PRN severe arm pain
_____	Fluticasone/salmeterol 250/50 mg one puff twice daily
	Albuterol one to two puffs q 4 h PRN wheezing
Allergic rhinitis	Loratadine 10 mg one tablet PO once daily
	Fluticasone intranasal spray two puffs each nostril once daily PRN allergies
	Acetaminophen 500 mg one to two tablets PRN headaches

The form is from *ASHP National Clinical Skills Competition Case Documents*, Copyright 2009, American Society of Health-System Pharmacists, Bethesda, MD (www.ashp.org). Adapted with permission.

Vital Signs, Laboratory Data, and Diagnostic Test Results			
Date	08/03/2010		
Weight (lb/kg)	162.8 (74)		
Temperature (°C)	37.9		
Blood pressure (mm Hg)	117/76		
Pulse	85		
Respiratory rate	16		
Na 135–145 mEq/L (135–145 mmol/L)	141		
K 3.3–4.9 mEq/L (3.3–4.9 mmol/L)	3.9		
Cl 97–110 mEq/L (97–110 mmol/L)	101		
CO_2/HCO_3 22–26 mEq/L (22–26 mmol/L)	25		
BUN 8–25 mg/dL (2.9–8.9 mmol/L)	5 (1.8)		
Creatinine (adult) Male 0.7–1.3 mg/dL; female 0.6–1.1 mg/dL (male 62–115 μmol/L; female 53–97 μmol/L)	0.5 (44)		
Creatinine clearance (adult) 85–135 mL/min (1.42–2.25 mL/s)	>120 (>2.00)		
Glucose (fasting) 65–109 mg/dL (3.6–6.0 mmol/L)	145 mg (8.0)		
Total Ca 8.6–10.3 mg/dL (2.15–2.58 mmol/L)			
Mg 1.3–2.2 mEq/L (0.65–1.10 mmol/L)			
PO_4 2.5–4.5 mg/dL (0.81–1.45 mmol/L)			
Hemoglobin Male 13.8–17.2 g/dL; female 12.1–15.1 g/dL (male 138–172 g/L; female 121–151 g/L; male 8.57–10.68 mmol/L; female 7.51–9.38 mmol/L)	15.0 (150; 9.31)		
Hematocrit Male 40.7–50.3%; female 36.1–44.3% (male 0.407–0.503; female 0.361–0.443)	43.7 (0.437)		
MCV 80.0–97.6 μm³ (80.0–97.6 fL)			
WBC 4–10 × 10³/mm³ (4–10 × 10⁹/L)	10.1		
Differential			
Platelet 140–440 × 10³/mm³ (140–440 × 10⁹/L)			
Albumin 3.5–5.0 g/dL (35–50 g/L)			
Total bilirubin 0.3–1.1 mg/dL (5.1–18.8 μmol/L)			
Direct bilirubin 0–0.3 mg/dL (0–5.1 μmol/L)			
AST 11–47 IU/L (0.18–0.78 μkat/L)			
ALT 7–53 IU/L (0.12–0.88 μkat/L)			
Alk phos (adult) 38–126 IU/L (0.63–2.10 μkat/L)			

Vital Signs, Laboratory Data, and Diagnostic Test Results			
ESR 0–20 mm/h (0–5.6 µm/s)	119 (33.1)		
CRP <0.8 mg/dL (<8 mg/L)	68 (680)		

Notes
Microbiology:
Blood culture (×2): Pending
Bone biopsy: Gram stain shows Gram-positive cocci in clusters; culture is pending
Imaging:
Plain radiograph: Positive for soft-tissue swelling
Radionuclide bone scan: Positive for increased uptake in left proximal humerus

DRUG THERAPY PROBLEM WORKSHEET

Type of Problem	Possible Causes	Problem List	Notes
Correlation between drug therapy and medical problems	Drugs without obvious medical indications		
	Medications unidentified	Sinus medication	
	Untreated medical conditions		
Need for additional drug therapy	New medical condition requiring new drug therapy	Acute osteomyelitis	Discontinue oral cephalexin
	Chronic disorder requiring continued drug therapy		
	Condition best treated with combination drug therapy		
	May develop new medical condition without prophylactic or preventative therapy or premedication		
Unnecessary drug therapy	Medication with no valid indication		
	Condition caused by accidental or intentional ingestion of toxic amount of drug or chemical		
	Medical problem(s) associated with use of or withdrawal from alcohol, drug, or tobacco		
	Condition is better treated with nondrug therapy		
	Taking multiple drugs when single agent as effective		
	Taking drug(s) to treat an avoidable adverse reaction from another medication		
Appropriate drug selection	Current regimen not usually as effective as other choices		
	Current regimen not usually as safe as other choices		
	Therapy not individualized to patient		
Wrong drug	Medical problem for which drug is not effective		
	Patient has risk factors that contraindicate use of drug		
	Patient has infection with organisms resistant to drug		
	Patient refractory to current drug therapy		
	Taking combination product when single agent appropriate		
	Dosage form inappropriate		
	Medication error		
Drug regimen	PRN use not appropriate for condition	Intranasal corticosteroid	Change from PRN to daily
	Route of administration/dosage form/mode of administration not appropriate for current condition		
	Length or course of therapy not appropriate		
	Drug therapy altered without adequate therapeutic trial		
	Dose or interval flexibility not appropriate		
Dose too low	Dose or frequency too low to produce desired response in this patient		
	Serum drug level below desired therapeutic range		
	Timing of antimicrobial prophylaxis not appropriate		
	Medication not stored properly		
	Medication error		
Dose too high	Dose or frequency too high for this patient		
	Serum drug level above the desired therapeutic range		
	Dose escalated too quickly		
	Dose or interval flexibility not appropriate for this patient		
	Medication error		

DRUG THERAPY PROBLEM WORKSHEET

Type of Problem	Possible Causes	Problem List	Notes
Therapeutic duplication	Receiving multiple agents without added benefit		
Drug allergy/ adverse drug events	History of allergy or ADE to current (or chemically related) agents		
	Allergy or ADE history not in medical records		
	Patient not using alert for severe allergy or ADE		
	Symptoms or medical problems that may be drug induced		
	Drug administered too rapidly		
	Medication error, actual or potential		
Interactions (drug–drug, drug–disease, drug–nutrient, drug–laboratory test)	Effect of drug altered due to enzyme induction/ inhibition from another drug patient is taking		
	Effect of drug altered due to protein-binding alterations from another drug patient is taking		
	Effect of drug altered due to pharmacodynamic change from another drug patient is taking		
	Bioavailability of drug altered due to interaction with another drug or food		
	Effect of drug altered due to substance in food		
	Patient's laboratory test altered due to interference from a drug the patient is taking		
Failure to receive therapy	Patient did not adhere with the drug regimen	In the past, several acute asthma exacerbations secondary to nonadherence to asthma medications	_____ _____
	Drug not given due to medication error		
	Patient did not take due to high drug cost/lack of insurance		
	Patient unable to take oral medication		
	Patient has no IV access for IV medication		
	Drug product not available		
Financial impact	The current regimen is not the most cost-effective		
	Patient unable to purchase medications/no insurance	Health insurance coverage through father	
Patient knowledge of drug therapy	Patient does not understand the purpose, directions, or potential side effects of the drug regimen		
	Current regimen not consistent with the patient's health beliefs	Cultural beliefs not known	

PHARMACOTHERAPY CARE PLAN

Medical Problem List	Current Drug Regimen	Drug Therapy Problems	Therapy Goals, Desired Endpoints	Therapeutic Recommendations	Rationale	Therapeutic Alternatives	Monitoring
Acute osteomyelitis	None (new diagnosis)	—— —— ——	Eradicate infection and prevent recurrence	—— —— —— —— Achieve steady-state vancomycin trough concentration of 15–20 mcg/mL (10.4–13.8 μmol/L) with goal AUC$_{24}$/MIC of >350–400	Appropriate therapy	IV alternatives include daptomycin and linezolid Oral alternatives include: —— ——	Monitor BUN/SCr, vancomycin troughs, CPR, and ESR weekly Monitor for: —— —— —— ——
—— ——	Ibuprofen 400 mg one tablet PO q 6 h PRN mild-to-moderate arm pain Hydrocodone/ acetaminophen 5/500 mg one tablet q 4 h PRN severe arm pain Cephalexin 500 mg one capsule PO q 6 h for 7 d	—— —— ——	Reduce symptoms of pain	Change ibuprofen to 400 mg one tablet q 6 h with food for 48 h and then switch to PRN Continue hydrocodone/ acetaminophen 5/500 mg PO PRN for pain not controlled with ibuprofen Discontinue cephalexin	—— —— ——	Dosage modification of ibuprofen and/or hydrocodone/ acetaminophen If severe pain, consider oxycodone/ acetaminophen	
Asthma	Fluticasone/ salmeterol 250/50 mg one puff twice daily Albuterol one to two puffs q 4 h PRN wheezing	—— —— —— ——	Reduce symptoms, maintain normal pulmonary function, and prevent acute exacerbations	—— —— —— ——	Patient asymptomatic when adheres to the current regimen	Dosage modification of fluticasone/ salmeterol	Self-monitor symptoms (dyspnea, cough, SOB) Pulmonary function tests
Allergic rhinitis	Loratadine 10 mg one tablet PO once daily Fluticasone intranasal spray two puffs each nostril once daily PRN allergies Acetaminophen 500 mg one to two tablets PO PRN headaches	Unidentified sinus medication; need to identify ingredients	Reduce symptoms	—— —— Change fluticasone to scheduled once daily rather than PRN —— ——	Fluticasone therapy will be optimized if utilized as scheduled rather than PRN	Different agent within the class of second-generation antihistamines or intranasal corticosteroids Decongestants —— ——	—— ——

Notes

Acute Osteomyelitis

- The reason for taking the intravenous antibiotic is to: _____
  _____.

- It is extremely important that you receive the antibiotic exactly as prescribed by your health care provider and for as long as prescribed by health care provider. If your bone infection is not cured, you are likely to have life-long recurring infections. Recurrent infections are much more difficult to treat and could even result in amputation of your arm.

- It is very important that you do not miss a single dose of your antibiotic. The bacteria causing the infection may become resistant to the medication you are taking and could result in recurrent infections.

- Blood tests will need to be done weekly to help the health care provider determine if your infection is responding to the antibiotic or if changes need to be made in either the drug or the dose.

- You should begin to feel better in _____
  _____.

- It is important to keep regularly scheduled appointments with your health care provider so that your infection and response to therapy can be carefully monitored.

Asthma

- It is important that you use the fluticasone/salbuterol inhaler every morning and every evening. If you take the medication twice daily as directed, your breathing should improve and you should have fewer visits to the emergency department for your asthma.

- _____.

- _____.

- Ask your friends not to smoke when you are with them and tell them how it worsens your breathing. Encourage them to not smoke so that they will not have breathing problems like you have.

Allergic Rhinitis

- Your nasal spray should work better if you use it every day. If you use it daily for 3 wk and your allergy symptoms are still present, contact your health care provider.

- _____.

Fractured Proximal Humerus

- Take the pain medication exactly as your health care provider directed. If your pain increases or has not decreased in 2 or 3 d, contact your health care provider.

- Avoid taking too much acetaminophen (Tylenol). _____.